External Disease and Cornea

Section 8

2005–2006

(Last major revision 2002–2003)

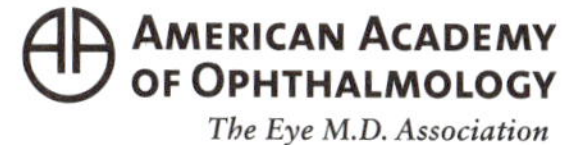

AMERICAN ACADEMY OF OPHTHALMOLOGY
The Eye M.D. Association

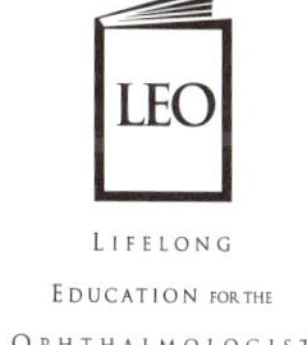

LEO

LIFELONG

EDUCATION FOR THE

OPHTHALMOLOGIST®

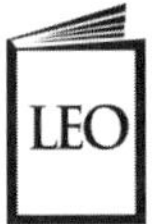

The Basic and Clinical Science Course is one component of the Lifelong Education for the Ophthalmologist (LEO) framework, which assists members in planning their continuing medical education. LEO includes an array of clinical education products that members may select to form individualized, self-directed learning plans for updating their clinical knowledge. Active members or fellows who use LEO components may accumulate sufficient CME credits to earn the LEO Award. Contact the Academy's Clinical Education Division for further information on LEO.

The Academy provides this material for educational purposes only. It is not intended to represent the only or best method or procedure in every case, nor to replace a physician's own judgment or give specific advice for case management. Including all indications, contraindications, side effects, and alternative agents for each drug or treatment is beyond the scope of this material. All information and recommendations should be verified, prior to use, with current information included in the manufacturers' package inserts or other independent sources, and considered in light of the patient's condition and history. Reference to certain drugs, instruments, and other products in this course is made for illustrative purposes only and is not intended to constitute an endorsement of such. Some material may include information on applications that are not considered community standard, that reflect indications not included in approved FDA labeling, or that are approved for use only in restricted research settings. The FDA has stated that it is the responsibility of the physician to determine the FDA status of each drug or device he or she wishes to use, and to use them with appropriate patient consent in compliance with applicable law. The Academy specifically disclaims any and all liability for injury or other damages of any kind, from negligence or otherwise, for any and all claims that may arise from the use of any recommendations or other information contained herein.

Basic and Clinical Science Course

Thomas J. Liesegang, MD, Jacksonville, Florida, *Senior Secretary for Clinical Education*

Gregory L. Skuta, MD, Oklahoma City, Oklahoma, *Secretary for Ophthalmic Knowledge*

Louis B. Cantor, MD, Indianapolis, Indiana, *BCSC Course Chair*

Section 8

Faculty Responsible for This Edition

John E. Sutphin, Jr, MD, *Chair*, Iowa City, Iowa
James Chodosh, MD, Oklahoma City, Oklahoma
M. Reza Dana, MD, MPH, Boston, Massachusetts
W. Craig Fowler, MD, Charlotte, North Carolina
James J. Reidy, MD, Buffalo, New York
Jayne S. Weiss, MD, Detroit, Michigan
Paul W. Turgeon, MD, Canton, Ohio
   Practicing Ophthalmologists Advisory Committee for Education

The authors state the following financial relationships:
Dr. Dana: Consultant—Allergan, Biogen, and Dai-ichi
Dr. Sutphin: Consultant—Santen

The other authors state that they have no significant financial interest or other relationship with the manufacturer of any commercial product discussed in the chapters that they contributed to this publication or with the manufacturer of any competing commercial product.

Recent Past Faculty

Michael W. Belin, MD

Vincent P. deLuise, MD

Steven P. Dunn, MD

Randy J. Epstein, MD

David J. Harris, Jr, MD

Andrew J.W. Huang, MD

David G. Hwang, MD

Jeffrey D. Lanier, MD

Carolyn M. Parrish, MD

Priscilla E. Perry, MD

Stephen C. Pflugfelder, MD

Ivan R. Schwab, MD

Kirk R. Wilhelmus, MD, MPH

Paul L. Wright, MD

In addition, the Academy gratefully acknowledges the contributions of numerous past faculty and advisory committee members who have played an important role in the development of previous editions of the Basic and Clinical Science Course.

Contents

PART II   Ocular Surface Disorders 45

3   Normal Physiology of the Ocular Surface   47

4   Diagnostic Approach to Ocular Surface Disease   53

5   Clinical Aspects of Ocular Surface Disorders   63

PART III Infectious Diseases of the External Eye and Cornea 101

6 Infectious Diseases of the External Eye: Basic Concepts 103

7 Infectious Diseases of the External Eye: Clinical Aspects 129

PART IV   Immune-Mediated Disorders of the External Eye and Cornea 181

8 Ocular Immunology. 183

9 Clinical Approach to Immune-Related Disorders of the External Eye 193

PART V   Neoplastic Disorders of the Eyelids, Conjunctiva, and Cornea   229

10   Tumor Cell Biology and Diagnostic Approaches to Ocular Surface Neoplasia   231

11   Clinical Approach to Neoplastic Disorders of the Conjunctiva and Cornea   239

PART VI Congenital Anomalies of the Cornea and Sclera 263

12 Basic Concepts of Congenital Anomalies of the Cornea and Sclera 265

13 Clinical Aspects of Congenital Anomalies of the Cornea and Sclera 271

General Introduction

The Basic and Clinical Science Course (BCSC) is designed to meet the needs of residents and practitioners for a comprehensive yet concise curriculum of the field of ophthalmology. The BCSC has developed from its original brief outline format, which relied heavily on outside readings, to a more convenient and educationally useful self-contained text. The Academy updates and revises the course annually, with the goals of integrating the basic science and clinical practice of ophthalmology and of keeping ophthalmologists current with new developments in the various subspecialties.

The BCSC incorporates the effort and expertise of more than 80 ophthalmologists, organized into 13 section faculties, working with Academy editorial staff. In addition, the course continues to benefit from many lasting contributions made by the faculties of previous editions. Members of the Academy's Practicing Ophthalmologists Advisory Committee for Education serve on each faculty and, as a group, review every volume before and after major revisions.

Organization of the Course

The Basic and Clinical Science Course comprises 13 volumes, incorporating fundamental ophthalmic knowledge, subspecialty areas, and special topics:

1. Update on General Medicine
2. Fundamentals and Principles of Ophthalmology
3. Clinical Optics
4. Ophthalmic Pathology and Intraocular Tumors
5. Neuro-Ophthalmology
6. Pediatric Ophthalmology and Strabismus
7. Orbit, Eyelids, and Lacrimal System
8. External Disease and Cornea
9. Intraocular Inflammation and Uveitis
10. Glaucoma
11. Lens and Cataract
12. Retina and Vitreous
13. Refractive Surgery

In addition, a comprehensive Master Index allows the reader to easily locate subjects throughout the entire series.

References

Readers who wish to explore specific topics in greater detail may consult the journal references cited within each chapter and the Basic Texts listed at the back of the book.

These references are intended to be selective rather than exhaustive, chosen by the BCSC faculty as being important, current, and readily available to residents and practitioners.

Related Academy educational materials are also listed in the appropriate sections. They include books, audiovisual materials, self-assessment programs, clinical modules, and interactive programs.

Study Questions and CME Credit

Each volume of the BCSC is designed as an independent study activity for ophthalmology residents and practitioners. The learning objectives for this volume are given on page 1. The text, illustrations, and references provide the information necessary to achieve the objectives; the study questions allow readers to test their understanding of the material and their mastery of the objectives. Physicians who wish to claim CME credit for this educational activity may do so by mail, fax, or online. The necessary forms and instructions are given at the end of the book.

Conclusion

The Basic and Clinical Science Course has expanded greatly over the years, with the addition of much new text and numerous illustrations. Recent editions have sought to place a greater emphasis on clinical applicability, while maintaining a solid foundation in basic science. As with any educational program, it reflects the experience of its authors. As its faculties change and as medicine progresses, new viewpoints are always emerging on controversial subjects and techniques. Not all alternate approaches can be included in this series; as with any educational endeavor, the learner should seek additional sources, including such carefully balanced opinions as the Academy's Preferred Practice Patterns.

The BCSC faculty and staff are continuously striving to improve the educational usefulness of the course; you, the reader, can contribute to this ongoing process. If you have any suggestions or questions about the series, please do not hesitate to contact the faculty or the editors.

The authors, editors, and reviewers hope that your study of the BCSC will be of lasting value and that each section will serve as a practical resource for quality patient care.

Objectives

Upon completion of BCSC Section 8, *External Disease and Cornea*, the reader should be able to:

- Describe the anatomy and molecular biology of the cornea

- Explain the pathogenesis of common disorders affecting the eyelid margin, conjunctiva, cornea, and sclera

- Recognize the distinctive signs of specific diseases of the ocular surface and cornea

- Describe how the environment can affect the structure and function of the ocular surface

- Outline the steps in an ocular examination for corneal or external eye disease and choose the appropriate laboratory and other diagnostic tests

- Summarize the developmental and metabolic alterations that lead to structural changes of the cornea

- Identify topographic changes of the cornea and describe the risks and benefits of corrective measures

- Assess the indications and techniques of surgical procedures for managing corneal disease, trauma, and refractive error

- Apply the results of recent clinical research to the management of selected disorders of the conjunctiva and cornea

- Integrate the discipline of corneal and external eye disease into the practice of ophthalmology

PART I

Basic and Clinical Concepts of Corneal and External Eye Disease

CHAPTER 1

Structure and Function of the External Eye and Cornea

The Outer Eye and Cornea in Health and Disease

The external eye is the most crucial part of the body exposed to the outside world. The normal structure and function of the healthy eye rely on homeostasis of the entire body for protection against an adverse environment. Genetics and nutrition determine the embryogenesis and growth of the eye. Intact vascular and nervous systems ensure stable metabolism, and the immune system maintains surveillance.

The cushioning effect of the periocular tissues and local barriers such as the orbital rim are needed to safeguard the globe. The eyebrows and eyelashes catch small particles, and the cilia also work as sensors to stimulate reflex eyelid closure. Blinking augments the lacrimal pump to rinse tears over the eye and flush off foreign material. The tear film also dilutes toxins and allergens and contains proteins that control the normal flora. Mucin stabilizes the tear film and demarcates the living cells of the ocular surface from the surrounding environment.

The epidermis and epithelium of healthy eyelids, conjunctiva, and cornea adhere tightly to their basement membranes. Regulation of cellular growth and metabolism are critical to the maintenance of an intact ocular surface and a transparent cornea. The underlying extracellular matrix of the eye's mucous membrane is rich in blood vessels and conjunctiva-associated lymphoid tissue (CALT). The anterior segment of the eye provides a clear, protected entrance for light that is to be processed by the visual pathways through the central nervous system.

Understanding the eye's innate defenses requires study of ocular histology and biochemistry and observation of many people, both healthy and ill. The practice of corneal and external eye disease builds on this understanding and extends from clinical examination to clinicopathologic problem solving, molecular medicine, and microsurgery. The reader should become familiar with ocular embryology, anatomy, physiology, and biochemistry (in BCSC Section 2, *Fundamentals and Principles of Ophthalmology*); ocular immunology (in BCSC Section 9, *Intraocular Inflammation and Uveitis*); and ophthalmic pathology (in BCSC Section 4, *Ophthalmic Pathology and Intraocular Tumors*).

Development of the Anterior Segment

The eye begins to develop during week 4 of gestation as an evagination from the *neuro-ectoderm*. Invagination of the optic vesicle forms the double-layered optic cup of neuro-ectoderm at week 5. At this time, the surface ectoderm forms the lens placode and gives rise to the corneal and conjunctival epithelium and the eyelid epidermis. Also at week 5, the first wave of *mesenchymal cells* from the *neural crest* of the surface ectoderm extends under the epithelium from the limbus to begin forming the corneal endothelium. A subsequent wave of mesenchymal cells of neural crest origin at week 6 begins forming the corneal stroma and sclera. Greater detail is available in Part II of BCSC Section 2.

At 2 months of gestation, the eyelids fuse and the conjunctiva begins to develop within the eyelid folds. The ocular surface epithelium differentiates shortly afterward. At 3 months, all corneal components are present except Bowman's layer, which appears in the fourth month as the scleral spur is also forming. The eyelids begin to open during the sixth month. At birth, the infant's globe is 80% of its adult size. The postnatal sclera and cornea are somewhat distensible, gradually becoming more rigid during the first 2 years of life. See also Chapter 12.

Anatomy

Eyelids

Eyelids are unique to vertebrates, and humans have one of the highest ratios of inter-palpebral fissure width to body mass. The eyelid skin blends into the surrounding per-iorbital skin, varying from 0.5 mm thick at the eyelid margin to 1 mm thick at the orbital rim. Except for fine vellus hairs, the only hairs of the eyelids are the eyelashes, or *cilia*, which are twice as numerous along the upper eyelid margin as along the lower. Cilia are replaced every 3–5 months; they usually regrow in 2 weeks when cut and within 2 months if pulled out.

The epidermis of the eyelids is similar to other facial skin. It abruptly changes to nonkeratinized stratified squamous epithelium at the mucocutaneous junction of the eyelid margin, along the row of *meibomian gland* orifices. Holocrine sebaceous glands and eccrine sweat glands are present in the eyelid skin. Near the eyelid margin are the apocrine sweat glands (the *glands of Moll*) and numerous sebaceous glands (the *glands of Zeis*) (Fig 1-1).

Sensory nerves from the first division of cranial nerve V (trigeminal) extend to the eyelids through the supraorbital nerve and its lacrimal, supratrochlear, and infratrochlear branches. Innervated by the zygomatic branch of cranial nerve VII (facial), the *orbicularis oculi* muscle closes the eyelids, whether by volition using its orbital and preseptal portions or by subconscious blinking using the pretarsal portion. Nonstressed healthy people blink about every 3–4 seconds when not concentrating on a visual task; conscious vision is turned off just before a blink starts. Besides moving toward each other, the eyelids also move medially during a blink, providing a pumping action within the lacrimal drainage

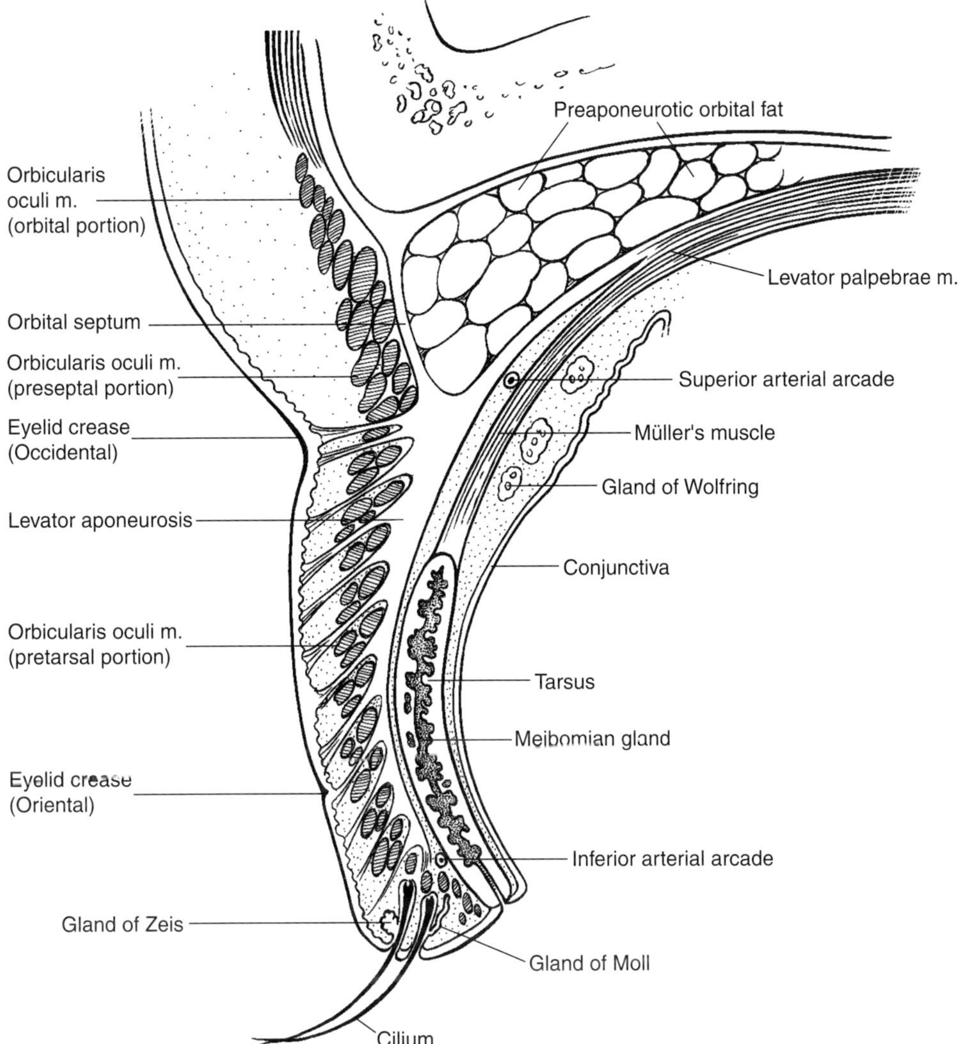

Figure 1-1 Cross section of the upper eyelid. *(Illustration by Christine Gralapp.)*

system. Maintaining eyelid closure during sleep involves active tonus of the orbicularis and sustained inhibition of the elevator muscle.

The blood supply of the eyelids comes chiefly from two sources: the *external carotid artery* through the facial, superficial, temporal, and infraorbital branches of the *facial artery;* and the *internal carotid artery* through the dorsal, nasal, frontal, supraorbital, and lacrimal branches of the *ophthalmic artery.* Venous drainage occurs through the anterior facial and superior *temporal veins* into the *jugular vein* and through the *ophthalmic vein* into the *cavernous sinus.* Lymphatics drain primarily to the *preauricular lymph node,* although the medial aspect of the eyelid and conjunctiva drain into the submandibular and submental nodes.

Tarsal plates are situated in the deep upper and lower eyelids, providing a structural foundation for attachment of muscles and the orbital septum. Each tarsus is 0.75 mm thick and measures approximately 10 mm in height in the upper eyelid and 4 mm in the lower. The orbital septum, which separates the orbicularis muscle from the orbital fat, extends from the tarsi to the periosteum of the orbital rim. The *meibomian glands* embedded within each tarsus are composed of multiple lobules that open in a common secretory duct.

Krachmer JH, Mannis MJ, Holland EJ, eds. *Cornea.* Vol 1. St Louis: Mosby; 1997:61–67.

Conjunctiva

The conjunctival sac includes the *bulbar conjunctiva,* a *fornix* on three sides and a medial *semilunar fold,* and the *palpebral conjunctiva.* Smooth-muscle fibers from the levator muscle maintain the superior fornix, and fibrous slips extend from the horizontal rectus tendons into the temporal conjunctiva and plica to form cul-de-sacs during horizontal gaze. The *caruncle* is a fleshy tissue mass containing hairs and sebaceous glands. The *tarsal conjunctiva* is tightly adherent to the underlying tarsus, and the bulbar conjunctiva is loosely adherent to Tenon's capsule. These tissues blend at the limbus, where a series of radiating ridges called the *palisades of Vogt* appear. This area contains corneal stem cells.

The cell morphology of the conjunctival epithelium varies from stratified cuboidal over the tarsus to columnar in the fornices to squamous on the globe. Multiple surface folds are present. Goblet cells account for up to 10% of basal cells of the conjunctival epithelium; they are most numerous in the tarsal conjunctiva and the inferonasal bulbar conjunctiva.

The *substantia propria* of the conjunctiva consists of loose connective tissue. Conjunctiva-associated lymphoid tissue (CALT) consisting of lymphocytes and other leukocytes is present, especially in the fornices. Lymphocytes interact with mucosal epithelial cells through reciprocal regulatory signals mediated by growth factors, cytokines, and neuropeptides.

The palpebral conjunctiva shares its blood supply with the eyelids. The bulbar conjunctiva is supplied by the anterior ciliary arteries branching off the ophthalmic artery. These capillaries are fenestrated and leak fluorescein just like the choriocapillaris. Sensory innervation is controlled by the lacrimal, supraorbital, supratrochlear, and infraorbital branches of the ophthalmic division of cranial nerve V.

Krachmer JH, Mannis MJ, Holland EJ, eds. *Cornea.* Vol 1. St Louis: Mosby; 1997:41–47.

Cornea

The cornea is a transparent, avascular tissue that measures 11–12 mm horizontally and 10–11 mm vertically. Its refractive index is 1.376, although a refractive index of 1.3375 is used in calibrating the keratometer to account for the combined optical power of the anterior and posterior curvatures of the cornea. The cornea is aspheric, although its radius of curvature is often recorded as a spherocylindrical convex mirror representing the central anterior corneal surface, also called the *corneal cap.*

The average radius of curvature of the central cornea is 7.8 mm (6.7–9.4 mm). The cornea thus contributes 74%, or 43.25 diopters (D), of the total 58.60 dioptric power of a normal human eye. The cornea is also the major source of astigmatism in the optical system. See Measurement of Corneal Topography in Chapter 2 for more information on corneal optics.

For its nutrition, the cornea depends on glucose diffusing from the aqueous humor and oxygen diffusing through the tear film. In addition, the peripheral cornea is supplied with oxygen from the limbal circulation.

The cornea has one of the body's highest densities of nerve endings, and the sensitivity of the cornea is 100 times that of the conjunctiva. Sensory nerve fibers extend from the long ciliary nerves and form a subepithelial plexus. Neurotransmitters in the cornea include acetylcholine, catecholamines, substance P, and calcitonin gene–related peptide.

Epithelium

The corneal epithelium is composed of stratified squamous epithelial cells and makes up about 5% (0.05 mm) of the total corneal thickness (Fig 1-2; see also Fig 2-1). The epithelium and tear film form an optically smooth surface. Tight junctions between superficial epithelial cells prevent penetration of tear fluid into the stroma. Continuous proliferation of perilimbal basal epithelial cells gives rise to the other layers that subsequently differentiate into superficial cells. With maturation, these cells become coated with microvilli on their outermost surface (which causes them to appear dark by scanning electron microscopy and bright by specular microscopy) and then desquamate into the

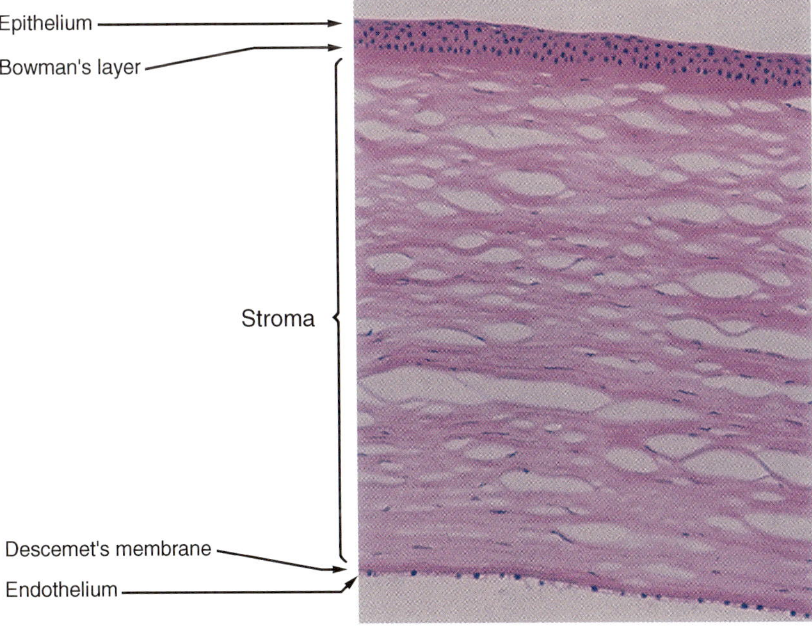

Figure 1-2 Normal cornea. The epithelium, normally five cell layers, will thicken to maintain a smooth surface (H&E ×32).

tears. This process of differentiation takes about 7–14 days. Basal epithelial cells secrete a continuous, 50 nm thick basement membrane, composed of type IV collagen, laminin, and other proteins.

Stroma

Optimal corneal optics requires a smooth surface with a healthy tear film and epithelium. Clarity of the cornea depends on tight packing of epithelial cells to produce a layer with a nearly uniform refractive index and minimal light scattering. The regular arrangement of stromal cells and macromolecules is also necessary for a clear cornea. Keratocytes vary in density and size throughout the stroma (Fig 1-3) and form a spiraling three-dimensional network throughout the cornea (Fig 1-4). These corneal fibroblasts continually digest and manufacture stromal molecules.

Beneath the acellular *Bowman's layer,* the corneal stroma is composed of an extracellular matrix formed of collagens and proteoglycans. Type I and type V fibrillar collagens are intertwined by filaments of type VI collagen. The major corneal proteoglycans are decorin (associated with dermatan sulfate) and lumican (associated with keratan sulfate). The concentrations and ratio of proteoglycans vary from anterior to posterior. Similarly, the posterior stroma is "wetter" than the anterior (3.85 mg H_2O/mg dry weight vs 3.04). Other water-soluble proteins, analogous to lens crystallins, may be secreted by keratocytes to control the optical properties of the cornea. The lamellae of the anterior stroma are short, narrow sheets with extensive interweaving between layers, while the posterior stroma has long, wide, thick lamellae extending from limbus to limbus with minimal interlamellar connections. The human cornea has little elasticity and stretches only 0.25% at normal intraocular pressures.

The lattice arrangement of collagen fibrils embedded in the extracellular matrix is partly responsible for corneal transparency. This pattern acts as a diffraction grating to reduce light scattering by means of destructive interference. Scattering is greater anteriorly, resulting in a higher refractive index that decreases from 1.401 at the epithelium to 1.380 in the stroma and 1.373 posteriorly. The cornea is transparent because the size of the lattice elements is smaller than the wavelength of visible light.

Transparency also depends on keeping the water content of the corneal stroma at 78%. Corneal hydration is largely controlled by intact epithelial and endothelial barriers

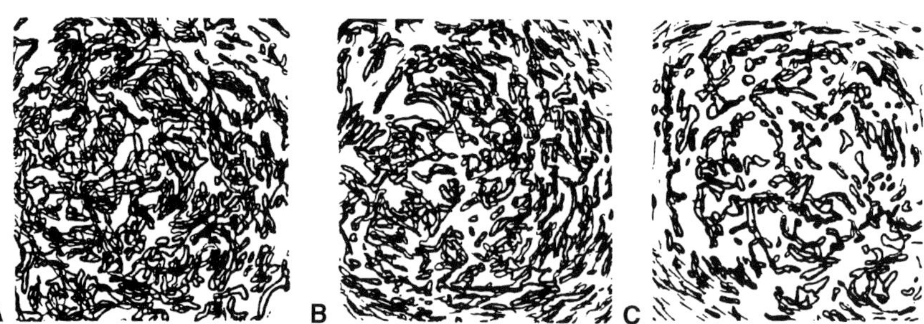

Figure 1-3 Organization of keratocytes in the corneal stroma. They change in density and shape but spiral in all layers. **A,** Anterior stroma; **B,** midstroma; **C,** posterior stroma. *(Reprinted with permission from Müller LJ, Pels L, Vrensen GFJM. Novel aspects of the ultrastructural organization of human corneal keratocytes. IOVS. 1995;36:2564.)*

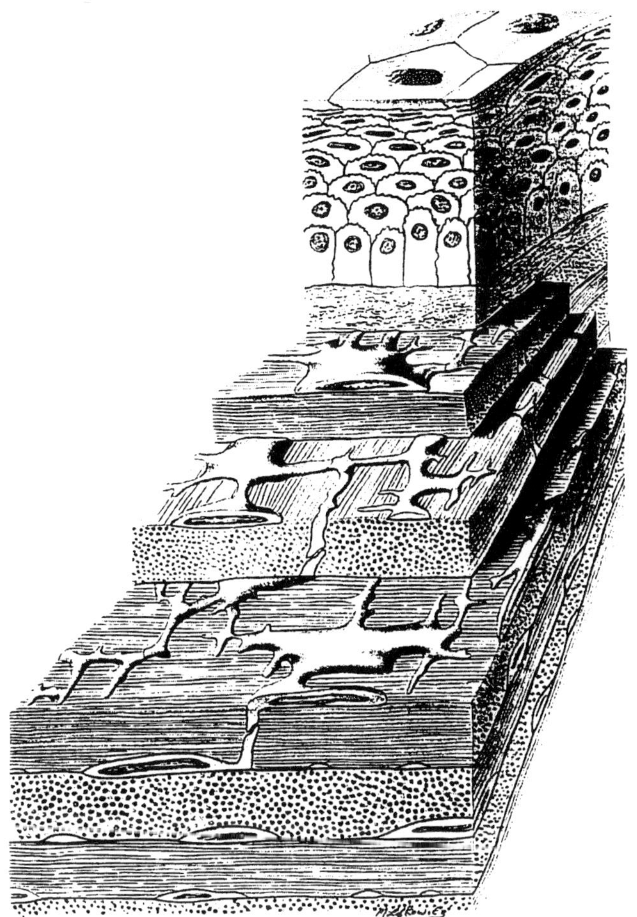

Figure 1-4 Organization of keratocytes in the corneal stroma, showing interconnection across lamellae. *(Reprinted with permission from Leibowitz HM, Waring GO III.* Corneal Disorders: Clinical Diagnosis and Management. *Philadelphia: Saunders; 1998:17.)*

and the functioning of the endothelial pump, which is linked to an ion-transport system controlled by temperature-dependent enzymes such as Na^+, K^+-ATPase. In addition, negatively charged stromal glycosaminoglycans tend to repel each other, producing a *swelling pressure* (SP). Because the intraocular pressure (IOP) tends to compress the cornea, the overall imbibition pressure of the corneal stroma is given as IOP − SP. The total transendothelial osmotic force is calculated by adding the imbibition pressure and the various electrolyte gradients produced by the endothelial transport channels. Corneal hydration varies from anterior to posterior with increasing wetness closer to the endothelium and resistance of movement of water laterally within the stroma. See also Part IV of BCSC Section 2.

Jester JV, Moller-Pedersen T, Huang J, et al. The cellular basis of corneal transparency: evidence for "corneal crystallins." *J Cell Sci.* 1999;112:613–622.

Endothelium

The endothelium is made up of closely interdigitated cells arranged in a mosaic pattern of mostly hexagonal shapes. Human endothelial cells do not proliferate in vivo. Cell loss results in enlargement and spread of neighboring cells to cover the defective area. Cell density varies over the endothelial surface; normally, the concentration is highest in the periphery.

Descemet's membrane is the basement membrane of the corneal endothelium. It increases in thickness from 3 μm at birth to 10–12 μm in adults as the endothelium gradually lays down a posterior amorphous nonbanded zone.

Krachmer JH, Mannis MJ, Holland EJ, eds. *Cornea.* Vol 1. St Louis: Mosby; 1997:3–27.

Smolin G, Thoft RA, eds. *The Cornea: Scientific Foundations and Clinical Practice.* 3rd ed. Boston: Little, Brown; 1994:3–67.

Sclera

The sclera is composed primarily of type I collagen and proteoglycans (decorin, biglycan, and aggrecan). Other components include elastin and glycoproteins such as fibronectin. Fibroblasts lie along collagen bundles. The long posterior ciliary nerves supply the anterior sclera. An intrascleral loop *(Axenfeld loop)* from a branch of one of these nerves sometimes forms a visible nodule over the ciliary body.

Normally a densely white tissue, sclera becomes more translucent when thinning occurs or the water content changes, falling below 40% or rising above 80%. For example, senile scleral plaques are areas of calcium phosphate deposits just anterior to the insertions of the medial and lateral rectus muscles that become dehydrated and reveal the blue color of the underlying uvea.

Krachmer JH, Mannis MJ, Holland EJ, eds. *Cornea.* Vol 1. St Louis: Mosby; 1997:29–40.

CHAPTER 2

Examination Techniques for the External Eye and Cornea

Examination of the patient begins the moment the examiner enters the room. Since the reader should already be familiar with the basic techniques of the complete ocular examination, this chapter will describe how to recognize abnormalities produced by disorders of the external eye and cornea. *Practical Ophthalmology: A Manual for Beginning Residents*, published by the American Academy of Ophthalmology, offers a concise review of examination techniques.

Vision

Visual acuity testing is an essential part of the examination, and the refraction of a patient with an abnormal cornea requires special attention. If visual acuity is reduced because of corneal irregularity, it may be necessary to use a rigid gas-permeable (RGP) contact lens with overrefraction. One method is to obtain keratometry readings and select a large-diameter hard contact lens with a base curve halfway between the two powers and with a power near the patient's spherical equivalent. Topical anesthesia helps reduce tearing as the spherical overrefraction is performed. The potential acuity meter provides another method for assessing visual acuity potential in a patient with focal corneal opacification or surface irregularity, but this instrument can give misleading results. BCSC Section 3, *Clinical Optics*, discusses these difficulties in detail in its appendix on prescribing cylinders.

External Examination

Physical examination of the eye begins with inspection, palpation, and occasionally auscultation. The examiner observes the patient's appearance and notes the condition of the skin, the position and action of the eyelids, the presence of preauricular lymph nodes, and the placement of the globes. Eversion of the eyelids permits examination of the palpebral conjunctiva. Infants and frightened patients may need to have their eyelids gently pried open with the thumbs or a retractor.

Common measurements include palpebral fissure height and levator function. The examiner should also measure any visible or palpable mass by its height and longest dimension. Tear production is measured with sterile filter-paper strips and may be done without anesthetic (Schirmer I test) or with anesthetic (basic secretion test).

External examination of the outer eye and adnexa begins with the examiner looking at the patient, preferably in daylight or bright room light, then proceeding to magnification with focal illumination. The simplest magnifying instruments are loupes and condensing lenses like those used for indirect ophthalmoscopy. Many handheld penlights and transilluminators are also available, and these tools are helpful at the bedside and for external surgical procedures.

Krachmer JH, Mannis MJ, Holland EJ, eds. Cornea. Vol 1. St Louis: Mosby; 1997:237–242.

Slit-Lamp Biomicroscopy

The slit-lamp biomicroscope has two rotating arms—one for the slit illuminator and the other for the biomicroscope—mounted on a common axis. The illumination unit is essentially a projector with a light beam that is adjustable in width, height, direction, intensity, and color. The biomicroscope is a binocular Galilean telescope with multiple magnifications. A headrest immobilizes the patient, and a joystick lever and adjustable eyepieces allow the examiner to focus the stereoscopic image.

The illumination and microscope arms are parfocal, arranged so that both focus on the same spot, with the slit beam centered in the field of view. This setup provides direct illumination, and purposeful shifting of alignment allows for indirect illumination. Variations of these illumination techniques, using both dark-field and bright-field contrast, are used to examine the anterior segment of the eye.

Leibowitz HM, Waring GO III, eds. Corneal Disorders: Clinical Diagnosis and Management.
2nd ed. Philadelphia: Saunders; 1998:34–81.

Direct Illumination Methods

Diffuse illumination

The light beam is broadened, reduced in intensity, and directed at the eye from an oblique angle. Diffuse illumination is usually used at low magnification to give an overview of the eyelids, conjunctiva, sclera, and cornea. Swinging the illuminator arm to produce highlights and shadows can enhance the visibility of surface changes.

Slit illumination

The light and the microscope are focused on the same spot, and the slit aperture is adjusted from wide to narrow. Broad-beam illumination, using a slit width of around 3 mm, can help the examiner visualize opaque lesions. Slit-beam illumination, using a beam width of about 1 mm or less, gives an optical section of the cornea (Fig 2-1). A very narrow slit beam helps identify refractive index differences in transparent structures as light rays pass through the cornea, anterior chamber, and lens. The examiner can reduce the height of a narrow beam to determine the presence and amount of cells and flare in the anterior chamber.

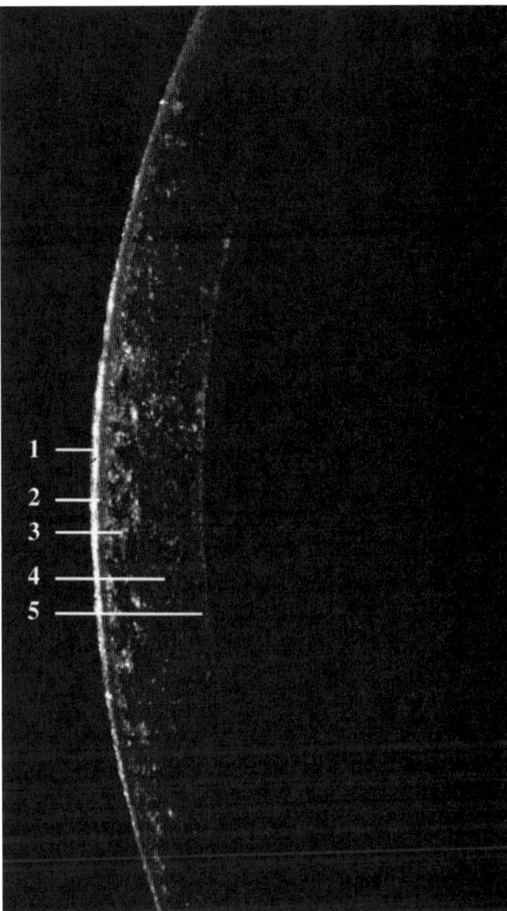

Figure 2-1 Slit section of normal cornea. **1,** Tear film. **2,** Epithelium. **3,** Anterior stroma with high density of keratocytes. **4,** Posterior stroma with lower density of keratocytes. **5,** Descemet's membrane and endothelium. *(Reproduced with permission from Krachmer JH, Mannis MJ, Holland EJ, eds.* Cornea. *Vol 1. St Louis: Mosby; 1997:249. ©CL Mártonyi, WK Kellogg Eye Center, University of Michigan.)*

Specular reflection

Specular reflections are normal light reflexes bouncing off a surface. An example is the bright round or oval spot seen reflected from the ocular surface in a typical flash photograph of an eye. These mirror images of the light source can be annoying, and it is tempting to ignore them during slit-lamp examination. However, the clarity and sharpness of these reflections from the tear film give clues to the condition of the underlying tissue.

A faint reflection also comes from the posterior corneal surface. The examiner can enhance this specular reflection by using a light beam at an appropriate angle, revealing the corneal endothelium (Fig 2-2). Following are the steps for examining the corneal endothelium with specular reflection.

1. Begin by setting the slit-beam arm at an angle of 60° from the viewing arm and using a short slit or 0.2 mm spot.
2. Identify the very bright mirror image of the lightbulb's filament and the paired epithelial and endothelial Purkinje light reflexes.

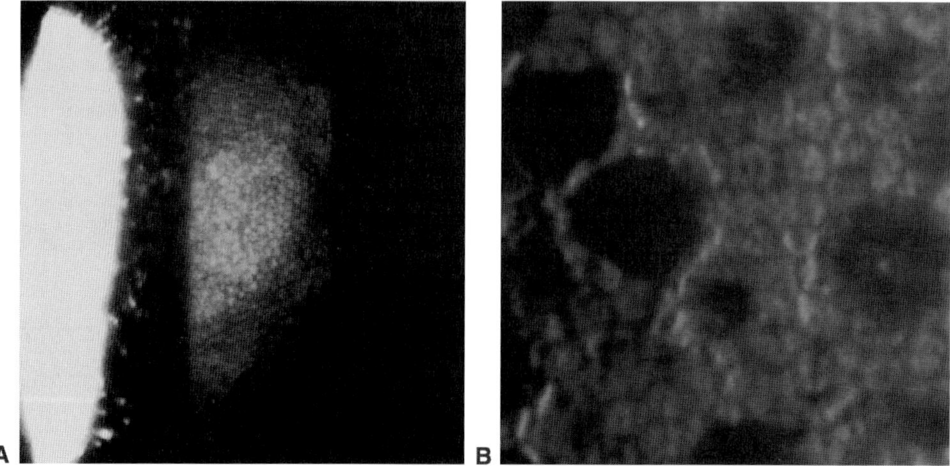

Figure 2-2 A, Corneal endothelium seen with specular reflection using the slit-lamp biomicroscope at ×40 magnification. *(Reproduced with permission from Krachmer JH, Mannis MJ, Holland EJ, eds. Cornea. Vol 1. St Louis: Mosby; 1997:255. ©CL Mártonyi, WK Kellogg Eye Center, University of Michigan.)* **B,** Fuchs endothelial dystrophy seen in specular microscopy showing guttata. *(Photograph courtesy of John E. Sutphin, Jr, MD.)*

3. Superimpose the corneal endothelial light reflex onto the filament's mirror image, giving a bright glare.
4. Use the joystick to move the biomicroscope slightly forward in order to focus the endothelial reflex.

Specular microscopy is monocular, and one eyepiece may require focusing. A setting of ×25 to ×40 is usually needed to obtain a clear view of the endothelial mosaic. Cell density and morphology are noted; guttae and keratic precipitates appear as nonreflective dark areas.

Indirect Illumination Methods

Proximal illumination

Turning a knob on the illumination arm slightly decenters the light beam from its isocentric position, causing the light beam and the microscope to be focused at different but adjacent spots. This technique highlights an opacity against deeper tissue layers and allows the examiner to see small irregularities that have a refractive index similar to their surroundings. Moving the light beam back and forth in small oscillations can help the examiner detect small three-dimensional lesions.

Sclerotic scatter

Total internal reflection in the cornea makes possible another form of indirect illumination. Decentering the isocentric light beam so that an intense beam shines on the limbus and scatters off the sclera causes a very faint glow of the cornea. Reflective opacities stand out against the dark field, while areas of reduced light transmission in the cornea are seen as shades of gray. This technique is effective in demonstrating epithelial edema and nebulae.

Retroillumination

This technique can be used to examine more than one area. Retroillumination from the iris is performed by displacing the beam tangentially while examining the cornea. The examiner observing the zone between the light and dark backgrounds can detect subtle corneal abnormalities. Retroillumination from the fundus is performed by aligning the light beam nearly parallel with the examiner's visual axis and rotating the light so it shines through the edge of the pupil. Opacities in the cornea or lens are highlighted against the red reflex, and iris defects are transilluminated. Retroillumination from light reflected off the retinal pigment epithelium is used with the Hruby lens or an indirect condensing lens to reveal vitreous floaters.

Farrell TA, Alward WLM, Verdick RE. *Fundamentals of Slit-Lamp Biomicroscopy* [videotape]. San Francisco: American Academy of Ophthalmology; 1993.

Clinical Use

Slit-lamp examination is performed in a logical sequence:

1. Eyelids
2. Eyelid margins
3. Tear film
4. Conjunctiva
5. Cornea
6. Aqueous humor
7. Iris
8. Lens
9. Vitreous

After adjusting the focus of the eyepieces, the clinician usually begins the examination with direct illumination of the eyelids, conjunctiva, and sclera. A broad beam illuminates the cornea and overlying tear film in optical section. Details are examined with a narrow beam. The clinician estimates the height of the tear meniscus and looks for mucin cells and other debris in the tear film. Discrete lesions are measured with a slit-beam micrometer or an eyepiece reticule. Retroillumination and indirect illumination accentuate fine changes. The examiner then uses specular reflection to inspect the endothelium and has the patient shift gaze in different directions so that each corneal quadrant can be surveyed. A slit beam is used to judge the corneal thickness and the depth of the anterior chamber. A short beam or spot will show flare or cells in the aqueous humor. Direct, slit, and retroillumination techniques are used to identify abnormalities of the iris and lens.

The experienced examiner actively controls the light beam with multiple illumination methods to sweep across the eye, using shadows and reflections to bring out details. Having the patient blink can also help the examiner to distinguish changes of the ocular surface from tiny opacities floating in the tear film. After initial low-power screening, much of the slit-lamp examination is performed using higher magnifications.

Except for the anterior vitreous humor, deeper and peripheral intraocular structures require special lenses. A contact lens permits examination of the intermediate and posterior portions of the eye and is often combined with angled mirrors and prisms for gonioscopy and peripheral fundus examination. A concave Hruby lens or a convex condensing lens allows diffuse and focal illumination of the posterior segment.

Stains

Hydroxyxanthene dyes such as fluorescein have been in clinical use for more than a century. They are commonly used to detect corneal epithelial lesions, to aid in applanation tonometry, and to evaluate lacrimal drainage and deficient tear flow. In clinical practice, fluorescein is used to detect disruption of intercellular junctions, and rose bengal is used to evaluate abnormal epithelial cells and ocular surface changes associated with insufficient tear film protection. Lissamine green strips are also available for diagnostic use.

Fluorescein

Topical fluorescein is a nontoxic, water-soluble dye that is available in several forms: as a 0.25% solution with an anesthetic (benoxinate or proparacaine), an antiseptic (povidone-iodine), and a preservative; as a 2% nonpreserved unit-dose eyedrop; and in impregnated paper strips. Fluorexon is a related macromolecular compound available as a 0.35% nonpreserved solution that will not stain most contact lenses. Fluorescence is easily detected with a cobalt blue filter.

Fluorescein is most commonly used for applanation tonometry and evaluation of the tear film. Tear breakup time is measured by instilling fluorescein, asking the patient to hold the eyelids open after one or two blinks, and counting the seconds until a dry spot appears. Fluorescein will stain punctate and macroulcerative epithelial defects (*positive staining*), and it can highlight nonstaining lesions that project through the tear film (*negative staining*). Different disease states can produce various punctate staining patterns (Fig 2-3). Fluorescein that collects in an epithelial defect will diffuse into the corneal stroma and cause a green flare in the anterior chamber. In the *dye disappearance test,* the tear meniscus is observed for the disappearance of fluorescein. Prolonged presence of dye suggests either blockage of the drainage system or decrease in tear flow consistent with lacrimal deficiency.

The *Seidel test* is used to detect seepage of aqueous humor through a corneal perforation. The examiner applies fluorescein using a moistened strip or concentrated drop to the site of suspected leakage and looks for a flow of clear fluid streaming through the orange dye under cobalt blue light.

Rose Bengal

Rose bengal is a halide derivative of fluorescein available in impregnated paper strips. This dye is routinely used for evaluation of tear deficiency states and detection of various epithelial lesions. Rose bengal stains cells that are devitalized or have lost their normal

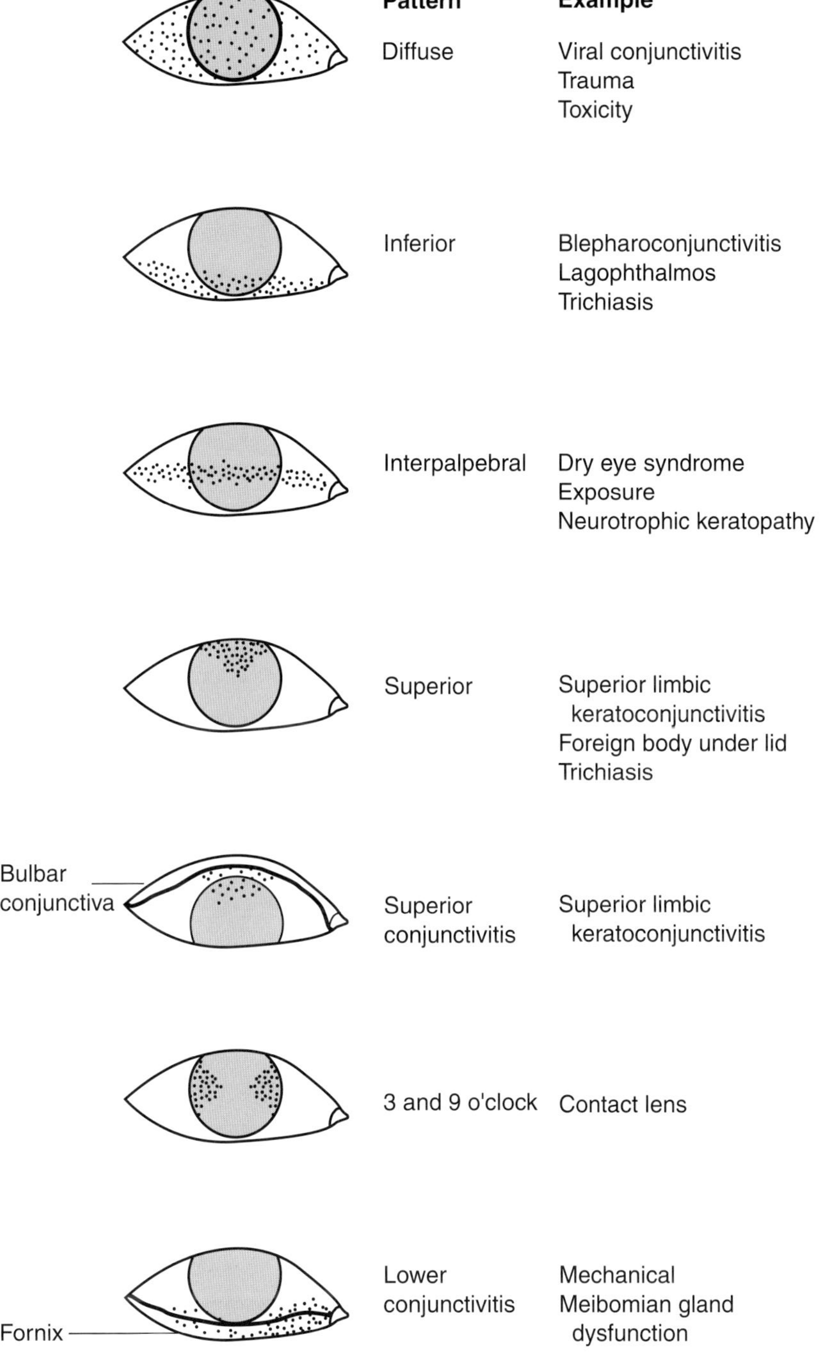

Figure 2-3 Punctate staining patterns of the ocular surface. *(Illustration by Joyce Zavarro.)*

mucin surface (eg, punctate epithelial keratitis). The red-free light filter accentuates its visibility. This dye is a photosensitizer and has antiviral and other toxic effects.

Krachmer JH, Mannis MJ, Holland EJ, eds. *Cornea.* Vol 1. St Louis: Mosby; 1997:243–273.

Clinical Evaluation of Ocular Inflammation

In clinical practice, it is helpful to use key distinctive features to categorize a patient's problem. The major disease mechanisms of the outer eye that the clinician should recognize by the history and examination are the following:

- Infection
- Immune alteration
- Neoplasia
- Maldevelopment
- Degeneration
- Trauma

These pathogenic categories are discussed in greater detail in individual chapters that follow. Because redness is often a feature of infection, allergy, neoplasia, injury, and other conditions, the following pages introduce the most common signs of ocular inflammation (see Table 2-1 for a summary of changes seen in the external eye and cornea).

Leibowitz HM, Waring GO III, eds. *Corneal Disorders: Clinical Diagnosis and Management.* 2nd ed. Philadelphia: Saunders; 1998:502–542.

Eyelid Signs of Inflammation

Individual skin changes should be described by their size, shape, and borders. Multiple lesions or a generalized skin eruption should be characterized by arrangement and distribution, using such terms as *disseminated, grouped,* or *confluent.* Several commonly encountered cutaneous lesions and their accompanying characteristics are described in Table 2-1.

Cellular infiltration and edema of the upper eyelid can cause eyelid drooping, called *mechanical blepharoptosis.* Protective ptosis is a result of ocular surface discomfort and photophobia.

Conjunctival Signs of Inflammation

Many forms of conjunctivitis heal without complications, but permanent changes may occur with severe or chronic inflammation. Keratinization of the ocular surface epithelium may occur over a chronically inflamed, indurated lesion. Chemosis may occur acutely or develop into conjunctivochalasis over time, with redundant folds that may even protrude over the lower eyelid. Conjunctival scarring can range from subepithelial reticular or lacy fibrosis to extensive symblepharon formation with eyelid distortion and secondary dry eye changes. Identification of the principal clinical feature of ocular inflammation can help in the differential diagnosis of common causes of conjunctivitis (see Table 2-2). Two common changes are papillae and follicles.

Table 2-1 Common Clinical Changes of the External Eye and Cornea

Tissue	Finding	Description
Eyelid	Macule	Spot of skin color change
	Papule	Solid, raised spot
	Vesicle	Blister filled with serous fluid
	Bulla	Large blister
	Pustule	Pus-filled blister
	Keratosis	Scaling from accumulated keratinizing cells
	Eczema	Scaly crust on a red base
	Erosion	Excoriated epidermal defect
	Ulcer	Epidermal erosion with deeper tissue loss
Conjunctiva	Hyperemia	Focal or diffuse dilation of the subepithelial plexus of conjunctival blood vessels, usually with increased blood flow; other changes include fusiform vascular dilations, saccular aneurysms, petechiae, and intraconjunctival hemorrhage
	Chalasis	Laxity of conjunctiva, sometimes with prolapse over the eyelid
	Chemosis	Conjunctival edema caused by a transudate leaking through fenestrated conjunctival capillaries as a result of altered vascular integrity (eg, inflammation and vasomotor changes) or hemodynamic changes (eg, impaired venous drainage or intravascular hyposmolarity)
	Tearing	Excess tears from increased lacrimation or impaired lacrimal outflow
	Mucous excess	Increased amount of mucin relative to aqueous component of tears
	Discharge	Exudate on the conjunctival surface, varying from proteinaceous (serous) to cellular (purulent)
	Papilla	Dilated, telangiectatic conjunctival blood vessels, varying from dotlike changes to enlarged tufts surrounded by edema and inflammatory cells
	Follicle	Focal lymphoid nodule with accessory vascularization
	Pseudomembrane	Inflammatory coagulum on the conjunctival surface that does not bleed during removal
	Membrane	Inflammatory coagulum suffusing the conjunctival epithelium that bleeds when stripped
	Granuloma	Nodule of chronic inflammatory cells with fibrovascular proliferation
	Phlyctenule	Nodule of chronic inflammatory cells, often at or near the limbus
	Punctate epithelial erosion	Loss of individual epithelial cells in a stippled pattern
	Epithelial defect	Focal area of epithelial loss
Cornea	Punctate epithelial erosion	Fine, slightly depressed stippling caused by altered or desquamated superfical epithelium
	Punctate epithelial keratitis	Swollen, slightly raised epithelial cells that can be finely scattered, coarsely grouped, or arranged in an arborescent pattern
	Epithelial edema	Swollen epithelial cells (intraepithelial edema) or intercellular vacuoles (microcystic edema)

(Continued)

Table 2-1 Common Clinical Changes of the External Eye and Cornea (Continued)

Tissue	Finding	Description
	Bulla	Fluid pocket within or under the epithelium
	Epithelial defect	Focal area of epithelial loss, caused by trauma (abrasion) or other condition
	Dendrite	Branching linear epithelial ridge with swollen cells, terminal end bulbs, and possible central ulceration
	Ulcer	Epithelial defect, stromal loss, stromal inflammation, or any combination of these changes
	Filament	Strand (filament) or clump (mucous plaque) of mucus and degenerating epithelial cells attached to an altered ocular surface
	Subepithelial infiltrate	Coin-shaped inflammatory opacity in the anterior portion of Bowman's layer
	Suppurative stromal keratitis	Focal yellow-white infiltrate composed of neutrophils
	Nonsuppurative stromal keratitis	Focal gray-white infiltrate of lymphocytes and other mononuclear cells; also called interstitial keratitis, especially when accompanied by stromal neovascularization
Sclera	Episcleritis	Focal or diffuse dilation of radial superficial episcleral vessels
	Nonnecrotizing scleritis	Dilated deep episcleral vessels with scleral edema
	Necrotizing scleritis	Area of avascular sclera

Table 2-2 Common Causes of Conjunctival Inflammation

Finding	Examples
Papillary conjunctivitis	Allergic conjunctivitis Bacterial conjunctivitis
Follicular conjunctivitis	Adenovirus conjunctivitis Herpes simplex virus conjunctivitis Molluscum contagiosum blepharoconjunctivitis Chlamydial conjunctivitis Drug-induced (eg, dipivefrin) conjunctivitis
Conjunctival pseudomembrane or membrane	Severe viral or bacterial conjunctivitis Stevens-Johnson syndrome Chemical burn
Conjunctival granuloma	Cat-scratch disease Sarcoidosis Foreign body reaction
Conjunctival erosion or ulceration	Stevens-Johnson syndrome Ocular cicatricial pemphigoid Graft-versus-host disease Factitious conjunctivitis

Papillae

Papillae are vascular changes seen most easily in the palpebral conjunctiva where fibrous septa anchor the conjunctiva to the tarsus (Fig 2-4). With progression, these dilated vessels sprout spokelike capillaries that become surrounded by edema and a mixed inflammatory cell infiltrate, producing raised elevations under the conjunctival epithelium.

A mild papillary reaction produces a smooth, velvety appearance (Fig 2-5A). Chronic or progressive changes result in enlarged vascular tufts that obscure the underlying blood vessels (Fig 2-5B). Connective tissue septa restrict inflammatory changes to the fibrovascular core, producing the appearance of elevated, polygonal, hyperemic mounds. Each papilla has a central red dot that represents a dilated capillary viewed end-on. The palpebral and forniceal conjunctiva beyond the tarsus is less helpful in revealing the nature of an inflammatory reaction because the anchoring septa become sparser toward the fornix and permit undulation of less adherent tissue. With prolonged, recurrent, or severe

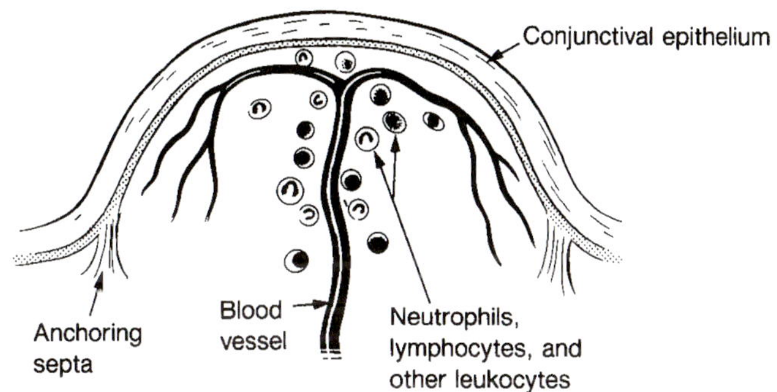

Figure 2-4 Cross-sectional diagram of conjunctival papilla with a central vascular tuft surrounded by acute and chronic leukocytes.

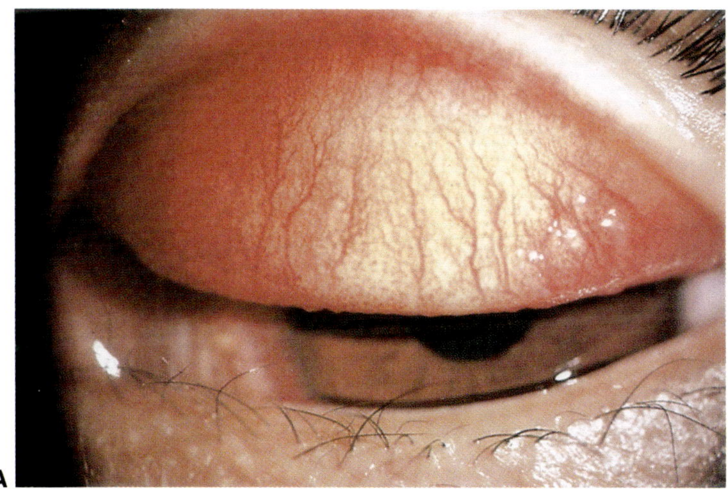

Figure 2-5 Papillary conjunctivitis. **A,** Mild papillae. *(Continues on next page.)*

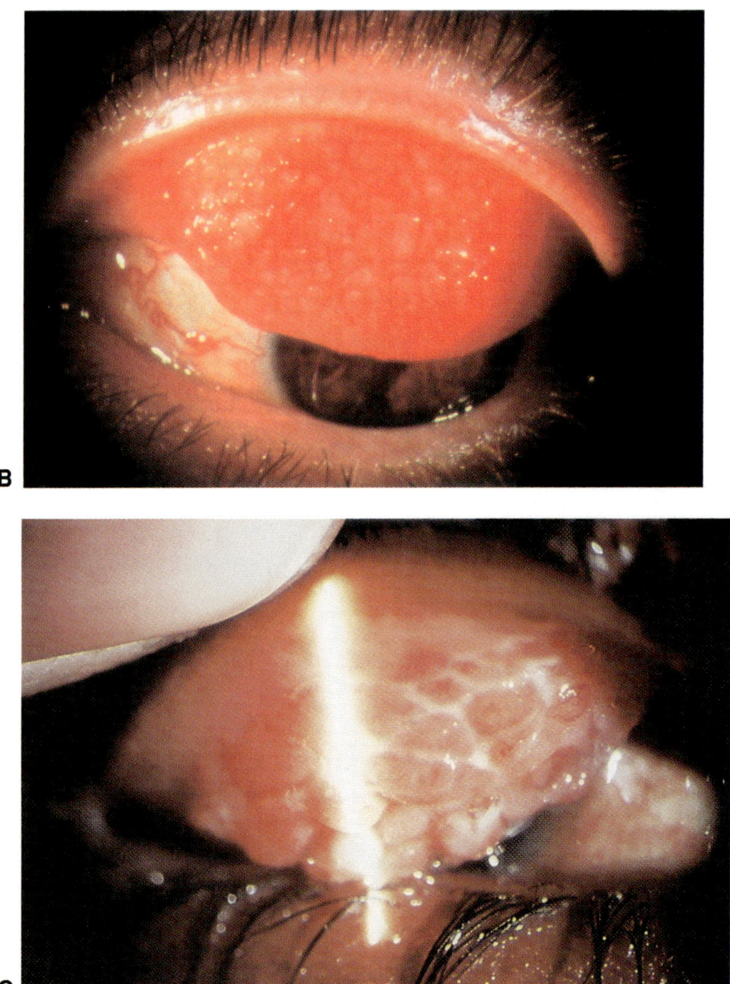

Figure 2-5 *(Continued)* **B,** Moderate papillae. **C,** Marked (giant) papillae.

conjunctival inflammation, the anchoring fibers of the tarsal conjunctiva stretch and weaken, leading to confluent papillary hypertrophy (Fig 2-5C). The furrows between these enlarged fibrovascular structures collect mucus and pus.

Follicles

Conjunctival lymphoid tissue is normally present within the substantia propria except in neonates, who do not have visible follicles. Conjunctival follicles are round or oval clusters of lymphocytes (Fig 2-6). Small follicles are often visible in the normal lower fornix. Clusters of enlarged, noninflamed follicles are occasionally seen in the inferotemporal palpebral and forniceal conjunctiva of children and adolescents, a condition known as *benign lymphoid folliculosis* (Fig 2-7).

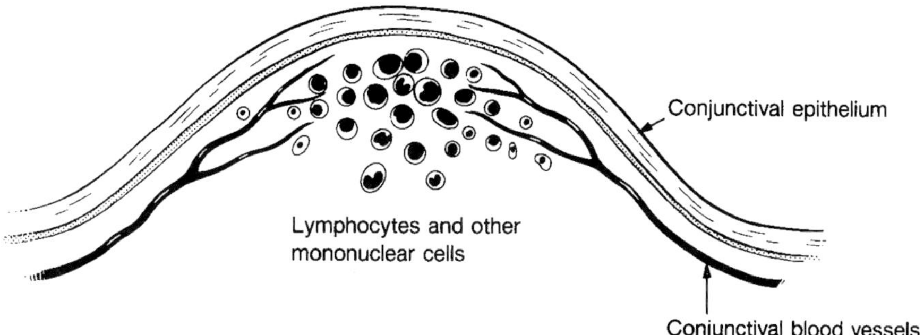

Figure 2-6 Cross-sectional diagram of conjunctival follicle with mononuclear cells obscuring conjunctival blood vessels.

Follicular conjunctivitis involves redness and new or enlarged follicles. Vessels surround and encroach on the raised surface of follicles but are not prominently visible within the follicle (Fig 2-8). Follicles can be seen in the inferior and superior tarsal conjunctiva and, less often, on the bulbar or limbal conjunctiva. They must be differentiated from cysts produced by tubular epithelial infoldings during chronic inflammation.

Corneal Signs of Inflammation

Inflammation can affect any layer of the cornea. The pattern of corneal inflammation, or *keratitis,* can be described according to the following:

- *Distribution:* diffuse, focal, or multifocal
- *Depth:* epithelial, subepithelial, stromal, or endothelial
- *Location:* central or peripheral
- *Shape:* dendritic, disciform, etc.

The clinician should also note any structural or physiologic changes associated with keratitis, such as ulceration or endothelial dysfunction.

Punctate epithelial keratopathy is a nonspecific term that includes a spectrum of biomicroscopic changes from punctate epithelial granularity to erosive and inflammatory changes (Fig 2-9).

A key feature of *stromal inflammation* is the presence of new blood vessels. Active corneal blood vessels most commonly come from the limbal vascular arcades and migrate into the peripheral cornea. Cells can also enter the stroma from the tear film through an epithelial defect or, less often, from direct interlamellar infiltration of leukocytes at the limbus. Inflammatory cells enter from aqueous humor in the presence of endothelial injury. In a vascularized cornea, inflammatory cells can emanate directly from infiltrating blood and lymphatic vessels.

Stromal inflammation is characterized as *suppurative* or *nonsuppurative* (Fig 2-10). It is further described by distribution (*focal* or *multifocal* infiltrates) and by location (*central, paracentral,* or *peripheral). Necrotizing* stromal keratitis is a severe form of infiltrate without the liquefaction associated with suppuration. The various morphological

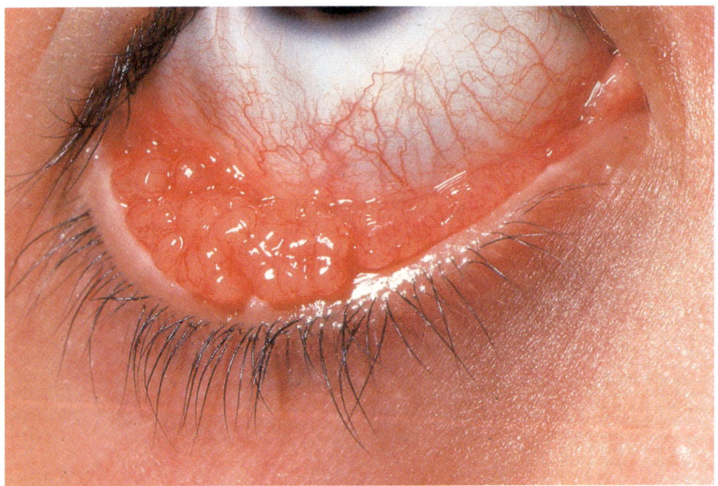

Figure 2-7 Benign folliculosis. *(Photograph courtesy of Kirk R. Wilhelmus, MD.)*

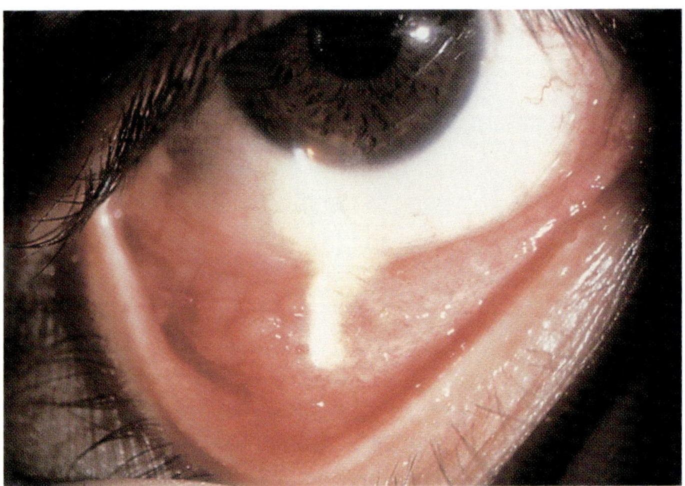

Figure 2-8 Follicular conjunctivitis.

changes of corneal inflammation, categorized by the principal clinical features, aid in differential diagnosis (Table 2-3).

Endothelial dysfunction often accompanies corneal stromal inflammation and contributes to epithelial and stromal edema. Swollen endothelial cells called *inflammatory pseudoguttae* are visible by specular reflection as dark areas of the normal mosaic pattern. *Keratic precipitates (KP)* are clumps of inflammatory cells on the back of the cornea that come from the anterior uvea during the course of keratitis or uveitis. The clinical appearance of KP depends on the composition:

- Fibrin and other proteins coagulate into small dots and strands

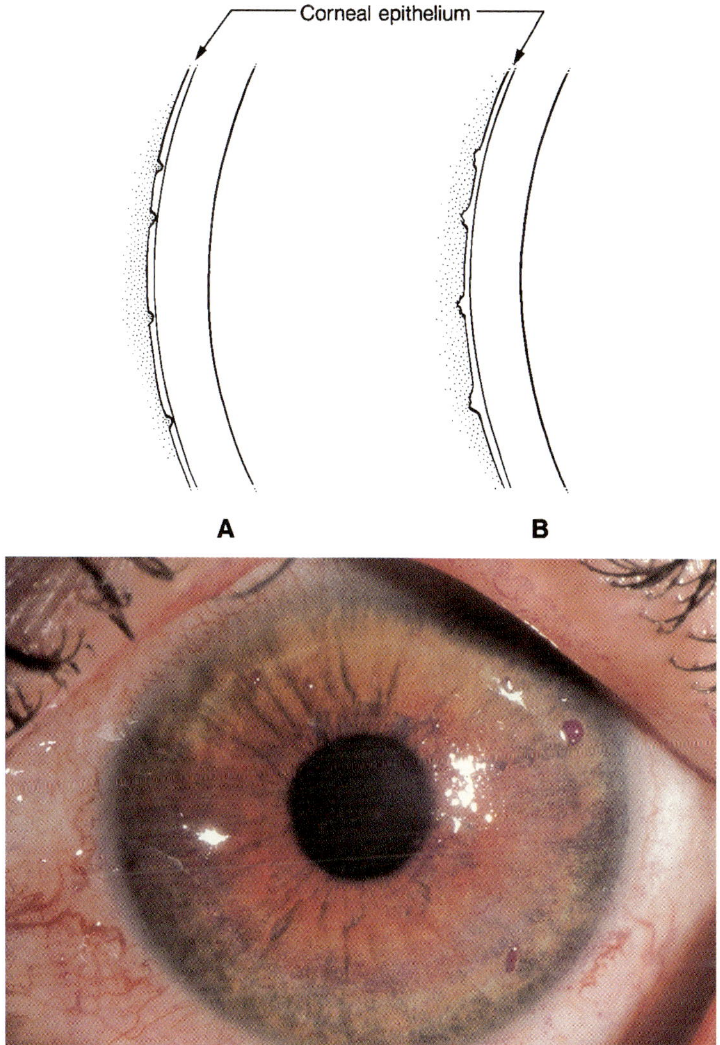

Figure 2-9 Punctate lesions of the corneal epithelium. **A,** Punctate epithelial erosions. **B,** Punctate epithelial keratitis. **C,** Punctate epithelial erosions. *(Continues on next page.)*

- Neutrophils and lymphocytes aggregate into punctate opacities
- Macrophages form larger "mutton-fat" clumps

Inflammation can lead to corneal opacification. Altered stromal keratocytes fail to produce some water-soluble factors and, consequently, make new collagen fibers that are disorganized, scatter light, and form a nontransparent scar. Scarring can also incorporate calcium complexes, lipids, and proteinaceous material. Dark pigmentation of a residual corneal opacity is often a result of incorporated melanin or iron salts.

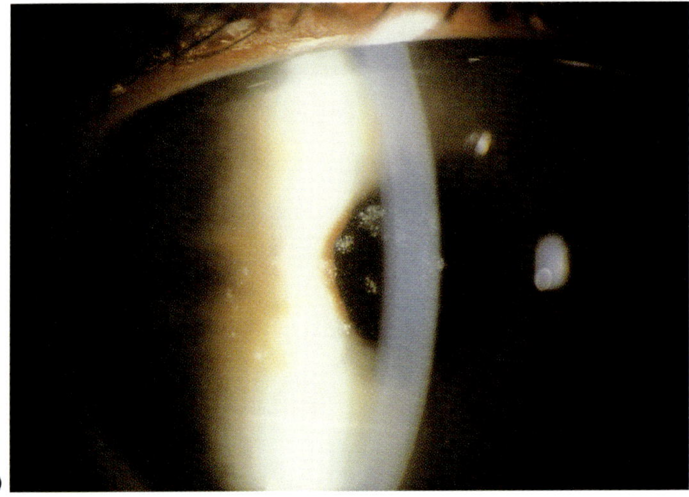

Figure 2-9 *(Continued)* **D,** Punctate epithelial keratitis.

Corneal inflammation can also lead to neovascularization. Superficial stromal blood vessels originate as capillary buds of limbal vascular arcades in the palisades of Vogt. New lymphatic vessels may also form but cannot be seen clinically. Subepithelial fibrous ingrowth into the peripheral cornea is called a *pannus* or vascularized pannus (Fig 2-11). Neovascularization may invade the cornea at deeper levels depending on the nature and location of the inflammatory stimulus. Any vessel tends to remain at a single lamellar plane as it grows unless stromal disorganization has occurred.

Leibowitz HM, Waring GO III, eds. *Corneal Disorders: Clinical Diagnosis and Management.* 2nd ed. Philadelphia: Saunders; 1998:432–479.

Scleral Signs of Inflammation

Episcleritis and scleritis may be *nodular* or *diffuse,* and anterior scleritis may be *necrotizing* or *nonnecrotizing.* The red-free light filter can help identify which layer of blood vessels is dilated. Areas of increased translucency *(scleromalacia)* are detected by direct observation and by transillumination.

Corneal Pachymetry

A corneal pachymeter measures corneal thickness, a sensitive indicator of endothelial physiology that correlates well with functional measurements such as aqueous fluorophotometry. The normal cornea has a central thickness of about 0.52 mm and becomes thicker in the paracentral zone (from about 0.52 mm inferiorly to 0.57 mm superiorly) and peripheral zone (from 0.63 mm inferiorly to 0.67 mm superiorly). The thinnest zone is about 1.50 mm temporal to the geographic center.

Optical pachymetry can be performed using a device that attaches to the slit-lamp biomicroscope, but it is somewhat imprecise. Ultrasonic pachymetry is both easier and

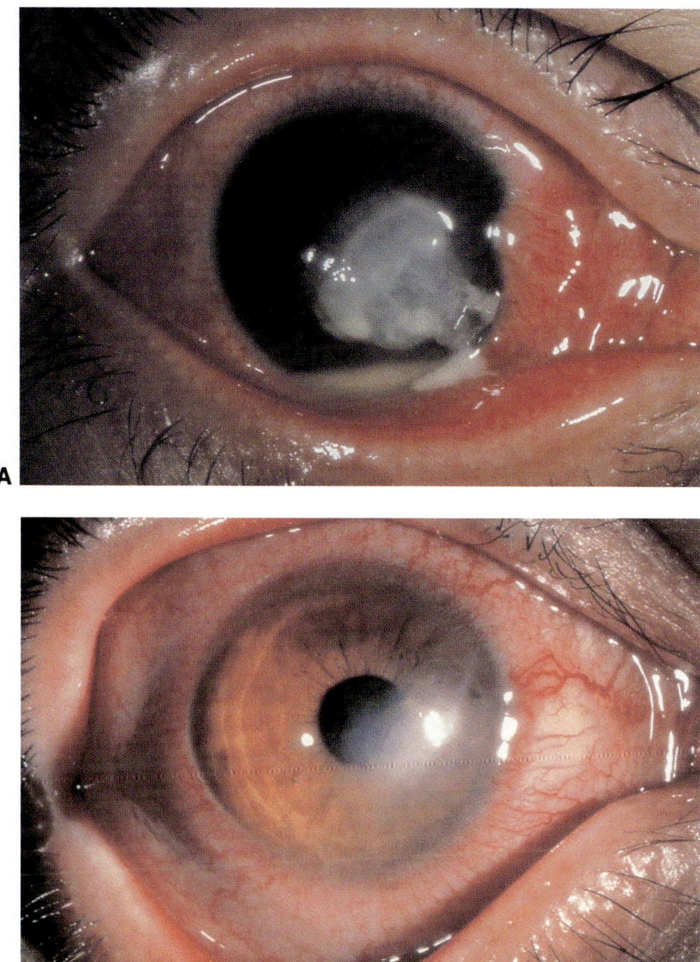

Figure 2-10 Inflammation of the corneal stroma. **A,** Suppurative keratitis. **B,** Nonsuppurative, nonnecrotizing (disciform) stromal keratitis.

more accurate. Instrumentation is based on the speed of sound in the normal cornea (1640 m/sec). The applanating tip must be perpendicular to the surface because errors are induced by tilting. Improved signal processing and other methods such as laser interferometry allow the examiner to map the corneal thickness very precisely.

Corneal pachymetry can aid in the diagnosis of corneal thinning disorders and can also be used to assess the function of the corneal endothelium. Folds in Descemet's membrane are first seen when corneal thickness increases by 10% or more; epithelial edema occurs when corneal thickness exceeds 0.70 mm. A central corneal thickness greater than 0.65 mm suggests a higher risk for symptomatic corneal edema after intraocular surgery.

Table 2-3 Common Causes of Corneal Inflammation

Finding	Examples
Punctate epithelial erosions	Dry eye syndrome Toxicity Atopic keratoconjunctivitis
Punctate epithelial keratitis	Adenovirus keratoconjunctivitis Herpes simplex virus epithelial keratitis Thygeson superficial punctate keratitis
Stromal keratitis, suppurative	Bacterial keratitis Fungal keratitis
Stromal keratitis, nonsuppurative	Herpes simplex virus stromal keratitis Varicella-zoster virus stromal keratitis Syphilitic interstitial keratitis
Peripheral keratitis	Blepharitis-associated marginal infiltrates Peripheral ulcerative keratitis caused by connective tissue diseases Mooren ulcer

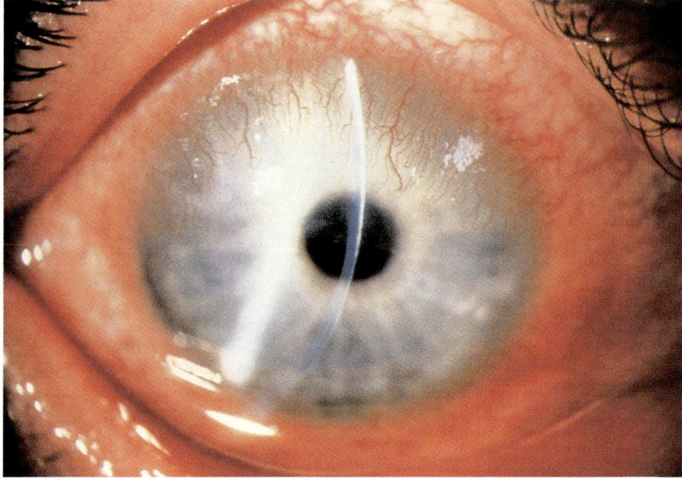

Figure 2-11 Corneal pannus. *(Photograph courtesy of Kirk R. Wilhelmus, MD.)*

Optical coherence tomography is a newer technique that can be used to image the cornea, including curvature and thickness, as well as the anterior segment.

Corneal Edema

The corneal endothelium maintains corneal clarity through two functions: by acting as a barrier to the aqueous humor and by providing a metabolic pump. Alteration of either function by damage or maldevelopment leads to corneal edema, a condition of abnormal homeostasis resulting in excess fluid within the corneal stroma and/or epithelium. Increased permeability and insufficient pump sites occur with an endothelial cell density lower than 500 cells/mm^2.

Acute corneal edema is often the result of an altered barrier effect of the endothelium or epithelium. *Chronic corneal edema* is usually caused by an inadequate endothelial pump. When functioning normally, the endothelial pump balances the leak rate to maintain the corneal stromal water content at 78% and the central corneal thickness at 0.52 mm. *Stromal edema* alters corneal transparency, but visual loss is most severe when epithelial microcysts or bullae occur. A *posterior collagenous layer,* or *retrocorneal membrane,* can arise after endothelial cell damage. The physiology of the endothelium is discussed in BCSC Section 2, *Fundamentals and Principles of Ophthalmology.*

Various traumatic, inflammatory, and dystrophic mechanisms can produce corneal edema (Table 2-4). The examiner can consider duration, laterality, and the presence of associated ocular disease in identifying the underlying etiology. Clinical examination should use the various illumination techniques of slit-lamp biomicroscopy. Early signs include patchy or diffuse haze of the epithelium, mild stromal thickening, faint deep stromal wrinkles *(Waite-Beetham lines),* Descemet's membrane folds, and a patchy or diffuse posterior collagenous layer. Endothelial alterations include reversible changes such as pseudoguttata and permanent alterations such as corneal guttae *(cornea guttata).*

Corneal thickness and intraocular pressure

It is important to be aware that corneal thickness can affect the measurement of intraocular pressure with Goldmann applanation tonometry. For example, patients with normal but thick corneas may have artifactually elevated IOP because of increased corneal rigidity and resistance to deformation. Conversely, increased IOP may cause compaction of the cornea and development of epithelial edema with a corresponding decrease in rigidity and resistance to deformation, leading to an artifactually lower IOP by Goldmann tonometry. Loss of endothelial function with development of stromal edema primarily in the posterior lamellae also results in artifactually reduced IOP when corneal strain is taken up by the relatively unaffected anterior lamellae only.

Doughty MJ, Zaman ML. Human corneal thickness and its impact on intraocular pressure measures: a review and meta-analysis approach. *Surv Ophthalmol.* 2000;44:367–408.

Esthesiometry

Esthesiometry is the measurement of corneal sensation, which is a function of the ophthalmic branch of cranial nerve V. Its primary use is in the evaluation of neurotrophic keratopathy. In most clinical circumstances, reduced corneal sensitivity can be diagnosed qualitatively without special instruments; but quantitative esthesiometry is useful in unusual cases and for research. Obviously, the examiner does not apply topical anesthesia (or any other topical agent, preferably) to the eye if corneal sensation is to be evaluated. In addition, the patient should be advised not to apply topical medications before the examination.

Corneal sensation is most easily tested in comparison to a normal fellow eye. A rolled wisp of cotton from a cotton-tipped applicator is touched lightly to corresponding quad-

Table 2-4 Causes of Corneal Edema

Type	Cause
Acute	Trauma (eg, epithelial defect, intraocular surgery)
	Inflammation (eg, infectious or immune-mediated keratitis, corneal graft rejection)
	Hypoxia (eg, contact lens overwear)
	Hydrops from ruptured Descemet's membrane (eg, keratoconus)
	Increased intraocular pressure
Chronic	Trauma or toxins (eg, intraocular surgery)
	Fuchs dystrophy
	Posterior polymorphous dystrophy
	Iridocorneal endothelial syndrome

rants of each cornea. The patient is asked to report the degree of sensation in the first eye relative to that of the fellow eye, and sensation is recorded as normal, reduced, or absent for each quadrant. This method can be used to detect most clinically relevant cases of reduced corneal sensation.

The handheld esthesiometer gives quantitative information about corneal sensation. This device contains a thin, flexible, retractable filament. The patient's cornea is touched with the filament extended to the full 6 cm. The filament is then retracted incrementally in 0.5 cm steps until it becomes rigid enough to allow the patient to feel its contact. This length is then recorded. Esthesiometry readings may vary with user technique, but in general a lower number, or shorter filament, indicates reduced corneal sensation. After the central cornea's sensitivity is measured, a map is produced of the cornea (and sometimes of the bulbar conjunctiva) by testing the superior, temporal, inferior, and nasal quadrants sequentially.

Krachmer JH, Mannis MJ, Holland EJ, eds. *Cornea.* Vol 1. St Louis: Mosby; 1997:275–281.

Anterior Segment Photography

External and Slit-Lamp Photography

External eye photography is usually performed with a single-lens reflex camera. Magnification up to 1:1 (life-size) can be obtained with a bellows, extension ring, or close-focusing lens. Digital or 35-mm cameras can be attached with an adapter to a slit lamp and will produce excellent quality images, particularly if used with a fill light.

Slit-lamp photography and videophotography allow a permanent record of most anterior segment conditions. A photo slit-lamp biomicroscope is an instrument with a fill light and an electronic flash.

Krachmer JH, Mannis MJ, Holland EJ, eds. *Cornea.* Vol 1. St Louis: Mosby; 1997:283–304.

Specular Photomicroscopy

Because slit-lamp illumination techniques are only semiquantitative and slit-lamp photography is difficult, specular photomicroscopes are available to photograph the endothelium for closer evaluation. Specular reflection permits visualization of the corneal endothelial mosaic. Wide-field specular microscopy can be performed throughout the entire cornea, permitting the study of regional variability. Specular microscopy can be an important diagnostic tool, especially for differentiating between difficult or overlapping diagnostic entities, such as the iridocorneal endothelial (ICE) syndrome and posterior polymorphous corneal dystrophy.

Most specular microscopy techniques involve the use of a photomicroscope attached to an applanating cone and a coupling fluid. They are best performed following the application of a topical anesthetic (although noncontact techniques also exist). A relatively clear cornea is generally required in order to obtain a good specular image. As fine focus is obtained, the endothelial mosaic comes into view (Fig 2-12). The stroma and epithelium can also be examined and photographed. Most instruments have a pachymeter attached to the focusing apparatus so that corneal thickness can be measured. The parameters that can be calculated from the image include the following. (Note that these parameters have implications for the cornea's response to surgical manipulation.)

- *Density.* The normal endothelial cell density decreases with age. Endothelial cell density normally exceeds 3500 cells/mm^2 in children and gradually declines with age to about 2000 cells/mm^2 in older eyes. An average value for adults is 2400 cells/mm^2 (1500–3500), with a mean cell size of 150–350 μm^2. Corneas with low cell density (eg, fewer than 1000 cells/mm^2) might not tolerate intraocular surgery; donor corneas for transplantation should have at least 2000 cells/mm^2.
- *Coefficient of variation.* The mean cell area divided by the standard deviation of the mean cell area gives the coefficient of variation of mean cell area, a unitless number normally less than 0.30. *Polymegethism* is increased variation in individual cell areas and is typically increased with contact lens wear. Corneas with significant polymegethism (greater than 0.40) might not tolerate intraocular surgery.
- *Percentage of hexagonal cells.* The percentage of cells with six apices should ideally approach 100%. Lower percentages indicate a diminishing state of health of the endothelium. *Pleomorphism* is increased variability in cell shape. Corneas with high pleomorphism (more than 50% nonhexagonal) might not tolerate intraocular surgery.

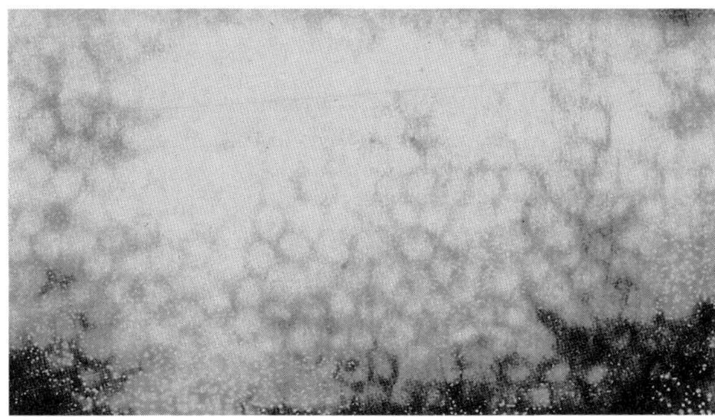

Figure 2-12 Specular photomicrograph of normal corneal endothelium, with cell density of 3300 cells/mm^2.

American Academy of Ophthalmology. *Corneal Endothelial Photography.* Ophthalmic Technology Assessment. 1996.

Krachmer JH, Mannis MJ, Holland EJ, eds. *Cornea.* Vol 1. St Louis: Mosby; 1997:313–334.

Leibowitz HM, Waring GO III, eds. *Corneal Disorders: Clinical Diagnosis and Management.* 2nd ed. Philadelphia: Saunders; 1998:83–122.

Anterior Segment Fluorescein Angiography

Anterior segment fluorescein angiography has occasionally been used to study the circulatory dynamics of normal and pathologic bulbar conjunctival, episcleral, scleral, and iris blood vessels. This technique is particularly applicable to patients who might have areas of vascular nonperfusion as in necrotizing scleritis and some forms of iritis.

Anterior Segment Echography

Echography of the anterior segment is occasionally required to detect foreign bodies, assess iris and ciliary body tumors, evaluate the extent of trauma, and determine the position of the crystalline lens or intraocular lens. Anterior segment echography may use an immersion technique, which involves inserting a small scleral shell between the eyelids and filling the shell with methylcellulose. This technique can be used to examine the cornea, anterior chamber, iris, lens, retrolental or retroiridal spaces, and ciliary body by A- and B-scan methods. The B-scan method called *ultrasound biomicroscopy* provides high resolution for examining the anterior segment structures. These 20–50 Hz instruments provide more detail of the angle, iris, and lens structure, but the higher frequency does not penetrate beyond 1.5–2.0 mm into the eye.

Confocal Microscopy

The scanning confocal microscope can be used to study cell layers of the cornea even in cases with edema and scarring. Confocal microscopy can detect infectious crystalline keratopathy, fungal keratitis, and amebic keratitis. It has also been used to follow refractive surgery patients to analyze haze formation and complications of LASIK flaps such as epithelial ingrowth.

Krachmer JH, Mannis MJ, Holland EJ, eds. *Cornea.* Vol 1. St Louis: Mosby; 1997:335–359.

Leibowitz HM, Waring GO III, eds. *Corneal Disorders: Clinical Diagnosis and Management.* 2nd ed. Philadelphia: Saunders; 1998:123–127.

Measurement of Corneal Topography

Zones of the Cornea

For more than 100 years the corneal shape has been known to be aspheric. Typically, the central cornea is about 3 D steeper than the periphery, a positive shape factor. Clinically, the cornea is divided into zones that surround fixation and blend into one another. The *central zone* of 1–2 mm closely fits a spherical surface. Adjacent to the central zone is a 3–4 mm doughnut with an outer diameter of 7–8 mm. Called the *paracentral zone*, this doughnut represents an area of progressive flattening from the center. Together, the paracentral and central zones constitute the *apical zone* as used in contact lens fitting. The central and paracentral zones are primarily responsible for the refractive power of the cornea (Fig 2-13). Adjacent to the paracentral zone is the *peripheral zone,* with an outer diameter of approximately 11 mm, and adjoining this is the *limbus,* with an outer diameter that averages 12 mm.

The peripheral zone is also known as the *transitional zone,* as it is the area of greatest flattening and asphericity of the normal cornea. The *limbal zone* lies adjacent to the sclera and is the area where the cornea steepens prior to joining the sclera at the limbal sulcus.

The *optical zone* is the portion of the cornea that overlies the entrance pupil of the iris; it is physiologically limited to approximately 5.4 mm because of the Stiles-Crawford effect. The *corneal apex* is the point of maximum curvature, typically temporal to the center of the pupil. The *corneal vertex* is the point located at the intersection of the patient's line of fixation and the corneal surface. It is represented by the corneal light reflex when the cornea is illuminated coaxially with fixation. The corneal vertex is the center of the keratoscopic image and does not necessarily correspond to the point of maximum curvature at the corneal apex (Fig 2-14).

Shape, Curvature, and Power

Three topographic properties of the cornea are important to its optical function: the underlying *shape,* which determines its *curvature* and hence its refractive *power.* Shape and curvature are *geometric* properties of the cornea, while power is the *functional* property. Historically, power was the first parameter of the cornea to be described, and diopters representing the refractive power of the central cornea were accepted as the basic unit of measurement. However, with the advent of contact lenses and refractive surgery, knowing the overall shape and the related property of curvature has become increasingly important.

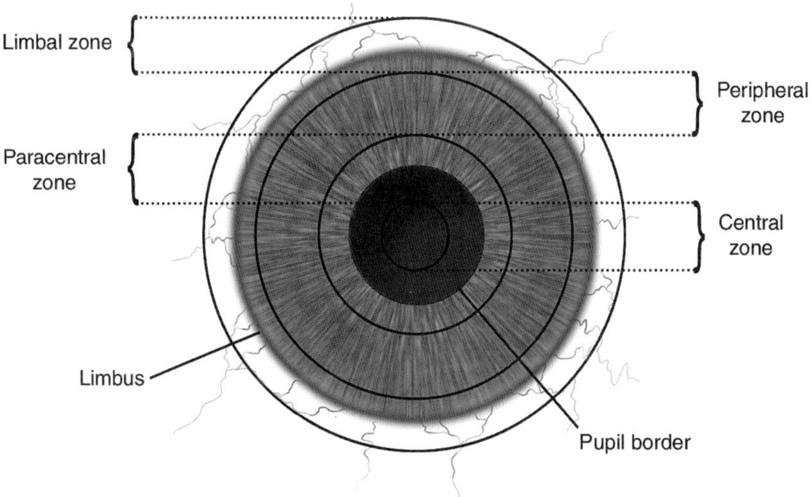

Figure 2-13 Topographic zones of the cornea. *(Illustration by Christine Gralapp.)*

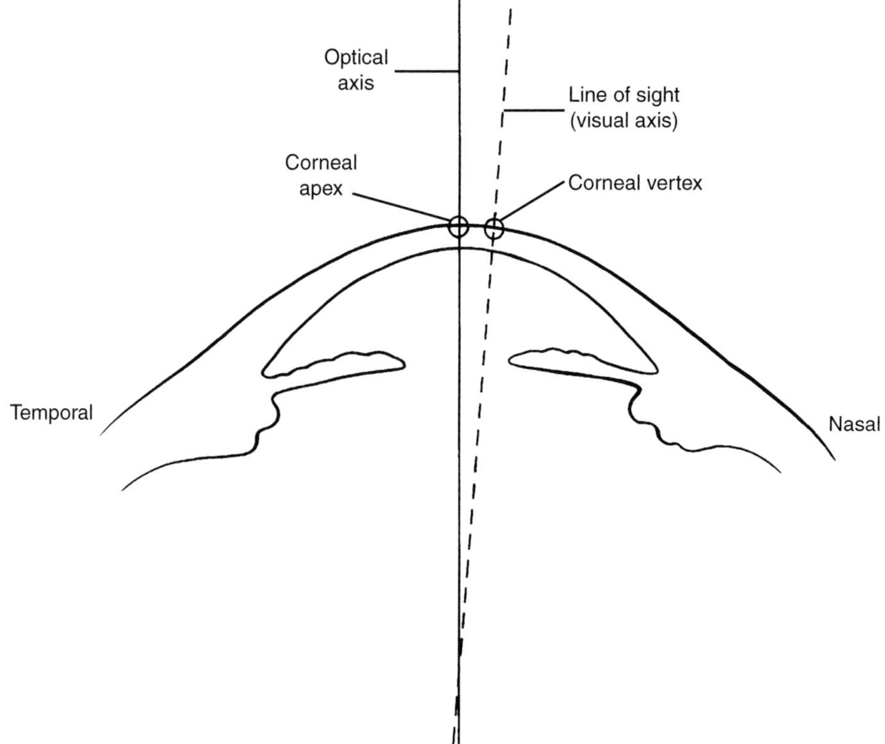

Figure 2-14 Corneal vertex and apex. *(Illustration by Christine Gralapp.)*

The refractive power of the cornea is determined by *Snell's law,* the *law of refraction.* Snell's law is based on the difference between two refractive indexes (in this case, of the cornea and of air), divided by the radius of curvature. The anterior corneal power using air and corneal stromal refractive indexes is higher than clinically useful because it does not take into account the negative contribution of the posterior cornea. Thus, for most clinical purposes, a derived corneal refractive index of 1.3375 is used in calculating central corneal power. This value was chosen to allow 45 D to equate to a 7.5 mm radius of curvature. Average refractive power of the central cornea is about +43 D, which is the sum of the refractive power at the air–stroma interface of +49 D minus the endothelium–aqueous power of 6 D. The refractive index of air is 1.000, aqueous and tears is 1.336, and corneal stroma is 1.376. Although the air–tear interface of the cornea is responsible for most of the eye's refraction, the difference between total corneal power based on stroma alone and with tears is only − .06 D.

BCSC Section 3, *Clinical Optics,* covers these topics in greater depth.

Keratometry

The ophthalmometer (keratometer) empirically estimates corneal power by reading four points of the central 2.8–4.0 mm zone. These points do not represent the corneal apex or vertex but are a clinically useful estimation of central corneal power. The radius of curvature is calculated from the simple vergence formula using the known circular object size and measuring the distance with doubling prisms to stabilize the image. The longer axis of the elliptical image is produced by the flattest portion of the cornea (ie, that part of the central cornea that has the longest radius of curvature and the lowest dioptric power). The axial radius of curvature is then used in computing the corneal power in this region. Results are reported as *radius of curvature* in millimeters or *refracting power* in diopters.

For most normal corneas, keratometry is sufficiently accurate for contact lens fitting or intraocular lens power calculation. Keratometry is also useful in detecting irregular astigmatism, in which keratometric images cannot be superimposed or are not regular ovals. However, in some circumstances, such as with keratoconus or after radial keratotomy, the optical properties of the cornea are affected by zones other than those measured by keratometry. Topographic keratometry can be performed with a special attachment to the instrument. See also BCSC Section 3, *Clinical Optics*.

Keratoscopy

Information about corneal curvature can be obtained with a variety of instruments that reflect the images of multiple concentric circles from the corneal surface. These devices allow analysis of corneal curvature in zones both central and peripheral to those measured by keratometry. In general, the reflected mires appear closer together on steeper parts of the cornea (Fig 2-15). The handheld *Placido disk* is a keratoscope with a flat target. *Collimating keratoscopes* use rings inside a column or a curve to maximize the area of the ocular surface that can reflect the target mires. Photokeratoscopy preserves the virtual image of concentric circles on film, and videokeratoscopy stores the images on video.

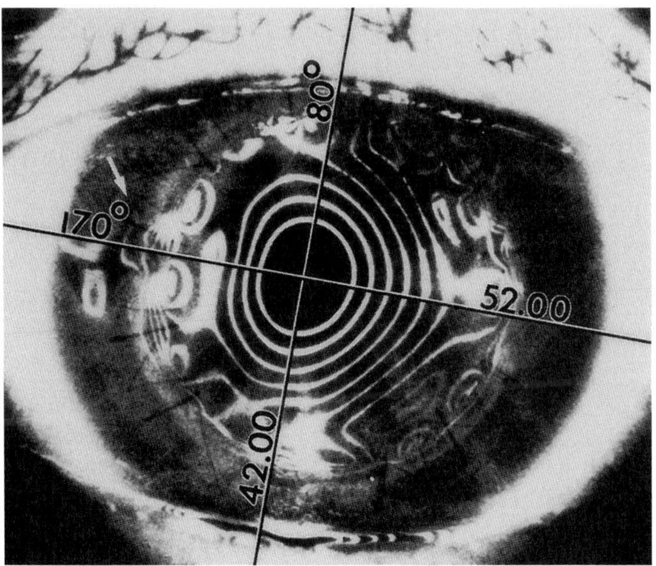

Figure 2-15 Photokeratoscopic mires are closer together in a zone of steep curvature *(arrow)* induced by a tight suture after penetrating keratoplasty. Keratometric values and meridians are superimposed.

Computerized Corneal Topography

Keratoscopy images can be digitally captured and analyzed with computers. Placido disk–based computerized topographers are the type most commonly available in the United States. These units assume the angle of incidence to be nearly perpendicular and the radius of curvature to be the distance from the surface to the intersection with the line of sight or visual axis of the patient *(axial distance)*. Some instruments determine the initial shape using triangulation or other methods and then calculate the power map from the shape.

These values *(axial curvature)* closely approximate the power of the central 1–2 mm of the cornea but fail to describe the true shape and power of the peripheral cornea. Ray tracing shows that corneal power must increase in the periphery based on Snell's law in order to refract the light into the pupil. Ellipsoidal surfaces will show aspheric power that increases in the periphery *(spherical aberration)*. Conventionally, normal corneas show decreasing diopters toward the periphery as displayed by the Placido disk. This instrument gives an intuitive sense of the normal flattening of the cornea but does not represent the true refractive powers or the true curvature of the cornea as inspection moves away from the center.

A second method of describing the corneal curvature is to use the *instantaneous radius of curvature* (also called *tangential power*) at a certain point. This radius is determined by taking a perpendicular path through the point in question from a plane that intersects the point and the visual axis but allowing the radius to be the length necessary to correspond to a sphere with the same curvature at that point. The instantaneous radius of curvature, with curvature given in diopters, is estimated by the difference between the corneal index of refraction and 1.000 divided by this tangentially determined radius. The tangential map typically shows better sensitivity to peripheral changes with less "smoothing" of the curvature than the axial maps (Fig 2-16). (In these maps, diopters are relative units of curvature and not the equivalent of diopters of corneal power.)

A third map, the *mean curvature map*, does not require the perpendicular ray to cross the visual axis, allowing for an infinite number of spheres to fit the curvature at

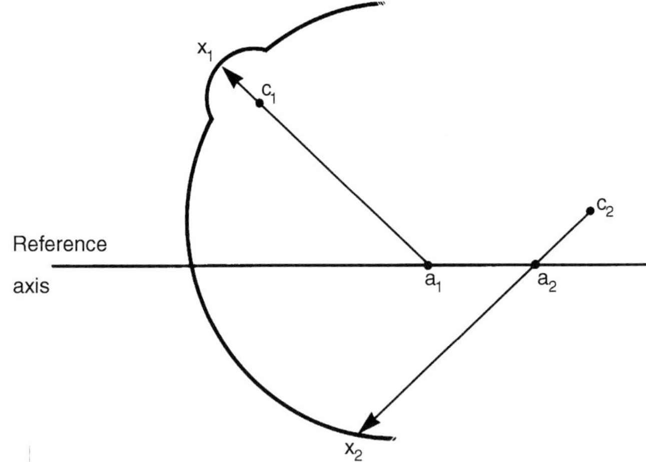

Figure 2-16 Axial and instantaneous corneal power (two dimensional). Axial curvature at points x_1 and x_2 is based on axial distances x_1 to a_1 and x_2 to a_2 Instantaneous curvature at points x_1 and x_2 is based on radii of curvature from x_1 to c_1 and x_2 to c_2. *(Illustration by Christine Gralapp.)*

that point (Fig 2-17). The algorithm determines a minimum and maximum size best-fit sphere and from their radii determines an average curvature (arithmetic mean of principal curvatures) known as the *mean curvature* for that point. These powers are then mapped using standard colors to represent diopter changes, allowing even more sensitivity to peripheral changes of curvature.

In addition to power maps, computerized topographic systems may display other data: pupil size and location, indexes estimating regular and irregular astigmatism, estimates of the probability of having keratoconus, simulated keratometry, and more.

All of the maps described above attempt to depict the underlying shape of the cornea by scaling curvature through the familiar dioptric notation instead of the less familiar millimeters of radius. Of course, a more accurate way to describe curvature would be to use the true shape of the cornea: some systems directly derive corneal shape by means of scanning slits or rectangular grids and then determine power from that shape.

In order to represent shape directly, maps may display a *z-height* from an arbitrary plane (iris plane, limbal plane, or frontal plane) using color maps. Just as viewing the curvature of the earth in an appropriate scale fails to show details of mountains and basins, these *z* maps do not show clinically important variations. Geographic maps show land elevation relative to sea level. Similarly, corneal surface maps are plotted to show

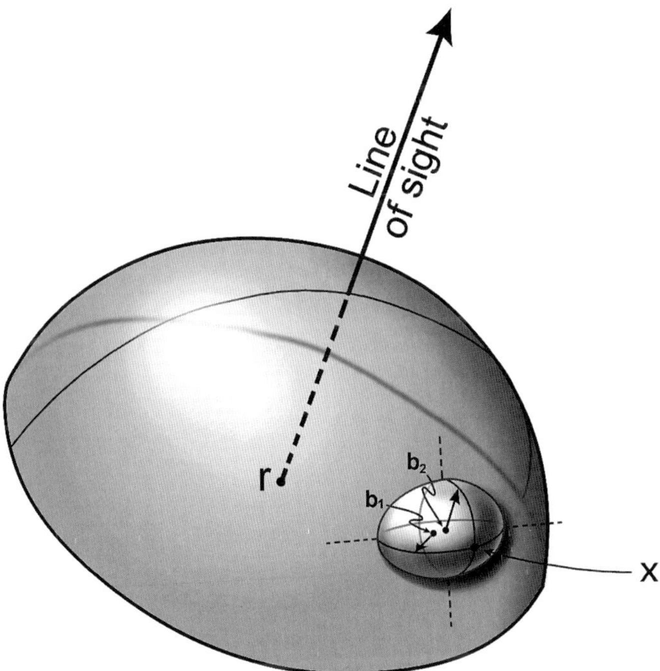

Figure 2-17 Mean corneal power (three dimensional). Power at point x of this outpouching from the basic spheroid is calculated by averaging the minimum curvature represented by radius of curvature from b_1 to x and the maximum curvature from b_2 to x. These two lines do not necessarily cross the reference axis. r is the center of rotation of the large sphere; b_1 and b_2 are the centers of rotation of the minimum and the maximum best-fit sphere. *(Illustration by Christine Gralapp.)*

differences from best-fit spheres or other objects that closely mimic the normal corneal shape (Fig 2-18).

Ideally, researchers hope to develop practical methods for accurately depicting the anterior and posterior surface shapes of the cornea and lens. Then, ray tracing can be used to plot an accurate refractive map of the eye to establish the normal effects of the cornea and lens surfaces on the wavefront of light. With such information, alterations to the shape of the eye structures can be planned to maximize the refractive effect and minimize the aberrations of keratorefractive and other surgeries. The American National Standards Institute (ANSI) in the United States is currently developing standards for the corneal topography industry to make the comparison of maps more uniform and to clarify the confusion of terminology.

Indications

About two thirds of patients with normal corneas have a symmetric pattern that is round, oval, or bowtie-shaped, as in Figure 2-19. The other patients are classified as having an asymmetric pattern: inferior steepening, superior steepening, asymmetric bowtie patterns, or nonspecific irregularity. However, many corneas are found to have a complex shape that is oversimplified by the use of such qualitative pattern descriptions.

Corneal topography detects irregular astigmatism from contact lens warpage, keratoconus and other thinning disorders, corneal surgery, trauma, and postinflammatory and degenerative conditions. Different values obtained at subsequent examinations can signal a change in corneal contour if the alignment of the eye and the instrument is the same. Computer-assisted topographic modeling systems allow the clinician to detect subtle and minor variations in power distribution of the anterior corneal surface.

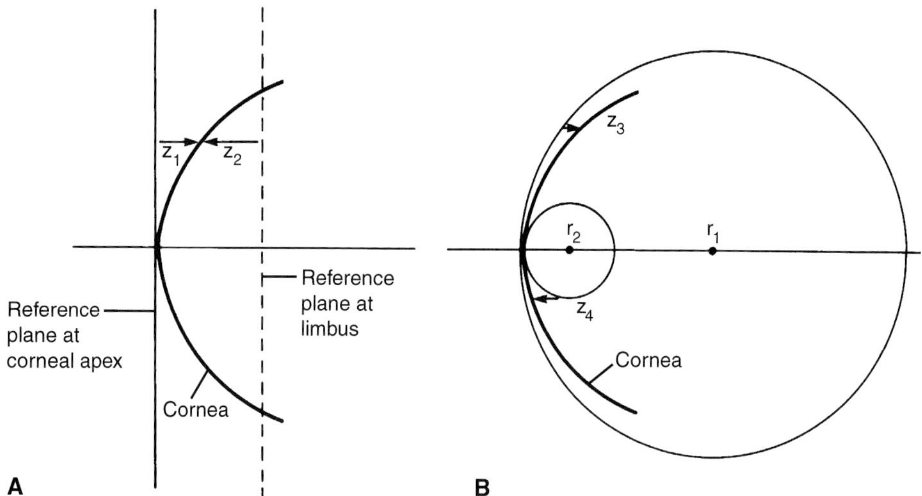

Figure 2-18 Height maps (typically in micrometers). **A,** Height relative to plane surface. z_1 is below surface parallel to corneal apex. z_2 is above surface parallel to corneal limbus. **B,** Height relative to reference sphere. z_3 is below a flat sphere of radius r_1. z_4 is above a steep sphere of radius r_2. *(Illustration by Christine Gralapp.)*

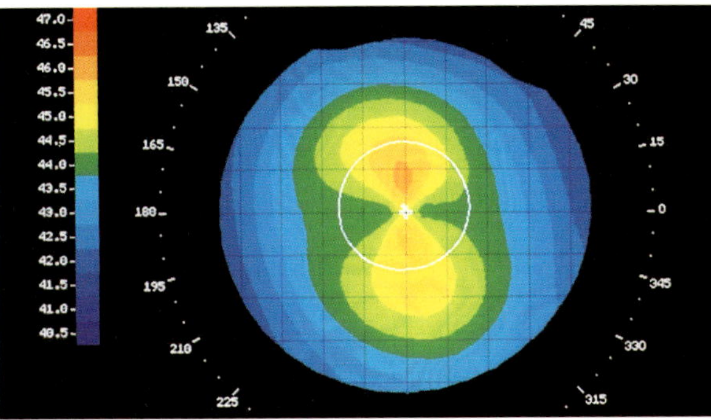

Figure 2-19 Keratography of normal cornea with regular astigmatism. White circle indicates pupil. *(Keratograph courtesy of Kirk R. Wilhelmus, MD.)*

Corneal topography is important in the preoperative evaluation of refractive surgery patients. Patients with corneal warpage (irregular astigmatism and/or peripheral steepening, distorted keratoscopic mires) should discontinue contact lens wear and allow the corneal map and refraction to stabilize prior to undergoing refractive surgery. Patients with keratoconus are not routinely considered for refractive surgery, as the thin cornea has an unpredictable response and reducing its thickness may lead to progression of keratoconus. The form fruste, or subclinical, keratoconus recognized by Placido disk–based topography requires caution on the part of the ophthalmologist and is now considered to be a contraindication to refractive surgery. However, studies are under way to determine suitability of keratorefractive procedures as an alternative to corneal transplant.

Corneal topography can also be used to show the effects of keratorefractive procedures. Pre- and postoperative maps may be algebraically subtracted to determine whether the desired effect was achieved. Corneal mapping may help to explain unexpected results including undercorrections, aberrations, induced astigmatism, or glare and haloes by detecting decentered surgery or inadequate surgery such as shallow incisions in radial keratotomy. Corneal topography also confirms the expected physiologic effects of refractive surgery. For example, in radial keratotomy, peripheral incisions lead to flattening of the central cornea from a relative peripheral steepening, as shown in this difference map (Fig 2-20).

Corneal topography is needed in the management of congenital and postoperative astigmatism, particularly following penetrating keratoplasty. Complex peripheral patterns may result in a refractive axis of astigmatism that is not aligned with topographic axes. Failure to correct the underlying shape by removing appropriate sutures or operating on the appropriate axis may lead to unexpected results. The appropriate axis depends on the type of surgery (incisional is done on the steep axis, compression sutures on the flat axis, and minus cylinder ablation on the flat axis. See also Chapter 25).

Finally, detection of irregular astigmatism by means of corneal topography can be used in the management of ocular surface disorders such as map-dot-fingerprint dystrophy.

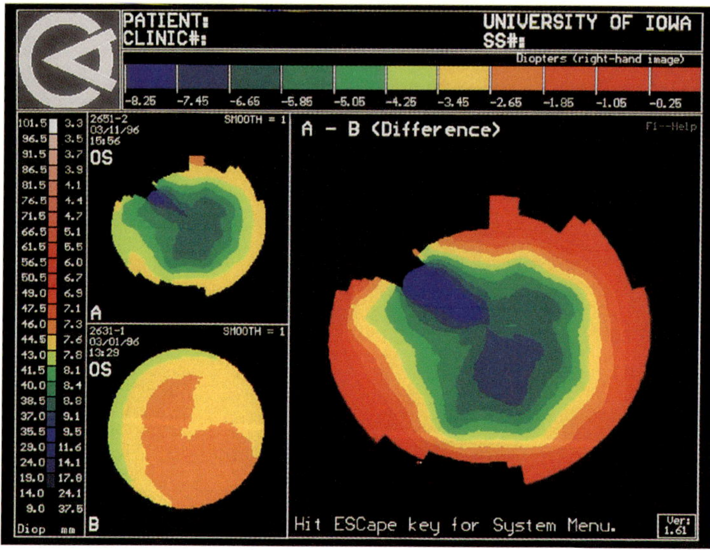

Figure 2-20 Difference map in radial keratotomy. Both central and peripheral flattening are seen in the postoperative image (A) and in the difference map on the right. B is the preoperative image.

Limitations

In addition to the limitations of the algorithms and variation in terminology by manufacturer, the accuracy of corneal topography may be affected by various potential problems:

- Misalignment
- Stability (test to test variation)
- Sensitivity to focus errors
- Tear film effects
- Distortions
- Area of coverage (central and limbal)
- Nonstandardized data maps
- Colors may be absolute or varied (normalized)

Corbett MC, O'Brart DPS. *Corneal Topography: Principles and Applications.* London: BMJ Books; 1999.

Maguire LJ. Computerized corneal analysis. In: *Focal Points: Clinical Modules for Ophthalmologists.* San Francisco: American Academy of Ophthalmology. 1996;vol 14, no 5.

Roberts C. Principles of corneal topography. In: Elander R, Rich LF, Robin JB, eds. *Principles and Practice of Refractive Surgery.* Philadelphia: Saunders; 1997:475–497.

Retinoscopy

Retinoscopy can detect irregular astigmatism by showing nonlinear or multiple reflexes that cannot be completely neutralized with a spherocylindrical lens. With a multifocal cornea, retinoscopy reveals multiple regular reflexes that move in different directions.

Irregular astigmatism and multifocal cornea can occur in keratoconus and after kerato-refractive surgery. Abnormalities found with retinoscopy can help explain why a patient with a clear cornea cannot see well. Additionally, retinoscopy can disclose disrupted light reflexes caused by disturbances of the corneal surface. In cases where retinoscopic findings exceed the corresponding slit-lamp findings, retinoscopy can help gauge the relative effect of corneal surface changes on vision.

Krachmer JH, Mannis MJ, Holland EJ, eds. *Cornea*. Vol 1. St Louis: Mosby; 1997:215–221.

Wavefront Analysis

The wave theory of light and its application in wavefront analysis is described and illustrated in BCSC Section 3, *Clinical Optics*. Presently, wavefront analysis can be performed clinically by four methods: Hartmann-Shack, Tscherning, thin-beam single ray tracing, and optical path difference (Nidek), which combines retinoscopy with corneal topography. Each of these results in a detailed report of higher order aberrations (irregular astigmatism). The utility of this information in explaining patients' symptoms and in aiding the calculation of custom ablations to correct problems or enhance vision is under review. At present, the ideal wavefront is not known.

Prevention Practices in Ophthalmology

Some corneal and external eye diseases can be prevented. Strategies for prevention include adequate hygiene and nutrition, aseptic surgical techniques, protective spectacles to minimize ocular trauma, and prophylactic antibiotics. Prevention begins with immunization. Practicing ophthalmologists should provide an opportunity for hepatitis B vaccination for their office staff and follow other regulations of the Occupational Safety and Health Administration. Universal precautions that safeguard the health of patients' eyes as well as the ophthalmologist and staff should be a part of daily practice.

Universal Precautions

Optimal infection control is based on the assumption that all specified human body fluids are potentially infectious. Many transmissible diseases of the external eye, such as adenoviral conjunctivitis, cause redness that immediately indicates infection. Other infectious agents, however, can be present on the ocular surface without causing inflammation. Human immunodeficiency virus (HIV), hepatitis B virus, hepatitis C virus, rabies virus, and the agent of Creutzfeldt-Jakob disease are not immediately obvious without systemic clues or laboratory testing. Every patient must be approached as potentially contagious. Guidelines for routine ophthalmic examinations include the following:

- Wash hands between patient examinations. Use disposable gloves if an open sore, blood, or blood-contaminated fluid is present. Using cotton-tipped applicators to manipulate the eyelids can also minimize direct contact.
- Avoid unnecessary contact. Eyedropper bottles used in the office should not directly touch the ocular surface of any patient. Individual sterile strips impregnated with dye are preferred where available.

- Disinfect all contact instruments after each use. Tonometer tips and pachymeter tips should be soaked in diluted bleach or hydrogen peroxide or cleansed with isopropyl alcohol after every use. Trial contact lenses must be disinfected between patients. BCSC Section 10, *Glaucoma,* discusses infection control in clinical tonometry in greater detail.
- Handle sharp devices carefully. Needles must always be discarded into puncture-resistant (sharps) containers.

Universal precautions are also discussed in BCSC Section 9.

Updated recommendations for ophthalmic practice in relation to the human immunodeficiency virus and other infectious agents. Information Statement. San Francisco: American Academy of Ophthalmology; 1992.

Public Health Ophthalmology

Nearly 150 million people worldwide are blind or have low vision. Corneal diseases, especially infection, are major causes of visual loss (Table 2-5). In the absence of an available vaccine for these conditions, specific programs are designed to reduce the risk of communicable diseases. Examples of such efforts are the following:

- Improved hygiene and mass distribution of antibiotics to interrupt hyperendemic trachoma
- Eradication of the insect vector to control onchocerciasis
- Vitamin A supplementation in communities with childhood xerophthalmia
- Education about contact lens disinfection in industrialized countries

International Ophthalmology, a BCSC companion book, discusses these and many other topics in public health ophthalmology at greater length.

Schwab L. *Eye Care in Developing Nations.* 3rd ed. San Francisco: American Academy of Ophthalmology; 1999.

Table 2-5 Ocular Infections of Global Importance

Disease	No. of Visually Disabled	High Regional Burden
Trachoma	5,800,000	Africa
Herpes simplex virus keratitis	1,000,000	Worldwide
Microbial keratitis	500,000	Worldwide
Toxoplasmosis	500,000	Latin America
Onchocerciasis	500,000	Africa, Latin America
Hansen disease	250,000	Southeast Asia
Neonatal conjunctivitis	200,000	Africa

(Modified from Wilhelmus KR. Epidemiology of ocular infections. In: Tasman W, Jaeger EA, eds. *Duane's Foundations of Clinical Ophthalmology.* Philadelphia: Lippincott Williams & Wilkins; 1998: chap 43.)

Ocular Surface Disorders

CHAPTER 3

Normal Physiology of the Ocular Surface

Problems of the ocular surface are diverse in their etiology, symptoms, and prognosis. They range from relatively minor irritations with excellent preservation of vision to devastating and potentially blinding chemical injuries with persistent epithelial defects and stromal ulceration. This discussion of the maintenance of ocular surface integrity begins with a review of normal physiology of the external eye.

Eyelids

The *ocular surface* encompasses the entire epithelial surface of the cornea, limbus, and conjunctiva. It is physically contiguous with the adjacent eyelids and adnexa and shares important functional relationships with the external eye. The eyelids have important protective functions for the globe, both voluntary and involuntary. The involuntary fright blink reflex that occurs in response to external stimuli without physical contact is mediated by the optic nerve or cranial nerve VIII (auditory) as the afferent arc and primarily by cranial nerve VII (facial) as the efferent arc. Neuronally controlled eyelid blinking, which occurs approximately every 5–10 seconds, mechanically spreads the tear film to lubricate the ocular surface. This subconscious blink reflex is mediated by the ophthalmic division of cranial nerve V (trigeminal) as afferent arc and CN VII as efferent arc.

The blinking movement protects the ocular surface from unwanted stimuli and allows the eyelids to spread the tear meniscus over the ocular surface. Impairment of this protective reflex mechanism may render the ocular surface susceptible to pathologic insults, as may be seen in neuroparalytic keratopathy. Through blinking and contraction of eyelid muscles, tears are removed from the ocular surface and drain through the puncta into the nasolacrimal system. BCSC Section 7, *Orbit, Eyelids, and Lacrimal System,* discusses and illustrates the functions of the eyelids and lacrimal system in depth. Ocular surface integrity can also be compromised by malfunctioning or malpositioning of the eyelid apparatus, as in entropion or ectropion of the eyelids.

Precorneal Tear Film

The normal ocular surface is covered by a layer of tear film. Because the precorneal tear film–air interface is the initial refractive surface of the eye, the maintenance of a stable, healthy tear film is of paramount importance to vision. Tears provide a moist environment for epithelial cells, lubricating the ocular surface while they dilute and remove noxious stimuli. The tear film provides the cornea with essential nutrients and oxygen, and leukocytes gain access to the cornea through the tear film. Numerous growth factors are also present in the tear film.

Specific proteins contained within the tear film, including lysozyme, lactoferrin, tear lipocalin, secretory IgA, and cystatin S, impart antimicrobial activity to the tear film. Lack of this physiologic lubricating fluid, as in tear deficiency states, may predispose the eye to microbial infections.

The exact structure of the tear film is controversial. Traditionally, the precorneal tear film has been thought to be tripartite, with a lipid superficial layer about 0.1 μm in thickness (with the eyelids open), an aqueous midphase 7 μm thick, and a mucin basal layer 20–50 nm thick. Although this is still the most prevalent concept, some recent evidence suggests that the tear film may be as thick as 40 μm and is largely made up of a mucin gel or partial mucin layer, with an increase in mucin content basally and without discrete separation of the aqueous and mucin layers (Fig 3-1). Various other concepts of the tear film have also been presented in recent years.

The most superficial layer of the tear film is the *lipid layer* produced by the meibomian glands. Its principal function is to retard tear evaporation and enhance stability, while maintaining the tear meniscus. Meibomian gland dysfunction (MGD) can lead to unstable tear film and associated ocular surface disorders. The *aqueous component* is produced by the main lacrimal glands, as well as the accessory lacrimal glands of Krause and Wolfring. The aqueous layer transports all of the water-soluble nutrients, and aqueous tear deficiency (ATD) is the most common cause of dry eye. The layer coating the

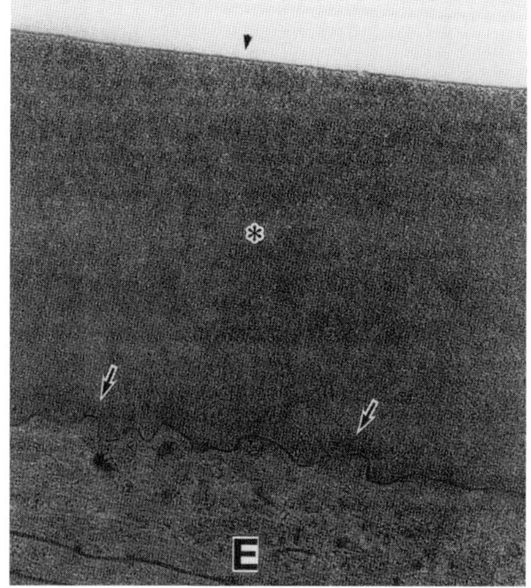

Figure 3-1 Cross section of the precorneal tear film, showing a homogeneous gel *(asterisk)* with a lipid surface film *(arrowhead)*. The superficial epithelium *(E)* had glycocalices *(arrows)* on its microvilli. *(Reproduced from Chen H-B, Yamabayashi S, Ou B, et al. Structure and composition of rat precorneal tear film: a study by an in vivo cryofixation. Invest Ophthalmol Vis Sci. 1997;38:383.)*

cornea is the *mucin layer*, which is produced by both conjunctival goblet cells and ocular surface epithelium. The mucin is hydrophilic, and this quality enhances the ability of the aqueous layer to spread over the corneal epithelium. The mucin layer also functions to trap various trophic factors, leukocytes, and cytokines. The loss of conjunctival goblet cells—for example in chemical burns—leads to xerosis of the ocular surface.

Normal tear film has a pH of about 7.2, an osmolarity of 302 mOsm per liter, and a volume of 7.0 µL in the precorneal film. It is produced at a rate of 1.2 µL per minute and has a refractive index of 1.336. BCSC Section 2, *Fundamentals and Principles of Ophthalmology,* discusses the tear film in detail.

Lipid Tear Secretion

The meibomian glands are richly innervated. The nerve fibers surrounding them are probably cholinergic since they contain cholinesterase, and cholinergic agonists such as pilocarpine stimulate release of meibomian oil. However, no evidence has yet been produced to show that meibomian gland secretion in humans is controlled by either parasympathetic or sympathetic innervation. Hormones may influence meibomian secretion: both estrogen and androgen receptors are present in the meibomian glands, similar to sebaceous glands elsewhere on the skin. These receptors may play a role in the modulation of meibomian secretion. Bacteria colonizing the eyelids also modify the lipid secretion in MGD.

Blinking is thought to be important in the release of meibomian gland lipid. It has been estimated that a gravitational force of 50–70 g is applied to the globe during a blink, and the globe is retroplaced on average 1.5 mm. When the eye is open, the muscle of Riolan surrounding the meibomian gland ducts contracts and compresses the ducts, thereby preventing outflow. The palpebral portion of the orbicularis may possibly act as an opponent by milking the glands on contraction. Blinking would lead to expression or jetting of the oil onto the precorneal tear film; between blinks, with the muscle of Riolan contracted and the orbicularis relaxed, secretion would be prevented. Cells in the acinar wall may act as valves to control lipid flow.

Aqueous Tear Secretion

Aqueous tear secretion is largely a reflex mechanism. Cranial nerve V is the afferent pathway in the reflex tear arc. Stimulation of receptors in the fifth nerve distribution in the cornea, conjunctiva, or nasal mucosa induces tear secretion from the lacrimal gland. The efferent pathway is more roundabout. Parasympathetic fibers leave cranial nerve VII in the greater superficial petrosal nerve and pass to the sphenopalatine ganglion. From there the lacrimal secretory nerve fibers travel with the zygomaticotemporal nerve of the maxillary division (V_2) and join the lacrimal (sensory) nerve of the ophthalmic division (V_1) of CN V before entering the lacrimal gland. Sympathetic efferent pathways may also be involved. Reduction of tear secretion and associated dry eye syndrome can be caused by diseases such as familial dysautonomia or, more commonly, by medications affecting the autonomic system.

Mucin Tear Secretion

Mucin-like glycoproteins are secreted by conjunctival goblet cells and by conjunctival and corneal epithelium. They make up the inner portion of the precorneal tear film and are essential for proper ocular surface wetting. The mucin components of the preocular tear film result in the formation of a hydrophilic layer over a hydrophobic ocular surface. A continuous aqueous tear film of 7–40 μm thickness can exist only on a hydrophilic surface. When mucin production is deficient, as occurs with chemical or inflammatory destruction of the ocular surface, poor wetting of the corneal surface with subsequent desiccation and epithelial damage may occur, even in the setting of sufficient aqueous tear production. The mechanisms controlling mucin secretion by the conjunctival goblet cells and ocular surface epithelium are not known.

Tear Breakup

Meibomian lipids cannot spread over mucin or an aqueous film surface containing surfactants, because the lipid would disperse and emulsify. Tear film breakup has been attributed to lipid contamination of the hydrophilic supporting solid, or mucin layer, rendering it hydrophobic. Polar lipids could diffuse into the mucin layer, causing focal disruption in the tear film, especially over irregularities in the surface epithelium, or during conditions of increased evaporation. This model has been questioned, however, and it is postulated that the key step in tear film breakup is instability and rupture of the mucin layer caused by van der Waals forces acting on the mucin layer. Precise biomechanical models of the tear film await further elucidation.

Decreased tear breakup time rapidly returns to normal once the meibomian glands are expressed. A decrease in secretion from the meibomian glands as a result of obstruction or reduced blinking could result in a compromised lipid layer and increased evaporation of the aqueous layer, with subsequent thinning of the tear film and greater contamination. Blinking can remove the lipid-contaminated mucin. Blinking increases to compensate for pathological conditions (such as blepharitis) associated with decreased tear breakup time resulting from greater tear evaporation. Incomplete blinking and abnormalities in eyelid congruity have similar effects.

The Ocular Surface

Epithelium

Corneal epithelium

Under the precorneal tear film lies the anterior surface of the cornea, which is made up of nonkeratinized, stratified squamous epithelium. This highly organized epithelium has plentiful desmosomes and tight junctions, thereby providing paracellular permeability barriers to limit nonionic solutes and to maintain the homeostasis of the intraocular milieu. Disruption of this physiologic barrier by the preservatives contained in many topical ocular medications may lead to a punctate epitheliopathy and compromised epithelial wound healing. Because the corneal epithelium is highly differentiated and renews itself rapidly, it depends on its stem cells for continual migration and replacement. Cumulative research and clinical evidence have indicated that the stem cells of the corneal epithelium are located in the basal layer of the limbal epithelium.

The limbus is a unique structure that acts as a junctional barrier to separate the cornea and conjunctiva. Phenotypical and biochemical characteristics of limbal epithelium have been shown to be intermediate between corneal and conjunctival epithelium. In humans, the limbal palisades of Vogt, representing specialized regions of epithelial structure, are the location of the limbal stem cells. The palisades are tightly attached to the underlying basement membrane and have a rich limbal vascular network to nourish the metabolically active stem cells. In the absence of these limbal stem cells, epithelial wound healing is compromised. Persistent epithelial defects or abnormal wound healing associated with the invasion of conjunctival goblet cells is often observed in conditions associated with limbal stem-cell deficiency.

Dua HS, Azuara-Blanco A. Limbal stem cells of the corneal epithelium. *Surv Ophthalmol.* 2000;44:415–425.

Tseng SC, Tsubota K. Important concepts for treating ocular surface and tear disorders. *Am J Ophthalmol.* 1997;124:825–835.

Conjunctival epithelium

Conjunctival epithelium varies from stratified to columnar and has numerous mucin-secreting goblet cells. The junctional structures of conjunctival epithelium are less developed than those of corneal epithelium, and increased epithelial permeability has been observed in conjunctiva. Conjunctival stem cells appear to be uniformly distributed over the ocular surface.

Near the eyelid margins, the epithelium of the conjunctiva merges with the keratinized, stratified squamous epithelium of the eyelid skin. A different transition occurs at the limbus, where the conjunctival epithelium merges with that of the cornea. The areas of stratified squamous epithelium at the eyelid margin and limbus correspond to the areas of most frequent contact and greatest pressure between the palpebral and bulbar surfaces. These mechanical factors of eyelid movement and appositional pressure have been suggested as the greatest stimulus for the formation of stratified squamous epithelium around the eyelid margin and the limbus. Such mechanical forces may be crucial in stimulating the limbal stem cells to maintain corneal epithelial proliferation and differentiation. Through such a mechanism, the eyelids also play an active role in regulating the surface epithelial turnover, in addition to their passive role in protecting the ocular surface.

Unlike the normal cornea, the conjunctival epithelium lacks an organized basement membrane and rests loosely on the fibrovascular tissue of the substantia propria. The conjunctiva is a complex element of the mucosal immune defense system that contains populations of immune-inflammatory cells such as dendritic cells, lymphocytes, polymorphonuclear leukocytes, plasma cells, and mast cells. This specialized conjunctival lymphoid tissue is known as *conjunctiva-associated lymphoid tissue (CALT).*

Blood Supply

Conjunctival blood vessels derived from anterior ciliary arteries maintain their superficial position, and deeper branches furnish blood to the peripheral corneal arcades, iris, and ciliary body. Inflammatory processes of the conjunctiva result in prominence of the superficial vessels, which increases away from the limbus. In contrast, inflammatory processes of the cornea, iris, or ciliary body result in prominence of the deep vessels, which increases toward the limbus. Clinically, this process manifests as ciliary flush at the limbus. Conjunctival blood vessels near the limbus provide nourishment for the peripheral cornea and limbus, the location of the corneal epithelial stem cells. In pathologic circumstances, these vessels transport inflammatory cells for combating infection (for example, polymorphonuclear cells). In other circumstances (such as peripheral ulcerative keratitis), inflammatory cells can release metalloproteases that result in corneal stromal degradation.

When the conjunctiva in the involved eye is relatively normal (eg, neurotrophic keratopathy or after microbial keratitis), a conjunctival flap may supply the necessary corneal vascularity to prevent further stromal degradation and support repair. In cases of ischemia-induced sterile stromal ulceration related to a severe chemical burn involving the cornea, limbus, and conjunctiva, advancement of adjacent conjunctiva or Tenon's tissue may restore the limbal vascular supply. Local resection of the limbal conjunctiva adjacent to an area of advancing peripheral ulcerative keratitis may be necessary to halt further proteolytic degradation of the cornea.

Normal cornea is avascular and angiostatic. A healthy cornea has an intact Bowman's layer and compact stroma. Inflammatory reactions or degenerative processes of the peripheral cornea often lead to breakdown of the basement membrane and perturbation of limbal barrier functions (limbal deficiency), and they can result in corneal vascularization and conjunctival ingrowth such as pterygium, which is discussed in detail in Chapters 17 and 21.

Mechanical Functions

In addition to their physiologic functions, the conjunctiva and especially the limbus also contribute mechanically to the maintenance of corneal epithelial integrity. For example, a smooth palpebral conjunctiva permits the eyelid to glide over the cornea, thereby affording protection, distribution of the tear film, and debridement of foreign matter. Diseases that produce keratinization of the palpebral conjunctiva (such as Stevens-Johnson syndrome) can cause significant mechanical damage to the corneal epithelium. Flexible conjunctival folds are essential for the proper movements of the globe and maintenance of the normal eyelid–globe relationship. Thus, conditions that produce conjunctival scarring (for example, ocular cicatricial pemphigoid) can obliterate the normal forniceal anatomy and lead to cicatricial entropion, trichiasis, and secondary corneal erosion and scarring.

CHAPTER 4

Diagnostic Approach to Ocular Surface Disease

Tear Film Evaluation

Tests for dry eye lend some degree of objectivity to what is essentially a clinical diagnosis, although no one test is sufficiently specific to permit an absolute diagnosis. The best approach is to combine information from the history and examination with the results of one or more of the following diagnostic tests. The tests described may be performed in the following sequence to minimize the potential for alteration of subsequent test results by preceding procedures. However, any of the tests may affect the outcome of subsequent ones.

Inspection

Inspection of the tear meniscus between the globe and the lower eyelid (normally 1.0 mm in height and convex) is a common starting point. A tear meniscus 0.3 mm or less is considered abnormal. *Tear breakup time* is determined by instilling fluorescein in the inferior cul-de-sac and then evaluating the stability of the precorneal tear film. Tear breakup time should be measured prior to the instillation of any eyedrops and before the eyelids are manipulated in any way. The examiner moistens a fluorescein strip with sterile saline and applies it to the tarsal conjunctiva. (Fluorescein-anesthetic combination drops are not suitable for this purpose.) After several blinks, the tear film is examined using a broad beam of the slit lamp with a blue filter. The time lapse between the last blink and the appearance of the first randomly distributed dry spot is the tear breakup time. Dry spots appearing in less than 10 seconds are considered abnormal.

The ocular surface can then be evaluated with lissamine green or rose bengal staining. The specific pattern of corneal and bulbar conjunctival staining can be very helpful in establishing the diagnosis. These patterns are described and illustrated in Chapter 2.

Tests of Tear Production

Aqueous tear production can be assessed in a variety of ways (Table 4-1). *Schirmer testing* is performed by placing a thin strip of filter paper in the inferior cul-de-sac (Fig 4-1). The amount of wetting can be measured to quantify aqueous tear production. The *basic secretion test* is performed following the instillation of a topical anesthetic, followed by lightly blotting residual fluid out of the inferior fornix. A thin filter paper strip (5 mm

Table 4-1 Tear Production Testing

Test	Topical Anesthesia	Time	Nasal Stimulation	Normal Value
Basic tear secretion	+	5 min	−	≥10 mm
Schirmer I	−	5 min	−	≥10 mm
Schirmer II	−	5 min	+	≥15 mm

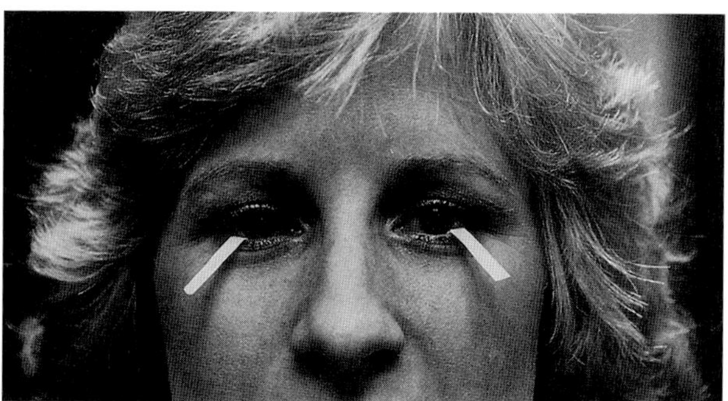

Figure 4-1 The Schirmer test uses the amount of wetting of the paper strips as a measure of tear flow. *(Reproduced with permission from Carr T, ed.* Ophthalmic Medical Assisting. *3rd ed. San Francisco: American Academy of Ophthalmology; 1999:93.)*

wide, 35 mm long) is placed at the junction of the middle and lateral thirds of the lower eyelids to minimize irritation to the cornea during the test. The eyes are then closed to limit the effect of blinking. Although normal measurements are quite variable, repeated measurements of less than 5 mm of wetting, with anesthesia, can be highly suggestive of aqueous tear deficiency, while 5–10 mm is equivocal. The *Schirmer I test*, which is similar to the basic secretion test *without* topical anesthesia, measures both basic and reflex tearing combined. Less than 10 mm of wetting after 5 minutes is diagnostic of aqueous tear deficiency. While this test is relatively specific, the level of sensitivity is poor. Using lower cutoff measurements increases the specificity of these tests but decreases their sensitivity. The *Schirmer II test*, which measures reflex secretion, is performed in a similar manner. However, after the filter paper strips have been inserted into the inferior fornices, a cotton-tipped applicator is used to irritate the nasal mucosa. Wetting of less than 15 mm after 5 minutes is consistent with a defect in reflex secretion. While an isolated abnormal result for any of these tests can be misleading, serially consistent results are highly suggestive. Schirmer testing is also useful in demonstrating to patients the presence of an aqueous tear deficiency.

Tear Composition Assays

Other procedures may be useful in supporting the diagnosis of aqueous tear deficiency. Cultures of the eyelid margins are rarely helpful, but they may provide useful information in selected cases. Additional tests include tear film osmolarity, tear lysozyme, and tear lactoferrin. In lacrimal gland dysfunction states, the normal production of proteins by the lacrimal gland is diminished. A decreased tear lysozyme or lactoferrin level is highly suggestive of dry eye. A commercial assay is available for the measurement of lactoferrin in tears. Tear film osmolarity has been shown to be increased in patients with aqueous tear deficiency as well as those with MGD. At the present time no consensus has been reached as to which of these tests is most sensitive and/or specific for the diagnosis of aqueous tear deficiency, and some are not readily available.

Ocular Cytology

An important step in the diagnosis of many infectious and inflammatory conditions is the examination of conjunctival or corneal specimens by light microscopy. Standard staining procedures are widely used to facilitate the detection of microbial and human cells. This chapter discusses the procedures used in these investigations and the implications that can be drawn from their results. See also BCSC Section 4, *Ophthalmic Pathology and Intraocular Tumors.*

Specimen Collection

Scraping or swabbing

Conjunctival scrapings are generally preferred to swabbings that harvest surface exudate. To obtain a conjunctival specimen for cytological examination, the clinician applies a topical anesthetic and everts the upper eyelid. The tarsal conjunctiva is lightly scraped with a sterile spatula. When epithelial cells are removed, the conjunctival surface should blanch slightly during scrapings, avoiding excessive bleeding. An alternative method of gathering conjunctival cells involves a cytobrush. After the conjunctiva is rubbed, the brush is dipped into buffer solution, and the floated cells are concentrated on a Millipore filter. Rapid immersion into fixative avoids excessive air drying of material on a glass slide or filter paper.

Ideally, conjunctival swabbings for culture are obtained before instillation of a topical anesthetic. Calcium alginate or Dacron swabs slightly moistened with liquid broth are preferable for collecting specimens of epithelial cells and microflora; cotton swabs may inhibit bacterial growth. Specimens can also be obtained from the contralateral conjunctiva for comparison.

Procedures for obtaining and culturing specimens for suspected infectious conditions are discussed further in Chapter 6.

Impression cytology

In impression cytology, a piece of filter paper is pressed against a specific area of the conjunctival or corneal surface to lift off superficial cells. This procedure can be considered a noninvasive superficial biopsy that provides a means to map specific cell changes topographically and to quantify surface abnormalities.

Preferred Practice Patterns Committee, Cornea Panel. *Conjunctivitis.* San Francisco: American Academy of Ophthalmology; 1998.

Tseng SC. Staging of conjunctival squamous metaplasia by impression cytology. *Ophthalmology.* 1985;92:728–733.

Interpretation of Ocular Cytology

Microscopic examination of material collected from the ocular surface can reveal cells, cellular elements, and microorganisms that can be helpful in diagnostic evaluation (Table 4-2). The staining procedures used in ocular cytology are described in Table 4-3.

Brinser JH, Burd EM. Principles of diagnostic ocular microbiology. In: Tabbara KV, Hyndiuk RA, eds. *Infections of the Eye.* 2nd ed. Boston: Little, Brown; 1996.

Human cells

A methylene blue-based dye such as the Giemsa or Wright stain is useful to highlight specific morphologic characteristics that aid in identifying the following cell types.

Normal conjunctival and corneal epithelial cells Slightly larger than leukocytes, epithelial cells have a central round nucleus (sometimes with a prominent nucleolus) and homogeneous cytoplasm (Fig 4-2). The usually flat squamous epithelial cells can appear cuboidal when smeared onto a glass slide, and they tend to clump together in sheets.

Degenerated or keratinized epithelial cells Degenerating epithelial cells have a faint, ghostlike appearance with faded or no nuclei (Fig 4-3). Keratinization is visualized as eosinophilic cytoplasmic granularity. Keratinized epidermal cells of the normal eyelid margin can also be seen, occasionally with adherent bacteria.

Goblet cells Conjunctival goblet cells contain a clump of pale staining mucus that displaces the cytoplasm and nucleus toward the edge of the cell membrane. Goblet cells may be found singly or in clusters. The cell can be identified by its mucin contents stained magenta by periodic acid–Schiff reagent (PAS) (Fig 4-4).

Table 4-2 Clinical Interpretation of Ocular Surface Cytology

Finding	Examples
Predominance of neutrophils	Bacterial conjunctivitis Early stage of severe viral conjunctivitis Severe allergic or atopic conjunctivitis
Predominance of lymphocytes and monocytes	Viral conjunctivitis Chronic toxic or allergic conjunctivitis
Eosinophils	Acute allergic conjunctivitis Parasitic conjunctivitis
Basophils or mast cells	Vernal conjunctivitis
Plasma cells and macrophages	Chlamydial conjunctivitis
Multinucleated cells	Herpes simplex blepharoconjunctivitis
Keratinized epithelial cells	Tear dysfunction states Pemphigoid Stevens-Johnson syndrome
Cytoplasmic inclusions	Chlamydial conjunctivitis

Table 4-3 Staining Procedures in Ocular Cytology

Gram staining
1. Flood the slide with crystal violet for 1 minute. Rinse gently with tap water.
2. Apply Gram's iodine for 1 minute. Rinse.
3. Tilt slide, and allow the decolorizing solvent to run over the slide until the purple color ceases to be washed off. Rinse.
4. Apply safranin solution for 1 minute. Rinse and blot dry.
5. Examine with oil-immersion light microscopy. Gram-positive cocci and rods stain blue-purple, and gram-negative bacteria stain pink-red.

Giemsa staining
1. Immerse slide in freshly prepared Giemsa stain solution for 1 hour.
2. Rinse briefly in ethanol and blot dry.
3. Examine by light microscopy. Leukocytes have lavender cytoplasm with purple nuclei. Neutrophilic granules stain pink-purple, and eosinophilic granules stain bright purple-red. Chlamydial inclusions, as well as bacteria and fungi, stain blue-purple.

Acridine orange staining
1. Apply acidic acridine orange dye to slide for 2 minutes.
2. Rinse and blot dry.
3. Examine by fluorescent microscopy. Bacteria and amoebae generally stain orange, and tissue cells and fungi stain green.

Calcofluor white staining
1. Apply several drops of calcofluor white–Evans blue solution, and apply a coverslip.
2. Examine by fluorescent microscopy. Fungi and amebic cysts stain green against a dark red background.

Acid-fast staining
1. Apply carbolfuchsin solution for 5 minutes. Rinse with tap water.
2. Decolorize with acid-alcohol.
3. Apply malachite green solution for 5 minutes. Rinse.
4. Examine by light microscopy. Most mycobacteria and nocardioforms stain red.

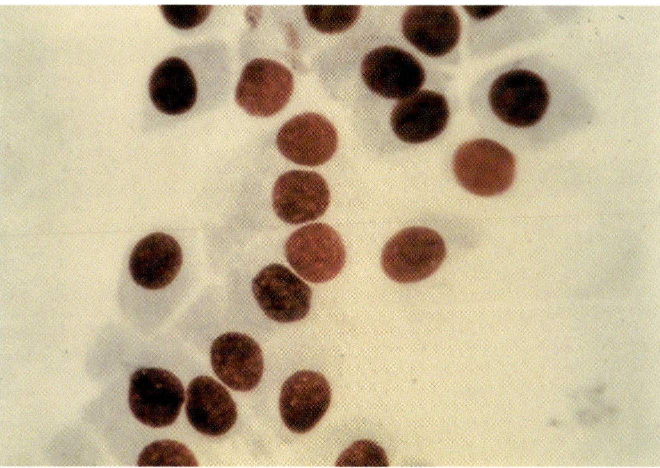

Figure 4-2 Normal conjunctival epithelial cells (Giemsa ×400).

Neutrophils Like other granulocytes that are derived from promyelocytes of the bone marrow, neutrophils are polymorphonuclear; that is, the nucleus is usually separated into distinct lobes connected by narrow strands (Fig 4-5). Less mature neutrophils *(band cells)* have an indented nucleus. About twice the size of erythrocytes, neutrophils have a fairly homogeneous cytoplasm that contains pale or nonstaining granules. Dark intracytoplasmic granules are sometimes visible in certain toxic and infectious conditions, and intracellular bacteria can be identified within phagolysosomes.

Eosinophils About the same size as neutrophils, eosinophils usually have a bilobed nucleus and eosinophilic, uniformly spherical granules that fill the cytoplasm (Fig 4-6). In chronic allergy, intact eosinophils may be less prominent than ruptured cells, extracellular granules, and Charcot-Leyden crystals.

Basophils and mast cells Basophilic leukocytes have banded or lobulated nuclei and dark, basophilic intracytoplasmic granules that are unevenly distributed and vary in size and shape.

Lymphocytes Lymphocytes vary somewhat in size depending on whether they are in a resting or an activated state. The cell contains a single large nucleus and scant, faintly staining cytoplasm that sometimes has scattered granules or vacuoles. Lymphocytes that are unusually round and larger can be compressed or ruptured.

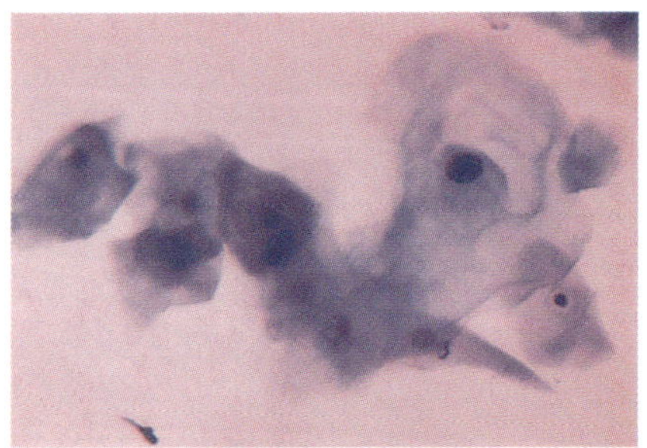

Figure 4-3 Degenerated epithelial cells (Giemsa ×1000).

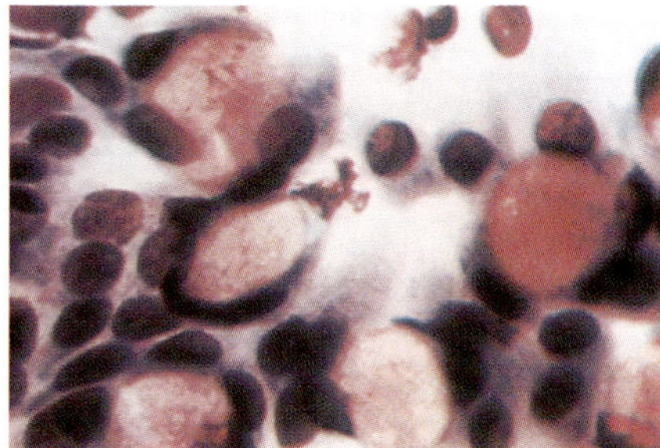

Figure 4-4 Conjunctival goblet cells (Giemsa ×1000).

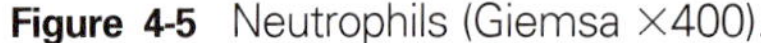

Figure 4-5 Neutrophils (Giemsa ×400).

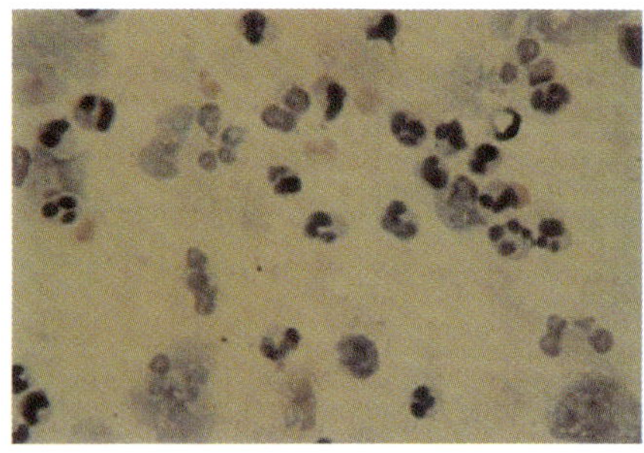

Monocytes and macrophages These large mononuclear cells can be difficult to distinguish from neutrophils and lymphocytes (Fig 4-7). Characteristic features of monocytes include dull coloration of the cytoplasm, blunt pseudopods, and a brainlike convolution of the nucleus. *Histiocytes* contain phagocytized particles and have pseudopods or shaggy cytoplasmic margins. Large engorged macrophages are sometimes referred to as *Leber* or *epithelioid cells.*

Plasma cells These large oval cells have eccentric nuclei and a velvety cytoplasm that is paler adjacent to the nucleus (Fig 4-8).

Erythrocytes Red blood cells are doughnut-shaped cells without nuclei that measure 7 μm across.

Multinucleated cells Multinucleated epithelial cells usually result from failure of the nucleus to divide during mitosis, but they can also arise from a syncytium of coalescent cells. Staining characteristics of these polykaryocytes resemble those of normal conjunctival epithelial cells (Fig 4-9). Giant cells produced by a granulomatous reaction can be identified in histopathologic sections but are rarely seen on conjunctival scrapings.

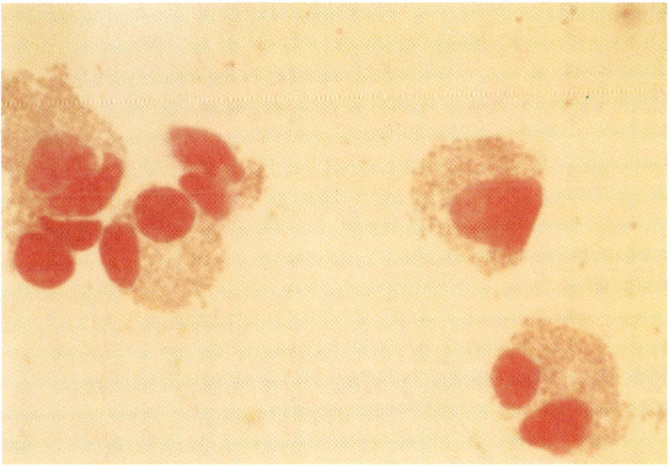

Figure 4-6 Eosinophils (Giemsa ×1000).

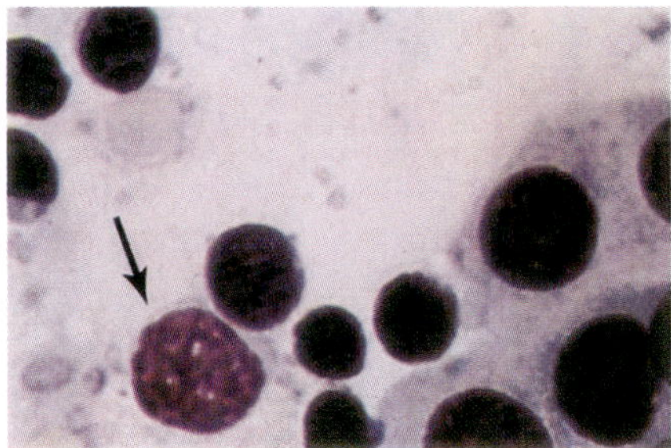

Figure 4-7 Mononuclear inflammatory response. Cells with large, deeply basophilic nuclei and scant, barely noticeable cytoplasm are lymphocytes. The cell with the larger violet nucleus and moderate amount of light blue cytoplasm is a monocyte *(arrow)*. Large, clustered cells at lower right are normal epithelial cells (Giemsa ×1000).

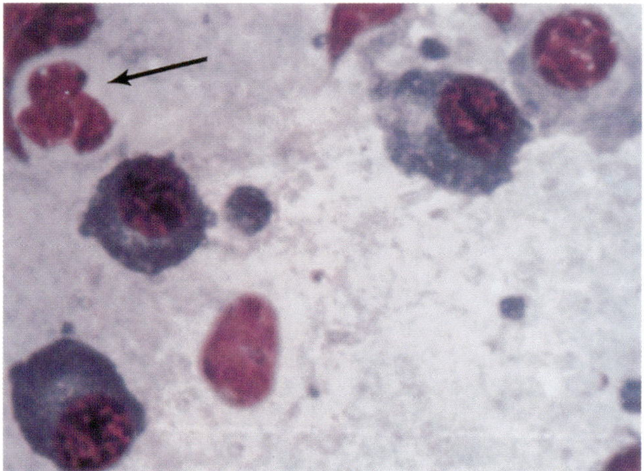

Figure 4-8 Plasma cells *(arrow)* (Giemsa ×1000).

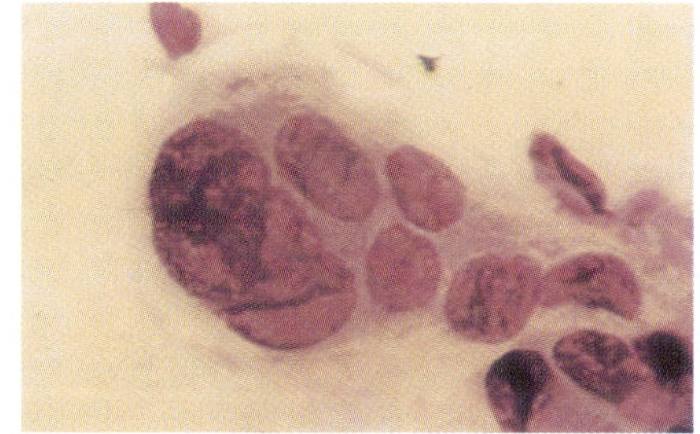

Figure 4-9 Multinucleated epithelial cell (Giemsa ×1000).

Cytoplasmic inclusions A basophilic inclusion within epithelial cells, typically capping the nucleus, is formed by a mass of *Chlamydia trachomatis* elementary bodies. These Halberstaedter-Prowazek inclusion bodies are more likely to be found in neonatal chlamydial conjunctivitis than in adult infection. At least 1000 epithelial cells should be present on the smear to permit adequate search for chlamydial inclusions (Fig 4-10). Extracellular elementary bodies are usually too small to be identified with cytologic stains but can be visualized by immunofluorescence.

Nuclear inclusions Eosinophilic intranuclear inclusions are detected more easily with Papanicolaou stain than with Giemsa stain. A pale halo surrounds the clump, the nucleolus is displaced, and nuclear chromatin is usually clumped or rimmed along the nuclear margins. *Lipschutz bodies,* classified as Cowdry type I inclusion bodies, are sometimes seen in herpes simplex and varicella-zoster viral blepharoconjunctivitis. Viral inclusions are difficult to identify without electron microscopy.

Pigment and other material Small pigment granules are sometimes visible within phagocytic inflammatory cells or scattered extracellularly (Fig 4-11). Melanin granules of the uvea are uniformly spherical, and pigment granules from the retinal pigment epithelium are ellipsoid. Mascara, carbon from the collecting device, and precipitated stain particles vary in size and shape. Remnants of extruded nuclei can clump into basophilic fragments. Basophilic mucin and eosinophilic fibrin strands are sometimes visible in the background.

Tumor cells Neoplastic cells can exhibit several features, including aberrant or multiple nuclei, variable cell shapes and sizes, and mitotic figures (Fig 4-12).

Microorganisms

Bacterial cocci and bacilli, fungi, and protozoa can be visualized with cytologic methods. Gram and acridine orange stains are used to facilitate detection and to highlight the morphology of these microorganisms (Fig 4-13). See Chapters 6 and 7 for further information.

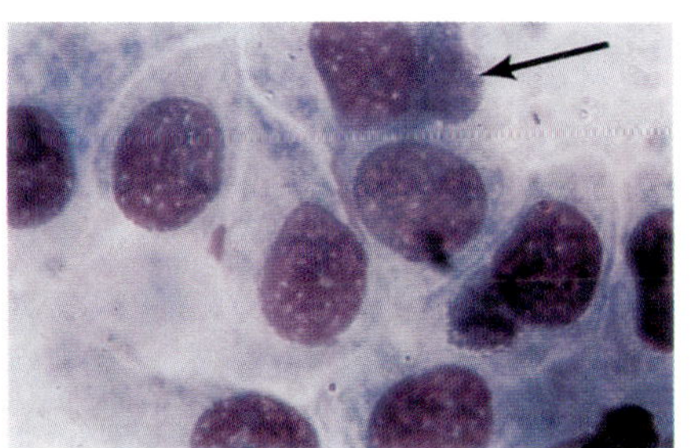

Figure 4-10 Chlamydial inclusion within conjunctival epithelial cell *(arrow)* (Giemsa ×1000). *(Photograph courtesy of Francis I. Proctor Foundation, San Francisco.)*

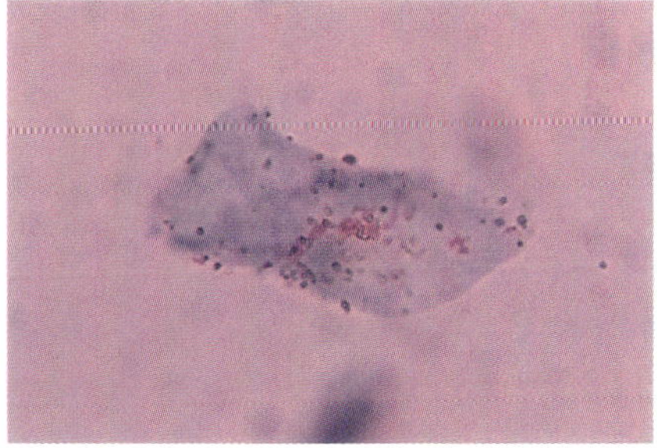

Figure 4-11 Melanin pigment granules on degenerated epithelial cell (Giemsa ×1000).

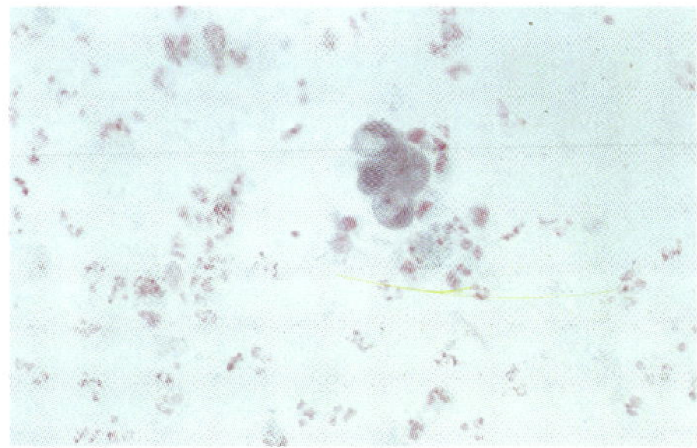

Figure 4-12 Sebaceous cell carcinoma (conjunctival impression cytology). *(Photograph courtesy of Andrew J.W. Huang, MD.)*

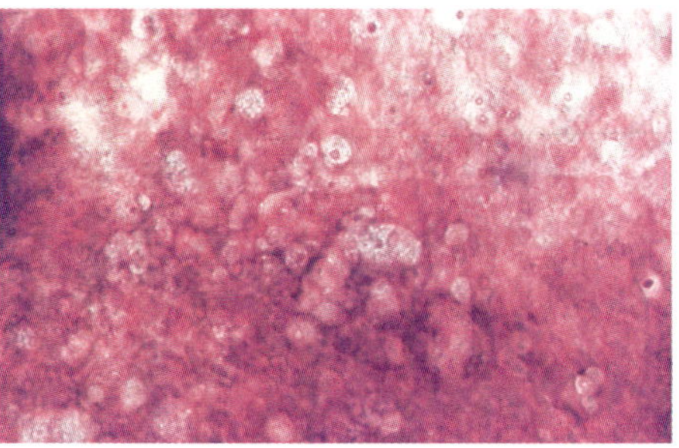

Figure 4-13 *Acanthamoeba* in the corneal epithelial cells (corneal impression cytology). *(Photograph courtesy of Andrew J.W. Huang, MD.)*

CHAPTER 5

Clinical Aspects of Ocular Surface Disorders

Dermatoses Affecting the Ocular Surface

Meibomian Gland Dysfunction

PATHOGENESIS Meibomian gland dysfunction (MGD) is now recognized as a very common yet frequently overlooked cause of ocular irritation. It can be broadly classified into obstructive and nonobstructive types. Patients with MGD develop lipid tear deficiency, which results in tear film instability, increased rate of tear film evaporation, and elevated tear osmolarity. Risk factors for MGD include rosacea and oral retinoid therapy.

CLINICAL PRESENTATION Symptoms consist of burning, foreign body sensation, redness of the eyelids and conjunctiva, filmy vision, and recurrent chalazia. Inflammation is usually confined to the posterior eyelid margins, conjunctiva, and cornea, although patients may occasionally have associated seborrheic changes on the anterior eyelid margin (Fig 5-1). The posterior eyelid margins are often irregular and have prominent, telangiectatic blood vessels *(brush marks)* coursing from the posterior to anterior eyelid margins. The meibomian gland orifices may pout or show metaplasia with a white plug of keratin protein extending through the glandular orifice. They also may become posteriorly displaced on the eyelid margin. Meibomian secretions in active disease may be turbid and have increased viscosity. Following years of meibomian gland inflammation, extensive atrophy of the meibomian gland acini may develop, and eyelid compression can no longer express the meibomian secretions. Atrophy of meibomian gland acini and derangement of glandular architecture can be demonstrated by transillumination of the eyelid as well as infrared photography.

Foam may appear in the tear meniscus along the lower eyelid. Patients frequently have an unstable tear film with rapid tear breakup times, particularly in long-standing disease with meibomian gland atrophy and reduced lipid production. Mild to severe ocular surface inflammation may accompany MGD, which may include the following manifestations:

- Bulbar and tarsal conjunctival injection
- Papillary reaction on the inferior tarsus
- Episcleritis

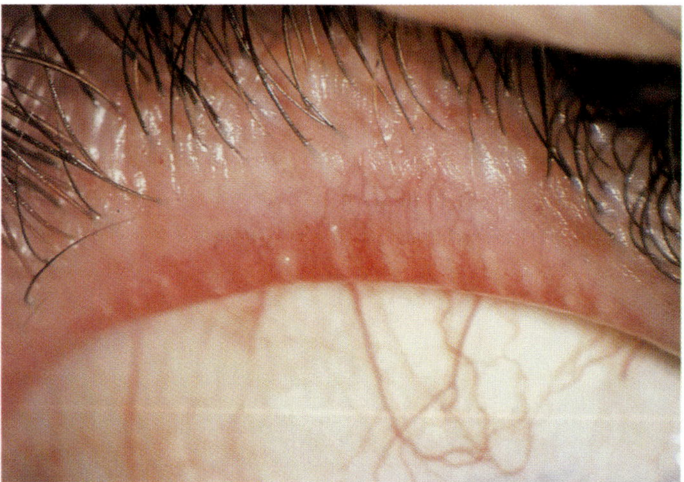

Figure 5-1 Meibomian gland dysfunction.

- Punctate epithelial erosions in the inferior cornea that stain with fluorescein and rose bengal
- Marginal epithelial and subepithelial infiltrates
- Corneal neovascularization and scarring *(pannus)*
- Corneal thinning

Patients with MGD are frequently noted as having one or more manifestations of rosacea, including facial telangiectasia in an axial distribution (forehead, cheeks, nose, and chin), persistent erythema, papules, pustules, hypertrophic sebaceous glands, and rhinophyma. Alterations of the chemical composition of the meibomian secretions have been observed in patients with MGD; however, the precise relationship between these changes and the disease process requires further elucidation.

MANAGEMENT Eyelid hygiene is the initial treatment for patients with blepharitis. These measures include the application of warm compresses to the eyelids for several minutes in order to liquefy thickened meibomian secretions and soften adherent incrustations on the eyelid margins. The application of heat should be followed by gentle massage of the eyelids to express retained meibomian secretions. Eyelid massage can be followed by cleansing the closed eyelid margin with a clean washcloth, a cotton ball, or a commercially available pad. A diluted solution of a nonirritating shampoo, or a commercially available solution designed for this purpose, may facilitate cleansing. Routine performance of eyelid hygiene measures, daily or several times per week, may improve the chronic symptoms of blepharitis.

If the signs and symptoms of MGD are not adequately controlled with eyelid hygiene, systemic tetracyclines can be very effective. Treatment may be initiated with tetracycline 250 mg orally every 6 hours for the first 3–4 weeks, followed by a tapering dose guided by clinical response (usually 250–500 mg daily). Because tetracycline must be taken on an empty stomach and requires more frequent dosing, doxycycline and minocycline are now used with increasing frequency. The dose of doxycycline and minocycline is 100 mg or 50 mg (respectively) every 12 hours for 3–4 weeks, tapering to 50–100 mg per day based on clinical response. It often takes 3–4 weeks to achieve a clinical response. Therapy must often be continued on a chronic basis. Erythromycin can be used as alternative therapy in patients with known hypersensitivity to tetracycline or in children, but its efficacy in treating MGD is not well established. Patients with MGD should be informed that therapy may control but not eliminate their condition.

Side effects of the systemic tetracyclines include photosensitization, gastrointestinal upset and, rarely, azotemia. Chronic use may lead to oral or vaginal candidiasis in susceptible patients. The use of tetracyclines is contraindicated during pregnancy, for women who are nursing, and in patients with a known hypersensitivity to these agents. These agents should be used with caution in women in the child-bearing age range. Tetracyclines may also reduce the efficacy of oral contraceptives. These antibiotics should also be avoided in children under 10 years of age because they deposit in bones and teeth.

Topical corticosteroids may be required for short periods in cases with moderate to severe inflammation, particularly those with corneal infiltrates and vascularization. Patients treated with topical steroids should be warned about the complications of chronic use, because this stubborn condition may prompt patients to become dependent.

Bron AJ, Benjamin L, Snibson GR. Meibomian gland disease. Classification and grading of lid changes. *Eye.* 1991;5:395–411.

Driver PJ, Lemp MA. Meibomian gland dysfunction. *Surv Ophthalmol.* 1996;40:343–368.

Rosacea

PATHOGENESIS Rosacea (sometimes called acne rosacea) is a chronic acneiform disorder that can affect both the skin and eyes. This disease has no proven cause. It is associated with cutaneous sebaceous gland dysfunction of the face, neck, and shoulders. Although rosacea has generally been thought to be more common in fair-skinned individuals, it may simply be more difficult to diagnose in persons with dark skin. It is infrequently diagnosed by ophthalmologists, in spite of its relatively frequent association with blepharitis and/or aqueous tear deficiency. Although alcohol can contribute to a worsening of this disorder because of its effect on vasomotor stability, not all patients with rosacea have a history of excessive alcohol intake. Recently, experimental studies based on immunohistochemical staining of inflammatory cell infiltrates have shown this disease to represent a delayed hypersensitivity reaction. Dysfunction of the meibomian and other lipid-producing glands of the eyelids and skin of the face is believed to be responsible for these infiltrates.

CLINICAL PRESENTATION A skin condition that frequently involves the eyes, rosacea is characterized by excessive sebum secretion with a frequently recalcitrant chronic blepharitis. Eyelid margin telangiectasia is very common, as are meibomian gland distortion, disruption, and dysfunction, which can lead to recurrent chalazia. Ocular involvement can also progress, leading to chronic conjunctivitis, marginal corneal infiltrates, sterile ulceration, episcleritis, or iridocyclitis (Fig 5-2). If properly treated, these lesions can resolve with few sequelae. Repeated bouts of ocular surface inflammation can bring about corneal neovascularization and scarring, often in a characteristic triangular configuration (Fig 5-3).

This disorder is generally found in patients aged 30–60, with a slight female preponderance. However, ocular rosacea can be encountered in younger patients and is often underdiagnosed. Facial lesions consist of telangiectasias, recurrent papules and pustules, and midfacial erythema (Fig 5-4). Rosacea is characterized by a malar rash with unpredictable flushing episodes, sometimes associated with the consumption of alcohol, coffee, or other foods. *Rhinophyma,* thickening of the skin and connective tissue of the nose, is a characteristic and obvious sign associated with this disorder, but such hypertrophic cutaneous changes occur relatively late in the disease process.

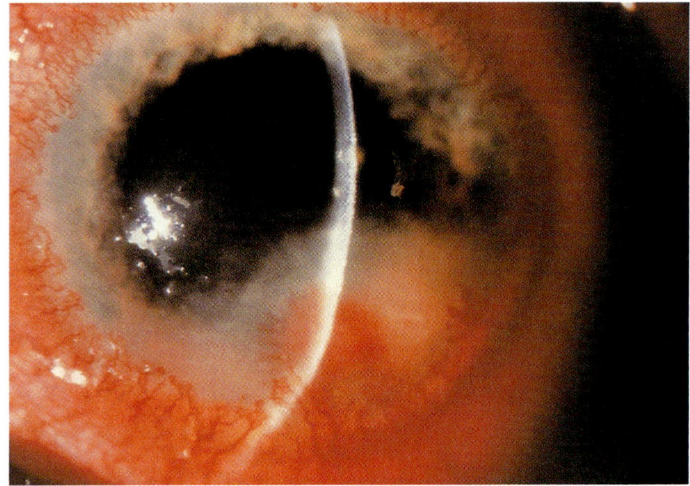

Figure 5-2 Marginal keratitis associated with rosacea.

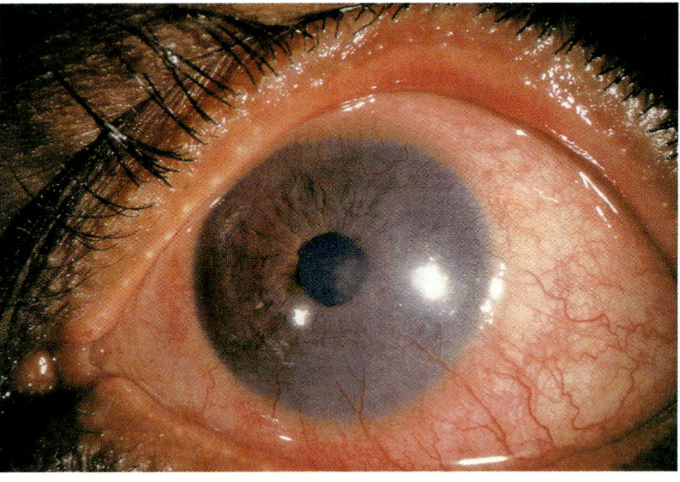

Figure 5-3 Rosacea with chronic superficial keratopathy and corneal neovascularization.

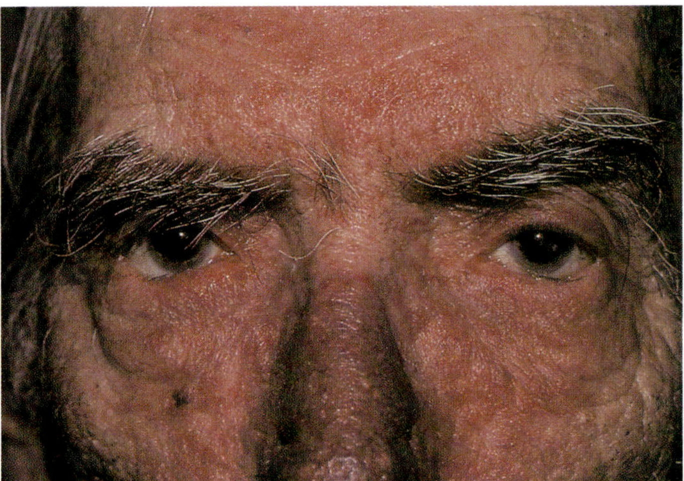

Figure 5-4 Facial changes of rosacea.

MANAGEMENT The ocular and systemic diseases are managed simultaneously, with systemic tetracyclines as the mainstay of therapy. These agents alter the nature of lipid production by the sebaceous glands, inhibit production of matrix metalloproteases, and may alter the interaction between the meibomian glands and the resident bacteria.

With time, oral therapy with doxycycline or minocycline can be tapered, although it is recommended that a low dose be continued indefinitely. In addition to oral therapy, application of topical metronidazole 0.75% gel (Metrogel) to the affected facial areas can significantly reduce facial erythema. Topical dermatologic therapy should also be continued indefinitely at a low dose.

Ulcerative keratitis can be associated with infectious agents in rosacea, or it may have a sterile inflammatory etiology. Once it is ascertained that ulceration is noninfectious, topical corticosteroids used judiciously can play a significant role in reducing sterile inflammation and enhancing epithelialization of the cornea. In advanced cases with scarring and neovascularization, conservative therapy is generally recommended. Penetrating keratoplasty in rosacea patients is a high-risk procedure that may have a poor prognosis if the ocular surface is severely compromised.

Bron AJ, Benjamin L, Snibson GR. Meibomian gland disease. Classification and grading of lid changes. *Eye.* 1991;5:395–411.

Browning DJ, Proia AD. Ocular rosacea. *Surv Ophthalmol.* 1986;31:145–158.

Macsai MJ, Mannis MS, Huntley AC. Acne rosacea. In: Mannis MJ, Macsai MS, Huntley AC, eds. *Eye and Skin Disease.* Philadelphia: Lippincott; 1996:335–341.

Seborrheic Blepharitis

CLINICAL PRESENTATION Seborrheic blepharitis may occur alone or in combination with staphylococcal blepharitis or MGD. Inflammation occurs primarily at the anterior eyelid margin, while a variable amount of crusting, typically of an oily or greasy nature, may be found on the eyelids, eyelashes, eyebrows, and scalp. Patients with seborrheic blepharitis often have increased meibomian gland secretions that appear opaque when expressed. Signs and symptoms include chronic eyelid redness, burning, and occasionally foreign body sensation. A small percentage of patients (approximately 15%) develop an associated keratitis or conjunctivitis. The keratitis is characterized by punctate epithelial erosions distributed over the inferior third of the cornea. Approximately one third of patients with seborrheic blepharitis have aqueous tear deficiency.

MANAGEMENT Eyelid hygiene is the primary treatment in patients with blepharitis. This regimen is detailed earlier, in the discussion of meibomian gland dysfunction. Concurrent treatment of scalp disease can also improve blepharitis.

If inflammation is a prominent component of the blepharitis, a brief course of topical steroid applied to the eyelid margins may be helpful. If blepharitis involves primarily the posterior eyelid margin (ie, meibomian gland dysfunction), systemic antibiotics such as doxycycline are the mainstay of treatment. Blepharitis caused by bacteria (eg, staphylococcus) often responds to the use of a topical antibiotic ointment such as bacitracin or bacitracin-polymyxin B. (Staphylococcal blepharitis is discussed further in Chapter 7.)

Chalazion

CLINICAL PRESENTATION A chalazion is a localized lipogranulomatous inflammation involving either the meibomian or Zeis glands. It usually develops spontaneously as a result of obstruction of one or more of the glands. The nodules develop slowly and are typically painless. The overlying skin is erythematous (Fig 5-5). The lesion disappears in weeks to months when the contents drain either externally through the eyelid skin or internally through the tarsus, or when the extruded lipid is phagocytosed and the granuloma dissipates. A small amount of scar tissue may remain. Occasionally, patients with a chalazion may experience blurred vision secondary to astigmatism induced by its pressure on the globe.

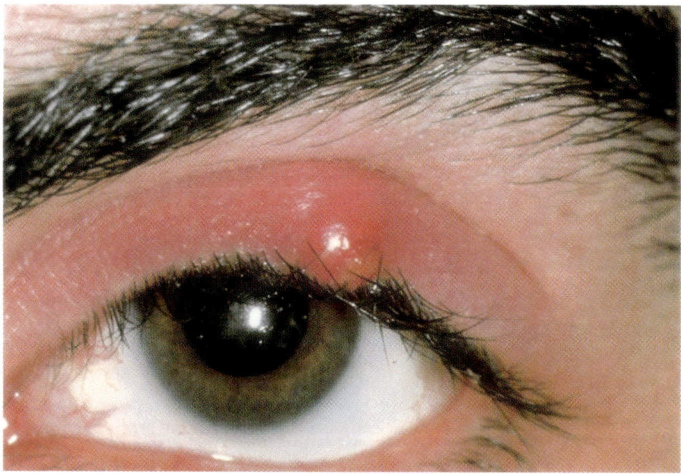

Figure 5-5 Chalazion. *(Photograph courtesy of Vincent P. deLuise, MD.)*

PATHOGENESIS AND LABORATORY EVALUATION Sebaceous material trapped in a plugged Zeis or meibomian gland extrudes into adjacent tissues, where it elicits a chronic granulomatous inflammation. A zonal granulomatous inflammation centered around lipid is seen histologically. As is typical of all granulomas, epithelioid cells are prominent. Also present are admixtures of other cells, including lymphocytes, macrophages, neutrophils, plasma cells, and giant cells. It must be emphasized that basal cell, squamous cell, or sebaceous carcinoma can be misdiagnosed as chalazia. The histopathologic examination of persistent, recurrent, or atypical chalazia is therefore quite important.

MANAGEMENT Because most chalazia are sterile, topical antibiotic therapy is of little or no value. Chalazia may be treated with hot compresses and attempted expression of the inflamed meibomian gland. Lesions that fail to respond to conservative therapy may be treated with intralesional injection of steroid (0.1–0.2 mL triamcinolone 10 mg/mL), incision and drainage, or a combination of both. In general, intralesional steroid injection works best with small chalazia, with chalazia on the eyelid margin, and with multiple chalazia. Intralesional steroid injection in patients with dark skin may lead to depigmentation of the overlying eyelid skin and thus should be used with caution.

Larger chalazia are best treated with surgical drainage and curettage. Internal chalazia require vertical incisions on the tarsal conjunctiva along the meibomian gland to facilitate drainage and avoid horizontal scarring of the tarsal plates. Surgical drainage usually requires perilesional anesthesia. Recurrent chalazia should be biopsied to rule out meibomian gland carcinoma. Systemic tetracyclines can be of benefit in patients with associated rosacea.

> Epstein GA, Putterman AM. Combined excision and drainage with intralesional corticosteroid injection in the treatment of chronic chalazia. *Arch Ophthalmol.* 1988;106:514–516.

Hordeolum

Hordeola are discussed in Chapter 7.

Sarcoidosis

A multisystem disorder of uncertain etiology, sarcoidosis is characterized by noncaseating granulomas in affected tissues. After pulmonary involvement, ocular involvement is the most common manifestation, seen in up to 50% of affected patients. Nontender small (millet seed) or large nodules may be seen in the eyelid skin and in the canthal region. Lacrimal gland involvement occurs in up to 25% of patients with ocular involvement, resulting in keratoconjunctivitis sicca. Concomitant enlargement of the lacrimal and salivary glands combined with the presence of keratoconjunctivitis sicca is known as *Mikulicz syndrome,* which can be confused with Sjögren syndrome. Patients with *Lofgren syndrome* present with erythema nodosum, hilar adenopathy, and iridocyclitis. Patients presenting with uveitis, fever, and facial nerve palsy (uveoparotid fever) have *Heerfordt syndrome.*

Conjunctival granulomas have been observed in approximately 7% of patients with ocular involvement. Such granulomas are often small and easily overlooked, and they may be difficult to distinguish from normal conjunctival follicles. The most common corneal finding is calcific band keratopathy, often associated with chronic uveitis or elevated serum calcium levels. Nummular keratitis, thickening of Descemet's membrane, and deep stromal vascularization as a result of chronic intraocular inflammation can be seen. Granulomatous uveitis with mutton-fat keratic precipitates and iris nodules occurs in as many as two thirds of patients with ocular involvement. Periphlebitis is the most common fundus finding. Chronic cystoid macular edema and exudative retinal detachment are related to intense and long-standing inflammation. Granulomatous involvement of the optic nerve is also seen.

See also BCSC Section 9, *Intraocular Inflammation and Uveitis,* for illustrations and further discussion of sarcoidosis.

Desquamating Skin Conditions

Ichthyosis

This spectrum of diverse skin disorders is characterized by excessively dry skin and accumulation of scale. *Ichthyosis vulgaris,* an autosomal dominant trait, is the most common hereditary scaling disorder, affecting 1 in 250–300 persons. Ocular involvement varies with the form of ichthyosis. Eyelid scaling, ectropion, and conjunctival thickening are common. Primary corneal opacities are seen in 50% of patients with *X-linked ichthyosis* but are rarely seen in ichthyosis vulgaris. Dots or filament-shaped opacities appear diffusely in pre-Descemet's membrane or in deep stroma and become more apparent with age without affecting vision. Nodular corneal degeneration and band keratopathy have been described. Secondary corneal changes such as vascularization and scarring from severe ectropion-related exposure can develop.

Ichthyosis is a prominent feature in several genetic disorders, including Sjögren-Larsson, Rud, and Conradi syndromes, congenital keratitis-ichthyosis-deafness (KID) syndrome, Refsum disease, and congenital hemidysplasia with ichthyosiform erythroderma and limb defects (CHILD). Vascularizing keratitis is a prominent feature of KID syndrome, and it may worsen with isotretinoin therapy. Treatment for the ichthyosis spectrum is aimed at hydrating the skin and eyelids, removing scale, and slowing the turnover of epidermis when appropriate. These disorders are not responsive to corticosteroids.

Ectodermal Dysplasia

This heterogeneous group of conditions is characterized by the following:

- Presence of abnormalities at birth
- Nonprogressive course
- Diffuse involvement of the epidermis plus at least one of its appendages (hair, nails, teeth, sweat glands)
- Various inheritance patterns

Many ocular abnormalities have been described in the ectodermal dysplasias, including sparse lashes and brows, blepharitis, ankyloblepharon, hypoplastic lacrimal ducts, diminished tear production, abnormal meibomian glands, dry conjunctivae, pterygia, corneal scarring and neovascularization, cataract, and glaucoma. These changes may be due to limbal stem-cell deficiency.

Anhidrotic ectodermal dysplasia is usually an X-linked disorder consisting of hypotrichosis, anodontia, and anhidrosis. Sweating is almost completely lacking, and hyperpyrexia is a common problem in childhood. Atopic disease is often an associated finding. The *ectodactyly-ectodermal dysplasial–clefting (EEC)* syndrome is an association of ectodermal dysplasia, cleft lip and/or palate, and a clefting deformity of the hands and/or feet ("lobster claw deformity").

Xeroderma Pigmentosum (XP)

XP is a recessively transmitted disease characterized by impaired ability to repair sunlight-induced damage to DNA. During the first or second decade of life, the patient's exposed skin develops areas of focal hyperpigmentation, atrophy, actinic keratosis, and telangiectasia as if the patient had received a heavy dose of radiation. Many cutaneous neoplasms appear later, including squamous cell carcinoma, basal cell carcinoma, and melanoma.

Ophthalmic manifestations include photophobia, tearing, blepharospasm, and signs and symptoms of keratoconjunctivitis sicca. The conjunctiva is dry and inflamed with telangiectasia and hyperpigmentation. Pingueculae and pterygia often occur. Corneal complications include exposure keratitis, ulceration, neovascularization, scarring, and even perforation. Keratoconus, band-shaped nodular corneal dystrophy, and gelatinous dystrophy have also been reported. Ocular neoplasms occur in 11% of patients, most frequently at the limbus. Squamous cell carcinoma is the most frequent histologic type seen, followed by basal cell carcinoma and melanoma, similar to the cutaneous tumors. The eyelids can be involved with progressive atrophy, madarosis, trichiasis, scarring, symblepharon, entropion, ectropion, and sometimes even loss of the entire lower eyelid.

Mannis MJ, Macsai MS, Huntley AC, eds. *Eye and Skin Disease.* Philadelphia: Lippincott; 1996:3–12, 39–44, 131–145.

Noninflammatory Vascular Anomalies of the Conjunctiva

Causes of conjunctival hyperemia include the following:
- *Inflammation:* infection, allergy, toxicity, neoplasia
- *Direct irritation:* foreign body, eyelash
- *Reflex response:* eyestrain, emotional weeping
- *Systemic or topical vasodilators:* alcohol, oxygen, carcinoid tumor
- *Autonomic dysfunction:* sympathetic paresis, sphenopalatine ganglion syndrome
- *Vascular engorgement:* venous obstruction, hyperviscosity

Conjunctival vascular tortuosities may result from trauma or from disorders such as rosacea that cause chronic conjunctival vascular dilation. Systemic conditions that cause sludging and segmentation of blood flow in conjunctival vessels, as well as conjunctival varicosities and aneurysms, include

- Hypertension
- Diabetes mellitus
- Sickle cell disease
- Multiple myeloma
- Polycythemia vera
- Old age

Causes of subconjunctival hemorrhage and, less commonly, of bloody tears are listed in Table 5-1. Hereditary causes of conjunctival telangiectasia and hemorrhage are hereditary hemorrhagic telangiectasia and ataxia-telangiectasia.

Hereditary Hemorrhagic Telangiectasia

Spontaneous hemorrhage from telangiectatic vessels of the palpebral and bulbar conjunctiva may occur in individuals with hereditary hemorrhagic telangiectasia *(Rendu-Osler-Weber disease)*, a vascular disorder that also involves the skin, nasal and oral mucous membranes, gastrointestinal tract, lungs, and brain. This dominantly inherited (but occasionally sporadic) disease is usually not apparent in early childhood, and its onset during early adult life may be subtle. Initial manifestations may be intermittent, painless gastrointestinal bleeding leading to iron deficiency anemia or recurrent epistaxis following minor trauma or occurring spontaneously.

Conjunctival hemorrhage may be associated with foreign body sensation, and it usually occurs spontaneously or after minor trauma, such as rubbing of the eyelids. The hemorrhage may extend into the subepithelial connective tissues or may be external (bloody tears). Conjunctival bleeding can be copious, but in most instances it can be controlled with local pressure. The conjunctival telangiectasias appear sharply circumscribed, are slightly elevated, and are composed of arborizing dilated channels. Typically, they involve the palpebral region, although lesions of the bulbar conjunctiva have also been reported.

Histologic study has shown superficial, dilated, thin-walled vascular channels. Similar findings have been noted in telangiectatic lesions of the skin and nasal and oral mucous membranes. It is likely that hemorrhage results from minor trauma to these superficial vessels; however, intravascular factors affecting bleeding time may also play a role.

Lymphangiectasia

This condition may be a developmental anomaly or may occur in association with trauma or inflammation. Unlike lymphangiomas, which are cellular proliferations of lymphatic

Table 5-1 Causes of Subconjunctival Hemorrhage

Ocular	Systemic
Conjunctival, orbital, or cranial trauma	Sudden venous congestion (Valsalva maneuver)
Acute viral or bacterial conjunctivitis	Vascular fragility
	Thrombocytopenia and impaired clotting
	Systemic febrile illness

channel elements, lymphangiectasias are irregularly dilated, periodically hemorrhage-filled, lymphatic channels of the bulbar conjunctiva. Surrounding conjunctival edema or subconjunctival hemorrhage may also be present, especially upon crying or exertion. Treatment is local excision or diathermy.

Lymphangiectasia must be distinguished from *ataxia-telangiectasia (Louis-Bar syndrome)*, in which the epibulbar and interpalpebral telangiectasia of the arteries lacks an associated lymphatic component. The conjunctival lesions of Louis-Bar syndrome are a marker for associated cerebellar and immunologic abnormalities (eg, hypogammaglobulinemia), which are conducive to sinopulmonary infection and lymphoreticular proliferations, particularly T-cell I leukemias. The epibulbar vascular lesions do not acquire a tumefactive characteristic (hamartia) because they are simple telangiectases that grow with the patient and the eyeball. No episodic events of hemorrhage or swelling are encountered. Ataxia-telangiectasia is discussed and illustrated in greater detail in BCSC Section 6, *Pediatric Ophthalmology and Strabismus.*

Tear Deficiency States (Dry Eye)

Dry eye affects 10%–15% of adults. This very common disorder of tear film results from either decreased tear production or excessive tear evaporation. The tear film becomes unstable with the loss of water, and a progressive deterioration of the ocular surface ensues. Interpretation of studies investigating risk factors, pathogenesis, and therapy of dry eye conditions has been complicated in the past by a lack of accepted diagnostic criteria and standardized, specific diagnostic tests. A diagnostic classification scheme for dry eye disorders has now been established, along with uniform guidelines for the evaluation of both the disorder and its response to therapy. The major subclassification in this scheme separates dry eye patients into those with aqueous tear deficiency and those with evaporative loss, predominantly patients with meibomian gland dysfunction (Table 5-2).

CLINICAL PRESENTATION The spectrum of aqueous tear deficiency ranges from mild irritation with minimal ocular surface disease to severe and disabling irritation, occasionally

---

Table 5-2 Classification of Dry Eye

Tear-deficient dry eye
  Non–Sjögren syndrome
    Lacrimal disease (primary or secondary)
    Lacrimal obstructive disease
    Decreased corneal sensation
    Other (e.g., multiple neuromatosis)
  Sjögren syndrome

Evaporative dry eye
  Blepharitis-associated
    obstructive meibomian gland disease
  Blink disorders
  Disorders of eyelid aperture and eyelid/globe congruity

associated with sight-threatening corneal complications. Advanced stages can include the development of corneal calcification, particularly in association with certain topical medications (especially antiglaucoma medications); band keratopathy; and keratinization of the cornea and conjunctiva.

Symptoms tend to be worse toward the end of the day, with prolonged use of the eyes, or with exposure to environmental extremes. Patients who live in temperate climates and are exposed to the lower levels of humidity associated with indoor heating systems during the winter tend to become particularly symptomatic. Foreign body sensation is a symptom frequently associated with punctate epithelial keratopathy. Associated complaints include burning, a dry sensation, photophobia, and blurred vision.

The signs of a dry eye include bulbar conjunctival vascular dilation, conjunctival pleating (redundancy of the bulbar conjunctiva), a decreased tear meniscus, irregular corneal surface, and increased debris in the tear film. Epithelial keratopathy, which can be fine and granular, coarse, or confluent, is best demonstrated following the instillation of lissamine green, rose bengal, or fluorescein. Fluorescein stains epithelial erosions and exposed basement membrane and may produce fine or coarse granular staining of the inferior or central cornea. Particularly useful in the evaluation of the dry eye patient is staining with either 1% rose bengal or lissamine green. Previously, rose bengal was thought to stain only dead and devitalized cells and mucus. It has recently been demonstrated that it may also stain epithelial cells that are inadequately protected by a mucin tear coating. Rose bengal and lissamine green staining can be more sensitive than fluorescein in revealing early or mild cases of keratoconjunctivitis sicca; the staining may be seen at the nasal and temporal limbus and/or inferior paracentral cornea *(exposure staining)* (Fig 5-6). Alternatively, it can be most prominent along the inferior cornea and inferior conjunctiva *(linear staining)*, as seen in MGD. Lissamine green has some advantages over rose bengal: it does not stain healthy conjunctival epithelium, it is far less irritating, and it does not inhibit viral growth as does rose bengal.

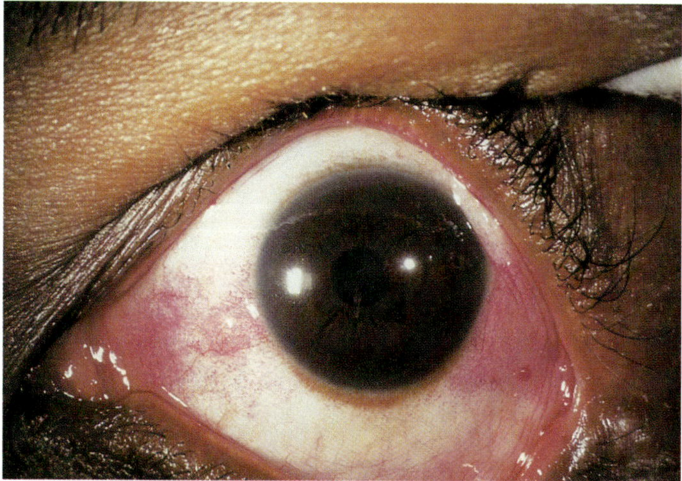

Figure 5-6 Keratoconjunctivitis sicca with punctate epithelial erosions, shown by rose bengal stain. *(Photograph courtesy of Vincent P. deLuise, MD.)*

In more severe dry eye states filaments and mucous plaques can be seen. *Filaments* represent strands of epithelial cells attached to the surface of the cornea over a core of mucus. Filamentary keratopathy can be quite painful, as these strands are firmly attached to the richly innervated surface epithelium (Fig 5-7). Marginal or paracentral thinning and even perforation can occur in more severe disease. Incomplete blinking is frequently noted. Associated local eye disease, such as blepharitis, MGD, and eyelid abnormalities, can contribute significantly to the patient's level of discomfort.

Aqueous Tear Deficiency (ATD)

Findings that are particularly indicative of ATD include, by definition, decreased aqueous tear production as measured by Schirmer testing. In addition, the characteristic exposure pattern of conjunctival and/or corneal staining with either lissamine green or rose bengal, corneal staining by fluorescein, and filamentary keratopathy support a diagnosis of ATD. There is increasing recognition that lacrimal gland secretory dysfunction results in the ocular surface condition known as *keratoconjunctivitis sicca (KCS)* and that the severity of aqueous tear deficiency is positively correlated with the severity of KCS. ATD can be congenital, as in Riley-Day syndrome (familial dysautonomia); congenital alacrima, or absence of the lacrimal gland; anhidrotic ectodermal dysplasia; Adie syndrome; and idiopathic autonomic dysfunction (Shy-Drager syndrome). Contact lens wear has also been associated with decreased tear production, possibly as a result of decreased corneal sensation. However, acquired ATD secondary to dysfunction of the lacrimal gland is the more frequently encountered clinical problem. Most commonly seen in association with inflammatory diseases of the main lacrimal gland, it can also be caused by trauma to the lacrimal gland, numerous anticholinergic medications (Table 5-3), and neuroparalytic hyposecretion. Decreased corneal sensation following either photorefractive keratectomy or laser in situ keratomileusis often results in dry eye symptoms lasting several months. These symptoms typically resolve following the restoration of normal corneal sensitivity.

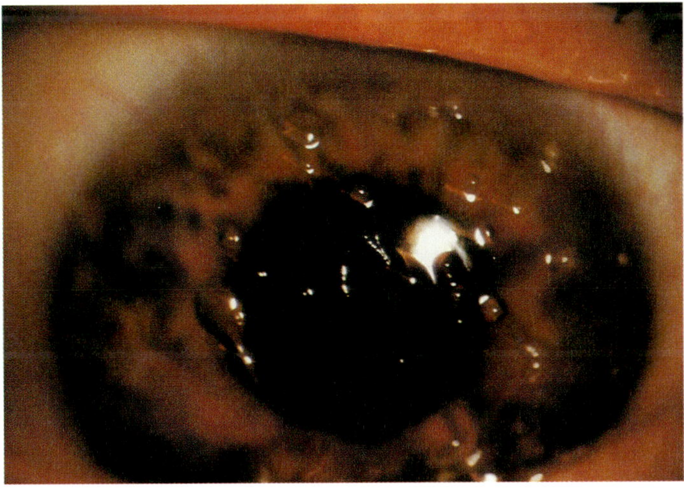

Figure 5-7 Filamentary keratopathy. *(Photograph courtesy of Vincent P. deLuise, MD.)*

Table 5-3 Medications With Anticholinergic Side Effects That Decrease Tear Production

Antihypertensives
  Clonidine (alpha$_1$ blocker)
  Prazosin (alpha$_1$ blocker)
  Propranolol (beta blocker)
  Reserpine
  Methyldopa, guanethidine

Antidepressants and psychotropics
  Amitriptyline, nortriptyline
  Imipramine, desipramine, clomipramine
  Doxepin
  Phenelzine, tranylcypromine
  Amoxapine, trimipramine
  Phenothiazines
  Nitrazepam, diazepam

Cardiac antiarrhythmia drugs
  Disopyramide
  Mexiletine

Parkinson disease medications
  Trihexyphenidyl
  Benztropine
  Biperiden
  Procyclidine

Antiulcer agents
  Atropine-like agents
  Metoclopramide, other drugs that decrease gastric motility

Muscle spasm medications
  Cyclobenzaprine
  Methocarbamol

Decongestants (nonprescription cold remedies)
  Ephedrine
  Pseudoephedrine

Antihistamines

Anesthetics
  Enflurane
  Halothane
  Nitrous oxide

Sarcoidosis and mumps can cause significant inflammation and dysfunction of the main lacrimal gland. Cicatricial conjunctivitis caused by ocular cicatricial pemphigoid, Stevens-Johnson syndrome, or trachoma can obliterate the lacrimal ducts in the superior conjunctival fornices, thereby blocking secretion.

Patients with ATD are considered to have *Sjögren syndrome (SS)* if they have associated xerostomia and/or evidence of collagen vascular disease. Sjögren syndrome can be subdivided into two clinical subsets. *Primary SS* includes those patients who either have ill-defined systemic immune dysfunction or lack any evidence of immune dysfunction or connective tissue disease. *Secondary SS* occurs in patients with a well-defined connective tissue disease. Secondary SS is most commonly associated with rheumatoid arthritis, although numerous other autoimmune diseases are also frequently encountered. Criteria for the diagnosis of SS are in Table 5-4. Additional systemic associations can include monocular exocrine gland dysfunction, atrophy of the gastric and vaginal mucosa, and lymphocytic infiltration of the kidney, lung, muscle, or visceral organs. Associated symptoms can include fever, fatigue, Raynaud's phenomenon, arthralgias, and myalgias.

Table 5-4 Criteria for the Classification of Sjögren Syndrome

1. Ocular symptoms
   Definition: A positive response to at least 1 of the following 3 questions:
   a. Have you had daily, persistent, troublesome dry eyes for more than 3 months?
   b. Do you have a recurrent sensation of sand or gravel in the eyes?
   c. Do you use tear substitutes more than 3 times a day?

2. Oral symptoms
   Definition: A positive response to at least 1 of the following 3 questions:
   a. Have you had a daily feeling of dry mouth for more than 3 months?
   b. Have you had recurrent or persistently swollen salivary glands as an adult?
   c. Do you frequently drink liquids to aid in swallowing dry foods?

3. Ocular signs
   Definition: Objective evidence of ocular involvement, determined on the basis of a positive result on at least 1 of the following 2 tests:
   a. Schirmer I test (=5 mm in 5 minutes).
   b. Rose bengal score (=4 Bijsterveld score)

4. Histopathologic features
   Definition: Focus score = 1 on minor salivary gland biopsy (*focus* defined as a conglomeration of at least 50 mononuclear cells; *focus score* defined as the number of foci in 4 mm² of glandular tissue).

5. Salivary gland involvement
   Definition: Objective evidence of salivary gland involvement, determined on the basis of a positive result on at least 1 of the following 3 tests:
   a. Salivary scintography
   b. Parotid sialography
   c. Unstimulated salivary flow (= 1.5 mL in 15 minutes)

6. Autoantibodies
   Definition: Presence of at least 1 of the following serum autoantibodies:
   a. Antibodies to Ro/SS-A or La/SS-B antigens
   b. Antinuclear antibodies
   c. Rheumatoid factor

Exclusion criteria: Preexisting lymphoma, acquired immunodeficiency syndrome, sarcoidosis, or chronic graft-versus-host disease.

Primary Sjögren syndrome: Presence of 4 out of 6 items (accepting only positive SS-A or SS-B as serologic parameters).

Probable primary Sjögren syndrome: Presence of 3 out of 6 items.

Secondary Sjögren syndrome: A combination of a positive response to item 1 or 2 plus a positive response to at least 2 items from among 3, 4, and 5.

Probable secondary Sjögren syndrome: A combination of a positive response to item 1 or 2 plus a positive response to at least 1 item from among 3, 4, and 5.

The precise cause of KCS in SS is unknown, although it is probably related to autoimmune infiltration of the lacrimal glands and salivary glands by lymphocytes. Viral infections such as Epstein-Barr virus and human immunodeficiency virus (HIV) have been implicated as the potential etiology, because ATD has been observed to develop in patients after mononucleosis or HIV infection. Lacrimal gland histology provides many insights into the pathogenesis of Sjögren syndrome. The histologic changes are usually identical to those noted in the salivary glands, with focal areas of glandular degeneration associated with infiltration by lymphocytes and plasma cells in the earliest stages. As the disease advances, fibrosis and replacement of the glandular tissue may occur. Immunoglobulin and complement are rarely detected within the glandular tissue. The lymphocytes are predominantly helper T cells, and the overall histology suggests a cell-mediated pathogenesis.

LABORATORY EVALUATION A lacrimal gland biopsy can be performed to aid the diagnosis, but because it can aggravate dry eye conditions, judicious use is recommended. Minor (labial) salivary gland biopsy is occasionally performed by oral surgeons to confirm the diagnosis of Sjögren syndrome. Finally, conjunctival impression cytology can be used to monitor the progression of ocular surface changes, beginning with decreased goblet cell density, followed by squamous metaplasia and, in later stages, keratinization.

Many patients with ATD have either circulating autoantibodies, including antinuclear antibody (ANA), or SS antibodies (SS-A and SS-B). The presence of these antibodies has been correlated with the severity of symptoms and ocular surface changes, including a higher incidence of sterile and bacterial keratitis, suggesting that a disturbance in immune regulation may play a role in pathogenesis. As previously noted, many systemic diseases have been associated with ATD (Table 5-5).

The psychological problems associated with a highly symptomatic, incurable, chronic disease can require considerable support. Organizations such as the Sjögren's Syndrome Foundation, Inc. (http://www.sjogrens.org) can provide valuable resources to these patients.

MEDICAL MANAGEMENT The selection of treatment modalities for patients with dry eye depends largely on the severity of their disease (Table 5-6). Mild cases of dry eye may require no more than the use of artificial tear solutions. Changing or discontinuing any topical or systemic medications that contribute to the condition should also be considered, although it is often not possible. Hot compresses with eyelid massage can also help by bolstering the lipid layer. If the condition is not sufficiently managed with artificial tears, the use of sustained-release ocular lubricants may be considered. It may also be appropriate to modify the patient's environment in an effort to reduce evaporation of the tear film; a humidifier and/or moisture shields on glasses can be helpful. Therapy for patients with severe dry eye syndrome includes all of the above measures as well as punctal occlusion and lateral tarsorrhaphy.

The mainstay of treatment for dry eye syndrome is the use of topical tear substitutes (eyedrops, gels, and ointments). Preservative-free tear substitutes are recommended to avoid toxicity in patients who use these agents frequently. Demulcents are polymers added to artificial tear solutions to improve their lubricant properties. Demulcent solutions are mucomimetic agents that can briefly substitute for glycoproteins lost late in the disease

Table 5-5 Systemic Diseases Associated With Dry Eye

Autoimmune disorders
Primary Sjögren syndrome
Secondary Sjögren syndrome associated with
    Rheumatoid arthritis
    Systemic lupus erythematosus
    Progressive systemic sclerosis (scleroderma)
    Polymyositis and dermatomyositis
    Primary biliary cirrhosis
Graft-versus-host disease
Immune reactions after radiation to head and neck

Infiltrative processes
Lymphoma
Amyloidosis
Hemochromatosis
Sarcoidosis

Infectious processes
HIV-diffuse infiltrative lymphadenopathy syndrome
Trachoma

Neuropathic dysfunction
Multiple sclerosis
Cranial neuropathies (Bell palsy, vasculitis)

Endocrine dysfunction
Androgen deficiency

Table 5-6 Recommended Treatment for Dry Eye

Severity	Therapeutic Options
Mild	Artificial tears with preservatives up to 4× daily Lubricating ointment at bedtime Hot compresses and eyelid massage
Moderate	Artificial tears without preservatives 4× daily to hourly Lubricating ointment at bedtime Reversible occlusion, lower puncta (plugs)
Severe	All of the above Punctal occlusion (lower and upper) Topical cyclosporine 0.05% (Restasis) Topical steroids (nonpreserved if available) Moist environment (humidifier, moisture shields) Tarsorrhaphy Bandage lenses (rarely)

process. Demulcents alone, however, cannot restore lost glycoproteins or conjunctival goblet cells, reduce corneal cell desquamation, or decrease osmolarity. Until relatively recently, all demulcent solutions contained preservatives. Preservative-free demulcent solutions were introduced after it was recognized that preservatives increased corneal desquamation. The elimination of preservatives from traditional demulcent solutions has led to improved corneal barrier function, and subsequent attempts have been made to improve the effect of preservative-free solutions on corneal barrier function by adding various ions to the solutions.

Topical cyclosporine A has been approved as a treatment for the inflammatory component of dry eye. Modulation of the inflammatory response might reduce destruction of lacrimal acini and increase neural responsiveness, thereby improving lacrimal secretion. Short courses of topical steroids such as methylprednisolone 1% have been used off label to interrupt the inflammatory cycle in dry eye patients. Other treatments that have been successfully used in the treatment of severe dry eye are dilute solutions of hyaluronic acid and autologous serum drops (both require special formulation). Pharmacologic stimulation of tear secretion has been attempted with many compounds, with varying degrees of success. Oral pilocarpine and cevimeline (Evoxac) have been shown to be effective in treating both xerostomia and dry eye in patients with Sjögren syndrome.

Treatment of filamentary keratopathy, which sometimes accompanies severe dry eye conditions, is best directed at controlling the underlying condition, particularly if ATD is responsible. Acetylcysteine 10%, dispensed in an eyedrop container, can be used as a mucolytic agent and is helpful in alleviating these symptoms. Wearing goggles, shields, or moisture bubbles can decrease the evaporation of tears, although these strategies are generally unacceptable to the patient. The surface area available for evaporation can also be decreased simply by fitting the patient with spectacles, which can be further augmented with plastic side shields. Soft contact lenses are used with a high degree of risk in dry eye patients, although gas-permeable lenses are frequently well tolerated. Scleral contact lenses may also be helpful in patients with severe dry eye symptoms.

A subgroup of patients with dry eye disorders also have glaucoma, and certain topical glaucoma medications can decrease conjunctival goblet cell density. The noncardioselective beta blockers (eg, timolol and levobunolol) have been associated with an increased incidence of systemic and ocular side effects including dry eye. Corneal sensitivity may decrease with the use of these topical agents. Oral administration of drugs such as carbonic anhydrase inhibitors such as acetazolamide and methazolamide can decrease tear production. See also BCSC Section 10, *Glaucoma*.

Many systemic medications—including diuretics, antihistamines, anticholinergics, and psychotropics—decrease aqueous tear production and increase dry eye symptoms. These drugs should be avoided as much as possible in patients with symptoms of ATD (see Table 5-3).

SURGICAL MANAGEMENT Surgical treatment is generally reserved for patients with severe disease for whom medical treatment is either inadequate or impractical. Patients with moderate to severe dry eyes may be helped by punctal occlusion. Tear drainage may be decreased with either temporary or permanent punctal occlusion. Temporary punctal occlusion can be performed in a number of ways, with varying degrees of effectiveness, using collagen implants or silicone punctal plugs (Fig 5-8). Collagen plugs usually dissolve within days and do not cause complete canalicular occlusion. Temporary occlusion can be used as a trial measure before permanent punctal occlusion. Punctal plugs are available in a variety of sizes and shapes for ease of insertion and removal. Instruments that assist in proper sizing of the punctal opening are commercially available. Overdilation of the puncta should be avoided. Silicone plugs will generally remain in place for months to

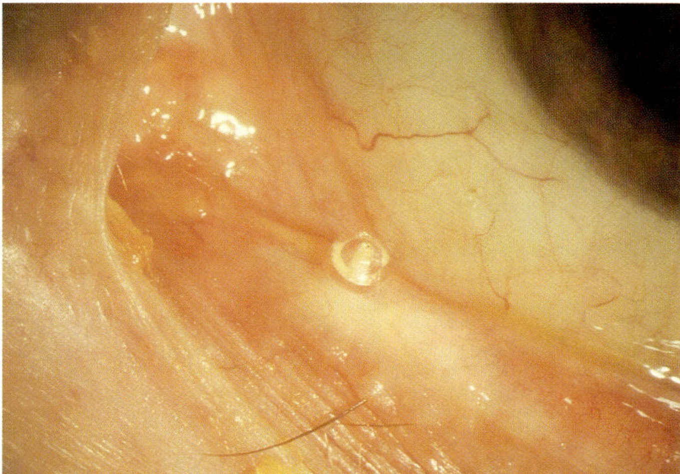

Figure 5-8 Nonabsorbable punctal plug. *(Photograph courtesy of Vincent P. deLuise, MD.)*

years unless they are loosely fit or manually displaced. Most silicone plugs are continuously visible at the slit lamp, making it obvious if they become displaced. One disadvantage of punctal plugs is that they can be inadvertently inserted into the nasolacrimal system and require surgical removal. One type of plug is designed for intracanalicular placement. If the plug protrudes from the punctum, conjunctival abrasions may occur. Granuloma formation at the punctal opening has been observed and requires removal of the plug.

When patients have successfully tolerated temporary punctal plugs, permanent punctal occlusion can be performed in the most cost-effective manner with either a hyfrecator tip or disposable cautery (Fig 5-9). The value of punctal occlusion for ocular surface disease other than dry eye is unproved. This procedure is recommended primarily for those patients in whom basal tear secretion is minimal and those with punctate keratopathy and without significant ocular surface inflammation, especially in elderly patients, in whom the risk of iatrogenically induced epiphora is minimal. Correction of eyelid malpositions such as entropion and ectropion may also be useful in managing patients with dry eye. Lateral and medial tarsorrhaphy can be performed in severe KCS when more conservative measures have failed.

Mucin Tear Deficiency

Systemic vitamin A deficiency is the most common cause of mucin deficiency worldwide. Conditions associated with goblet cell dysfunction can also cause mucin deficiency, including severe dry eye, chemical burns, cicatricial pemphigoid, Stevens-Johnson syndrome, and trachoma. Signs indicative of mucin deficiency include increased tear breakup time, which is also indicative of lipid tear deficiency, as well as conjunctival and eyelid changes associated with cicatricial conditions. The treatment of patients with mucin or lipid (see below) deficiency requires controlling the underlying condition. The measures described above for treatment of aqueous tear deficiency are also employed.

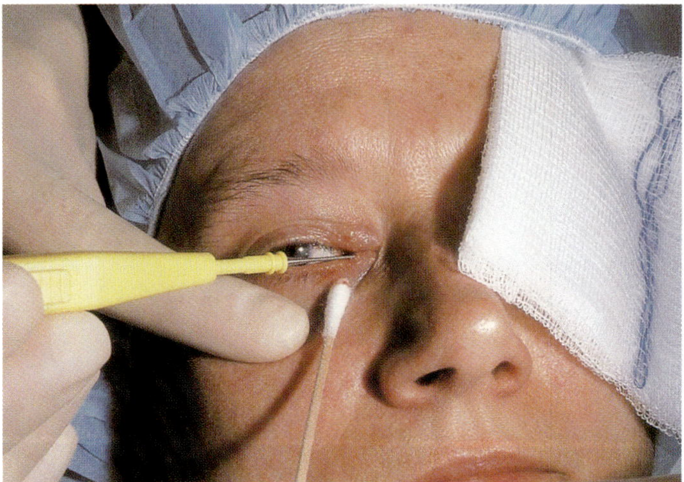

Figure 5-9 Cautery of punctum.

Lipid Tear Deficiency

Lipid tear deficiency states can be manifested by increased tear breakup time, meibomian gland dysfunction, abnormal aqueous tear production, and a characteristic linear pattern of rose bengal staining of the inferior conjunctiva and/or cornea. Conditions that cause MGD, such as rosacea or therapy with oral isotretinoin, can also lead to abnormalities of the lipid layer.

Lemp MA. Report of the National Eye Institute/Industry Workshop on Clinical Trials in Dry Eye. *CLAO J.* 1995;21:221–232.

Pflugfelder SC, Solomon A, Stern ME. The diagnosis and management of dry eye: a twenty-five-year review. *Cornea.* 2000;19:644–649.

Pflugfelder SC, Whitcher JP, Daniels TG. Sjögren syndrome. In: Pepose JS, Holland GN, Wilhelmus KR, eds. *Ocular Infection and Immunity.* St Louis: Mosby; 1996:313–333.

Preferred Practice Patterns Committee, Cornea Panel. *Blepharitis.* San Francisco: American Academy of Ophthalmology; 1998.

Preferred Practice Patterns Committee, Cornea Panel. *Dry Eye Syndrome.* San Francisco: American Academy of Ophthalmology; 1998.

Vitali C, Bombardieri S, Moutsopoulos HM, et al. Preliminary criteria for the classification of Sjögren's syndrome. Results of a prospective concerted action supported by the European community. *Arthritis Rheum.* 1993;36:340–347.

Nutritional and Physiologic Disorders

Vitamin A Deficiency

PATHOGENESIS Vitamin A is an essential fat-soluble vitamin. Human disease can be caused by too little or too much vitamin A intake. Table 5-7 presents an overview of vitamin A metabolism.

Table 5-7 Metabolism of Vitamin A

Level	Metabolite
Diet	Plant (carotenoids) and animal (retinyl-palmitate and retinol) foods
Intestine	Retinol-micelle
Portal circulation	Retinyl-palmitate
Liver	Retinol–retinol-binding protein
Target tissues	Retinoic acid (epithelium, epidermis, and lymphocytes)
	Retinal (rod photoreceptors)

Vitamin A deficiency xerosis, associated with loss of mucus production by the goblet cells, can occur in epithelial cells of the gastrointestinal, genitourinary, and respiratory tracts. The ocular consequence is the *Bitôt spot*, a superficial foamy, gray triangular area on the bulbar conjunctiva that appears in the palpebral aperture (Fig 5-10). This spot consists of keratinized epithelium, inflammatory cells, debris, and *Corynebacterium xerosis*. These bacilli metabolize the debris and produce the foamy appearance.

Vitamin A deficiency leads to *xerophthalmia*, which is responsible for at least 20,000–100,000 new cases of blindness worldwide each year. At greatest risk of xerophthalmia are malnourished infants and babies born to vitamin A–deficient mothers, especially infants who have another biological stress such as measles or diarrhea. Superficial concurrent infections with herpes simplex, measles, or bacterial agents probably further predispose the child to keratomalacia and blindness. Although xerophthalmia usually results from low dietary intake of vitamin A, decreased absorption of vitamin A may also be responsible. When vitamin A deficiency and xerophthalmia occur in countries with a low rate of malnutrition, the condition is usually caused by unusual self-imposed dietary practices, chronic alcoholism, or lipid malabsorption (particularly cystic fibrosis, biliary cirrhosis, and bowel resection).

CLINICAL PRESENTATION *Nyctalopia* (night blindness) is often the earliest symptom of hypovitaminosis A, but retinal function does not always correlate with anterior segment findings. *Xerophthalmic fundus,* a rare associated abnormality, features yellow-white spots in the peripheral retina.

Prolonged vitamin A deficiency leads to involvement of the external eye, including xerosis (dryness of the conjunctiva and cornea), metaplastic keratinization of areas of the conjunctiva (Bitôt spots), corneal ulcers and scars, and eventually diffuse corneal necrosis (keratomalacia). The World Health Organization classifies the ocular surface changes into three stages:

- Conjunctival xerosis, without (X1A) or with (X1B) Bitôt spots
- Corneal xerosis (X2)
- Corneal ulceration, with keratomalacia involving less than one third (X3A) or more than one third (X3B) of the corneal surface

Patients with chronic alcoholism may present with persistent epithelial defect and corneal ulceration unresponsive to antimicrobial therapy. Night blindness with an ab-

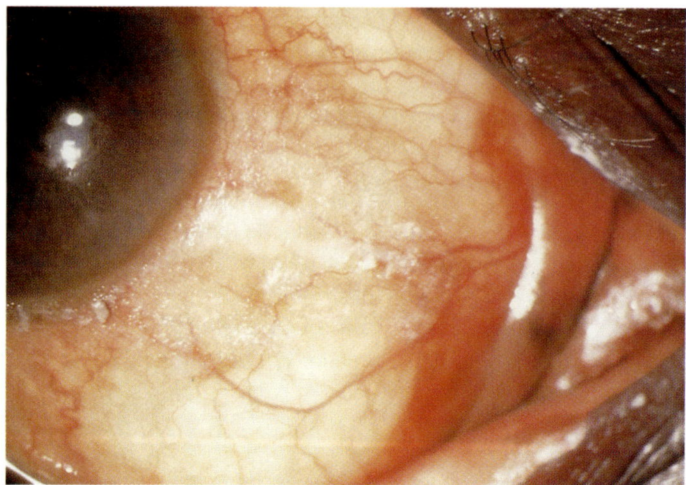

Figure 5-10 Conjunctival xerosis with focal keratinization (Bitôt spot) as a result of vitamin A deficiency. *(Photograph courtesy of Vincent P. deLuise, MD.)*

normal electroretinogram and conjunctival xerosis or Bitôt spots may be the presenting manifestation of the chronic malabsorption syndromes mentioned above. Laboratory diagnosis of low serum level of vitamin A or retinol-binding proteins is usually used to confirm the clinical suspicion.

MANAGEMENT Systemic vitamin A deficiency, best characterized by keratomalacia, is a medical emergency with an untreated mortality rate of 50%. While the administration of oral or parenteral vitamin A will address the acute manifestations of keratomalacia, these patients are usually affected by a much larger protein-energy malnutrition and should be treated with both vitamin and protein-calorie supplements. Problems with malabsorption may prevent oral administration from being effective in patients with acute vitamin A deficiency. Maintenance of adequate corneal lubrication and prevention of secondary infection and corneal melting are essential steps in treating keratomalacia, but identification and proper treatment of the underlying causes are vital to successful clinical management of the ocular complications.

As a result of the beneficial effects of systemic retinoids in xerophthalmia, studies were undertaken to determine if topical retinoids would be useful in reversing the squamous metaplasia and symptoms associated with dry eye syndromes. Although double-blind, placebo-controlled studies failed to demonstrate the efficacy of topical therapy for patients with dry eye alone, subsequent studies revealed that topical retinoids were primarily useful in conditions with conjunctival keratinization, such as Stevens-Johnson syndrome, cicatricial pemphigoid, radiation-induced dry eye, drug-induced pseudopemphigoid, and toxic epidermal necrolysis. Currently, an effective ophthalmic preparation of topical retinoids is not readily available for general clinical use.

Harris EW, Loewenstein JI, Azar D. Vitamin A deficiency and its effects on the eye. *Int Ophthalmol Clin.* 1998;38:155–162.

Sommer A, West KP. *Vitamin A Deficiency: Health, Survival, and Vision.* New York: Oxford University Press; 1996.

Vitamin C Deficiency

Ascorbic acid, or vitamin C, is an essential vitamin for humans because we lack its synthetic enzyme, L-gulonolactone oxidase. A major action mechanism of ascorbic acid is its effect as a cofactor on the hydroxylation of lysine and proline in ribosomal collagen synthesis. Impairment of hydroxylation secondary to ascorbic acid deficiency results in unstable collagen fiber formation.

Following transport through the ciliary epithelium, ascorbic acid is about 15–20 times more concentrated in aqueous humor than in plasma. In scurvy, subconjunctival and orbital hemorrhage may occur. In a vitamin C–deprivation trial extending over approximately 3 months, some subjects developed xerosis. In animal studies, scorbutic guinea pig corneas subjected to injury showed impaired wound healing. Animal studies also suggest that the alkali-burned cornea represents a localized scorbutic state in which adequate collagen cannot be synthesized for stromal wound repair. In rabbit eyes, topical and subcutaneous ascorbate can restore the ascorbate level in aqueous humor after an alkali burn and significantly reduce the incidence of corneal ulcer and perforation.

Neurotrophic Keratopathy

PATHOGENESIS Neurotrophic keratopathy results from damage to cranial nerve V, causing corneal hypoesthesia or anesthesia. This damage may be caused by surgical trauma (ablation of the trigeminal ganglion), cerebrovascular accidents, aneurysms, multiple sclerosis, tumors (such as neurofibroma or angioma), herpes zoster ophthalmicus, herpes simplex keratitis, Hansen disease (leprosy), or topical anesthetic abuse. Hereditary causes include hereditary sensory neuropathy and familial dysautonomia (Riley-Day syndrome), both of which are autosomal recessive disorders.

A recently reported animal model demonstrated that tear film osmolarity increased following corneal denervation. This study showed that, in addition to the ocular surface findings associated with ATD as a result of depressed tearing reflex, an additional mechanism for corneal disease was at work, related to the trophic influence of cranial nerve V.

CLINICAL PRESENTATION Neurotrophic keratopathy generally involves the central or inferior paracentral cornea as a result of corneal denervation or damage to cranial nerve V. *Herpes zoster ophthalmicus* can lead to a severe neurotrophic keratopathy. A patient showing other signs of herpes zoster ophthalmicus should undergo an assessment of corneal sensation in order to determine the relative level of risk. Corneal sensation may return to some extent during healing but usually remains permanently depressed. Neurotrophic keratopathy resulting from herpes simplex keratitis can result in persistent epithelial defects in the absence of replicating virus or active corneal inflammation. These epithelial defects stain intensely with fluorescein and are surrounded by raised, rolled-up gray edges (Fig 5-11). Progressive sterile ulceration or superinfection can result in perforation and loss of the eye.

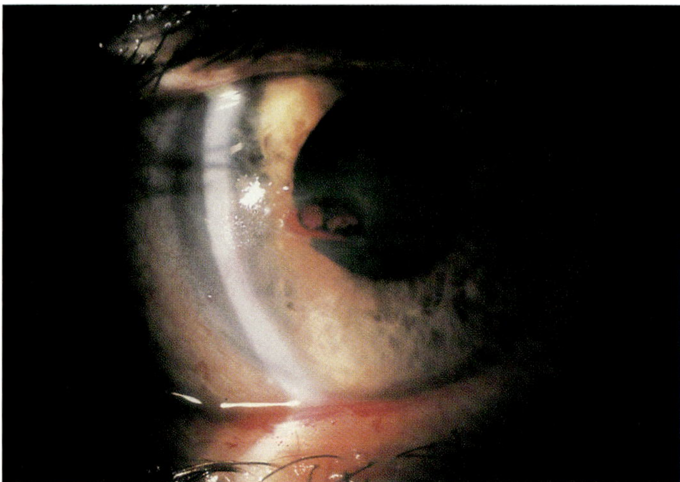

Figure 5-11 Neurotrophic ulcer.

In *hereditary sensory neuropathy* there is a reduction in small myelinated nerve fibers. This condition can lead to dramatic, persistent, nonhealing epithelial defects in infants in association with other defects of sensory nerves. In *familial dysautonomia (Riley-Day syndrome)*, patients usually present with emotional instability, skin blotching, transient but marked hypertension, excessive sweating and salivation, insensitivity to pain, failure to thrive, postural hypotension, and recurrent respiratory tract infection. Constantly diminished tear production while crying and corneal hypoesthesia are the most consistent ophthalmic findings. The autonomic dysfunction affects tear production by the lacrimal gland and leads to secondary conjunctival xerosis. Affected individuals frequently develop keratitis ranging in severity from mild punctate stippling of the lower portion of the corneal epithelium to frank neurotrophic ulcerations. This condition is seen predominantly but not exclusively in Jewish families of eastern European origin (Ashkenazi).

MANAGEMENT Management of neurotrophic keratopathy includes treatment of the underlying disease and use of the full spectrum of approaches outlined earlier for dry eye and below for exposure keratopathy. It is particularly important to choose ointments or eyedrops without potentially toxic preservatives such as benzalkonium chloride (BAK) for patients with neurotrophic keratopathy. Management of toxic ulcerative keratopathy includes discontinuation of the offending agent, patching, and the use of nonpreserved medications. Rarely, therapeutic contact lenses or collagen shields are used.

Lateral and/or medial tarsorrhaphy is frequently required in order to prevent surface desiccation. Tarsorrhaphy decreases tear film evaporation and tear film osmolarity. Presumably, reducing the surface area of corneal exposure accounts for the efficacy of tarsorrhaphy. Penetrating keratoplasty, although generally hazardous in cases of neurotrophic keratopathy, has recently been used with increasing success in patients with residual scarring from clinically inactive herpes zoster keratopathy. Concomitant lateral tarsorrhaphy and punctal occlusion appear to improve the long-term survival of the corneal graft. Surgical fixation of preserved amniotic membrane has been reported to encourage healing of persistent epithelial ulcerations. Partial or total conjunctival flaps will prevent corneal melting, but they should be used as a last resort in order to preserve the eye.

A recent small clinical trial evaluating the efficacy of topical nerve growth factor on chronic epithelial ulcerations demonstrated improved healing. This therapy is not currently available.

> Donaghy M, Hakin RN, Bamford JM, et al. Hereditary sensory neuropathy with neurotrophic keratitis. Description of an autosomal recessive disorder with a selective reduction of small myelinated nerve fibers and a discussion of the classification of the hereditary sensory neuropathies. *Brain.* 1987;110:563–583.

Structural and Exogenous Disorders

Exposure Keratopathy

PATHOGENESIS Exposure keratopathy can result from any disease process that limits eyelid closure. Lagophthalmos can be caused by the following:

- Neurogenic diseases such as seventh nerve palsy
- Degenerative neurologic conditions such as Parkinson disease
- Cicatricial or restrictive eyelid diseases such as ectropion
- Drug abuse
- Blepharoplasty
- Skin disorders such as Stevens-Johnson syndrome or xeroderma pigmentosum

Proptosis caused by thyroid orbitopathy or other inflammatory or infiltrative orbital diseases can also result in exposure keratopathy.

CLINICAL PRESENTATION Exposure keratopathy is characterized by a punctate epithelial keratopathy that usually involves the inferior third of the cornea, although the entire corneal surface can be involved in more severe cases. Large, coalescent epithelial defects may result, which may lead to ulceration, melting, and perforation. Symptoms are similar to those associated with dry eye, including foreign body sensation, photophobia, and tearing, unless there is an associated neurotrophic component resulting in corneal anesthesia.

MANAGEMENT Therapy is similar to that described for severe dry eye. In the earliest stages, nonpreserved artificial tears during the day and ointment at bedtime may suffice. Taping the eyelid shut at bedtime can be helpful if the problem is primarily one of nocturnal exposure. The use of bandage contact lenses can be hazardous in these patients because of a high incidence of desiccation and infection. In cases in which the problem is likely to be temporary or self-limited, a temporary tarsorrhaphy using tissue adhesive or sutures should be performed. However, if the problem is likely to be long-standing, definitive surgical therapy to correct the eyelid position is mandated. Correction of any associated eyelid abnormalities, such as ectropion and/or trichiasis, is also indicated.

Most commonly, surgical management consists of permanent lateral and/or medial tarsorrhaphy. Insertion of gold weights into the upper eyelid is also an effective technique to promote eyelid closure. Implantation of a gold weight does not alter the dimension of the horizontal eyelid fissure and thus creates a less obvious cosmetic change than does a lateral tarsorrhaphy. Reported complications of gold weight implants include infection, shifting, extrusion, induced astigmatism, unacceptable ptosis, and noninfectious inflammatory response to the gold. The weights remain stable when exposed to MRI. In cases of paralytic ectropion of the lower eyelid, a horizontal tightening procedure may also be beneficial in correcting the flaccid lower eyelid.

See BCSC Section 7, *Orbit, Eyelids, and Lacrimal System,* for further discussion of lagophthalmos and proptosis.

Donzis PB, Mondino BJ. Management of noninfectious corneal ulcers. *Surv Ophthalmol.* 1987;32:94–110.

Floppy Eyelid Syndrome

This syndrome of chronic ocular irritation and inflammation typically occurs in obese individuals. Patients have a flimsy, lax upper tarsus that everts with minimal upward force applied to the upper eyelid. Clinical findings include small to large papillae on the upper palpebral conjunctiva, mucous discharge, and corneal involvement ranging from mild punctate epitheliopathy to superficial vascularization (Fig 5-12). Keratoconus has also been reported in patients with floppy eyelid syndrome. The problem may result from spontaneous eversion of the upper eyelid when it comes into contact with the pillow or other bedclothes during sleep. Direct contact of the upper eyelid with bed linens may traumatize the upper tarsal conjunctiva and induce inflammation and chronic irritation. The condition may be unilateral if the patient always sleeps in the same position. Treatment consists of covering the affected eye(s) with a metal shield or taping eyelids closed at night or performing surgical eyelid-tightening procedures. Differential diagnosis includes vernal conjunctivitis, giant papillary conjunctivitis, atopic keratoconjunctivitis,

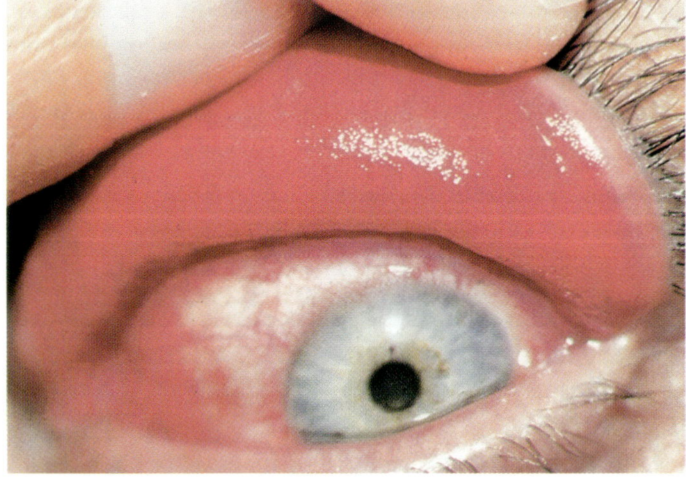

Figure 5-12 Floppy eyelid syndrome with papillary response on superior tarsus. *(Photograph courtesy of Vincent P. deLuise, MD.)*

bacterial conjunctivitis, and toxic keratopathy. See also BCSC Section 7, *Orbit, Eyelids, and Lacrimal System.*

Culbertson WW, Ostler HB. The floppy eyelid syndrome. *Am J Ophthalmol.* 1981;92:568–575.

Superior Limbic Keratoconjunctivitis (SLK)

PATHOGENESIS The pathogenesis of superior limbic keratoconjunctivitis has not been established, although it is thought to result from mechanical trauma transmitted from the upper eyelid to the superior bulbar and tarsal conjunctiva. Some patients have a history of thyroid dysfunction, and associated bulbar conjunctival edema may increase friction between the superior eyelid and the globe.

CLINICAL PRESENTATION SLK is a chronic, recurrent condition of ocular irritation and redness. The condition typically develops in adult women 20–70 years of age. SLK may recur over a period of 1–10 years. The condition usually resolves spontaneously. It is often bilateral, although one eye may be more severely affected than the other. SLK can be associated with aqueous tear deficiency or blepharospasm. Ocular findings may include the following:

- A fine papillary reaction on the superior tarsal conjunctiva
- Injection and thickening of the superior bulbar conjunctiva (Fig 5-13)
- Hypertrophy of the superior limbus
- Fine punctate fluorescein and rose bengal staining of the superior bulbar conjunctiva above the limbus and superior cornea just below the limbus (Fig 5-14)
- Superior corneal filamentary keratopathy

LABORATORY EVALUATION Hyperproliferation, acanthosis, loss of goblet cells, and keratinization are seen in histologic sections of the superior bulbar conjunctiva. The condition can often be diagnosed by clinical signs; however, scrapings or impression cytology of

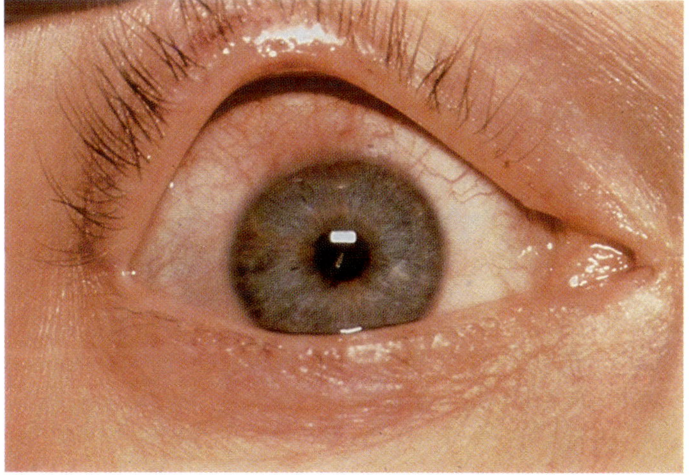

Figure 5-13 Superior limbic keratoconjunctivitis. *(Photograph courtesy of Vincent P. deLuise, MD.)*

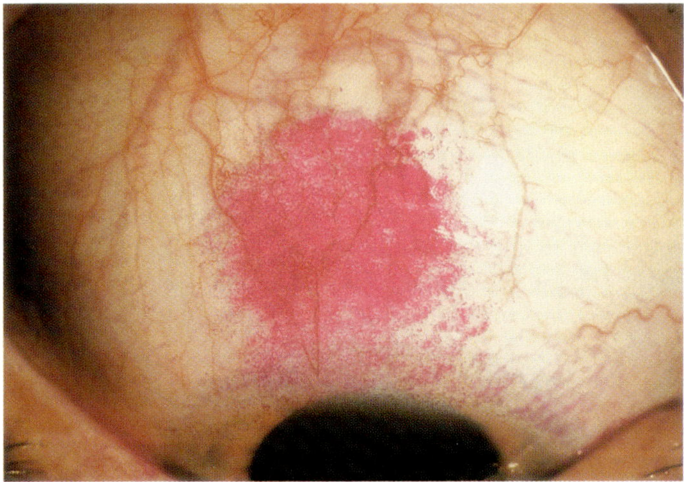

Figure 5-14 Rose bengal dye staining pattern in superior limbic keratoconjunctivitis. *(Photograph courtesy of Vincent P. deLuise, MD.)*

the superior bulbar conjunctiva showing characteristic features of nuclear pyknosis with "snake nuclei," increased epithelial cytoplasm-to-nucleus ratio, loss of goblet cells, and keratinization may be helpful in diagnosing mild or confusing cases. Patients with SLK should have thyroid function tests including T_4, TSH, and antithyroid antibody levels.

MANAGEMENT A variety of therapies have been reported to provide temporary or permanent relief of symptoms. Treatments include chemical cauterization of superior bulbar conjunctiva and superior tarsal conjunctiva with 0.5%–1.0% silver nitrate solution (silver nitrate solution in wax ampoules, not silver nitrate cauterization sticks), large-diameter bandage contact lenses, topical vitamin A ointment (0.1% transretinoic acid), superior punctal occlusion, thermocauterization of the superior bulbar conjunctiva, and resection of the bulbar conjunctiva superior to the limbus.

Theodore FH, Ferry AP. Superior limbic keratoconjunctivitis. Clinical and pathological correlations. *Arch Ophthalmol.* 1970;84:481–484.

Yang HY, Fujishima H, Toda I, et al. Lacrimal punctal occlusion for the treatment of superior limbic keratoconjunctivitis. *Am J Ophthalmol.* 1997;124:80–87.

Recurrent Corneal Erosion

PATHOGENESIS Recurrent erosions typically occur in eyes that have suffered either a sudden, sharp, abrading injury (fingernail, paper cut, tree branch) or in patients with preexisting epithelial basement membrane dystrophy. The superficial injury produces an epithelial abrasion that heals rapidly, frequently leaving no clinical evidence of damage. Some patients even fail to recall the original injury. After an interval varying from days to years, symptoms suddenly recur without any obvious precipitating event. Symptoms subside spontaneously in most cases, only to recur periodically. In contrast to shearing injuries, small superficial lacerating injuries involving the cornea rarely result in recurrent erosions. Poor adhesion of the epithelium is thought to be caused by underlying abnormalities in the epithelial basement membrane and its associated filament network. The precise nature of these abnormalities has yet to be fully elucidated.

Recent reports have observed that gelatinase activity (MMP-2 and -9) was up-regulated in epithelial specimens in patients with recurrent corneal erosions. Gelatinases alter the epithelial basement membrane during wound healing by cleaving collagen types IV, V, VII, and X. They also act on the adhesive macromolecules fibronectin and laminin that are thought to mediate attachment of the basal epithelial cells to the basement membrane. Activation of MMPs on a chronic basis may either be a result of, or the cause of, poor epithelial adherence that leads to the symptoms of recurrent corneal erosion. Some patients with recurrent corneal erosions have been noted to have meibomian gland dysfunction, and increased levels of MMPs have been observed in the tear film of patients with MGD.

CLINICAL PRESENTATION Recurrent corneal erosions are characterized by the sudden onset of eye pain, usually at night or upon first awakening, accompanied by redness, photophobia, and tearing. Individual episodes may vary in severity and duration. Minor episodes usually last from 30 minutes to several hours and typically have an intact epithelial surface at the time of examination. More severe episodes may last for several days and are often associated with greater pain, eyelid edema, decreased visual acuity, and extreme photophobia. Minor episodes resolve rapidly; often, when the patient is examined within hours of an acute recurrence, no abnormality is discernible on slit-lamp examination. Many patients seem to suffer from ocular discomfort that is out of proportion to the amount of observable pathology. However, slit-lamp examination using retroillumination can frequently reveal subtle corneal abnormalities. The corneal epithelium is loosely attached to the underlying basement membrane and Bowman's layer, both at the time of a recurrent attack and between attacks when the cornea appears to be entirely healed. During the acute attack, the epithelium in the involved area frequently appears heaped up and edematous. While no frank epithelial defect may be present, significant pooling of fluorescein over the affected area is often visible.

LABORATORY EVALUATION The key to making the distinction between a posttraumatic erosion and a dystrophic erosion in a patient who has no clear-cut history of superficial trauma lies in careful examination of the contralateral eye following maximal pupillary dilation. Occasionally, subtle areas of loosely adherent epithelium can be identified by gentle pressure with a surgical sponge following the instillation of topical anesthetics. The presence of basement membrane changes in the *unaffected* eye implicates a primary basement membrane defect in the pathogenesis, while the absence of such findings strongly suggests a posttraumatic etiology. Other clinical conditions with associated abnormalities of the epithelial basement membrane include diabetes mellitus and dystrophies of the stroma and Bowman's layer (see also Chapter 15 on corneal dystrophies).

MANAGEMENT Conservative therapy for this condition in the acute phase consists of frequent lubrication with antibiotic ointments and cycloplegia, followed by use of nonpreserved lubricants or hypertonic saline solution (5% NaCl) during the day and ointment at bedtime for 6–12 months to promote proper epithelial attachment. Hypertonic agents provide lubrication and may transiently produce an osmotic gradient, drawing fluid from the epithelium and theoretically promoting the adherence of epithelial cells to the underlying tissue. Some patients find hypertonic medications unacceptably irritating, although many others do quite well with this therapy indefinitely. Theoretically, systemic tetracyclines and topical steroids could be of some benefit by reducing MMP production.

Although use of a therapeutic bandage contact lens may be helpful, proper patient education and judicious monitoring are crucial. The ideal therapeutic lens should have a flat base curve and high oxygen transmissibility (Dk). New-generation soft contact lenses with surface treatments that decrease bacterial adherence may offer a better safety profile. Concomitant use of a topical broad-spectrum antibiotic four times daily may reduce the possibility of secondary infection. Application of preservative-free topical ketorolac four times daily may improve patient comfort in the first 24 hours. Occasionally, judicious use of topical corticosteroids is necessary to treat associated secondary keratitis or uveitis.

It is best to approach the management of patients with recalcitrant disease using a stepwise sequence of interventions. When consistent conservative management fails to control the symptoms, more invasive surgical therapy may be indicated. In patients with posttraumatic recurrent erosions, *anterior stromal micropuncture* can be very effective (Fig 5-15). Using a specially designed bent 25-gauge needle, the clinician makes numerous superficial puncture wounds in the involved area, producing a firm adhesion between the epithelium and the underlying stroma. This procedure should be used with caution in the visual axis. Rarely is a significant scar visible for more than a few months after this procedure. The treatment may need to be repeated in patients who were at first adequately controlled but later become symptomatic, usually because the area of treatment was inadequate. Histologic studies have revealed that the lesions produced by this procedure create subepithelial scars. Use of diathermy to create similar lesions in experimental animals has shown that the efficacy of these procedures is related to their ability to stimulate the formation of new basement membrane complexes.

In patients with dystrophic, degenerative, or other severe secondary basement membrane disorder–related recurrent erosions, the procedure of choice is *epithelial debridement,* which can easily be performed at the slit lamp. Following adequate application of topical anesthetic, loosely adherent epithelium is debrided using a surgical sponge, a spatula, or a surgical blade. Care must be taken not to damage the underlying Bowman's layer. Light application of an ophthalmic diamond burr to Bowman's layer in the affected area (outside the visual axis) may be effective in reducing recurrences in resistant cases.

Because a significant amount of discomfort can be expected for 3–4 days following this procedure, the patient will likely be more tolerant if debridement is performed at the time of a painful recurrent episode. Topical antibiotic ointment, cycloplegia, and, in some cases, bandage contact lenses are used until reepithelialization is complete. Oral analgesics are often necessary in the first 24 hours.

Excimer laser phototherapeutic keratectomy has recently emerged as an alternative modality for the treatment of patients with recalcitrant recurrent erosions, particularly the dystrophic variant. By creating a large, shallow zone of ablation, this procedure can minimize the refractive effects, or it can be used to correct an associated myopic refractive

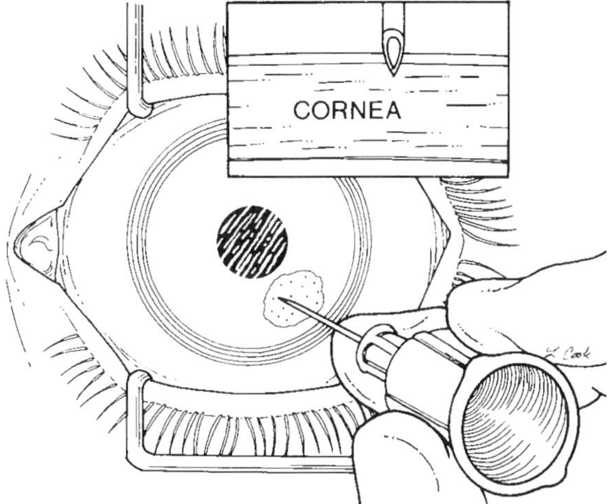

Figure 5-15 Anterior stromal puncture. The needle is used to encourage microcicatrization between epithelium, Bowman's layer, and stroma. *(Reproduced with permission from Kenyon KR, Wagoner MD. Therapy of recurrent erosion and persistent defects of the corneal epithelium. In:* Focal Points: Clinical Modules for Ophthalmologists. *San Francisco: American Academy of Ophthalmology; 1991: vol 9, no 9. Illustration by Laurel Cook.)*

error as well. The mechanism of action of this procedure for this condition has yet to be established. (See Part XII for further discussion.)

> Reidy JJ, Paulus MP, Gona S. Recurrent erosions of the cornea: epidemiology and treatment. *Cornea.* 2000;19:767–771.

Persistent Corneal Epithelial Defect

PATHOGENESIS Persistent corneal epithelial defects are generally related to some underlying disease process. Common causes of these defects include

- Herpetic corneal disease
- Delayed postsurgical epithelial healing
- Chemical burns
- Recurrent corneal erosions
- Dry eye syndromes
- Infections
- Neuroparalytic keratopathy
- Anterior segment necrosis

In many cases, the drugs used to treat some of these conditions impair epithelial wound healing and perpetuate the epithelial defect. A study has highlighted the drugs most frequently implicated and the characteristic clinical appearance of the resulting defects. The authors called this condition *toxic ulcerative keratopathy*. It usually occurs secondary to administration of ocular medications and/or their preservatives. This clinical problem, which is commonly encountered and frequently unrecognized, can begin as a diffuse punctate keratopathy. The nonhealing pseudogeographic defects that may result can be misinterpreted as a worsening of the underlying disease and thus may lead to even larger doses of the offending medication. Not infrequently, topical anesthetic abuse has been implicated. Frank ulceration can result as sterile inflammation ensues.

CLINICAL PRESENTATION Persistent corneal epithelial defects are characterized by central or paracentral areas of chronic nonhealing epithelium that resist maximal therapeutic endeavors. They frequently have elevated, rounded edges and may be associated with significant underlying stromal inflammation. Corneal anesthesia is frequently an accompanying sign, and it should always be evaluated. Left untreated, this condition can progress to vascularization and corneal opacification or scarring. Alternatively, progressive inflammation can lead to necrosis and thinning of the stroma, occasionally resulting in perforation.

LABORATORY EVALUATION The diagnosis is based upon careful history taking, paying particular attention to the preservatives present in any ophthalmic medications being administered. The lesions are frequently round or oval epithelial defects with grayish edges that are rolled under without heaped margins. The defects tend to be inferior or inferonasal and can be associated with an intense, coarse superficial keratitis. The inferonasal predilection of these lesions may be a result of the area's easy access and the protective effect of Bell's phenomenon on the superior cornea. Keratoconjunctivitis sicca is a frequently accompanying disease. Other associated conditions include corneal hypoesthesia as a result of previous cataract extraction or keratoplasty and prior herpes zoster or herpes simplex infections.

MANAGEMENT In addition to removing the offending stimulus or aggravating drugs or treating the underlying condition, a number of strategies have been employed in the management of persistent epithelial defects. Pharmacologic therapies have included systemic tetracycline, chosen for its anticollagenolytic effect, unrelated to the drug's antimicrobial properties. Other therapies, including use of nerve growth factor, have met with some success and are under investigation.

Generally, conventional therapies can be effective in promoting closure of the epithelial defect. These include frequent lubrication with nonpreserved ointments and, if necessary, temporary tarsorrhaphy or permanent lateral canthoplasty to encourage epithelial migration and minimize mechanical trauma from exposure and desiccation.

Persistent epithelial defects often occur in patients with diabetic retinopathy following epithelial debridement during vitreoretinal procedures. Diabetic neuropathy is thought to be a potential cause of neurotrophic keratopathy and nonhealing epithelial defects; further, abnormal metabolism of aldose reductase has been implicated in the pathogenesis of persistent epithelial defects in these patients. A clinical trial is currently investigating the efficacy of a topical aldose reductase inhibitor for persistent epithelial defects in patients with diabetes.

For more extensive insults, such as alkali injuries or other causes of devastating ocular surface trauma, damage to limbal stem cells cannot be overcome by conventional conservative therapies. Various strategies using healthy conjunctiva or limbal stem cells have been employed in ocular surface reconstruction with success. (Limbal stem-cell dysfunction is discussed at the end of this chapter; surgery of the ocular surface is covered in Chapters 20–22.)

Cavanagh HD, Pihlaja D, Thoft RA, et al. The pathogenesis and treatment of persistent epithelial defects. *Trans Am Acad Ophthalmol Otolaryngol.* 1976;81:754–769.

Trichiasis and Distichiasis

Trichiasis refers to an acquired condition in which lashes emerging from their normal anterior origin are curved inward toward the cornea. Most cases are probably the result of subtle cicatricial entropion of the eyelid margin. Trichiasis can be idiopathic or secondary to chronic inflammatory conditions.

Distichiasis is a congenital (often autosomal dominant) or acquired condition in which an extra row of lashes emerges from the ducts of meibomian glands. These lashes can be fine and well tolerated or coarser and a threat to corneal integrity.

Aberrant lashes emerge from the tarsus as a result of chronic inflammatory conditions of the eyelids and conjunctiva such as trachoma, ocular cicatricial pemphigoid, Stevens-Johnson syndrome, blepharitis, or chemical burns.

Aberrant lashes and poor eyelid position and movement should be corrected. Aberrant lashes may be removed by epilation, electrolysis, or cryotherapy. Mechanical epilation is temporary because the lashes will normally regrow within 2–3 weeks. Electrolysis works well only for removing a few lashes, although it can be preferred for cosmetic reasons in younger patients. Cryotherapy is still a common treatment for aberrant eyelashes, but freezing can result in eyelid margin thinning, loss of adjacent normal lashes, and persistent lanugo hairs that may continue to abrade the cornea. Treatment at −20°C should be limited to less than 30 seconds to minimize complications. The preferred surgical technique for aberrant eyelashes is a tarsotomy with eyelid margin rotation. For further discussion, see BCSC Section 7, *Orbit, Eyelids, and Lacrimal System.*

Factitious Ocular Surface Disorders

Factitious disorders include a spectrum of self-induced injuries with symptoms or physical findings intentionally produced by the patient in order to assume the sick role. Factitious conjunctivitis usually shows evidence of mechanical injury to the inferior and nasal quadrants of the cornea and conjunctiva. The areas of involvement show sharply delineated borders. Patients often have medical training or work in a medical setting, and they generally show an attitude of serene indifference. The detached conjunctival tissues usually show no evidence of inflammation by pathologic examination. Other types of noncorneal factitious ocular disorders include self-induced solar retinopathy, eyelid ulceration, and anisocoria.

Mucus-fishing syndrome

This condition is characterized by a well-circumscribed pattern of rose bengal or lissamine green staining on the nasal and inferior bulbar conjunctiva. All patients have a history of increased mucus production as a nonspecific response to ocular surface damage. The inciting event is typically keratoconjunctivitis sicca. Patients usually demonstrate vigorous eye rubbing and compulsive removal of the mucus strands from the fornix (mucus fishing). The resultant epithelial injury heightens the ocular surface irritation which, in turn, stimulates additional mucus production resulting in a vicious cycle.

Topical anesthetic abuse

Clinical application of topical anesthetics has become an integral part of the modern practice of ophthalmology. However, indiscriminate use of topical anesthetics can cause serious ocular surface toxicity and complications. Local anesthetics are known to inhibit epithelial migration and division. Loss of microvilli, reduction of desmosomes and other intercellular contacts, and swelling of mitochondria and lysosomes have been reported in ultrastructural studies. The clinical features of anesthetic abuse are characterized by the failure of the presenting condition, such as corneal abrasions or infectious keratitis, to respond to appropriate therapy.

Initially, a punctate keratopathy is seen. As the abuse continues, the eye becomes more injected and epithelial defects appear or take on a neurotrophic appearance. As the process goes on, keratic precipitates and hypopyon develop, thus mimicking an infectious course. Diffuse stromal edema, dense stromal infiltrates, and a large ring opacity are common presenting signs (Fig 5-16). Stromal vascularization may take place in chronic abuse, and secondary infection may ensue. Because of the presence of corneal infiltrates and anterior segment inflammation, infectious keratitis must be ruled out through corneal scraping, culture, or biopsy.

Differential diagnosis includes bacterial, fungal, herpetic, and amebic keratitis. Suspicion should be maintained in the face of negative cultures in any patient who is not responding to appropriate therapy. Many times the diagnosis is made only when the patient is discovered concealing the anesthetic drops. Once the diagnosis is made and infectious keratitis is ruled out, corneal healing usually occurs if all exposure to anesthetics is removed. In advanced cases permanent corneal scarring or perforation may occur. Occasionally, anesthetic abuse may continue after surgery. Psychiatric counseling is sometimes helpful.

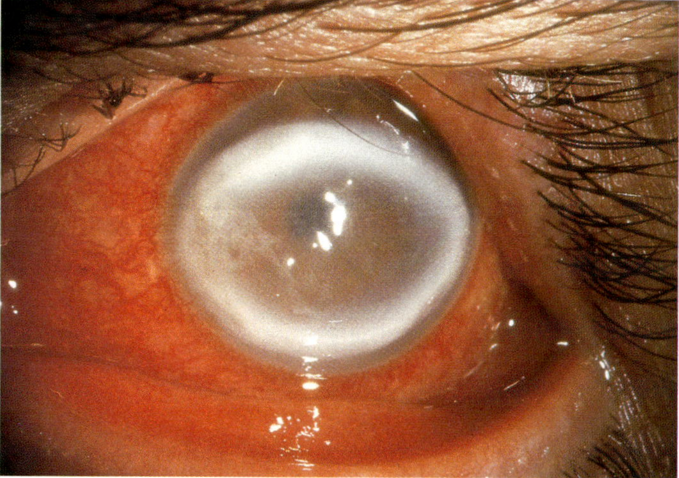

Figure 5-16 Topical anesthetic overuse with persistent corneal epithelial defect and necrotic ring opacity. *(Photograph courtesy of Kirk R. Wilhelmus, MD.)*

Dellen

Desiccation of the epithelium and subepithelial tissues occurs at or near the limbus adjacent to surface elevations such as those produced by pterygia, large filtration blebs, or dermoids. Because the tear film is interrupted by these surface elevations, normal blinking does not wet the involved area properly. Clinically, dellen are saucer-like depressions in the corneal surface. The epithelium exhibits punctate irregularities overlying a thinned area of dehydrated corneal stroma. Treatment with frequent ocular lubrication or pressure patching will accelerate the healing process and restore stromal hydration.

The orbital and conjunctival tissues surrounding the sclera also play a role in maintaining scleral hydration. This function becomes especially evident during surgical procedures, when the conjunctiva and extraocular muscles are removed from the scleral surface. The exposed sclera becomes thinner and partially translucent unless it is continually remoistened. Removal of the perilimbal conjunctiva and interference with the wetting effect of the tear film (as after excision of a pterygium by the bare sclera technique) can cause the underlying sclera to become markedly thinned and translucent, forming a scleral delle.

Ocular Surface Problems Secondary to Contact Lens Wear

Metabolic epithelial damage

Contact lens overwear syndromes can be manifested in several forms. Central epithelial edema (Sattler's veil) is found after many hours of wear, more commonly with hard contact lenses. This epithelial edema causes blurred vision that may persist for many hours or even progress to acute epithelial necrosis. Although acute epithelial necrosis is rarely seen, central epithelial edema can create epithelial erosions or frank ulceration. Physiologic stress as a result of hypoxia with lactate accumulation and impaired carbon dioxide efflux is responsible for these complications.

Microcystic epitheliopathy, another condition caused by impaired metabolic activities in epithelium, shows fine epithelial cysts best seen with retroillumination. This condition has been observed most commonly in patients using extended-wear soft contact lenses. These cysts may be either asymptomatic or cause recurrent brief episodes of pain and epiphora. It takes up to 6 weeks following discontinuation of contact lens wear for the cysts to resolve.

Toxic conjunctivitis

Conjunctival injection, epithelial staining, punctate epithelial keratopathy, erosions, and microcysts are all potential signs of conjunctival or corneal toxicity from contact lens solutions. Any of the proteolytic enzymes or chemicals used for cleaning contact lenses, or the preservative-containing soaking solution, can be the culprit. Cleaning agents such as benzalkonium chloride, chlorhexidine, hydrogen peroxide, and other substances used for chemical sterilization, if not properly removed from contact lenses, can cause an immediate, severe epitheliopathy with accompanying pain. See Chapter 19.

Allergic reactions

The preservative thimerosal can produce a delayed hypersensitivity response, resulting in conjunctivitis, keratitis with epithelial involvement, and even coarse epithelial and subepithelial opacities. Thimerosal may also be implicated in contact lens–induced superior limbic keratoconjunctivitis. The ocular signs of this disorder include injection of the superior bulbar conjunctiva, epitheliopathy of the cornea and conjunctiva, papillary conjunctivitis, and some superficial pannus (Fig 5-17). This condition has declined in prevalence, probably as a result of the replacement of thimerosal by other preservatives in the contact lens solutions.

Neovascularization

Neovascular ingrowth into the peripheral cornea *(micropannus)* is common in soft contact lens wearers. Less than 2 mm of such growth is believed to be acceptable, but contact lens wear should be discontinued if the neovascularization extends farther than 2 mm into the cornea. Superficial pannus is rarely associated with hard or rigid gas-permeable (RGP) contact lens wear but is encountered more frequently in patients using soft lenses. This type of neovascularization is probably caused by hypoxia and chronic trauma to the limbus, which leads to the release of angiogenic mediators. Other causes of pannus such as staphylococcal or chlamydial keratoconjunctivitis should be considered in the presence of appropriate accompanying signs.

Deep stromal neovascularization has been associated with extended-wear contact lenses, especially in aphakia. This condition is not usually symptomatic unless there is secondary lipid deposition. Deep neovascularization of the cornea is often irreversible and is best managed by discontinuing contact lens wear and resorting to other alternatives such as secondary intraocular lens implantation.

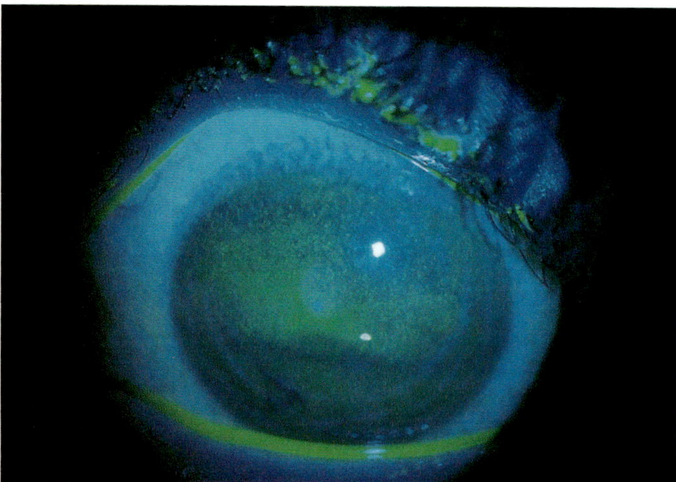

Figure 5-17 The superficial punctate epithelial keratopathy of contact lens–induced superior limbic keratoconjunctivitis often extends over the superior and middle thirds of the cornea.

Stapleton F, Dart J, Minassian D. Nonulcerative complications of contact lens wear. Relative risks for different lens types. *Arch Ophthalmol.* 1992;110:1601–1606.

Stein RM, Stein HA. Corneal complications of contact lenses. In: *Focal Points: Clinical Modules for Ophthalmologists.* San Francisco: American Academy of Ophthalmology; 1993: vol 11, no 2.

Limbal Stem-Cell Deficiency

PATHOGENESIS The ocular surface is composed of permanently renewing populations of epithelial cells. These epithelial cells are replaced through proliferation of a distinct sub-population of cells known as *stem cells.* The *corneal stem cells* are located in the basal cell layer of the limbus, whereas the *conjunctival stem cells* appear to be uniformly distributed throughout the bulbar surface. Stem cells have an unlimited capacity for self-renewal and are slow cycling (low mitotic activity). Once stem-cell differentiation begins, it is irreversible. The process of differentiation occurs by means of transit amplification. Transit-amplifying cells, which have a limited capacity for self-renewal, can be found at the limbus as well as the basal layer of the corneal epithelium. Each of these cells is able to undergo a finite number of cell divisions. Corneal and conjunctival stem cells can be identified only by indirect means such as clonal expansion and identification of slow cycling.

Approximately 25%–33% of the limbus must be intact in order to ensure normal ocular resurfacing. The normal limbus acts as a barrier against corneal vascularization from the conjunctiva and invasion of conjunctival cells from the bulbar surface. When the limbal stem cells are congenitally absent, injured, or destroyed, conjunctival cells migrate onto the ocular surface, often accompanied by superficial neovascularization. The absence of limbal stem cells reduces the effectiveness of epithelial wound healing, as evidenced by compromised ocular surface integrity with irregular ocular surface and recurrent epithelial breakdown.

CLINICAL PRESENTATION Clinically, stem-cell deficiency of the cornea can be observed in several ocular surface disorders. Patients usually suffer from recurrent ulceration and decreased vision as a result of the irregular corneal surface. Corneal neovascularization is invariably present in the involved cornea. A wavelike irregularity of the ocular surface emanating from the limbus can be more easily observed following the installation of topical fluorescein. In some cases, increased epithelial permeability can be observed clinically by diffuse permeation of topical fluorescein into the anterior stroma.

Stem-cell deficiency states can be divided into primary and secondary causes. Primary causes include congenital aniridia, ectodermal dysplasia, sclerocornea, KID syndrome, and congenital erythrokeratodermia. Secondary causes include chemical burns, thermal burns, contact lens wear, ocular surgery, and chronic cicatricial conjunctivitis (cicatricial pemphigoid, trachoma, Stevens-Johnson syndrome), pterygia, and dysplastic or neoplastic lesions of the limbus.

LABORATORY EVALUATION Impression cytology of the involved corneal surface usually shows the presence of goblet cells and conjunctival epithelium. There are no practical diagnostic tests for limbal stem-cell deficiency at this time; however, it is likely that such tests will be developed in the near future.

MANAGEMENT Replacement of stem cells by limbal transplantation seems to be the logical choice for ocular surface reconstruction in diseases associated with limbal stem-cell deficiency. When the limbus is focally affected in one eye, as with a pterygium, a limbal or conjunctival autograft can be obtained from the ipsilateral eye. For unilateral moderate or severe chemical injuries, a limbal autograft can be obtained from the healthy fellow eye. For bilateral limbal deficiency, as with Stevens-Johnson syndrome or bilateral chemical burns, a limbal allograft from an HLA-matched living related donor (or, if unavailable, an eye bank donor eye) can be considered. Systemic immune suppression is required following limbal allograft transplantation. Dramatic restoration of the ocular surface with limbal reconstruction has been reported in selected cases with desperate clinical situations. (See the discussion of ocular surface surgery in Chapters 20–21.)

PART III

Infectious Diseases of the External Eye and Cornea

Infectious Diseases of the External Eye: Basic Concepts

Defense Mechanisms of the External Eye

The external eye contains diverse tissues intricately linked to subserve visual function. The ocular adnexa—periorbita, eyelids and lashes, lacrimal and meibomian glands—produce, spread, and drain the preocular tear film, physically protect the sensitive ocular mucosa, and cushion the globe. The redundant conjunctiva with its low-viscosity tear film allows rapid multidirectional eye movements. Lymphoid tissues within the conjunctiva, lacrimal glands, and lacrimal drainage tract furnish acquired immune defense. The cornea and tear film fashion the major refractive surface of the eye. The sclera forms an external scaffold to maintain the position of the cornea, lens, and uveal tissues. Thus, the external eye and its adnexa maintain corneal clarity and comfort and act as a barrier to insult.

The bony orbit and eyelids protect the eye from external injury. Normal eyelid position and function prevent desiccation of the ocular surface and promote tear turnover by periodic closure. Eyelid blinking pumps tears from the lacrimal gland onto the ocular surface and into the lacrimal sac. Tear turnover dilutes and removes microbes from the tear film. In addition, soluble macromolecules secreted by the lacrimal gland exert antimicrobial properties. Tear lysozyme degrades bacterial cell walls, while β-lysin in the tears disrupts bacterial plasma membranes. Tear lactoferrin inhibits bacterial metabolism by scavenging free iron, augments tear antibody function, and may influence complement activation. Immunoglobulins in the tear film, particularly secretory IgA, mediate antigen-specific immunity at the ocular surface. Components of both the classic and alternative complement pathways are also found in the tear film. Meibomian gland–derived lipids reduce evaporation of the tear film and indirectly protect the corneal epithelium from desiccation and injury. Mucin expression by ocular surface cells as well as goblet cell–derived mucin inhibits attachment of microbes to ocular surface epithelium. Recent evidence also points to the presence of cytokines in the tears, including epidermal growth factor (EGF), transforming growth factor β (TGF-β), and hepatocyte growth factor (HGF). The contribution of these cytokines to ocular surface defense is a promising area of basic investigation. BCSC Section 2, *Fundamentals and Principles of Ophthalmology*, discusses the biochemistry and metabolism of the tear film and cornea in detail.

Lamberts DW. Physiology of the tear film. In: Smolin G, Thoft RA, eds. *The Cornea: Scientific Foundations and Clinical Practice.* 3rd ed. New York: Little Brown; 1994:439–455.

Mannis MJ, Smolin G. Natural defense mechanisms of the ocular surface. In: Pepose JS, Holland GN, Wilhelmus KR, eds. *Ocular Infection and Immunity.* St Louis: Mosby; 1996:185–199.

Pflugfelder SC, Solomon A, Stern ME. The diagnosis and management of dry eye: a twenty-five-year review. *Cornea.* 2000;19:644–649.

The epithelium of the ocular surface forms a mechanical barrier against microbial invasion. Phagocytosis and subsequent digestion of bacteria within intracellular phagosomes, combined with rapid cycling and the normal periodic sloughing of surface epithelial cells, aid in the removal of microbes that have attached to or invaded superficial corneal cells. Antigen-presenting cells such as Langerhans cells in the conjunctiva carry antigen to regional lymphatic tissue and facilitate an acquired immune response. In response to microbial invasion, ocular surface epithelial cells secrete interleukin-1 and other proinflammatory cytokines that boost the local immune response through the enhancement of immune-cell migration, adhesion, and activation.

Human conjunctiva contains a complete spectrum of immunologically competent cell types. Uninfected conjunctival epithelium possesses $CD8^+$ cytotoxic/suppressor T lymphocytes and Langerhans cells. Conjunctival substantia propria contains $CD4^+$ helper T cells and $CD8^+$ T cells in roughly equal numbers, along with natural killer T cells, mast cells, B lymphocytes, plasma cells, macrophages, and occasional polymorphonuclear leukocytes. Conjunctival lymphoid follicles, organized aggregates of lymphocytes and other immune cells, typically reside in the conjunctival fornices. Hyperplasia of conjunctival follicles and painful swelling of draining preauricular lymph nodes accompanies conjunctival infection by viruses, *Chlamydia*, and *Neisseria* species, suggesting that the conjunctiva participates in the immune response to these infections. The vascular and lymphatic channels of the conjunctiva transport humoral and cellular immune components to and from the eye. During an infection, inflammatory mediators promote vascular dilation, permeability, and diapedesis from conjunctival blood vessels.

The healthy cornea has classically been considered devoid of leukocytes, but activated Langerhans cells and other dendritic cells normally present in the peripheral corneal epithelium can migrate rapidly to the central cornea. Upon infection, the constitutive cells of the cornea, the keratocytes in particular, augment the inflammatory cascade by the secretion of proinflammatory cytokines. Lymphocytes and neutrophils are recruited into the cornea from the tear film, the limbal vascular arcades, and the anterior chamber.

For a more extensive, illustrated discussion of ocular immunology, see BCSC Section 9, *Intraocular Inflammation and Uveitis.*

Normal Ocular Flora

Bacterial colonization of the eyelid margin and conjunctiva is normal and beneficial for the eye. Interactions between ocular surface mucosa and resident nonpathogenic bacteria reduce opportunities for pathogenic strains to gain a foothold. The spectrum of normal ocular flora varies with the age and even the geographic locale of the host. Following vaginal birth, the infant's eye commonly harbors multiple bacterial species, including *Staphylococcus aureus, S epidermidis,* streptococci, and *Escherichia coli.* During the first two decades of life, streptococci and pneumococci predominate. With increasing age, gram-negative bacteria are more commonly isolated, but the most commonly isolated bacteria remain *S epidermidis* and other coagulase-negative staphylococci, *S aureus,* and diphtheroids (Table 6-1). Under the appropriate culture conditions, *Propionibacterium acnes, Malassezia furfur,* and *Candida* species may also be cultured from the eye. The parasites *Demodex folliculorum* and *Demodex brevis* are detected on the eyelid margins of normal healthy individuals, and with advancing age become almost ubiquitous. Clinically, the use of antibiotics or topical corticosteroids, or a condition such as dry eye that prevents normal tear turnover, may alter the spectrum of eyelid and conjunctival flora.

Osato MS. Normal ocular flora. In: Pepose JS, Holland GN, Wilhelmus KR, eds. *Ocular Infection and Immunity.* St Louis: Mosby; 1996:191–199.

Pathogenesis of Ocular Infections

Infection of the ocular surface can follow transplacental passage of the pathogen to the fetus; direct contact in the birth canal during delivery; exposure from fomites, fingers, airborne particles, or sexual contact; hematogenous seeding (rare); extension from contiguous adnexal disease; and spread from the upper respiratory tract through the nasolacrimal duct. The most common route of ocular surface infection is external via ocular surface epithelium.

The acquisition of infection is enhanced by circumstances that facilitate contact with the pathogen. Epidemic adenoviral conjunctivitis develops after mucosal contact with secretions from an infected person. Sexually transmitted ocular infections such as gonococcal and chlamydial conjunctivitis are spread through ocular contact with infected

Table 6-1 Relative Prevalence of the Normal Flora of the Outer Eye

Microorganisms	Normal Conjunctiva	Normal Eyelid Margin
Staphylococcus epidermidis	+ + +	+ + +
Straphylococcus aureus	+ +	+ +
Micrococcus spp	+	+ +
Corynebacterium spp (diphtheroids)	+ +	+ +
Propionibacterium acnes	+ +	+ +
Streptococcus spp[*]	+	±
Haemophilus influenzae[*]	±	−
Moraxella spp	±	−
Enteric gram-negative bacilli	±	−
Bacillus spp	±	−
Anaerobic bacteria	+	±
Yeasts (*Malassezia furfur, Candida* spp, etc)	−	+
Filamentous fungi	±	−
Demodex spp	−	+ +

* More common in children.

genital secretions during sexual activity. Zoonotic infections such as cat-scratch disease or Lyme disease are transmitted by contact with an infected animal host or vector. The risk of opportunistic infection by environmental pathogens may be enhanced by use of chemically disinfected but not fully sterilized surgical instruments *(Mycobacterium chelonei)*, use of homemade saline or tap water for contact lens hygiene *(Acanthamoeba)*, or trauma with soil or vegetable matter *(Bacillus cereus,* various fungi). The initiation, severity, and characteristics of subsequent infection are influenced by the interplay between the virulence of the pathogen, the size of the inoculum, and the competence and nature of host defense mechanisms.

Virulence

Successful infection of ocular tissues requires microorganisms to adhere, evade, invade, replicate, and in some instances, persist. Microbial virulence factors represent evolutionary adaptations by each microorganism that increase the odds of infection and organism survival.

Adherence

For those ocular surface infections acquired externally, adherence of organisms to ocular surface epithelium is the first step. Many bacteria express *adhesins,* which are microbial proteins that bind with high affinity to host cell surface molecules. *Candida albicans* expresses surface proteins that mimic mammalian *integrins* (transmembrane proteins that mediate cell–cell and cell–extracellular matrix interactions). Viruses typically express surface proteins or glycoproteins that attach to constitutive cell surface molecules such as heparan sulfate (herpes simplex virus) or sialic acid (adenovirus).

Evasion

Adherent bacteria evade interaction with unfavorable elements of their physical environment, such as immunologic cells or antibacterial molecules in the tears, by the expression of exopolysaccharide organized into a *biofilm,* a three-dimensional structure that allows interbacterial communication and signaling and interferes with phagocytosis. For viruses, evasion of the immune response involves multiple strategies. For example, a herpes simplex virus–encoded protein (ICP47) successfully competes with antigenic viral peptides for transport into the endoplasmic reticulum, where peptides are loaded onto the MHC complex. Thus, herpes simplex virus–infected cells can be resistant to lysis by cytotoxic T cells.

Watnick P, Kolter R. Biofilm, city of microbes. *J Bacteriol.* 2000;182:2675–2679.

Invasion

Neisseria gonorrhoeae, Neisseria meningitidis, Corynebacterium diphtheriae, and *Shigella* species each can overcome an intact corneal epithelium, but most bacteria must rely on a break in epithelial barrier function. Microbial invasion may be facilitated by microbial proteases that induce cell lysis and degrade the extracellular matrix. Bacterial exotoxins, such as those produced by streptococci, staphylococci, and *P aeruginosa,* can induce corneal cell necrosis. *Acanthamoeba* species and certain fungi secrete collagenases, while *Pseudomonas* elastase and alkaline protease destroy collagen and proteoglycan components of the cornea and degrade immunoglobulins, complement, interleukins, and other inflammatory cytokines. Microbial proteases also activate corneal matrix–derived metalloproteinases that in turn participate in autodigestion. For viruses, adherence interactions facilitate invasion by the appropriation of host cell mechanisms. For example, the interaction between adenovirus capsid proteins and host cell integrins mediates internalization of the adenovirus by means of an intracellular signaling cascade that culminates in actin polymerization and endocytosis of the virus.

Replication and persistence

Most organisms are cleared from the site of infection following acute infection. Some microorganisms persist in the host indefinitely. For example, following primary infection, herpes simplex and varicella-zoster viruses establish latency in trigeminal ganglion cells. *Chlamydia* survives and causes local chronic disease by persistence within intracellular phagosomes. Biofilm formation by streptococci within the corneal stroma inhibits recognition of the bacteria by the immune system and accounts for the relative paucity of inflammation and chronic nature characteristic of crystalline keratopathy caused by this organism.

Inoculum

Different species and strains of microorganisms vary intrinsically in their capacity to induce infection in the host. For example, experimental bacterial keratitis in an animal model can be established with an inoculum of *P aeruginosa* smaller than that required of *S aureus*. The status of host defense mechanisms further determines the threshold of inoculum at which infection occurs.

Host Defense

Intrinsic anatomic mechanisms

Lagophthalmos, ectropion, exophthalmos, a reduced blink reflex due to parkinsonism, and keratoconjunctivitis sicca can all lead to desiccation of the ocular surface epithelium and can predispose the cornea to infection. Microtrauma to the epithelium occurs with trichiasis, contact lens wear, use of an ocular prosthesis, prolonged or intense administration of preservative-containing topical medications, and exposure to a free surgical suture. Acute traumatic abrasion, bullous keratopathy, recurrent corneal erosion, recurrent epithelial disruption secondary to corneal epithelial and anterior stromal dystrophies, retained foreign body, or corneal surgery similarly can predispose to infection. Persistent epithelial defects due to neurotrophic mechanisms such as postherpetic hypoesthesia, diabetic neuropathy, or traumatic injury to cranial nerve V also may precede microbial keratitis. Any surgery in which the conjunctival epithelium is disrupted, including strabismus and cataract surgery, can lead to infection of the conjunctiva and the underlying scleral wound.

Immunologic competence

Local or systemic immune compromise predisposes to ocular infection. The use of topical corticosteroids is a frequent contributing factor in the pathogenesis of postoperative infections. Preexisting corneal or conjunctival pathology may cause structural and functional alterations that affect normal tissue responses to injury, inflammation, or infection. The propensity for development of ocular infection also increases with systemic immune compromise in hosts with acquired immunodeficiencies such as those with AIDS and other chronic debilitating diseases or on systemic chemotherapy; in such patients, normally nonpathogenic organisms may cause disease.

O'Brien TP, Hazlett LD. Pathogenesis of ocular infection. In: Pepose JS, Holland GN, Wilhelmus KR, eds. *Ocular Infection and Immunity.* St Louis: Mosby; 1996:200–214.

Ocular Microbiology

Of the many potentially pathogenic microorganisms capable of causing infectious external eye disease, those encountered most often are listed in Table 6-2. The clinical manifestations of each of the organisms below are described in Chapter 7.

Virology

Viruses are small (10–400 μm in diameter) infectious units consisting of a single- or double-stranded nucleic acid genome and a protein capsid shell, with or without an external lipid envelope. In generating a virus taxonomy, the International Committee on Taxonomy of Viruses (ICTV) considers multiple virus traits including morphology, physical properties, nucleic acid type and strandedness, physical state of the genome, proteins expressed, antigenic properties, and serologic cross-reactivity, as well as biologic effects of infection. Viruses lack the independent means for energy metabolism, molecular biosynthesis, or replication. Viral genes are transcribed and viral progeny produced only inside a permissive host cell.

Viral nucleic acid consists of either RNA or DNA. RNA viral genome may be either single- or double-stranded and, in the case of single-stranded viruses, either positive-sense (same polarity as mRNA) or negative-sense (opposite polarity to mRNA). Transcription of viral nucleic acid to produce the enzymatic and structural proteins necessary for replication varies with the type of viral genome. With the exception of the positive-sense single-stranded RNA viruses, it is necessary to first transcribe an mRNA. DNA viruses that replicate in the cell nucleus are able to utilize cell-derived polymerases. Otherwise, generation of a viral-encoded RNA polymerase is required. Antiviral medications typically target viral gene transcription. Therefore, the clinical significance of the nucleic acid type lies principally in differences in susceptibility to antiviral medications.

The *viral capsid* is a protein shell that surrounds the viral nucleic acid. The capsid interacts internally with the genome to stabilize it, protects the genome from the external environment, and in the case of nonenveloped viruses, expresses on its surface the ligand for virus–host cell binding. Viral capsid proteins also assist in delivery of the viral genome to the intracellular site of viral replication. Thus, viral capsid structure is integrally related to many viral functions, in particular, transmission, attachment, and entry into host target cells, but also virion assembly and egress.

For some virus families, a host cell–derived lipid bilayer or envelope surrounds the protein capsid. Viral genome–encoded glycoproteins bound to the membrane act as

Table 6-2 Principal Causes of External Ocular Infections

Condition	Viruses	Bacteria	Fungi	Parasites
Dermatoblepharitis	Herpes simplex Varicella-zoster	*Staphylococcus aureus* *Streptococcus* spp		
Blepharitis	Herpes simplex Molluscum contagiosum	*Staphylococcs* spp *Moraxella* spp		*Phthirus pubis*
Conjunctivitis	Adenovirus Herpes simplex	*Chlamydia trachomatis* *Staphylococcus aureus* *Steptococcus* spp *Neisseria gonorrhoeae* *Haemophilus influenzae* *Moraxella* spp		
Keratitis	Herpes simplex	*Pseudomonas aeruginosa* *Staphylococcus aureus* *Staphylococcus epidermidis* *Streptococcus pneumoniae* *Moraxella* spp	*Fusarium* spp *Aspergillus* spp *Candida albicans*	*Acanthamoeba* spp
Dacryoadenitis	Epstein-Barr virus Mumps	*Staphylococcus aureus* *Streptococcus pneumoniae*		
Canaliculitis		Actinomycetes		
Dacryocystitis		*Staphylococcus* spp *Streptococcus* spp		

ligands (antigens) for neutralizing antibodies directed against the virus. In the initial stages of infection, envelope glycoproteins mediate attachment of the virus to its receptor on the host cell surface and fusion of the viral envelope with the host cell membrane. Later during viral replication, viral-encoded glycoproteins are targeted on a molecular level to specific membranes in the host cell in order to serve as sites of interaction between the viral nucleocapsid and the host cell membrane prior to budding. The viral envelope lipid bilayer is vulnerable to damage by ultraviolet light, detergents, alcohols, and general-use antiseptics.

Enveloped viruses such as herpes simplex virus and human immunodeficiency virus are therefore intrinsically susceptible to the external environment, and their infectivity is short-lived outside the host. Enveloped viruses are difficult to transmit via fomites or medical instruments, and alcohol treatment of medical instrumentation is generally sufficient to prevent iatrogenic infection.

In contrast, *nonenveloped viruses* such as adenoviruses are relatively resistant to environmental insult and, in some cases, can persist for weeks outside the human host. The application of dilute (1%) bleach to tonometer tips for at least 10 minutes is recommended to prevent transmission of adenoviruses, but care must be taken to clean residual bleach from the tonometer tip prior to use.

CDC National Prevention Information Network. HIV/AIDS Prevention FAQs [website]. http://www.cdcnpin.org/hiv/faq/prevention.htm.

Chodosh J, Stroop WG. Introduction to viruses in ocular disease. In: Tasman W, Jaeger EA, eds. *Duane's Foundations of Clinical Ophthalmology.* Philadelphia: Lippincott Williams & Wilkins; 1998:chapter 85, pp 1–10.

DNA viruses

Herpesviruses The structure of all herpesviruses includes a core of linear double-stranded DNA genome, surrounded by an icosahedral protein capsid, an amorphous-appearing protein tegument, and finally an envelope studded with viral glycoproteins. Out of the eight known human herpesviruses, those that affect the eye include herpes simplex virus (HSV) types 1 and 2, varicella-zoster virus (VZV), Epstein-Barr virus (EBV), cytomegalovirus (CMV), and Kaposi sarcoma–associated herpesvirus/human herpesvirus 8 (KSHV). The production of viral progeny invariably destroys the infected cell. All herpesviruses establish latency in their natural hosts, but the site of latency varies. For example, while HSV types 1 and 2 and VZV establish latent infections in dorsal root ganglia such as the trigeminal ganglion, Epstein-Barr virus latency occurs in B lymphocytes.

Roizman B. Herpesviridae. In: Fields BN, Knipe DM, Howley PM, eds. *Fields Virology.* Philadelphia: Lippincott-Raven; 1996:chapter 71, pp 2221–2230.

Adenoviruses The *Adenoviridae* are double-stranded DNA viruses associated with significant human disease and morbidity. Forty-nine serotypes subdivide into six distinct subgroups (A–F) on the basis of genetic sequencing. Adenovirus subgroups associate broadly with specific clinical syndromes. For instance, subgroup D adenoviruses are strongly associated with epidemic keratoconjunctivitis. The nonenveloped protein capsid of the adenovirus forms a regular icosahedron. For most adenoviral subgroups, a projecting capsid protein serves as the ligand for the cellular adenovirus receptor, and the interaction of an adjacent capsid protein with cell surface integrins mediates internalization of the virus.

Horwitz MS. Adenoviruses. In: Fields BN, Knipe DM, Howley PM, eds. *Fields Virology.* Philadelphia: Lippincott-Raven; 1996:chapter 68, pp 2149–2171.

Poxviruses The *Poxviridae* encompass a large family of enveloped, double-stranded DNA viruses, with a distinctive brick or ovoid shape and a complex capsid structure. The best-known poxviruses are smallpox (variola) virus and vaccinia virus. Members of this family with the potential to cause human eye disease today include molluscum contagiosum virus and orf virus. *Molluscum contagiosum virus* is an obligate human virus that produces an umbilicated, wartlike lesion of the eyelid skin as a result of intradermal viral proliferation. Histopathologic examination of an expressed or excised nodule shows eosinophilic, intracytoplasmic inclusions *(Henderson-Patterson bodies)* within epidermal cells. The clinical aspects of molluscum contagiosum are described in Chapter 7. Another poxvirus, *orf virus,* is typically acquired from sheep and goats by shearers and handlers and causes pustular vesicular lesions of the skin that may involve the eyelid and occasionally the conjunctiva.

Papovaviruses Human papillomaviruses (HPV) are small, nonenveloped, double-stranded DNA viruses with an icosahedral capsid. Persistent viral infection of susceptible epithelial cells induces cellular proliferation and can lead to malignant transformation. Papillomavirus proteins can induce transformation of the cell and loss of senescence. Human papillomavirus subtypes 6 and 11 are maintained in a latent state within basal epithelial cells as circular episomes with very limited viral gene transcription and low copy number. Early viral gene products stimulate cell growth and lead to a skin wart or a conjunctival papilloma. As HPV-containing basal epithelial cells mature and differentiate into superficial epithelial cells, they become permissive for complete viral gene expression and produce infectious virus. Neoplastic transformation due to HPV 6 or 11 is very rare. In contrast, HPV 16 and 18 stereotypically integrate their viral genome into host chromosomal DNA, and this in turn is associated with malignant transformation and squamous cell carcinoma.

RNA viruses

Picornaviruses These negative-sense single-stranded RNA viruses have an icosahedral capsid and no envelope. Picornaviridae family members include the *enteroviruses* (poliovirus, coxsackievirus, echovirus, and enterovirus) and the *rhinoviruses,* the single most common etiology of the common cold.

Togaviruses These viruses contain positive-sense single-stranded RNA and have no envelope. Togaviruses with general medical and ophthalmic importance include rubella, encephalomyelitis, yellow fever, and dengue viruses.

Orthomyxoviruses and paramyxoviruses Orthomyxoviruses such as influenza virus are negative-sense, single-stranded RNA viruses with an enveloped helical icosahedral capsid. Structurally similar to the orthomyxoviruses, paramyxoviruses of ocular importance include mumps virus, measles (rubeola) virus, parainfluenza virus, respiratory syncytial virus, and Newcastle disease virus, the latter a cause of follicular conjunctivitis in poultry handlers. Paramyxovirus envelope contains hemagglutinin-neuraminidase protein spikes and a hemolysin, which mediate viral fusion with the host cell membrane.

Retroviruses These positive-sense single-stranded enveloped RNA viruses encode a viral enzyme, *reverse transcriptase,* that assists in conversion of the single-stranded RNA genome into a circular double-stranded DNA molecule. The viral nucleic acid then integrates into host cell chromosomal DNA.

The retrovirus of greatest medical importance is *human immunodeficiency virus (HIV),* the etiologic agent of acquired immunodeficiency syndrome (AIDS). HIV enters the human host via sexual contact at mucosal surfaces, through breast feeding, or via blood-contaminated needles. Sexually transmitted infection is facilitated by uptake of HIV by dendritic cells at mucosal surfaces. CD4$^+$ T lymphocytes are a primary target of the virus, as are dendritic cells and monocyte-macrophages. Infection of these cell types induces predictable defects of innate and acquired (both humoral and cellular) immunity. Primary viremia results in an infectious mononucleosis–like HIV prodrome, followed by seeding of the peripheral lymphoid organs and development of a measurable immune response. Infected patients may remain otherwise asymptomatic for several years, but CD4$^+$ T lymphocytes are progressively depleted. Clinical immunodeficiency eventually develops.

AIDS-related ocular disorders include herpes zoster ophthalmicus, molluscum contagiosum, keratoconjunctivitis sicca, microsporidial keratoconjunctivitis, HIV neuropathy, cryptococcal optic neuritis, retinal microvasculopathy, and choroiditis and retinitis due to syphilis, mycobacteria, pneumocystosis, toxoplasmosis, cytomegalovirus, herpes simplex virus, and varicella zoster virus.

AIDS is associated with a remarkably increased risk of Kaposi sarcoma (relative risk >10,000) and non-Hodgkin lymphoma (relative risk >100), and both of these disorders may affect the eyelids, conjunctiva, and orbit. When the CD4$^+$ T-cell count falls below a critical threshold, opportunistic diseases become more likely. For example, patients are at particular risk for CMV retinitis when their CD4$^+$ T lymphocyte count falls below 50 cells per cubic millimeter.

Anti-HIV antibody testing by enzyme immunoassay with confirmation by gel electrophoresis (Western blot) is used to establish HIV infection, and p24 antigen capture is used to show viremia. Viral mRNA load in the plasma can be assessed to determine the response to therapy. Highly active antiretroviral therapy (HAART) has resulted in clinical remission, a reduction in opportunistic infections, and plasma viral levels below the limit of detection (50 copies/mL); but natural reservoirs of HIV (including the central nervous system, male urogenital tract, and most important, latently infected resting memory CD4$^+$ T lymphocytes) have so far prevented complete eradication of infection. For more information regarding HIV, see BCSC Section 1 *(Update on General Medicine)* and Section 9 *(Intraocular Inflammation and Uveitis).*

Cunningham ET Jr, Margolis TP. Ocular manifestations of HIV infection. *N Engl J Med.* 1998;339:236–244.

Goedert JJ. The epidemiology of acquired immunodeficiency syndrome malignancies. *Semin Oncol.* 2000;27:390–401.

Bacteriology

Bacteria are round or rod-shaped cells with a wide range of sizes but are most commonly several micrometers in length. In bacteria, the genetic material is not separated from the cytoplasm by a nuclear membrane; hence, these organisms are referred to as *prokaryotic* cells in contrast to *eukaryotic* cells, which have a membrane-bound nucleus. In prokaryotes, a plasma membrane encloses a single cytoplasmic compartment containing DNA, RNA, and protein in an ultrastructurally amorphous matrix without membrane-bound cellular organelles. Most bacterial genes exist as part of a single circular chromosome, but other genes are present on smaller extrachromosomal circles called *plasmids.* Plasmid DNA typically determines inheritance of one or a few characteristics such as antibiotic resistance, and it represents an important mechanism by which traits are passed between different bacterial strains and sometimes between bacterial species. As a group, prokaryotes are able to adapt to and thrive in environments that may be too extreme for eukaryotes. Bacterial classification is determined by the International Committee for Systemic Bacteriology (ICSB). Classification is based on microscopic and colony morphology, enzyme activity, biochemical tests, DNA fingerprinting, and genomic sequence (when known).

Prokaryote structure determines many aspects of infection pathogenesis. The protective coat or cell wall surrounding the plasma membrane of bacteria imparts shape and rigidity to the cell and mediates interactions with the environment, other bacteria, and bacterial viruses. The cell wall also forms the basis of Gram stain reaction. Bacteria stain violet (gram-positive) or red (gram-negative) based on the structure and biochemical composition of their cell wall. Some bacteria that stain poorly with Gram stain, including *Mycobacteria* and *Nocardia asteroides,* can be visualized with acid-fast stain. Gram-positive bacterial cell walls contain predominantly peptidoglycan and teichoic acid. The latter serves as a major surface antigen, for example, the M protein of *Streptococcus pyogenes.* Gram negative cell walls are complex and have a thin peptidoglycan layer and an external lipid membrane containing lipopolysaccharide (LPS), also referred to as *endotoxin.* Gram staining of clinical specimens is important not only because it helps to classify a pathogenic organism but also because gram-positive and gram-negative bacteria are typically susceptible to different classes of antibiotic drugs.

Specialized structures external to the cell wall uniquely facilitate bacterial interactions with a diverse environment. External *flagella* enable some bacteria to negotiate a liquid environment. Thinner appendages on many gram-negative bacteria include pili and fimbriae. *Pili* are involved in bacterial conjugation (transfer of bacterial DNA from one bacterial cell to another). *Fimbriae* mediate adherence of one bacteria to another and to eukaryotic cells. Bacterial adhesins are specific surface-associated molecules or fimbriae that mediate attachment of bacteria to mucosal surfaces.

Bacteria replicate by binary fission, and under optimal conditions, a single bacterium can divide approximately every 20 minutes. This innate ability to replicate quickly permits rapid adaptation to environmental changes. The extreme variety of environmental niches also encourages bacterial survival strategies including the engagement of different enzymatic machinery (metabolic pathways) in response to changes in pH, access to oxygen, and availability of specific organic molecules as energy sources; the development of local bacterial ecosystems (biofilms); and the capacity to transmit genetic elements (plasmids) from one bacterial cell to another and, occasionally, from one bacterial species to another. Thus, the apparent simplicity of bacterial structure belies their diversity.

Gram-positive cocci

Staphylococcus species Staphylococci inhabit the skin, skin glands, and mucous membranes of healthy mammals. Staphylococci grow in grapelike clusters in culture but may be seen singly, in pairs, or in short chains on smears from ocular specimens (Fig 6-1). Staphylococci produce an external biofilm that interferes with phagocytosis and secrete a variety of extracellular proteins—including toxins, enzymes, and enzyme activators—that facilitate both colonization and disease. Staphylococci also produce *lantibiotics*, small polypeptides that exert antibacterial effects on other bacteria competing for the same natural habitat. Staphylococci adapt quickly and effectively to administered antibacterial agents and may develop resistance to beta lactams, macrolides, tetracyclines, and quinolones.

Streptococcus species Streptococci inhabit the mucous membranes of the normal upper respiratory tract and female genital tracts. Streptococci grow in pairs and chains. The historical classification of streptococci based on their ability to hemolyze blood-containing agar media is useful for initial recognition of clinical isolates. Other historical means of classification included serologic grouping based on cell wall carbohydrates (Lancefield groups), but these methods are used less today given the availability of genetic sequence data.

Disease-causing factors of the highly pathogenic β-hemolytic *S pyogenes* and other pyogenic streptococci include the M and M-like proteins, pyrogenic exotoxins, streptolysin, C5a peptidase, and hyaluronidase. M proteins anchor in the cytoplasmic membrane and extend externally through the bacterial cell wall to help the organism resist phagocytosis by neutrophils. Streptolysin lyses erythrocytes, platelets, and neutrophils. C5a peptidase cleaves and destroys the function of C5a, an important chemoattractant of neutrophils. Hyaluronidase is believed to act as a tissue invasion factor.

S pneumoniae appear in smears as lancet-shaped diplococci and express a polysaccharide capsule that resists phagocytosis by macrophages and neutrophils. The toxin pneumolysin is liberated by autolysis and inhibits neutrophil chemotaxis, phagocytosis, lymphocyte proliferation, and antibody synthesis.

Enterococcus species Enterococci are gram-positive cocci that may be seen in pairs or in short chains. They are capable of survival in harsh environments but, in humans, are commensal in the gastrointestinal and genitourinary tracts. *E faecalis*, an important cause of endophthalmitis, utilizes a unique mechanism of plasmid exchange involving the expression of sex pheromones. These chemicals, when expressed on the surface of enterococci, induce a bacterial mating response and exchange of genetic material, a means by which enterococci acquire antibiotic resistance. Enterococci also produce a cytolysin with potent effects on eukaryotic cell membranes.

Gram-negative cocci

Neisseria species *N gonorrhoeae* causes urogenital, rectal, and pharyngeal infections, as well as hyperacute conjunctivitis, and can invade intact corneal epithelium, induce keratolysis of the corneal stroma, and perforate the cornea. *N gonorrhoeae* is always a pathogen, while the closely related species, *N meningitidis*, may be commensal in the pharynx without causing disease. A bean-shaped gram-negative diplococcus usually seen within neutrophils on a clinical smear from ocular or genital sites (Fig 6-2), *N gonorrhoeae* grows well on chocolate agar and Thayer-Martin media.

Gram-positive rods

***Corynebacterium* species** These pleomorphic bacilli produce palisading or cuneiform patterns on smears. *C diphtheriae* is an exotoxin-producing cause of acute membranous conjunctivitis. Other *Corynebacterium* species are referred to as diphtheroids and are

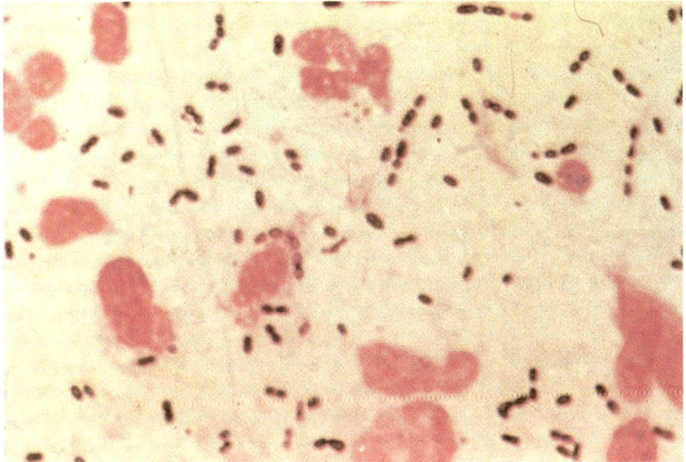

Figure 6-1 Gram-positive cocci (*Streptococcus pneumoniae*. Gram ×1000). *(Photograph courtesy of James Chodosh, MD.)*

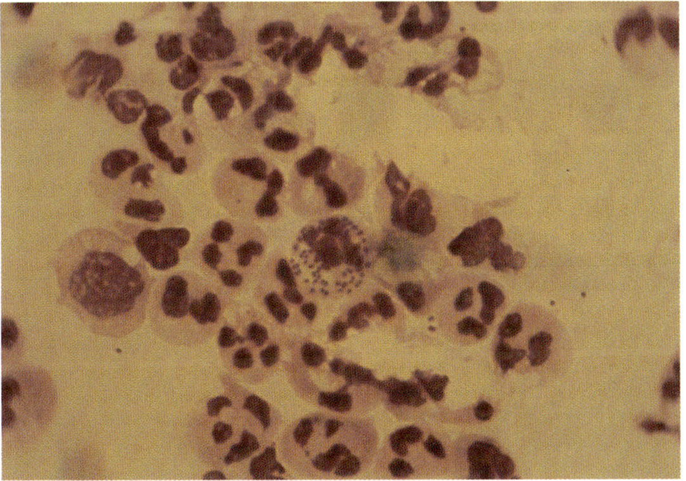

Figure 6-2 Gram-negative cocci (*Neisseria gonorrhoeae*. Gram ×1000).

routinely isolated from the external eye in the absence of clinical infection. *C xerosis* is commonly seen on histologic sections of vitamin A deficiency–associated conjunctival Bitôt spots, but its significance in conjunctival xerosis is unknown.

***Propionibacterium* species** *P acnes* and related species are normal inhabitants of human skin. They are aerotolerant but prefer an anaerobic environment. These slender, slightly curved gram-positive rods sometimes have a beaded appearance (Fig 6-3). *P acnes* is a major cause of chronic postoperative endophthalmitis and a rare cause of microbial keratitis.

***Bacillus* species** These ubiquitous gram-positive or gram-variable rods are commonly found in soil and are characterized by the production of spores, a form of the bacteria that allows survival for extended periods of time under extremely harsh conditions. *Bacillus* species are typically motile, and this feature may play a role in the explosive character of *Bacillus cereus*–induced posttraumatic endophthalmitis. *B cereus* produces a number of toxins that may rapidly damage ocular tissues. The closely related genus *Clostridium* is anaerobic while *Bacillus* species are aerobes or facultative anaerobes.

Gram-negative rods

Pseudomonas aeruginosa are slender gram-negative rods (Fig 6-4) commonly found as contaminants of water. *P aeruginosa* ocular infections are among the most fulminant. Permanent tissue damage and scarring is the rule following corneal infection. Structural virulence factors of *P aeruginosa* include polar flagella, adhesins, and surface pili. *P aeruginosa* secrete a number of toxins that disrupt protein synthesis and damage cell membranes of ocular cells, and proteases that degrade the corneal stromal extracellular matrix.

Enterobacteriaceae This family includes multiple genera of enteric non–spore-forming gram-negative rods, including *Escherichia coli, Klebsiella, Enterobacter, Citrobacter, Ser-*

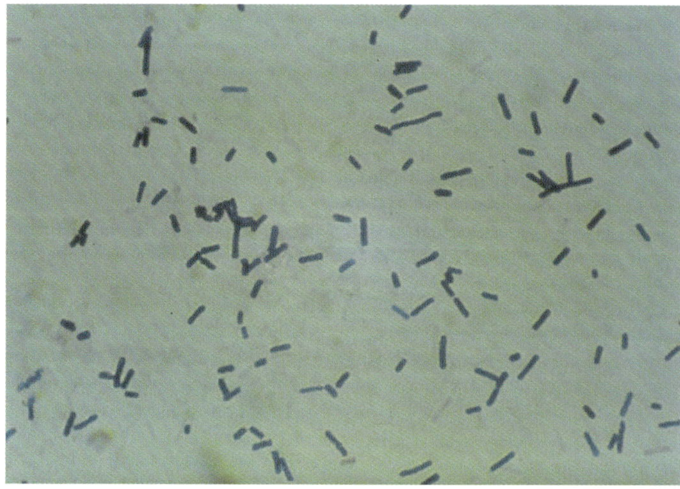

Figure 6-3 Gram-positive rods (*Propionibacterium acnes.* Gram ×1000).

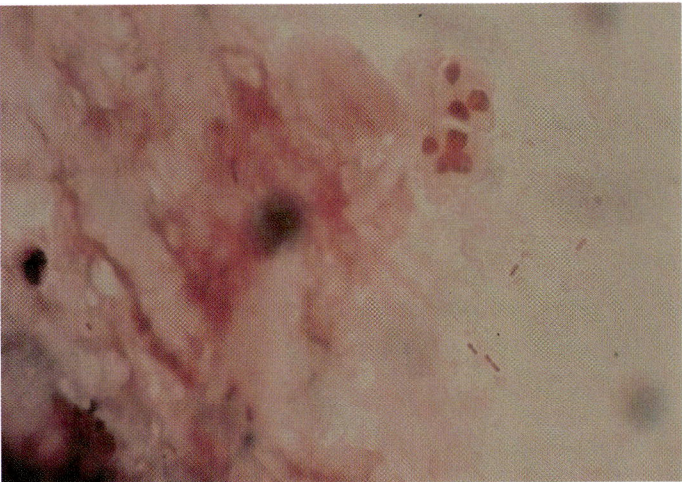

Figure 6-4 Gram-negative rods (*Pseudomonas aeruginosa.* Gram ×1000).

ratia, Salmonella, Shigella, and *Proteus.* In particular, *Klebsiella, Enterobacter, Citrobacter, Serratia,* and *Proteus* are important causes of keratitis. Pathogenetic factors include pili, adhesins, cytolysins, and toxins. Enteropathogenic *E coli* express a protein similar to cholera toxin. Organisms in this family are typically highly sensitive to aminoglycosides, but *Serratia marcescens* is unique in its variable resistance to specific aminoglycosides such as tobramycin. *S marcescens* may be able to survive preserved contact lens disinfection solutions.

***Haemophilus* species** *Haemophilus* species vary in morphology from coccobacilli to short rods. Culture isolation requires enriched media such as chocolate agar. *Haemophilus* species are obligate parasites of mammalian mucous membranes, commonly inhabit the human upper respiratory tract and mouth, and along with streptococci are important agents of bleb infections following glaucoma filtering surgery. *H influenzae* can be divided into biotypes based on biochemical reactions, and encapsulated strains are further divided into serotypes based on their capsular polysaccharides. *H influenzae* type b (Hib) is the primary human pathogen, and its capsule is a major virulence factor. *H influenzae* preseptal cellulitis may predispose children to a fulminant meningitis in which up to 20% of patients who recover have long-term neurological sequelae. The incidence of infection has been reduced by a vigorous program of vaccination against Hib.

Bartonella henselae The etiologic agent of cat-scratch disease, *B henselae* appear as gram-negative aerobic rods, best seen by Warthin-Starry staining of tissue biopsies. *B henselae* infection can be confirmed by culture, by polymerase chain reaction, by immunocytologic staining of histological specimens, and by serology. Cats act as the natural reservoir of *B henselae.* Infection may be transmitted by a cat scratch or by contact with fleas.

Gram-positive filaments

Mycobacterium species Mycobacteria are nonmotile, aerobic, weakly gram-positive, but acid-fast, and appear on smears as straight or slightly curved rods. Löwenstein-Jensen media is most commonly used for culture isolation. Mycobacteria are obligate intracellular pathogens and fall into two main groups based on growth rate. *M tuberculosis* and *M leprae* are slow growers. Ocular infection by *M tuberculosis* is uncommon, but it can manifest as a posterior uveitis. The fast-growing atypical mycobacteria, including *M fortuitum* and *M chelonei*, more commonly cause ulcerative keratitis and have been associated with keratitis acquired during refractive surgery.

Nocardia species *N asteroides* and related filamentous bacilli are gram-variable or gram-positive and weakly acid-fast. They may cause keratitis clinically similar to that caused by the atypical mycobacteria.

Actinomyces species Actinomycetes are gram-positive, non–acid-fast anaerobic bacteria that colonize the mouth, intestines, and genital tract. They are an important cause of canaliculitis.

Chlamydia

Chlamydiae are spherical or ovoid obligate intracellular parasites of mucosal epithelium with a dimorphic life cycle. The infectious form is the *elementary body* (EB), which develops within an infected host eukaryotic cell into the intracellular replicating form, the *reticulate body* (RB). Only the EB survives outside the host, and only the EB is infectious. Reticulate bodies divide by binary fission to produce one or more elementary bodies within a cytoplasmic vacuole, seen on light microscopy as a cellular inclusion. *C trachomatis*, a common agent of infectious external eye disease, is serotyped by its major outer membrane protein antigens. Repeated ocular infection with serotypes A through C are associated with trachoma. Types D through K cause genital infection and keratoconjunctivitis, the latter in sexually active adults or in neonates infected via the birth canal. *C trachomatis* can be demonstrated by immunodiagnostic methods or culture isolation using McCoy cells and others.

Spirochetes

Spirochetes are characterized by the periplasmic location of their flagella *(endoflagella)*. Spirochetes are too narrow to be seen by light microscopy. Visualization in fresh clinical specimens requires dark-field illumination. Silver staining or immunocytology can aid identification in histopathologic specimens.

Treponema pallidum causes venereal syphilis. By dark-field illumination, *T pallidum* appear fine and corkscrew shaped, with rigid, uniform spirals. Aside from direct identification of *T pallidum* by dark-field techniques, the diagnosis of syphilis is based on specific serologic tests. The serologic microhemagglutination assay for *T pallidum* (MHA-TP) and fluorescent treponemal antibody absorption (FTA-ABS) test are specific, but not reliable for testing cerebrospinal fluid. The rapid plasma reagin (RPR) and Venereal Disease Research Laboratory (VDRL) assays are nonspecific but are useful for assay of cerebrospinal fluid in patients with suspected neurosyphilis. The MHA-TP and FTA-ABS tests remain reactive for life, while the VDRL and RPR titers drop with antibiotic therapy and thus can be used to assess the response to therapy. In clinical practice, MHA-TP or FTA-ABS reactivity is used to confirm the clinical suspicion of syphilis, and the quantitative RPR (or VDRL) test is performed to determine disease activity and to compare with subsequent testing following treatment. For further discussion of syphilis, see BCSC Section 1 *(Update on General Medicine)* and Section 9 *(Intraocular Inflammation and Uveitis)*.

Borrelia burgdorferi *Borrelia* species are obligate parasites, best visualized with Giemsa stain. *B burgdorferi,* the etiologic agent of Lyme disease and associated Lyme uveitis, is transmitted to humans by tick bites. The preferred hosts for subadult ticks are rodents, while adult ticks feed on deer. *B burgdorferi* infection of migrating birds may account for the wide distribution of the organism. Although the organism can be cultured from biopsies of erythema migrans skin lesions, it is difficult to recover from blood or synovial fluid. In general, the diagnosis of Lyme disease is determined by serology and typical clinical findings. Pathogenetic factors of *B burgdorferi* include the expression of proteinases that facilitate tissue invasion, induction of proinflammatory cytokines upon binding to phagocytes, and activation of the complement cascade. See also BCSC Sections 1 and 9.

Mycology

Fungi are eukaryotes that develop branching filaments and reproduce by means of sexually or asexually produced spores. Fungal cell walls are rigid and contain chitin and polysaccharides. Fungi are classically divided into two groups: *yeasts* are round or oval fungi that reproduce by budding and sometimes form pseudohyphae by elongation during budding; and *molds* are multicellular fungi composed of tubular hyphae, either septate or nonseptate, that grow by branching and apical extension. Yeasts may also form hyphae under certain circumstances. The branching hyphae of molds can form a *mycelium,* an interconnected network of hyphae. *Septate fungi* are distinguished by walls that divide the filaments into separate cells, each containing one or more nuclei (Fig 6-5). *Dimorphic fungi* grow in two distinct forms as a result of changes in cell wall synthesis in different environments. Such fungi may appear as yeast in the host and as molds in a room-temperature laboratory. Dimorphic fungi may be highly virulent pathogens. Fungal cells walls stain with Gomori methenamine silver but, except for *Candida,* do not take up Gram stain. Classification of filamentous fungi is based on microscopic features of *conidia* (fungal elements that form asexually) and *conidiophores* (the specialized hyphae where conidia are formed). Most antifungal medications target the sterol-containing cell membrane within the fungal cell wall.

Yeasts

***Candida* species** The incidence of mycotic infections in general and yeasts in particular has risen concomitantly with the advent of extensive antibiotic usage in the general population and is closely associated with immunosuppression, whether due to disease or medical therapy. *Candida* species are ubiquitous in the environment and can be isolated in the absence of clinical disease from the gastrointestinal and genitourinary tracts, the oropharynx, and the skin. *C albicans* is the yeast most commonly isolated from each of these sites. *C albicans* (Fig 6-6) and other *Candida* species cause ocular infections in immunocompromised hosts and in corneas with chronic ulceration from other causes. Ocular topical corticosteroids reduce local cell-mediated immunity and may predispose the cornea to fungal infection. *Candida* species can be isolated on blood agar and common fungal growth media.

Binding to host tissues is a prerequisite for infection; and *C albicans* mannan protein, fibrinogen-binding protein, and a primitive integrin-like protein facilitate adhesion to target tissues. The transformation to a hyphal form and the expression of aspartyl pro-

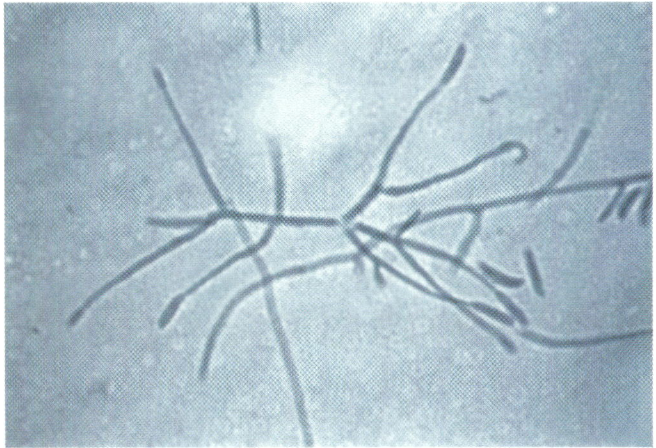

Figure 6-5 Septate hyphae of filamentous fungus (*Fusarium solani.* Gram ×1000). *(Photograph courtesy of Vincent P. deLuise, MD.)*

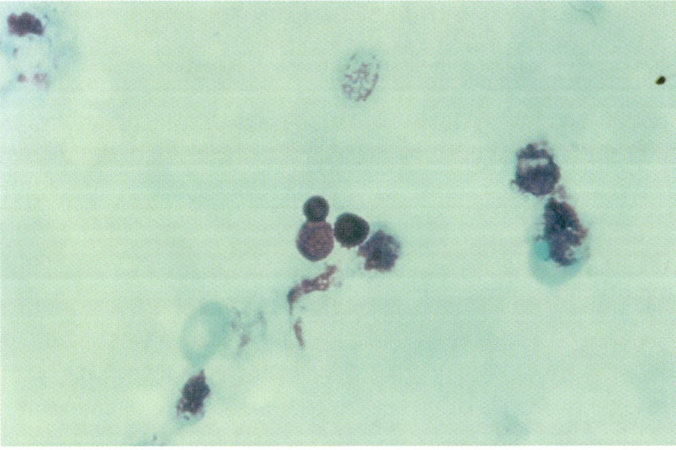

Figure 6-6 Yeasts (*Candida albicans.* Gram ×1000). *(Photograph courtesy of James Chodosh, MD.)*

teases and phospholipases (the latter at the hyphal tip) facilitate penetration of *C albicans* through tissue barriers.

Cryptococcus neoformans is acquired through inhalation and causes subclinical infection of the pulmonary tract. Clinical cryptococcal disease in the brain and optic nerve, eye, lung, skin, and prostate occur in immunosuppressed patients.

Rhinosporidium seeberi organisms are present in soil and groundwater and presumably infect humans through contact with these sources. Ocular rhinosporidiosis manifests as sessile or pedunculated papillomatous or polypoid lesions in the conjunctiva, which may be associated with similar lesions in the nose and nasopharynx.

Septate filamentous fungi

Fusarium species such as *F solani* and *F oxysporum* are encountered in warm, humid environments and can cause a fulminant keratitis. Most other filamentous fungal corneal infections are more indolent. Among the genera that have been isolated from the external eye are *Aspergillus*, *Curvularia*, *Paecilomyces*, and *Phialophora*. Most cases of oculomycosis follow trauma with vegetative matter. Isolation of filamentous fungi may be achieved on blood agar and other standard media, but room-temperature incubation of specimens on Sabouraud agar or brain–heart infusion broth allows better morphologic classification. Several weeks may be required to cultivate some slow-growing fungi.

Nonseptate filamentous fungi

These include the *Mucor, Rhizopus,* and *Absidia* species in class Zygomycetes, order Mucorales, family Mucoraceae. These ubiquitous fungi cause life-threatening infections of the paranasal sinuses, brain, and orbit in immunocompromised patients, with particular predilection for those with failure of normal phagocytic responses due to acidosis from diabetes mellitus or renal failure. Fungal invasion of blood vessels results in ischemic necrosis of affected tissues.

Pneumocystis carinii was formerly classified as a protozoa, but gene sequencing placed the organism firmly in the Fungi kingdom. Pneumocystosis remains one of the primary conditions associated with HIV infection and is an important cause of choroiditis in affected individuals.

> Wilson LA, Ajello L. Agents of oculomycosis: fungal infections of the eye. In: Collier L, Balows A, Sussman M, eds. *Topley & Wilson's Microbiology and Microbial Infections.* Volume 4, *Medical Mycology,* edited by Ajello L, Hay RJ. London: Arnold; 1998:chapter 28, pp 525–567.

Parasitology

Protozoa

Acanthamoeba species are aquatic protozoa (unicellular eukaryotes) that infect the human cornea and brain with potentially devastating results. The *Acanthamoeba* life cycle includes the motile trophozoite (15–45 μm in diameter) and the dormant cyst (10–25 μm in diameter) forms (Fig 6-7). Free-living amoebae are found in both forms, but only the trophozoite is infectious. Both forms are found in infected human tissues. Cysts are double walled and very resistant to environmental stressors. *Acanthamoeba* species are

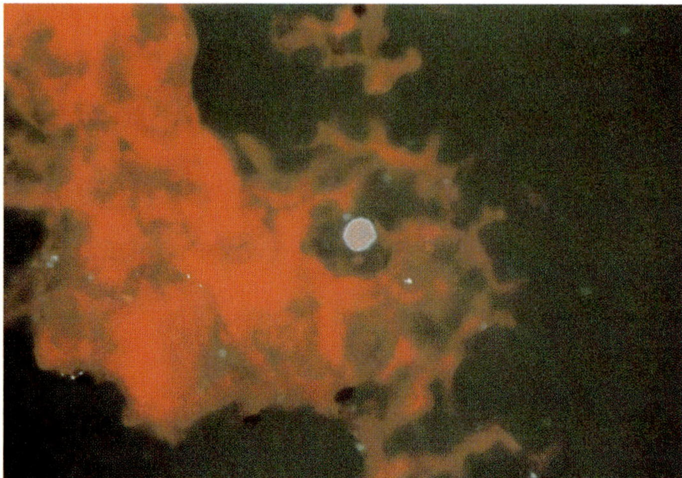

Figure 6-7 Amebic cyst (*Acanthamoeba polyphaga.* Calcofluor white ×1000).

differentiated from one another on the basis of their cyst morphology and antigenic composition.

Laboratory diagnosis of *Acanthamoeba* depends on recovery and identification of organisms with appropriate morphology, size, and staining characteristics. Either corneal scrapings (for chemical stain and culture) or corneal biopsy (for histochemistry) can be used. *Acanthamoebae* grow on many standard media including blood agar, but isolation is facilitated by the use of nonnutrient agar with an overlay of heat-killed *E coli.* Careful inspection of agar plates may reveal trophozoite tracks across the surface of the media. *Acanthamoeba* organisms are identified under a fluorescent microscope after staining of corneal epithelial scrapings with calcofluor white (cysts) or acridine orange (cysts and trophozoites), but can also be visualized with hematoxylin-eosin or periodic acid–Schiff (PAS) stains and, less commonly, on a Gram or Giemsa stain.

Microsporida are obligate intracellular parasites with a unique means of infection. *Microsporida* spores enter eukaryotic cells through a polar tube that opens a hole in the eukaryotic cell membrane and allows the infectious sporoplasm to enter the cell. Growth and differentiation of the sporoplasm result in the formation of intracellular spores that may be liberated by lysis of the host cell. Microsporidial epithelial keratitis occurs almost exclusively in immunosuppressed patients, most commonly in association with AIDS. Although the spores may stain with commonly used chemical stains, including Gram and Giemsa, electron microscopy of corneal scrapings is the most reliable way to definitively demonstrate *Microsporida.*

Toxoplasma gondii causes one of the most common parasitic infections of humans and is a common cause of chorioretinitis (see BCSC Section 9). Cats shed oocysts in their feces after ingestion of *T gondii.* Oocysts may be ingested by human food animals such as swine, and the cyst-containing meat of these animals eaten by humans. Alternatively, cysts may be ingested directly by human contact with cat feces or feces-contaminated water. Transplacental transmission to the fetus of *T gondii* tachyzoites can result in a devastating fetal infection. See BCSC Section 6, *Pediatric Ophthalmology and Strabismus*, for discussion of the consequences of maternal transmission of toxoplasmosis.

***Leishmania* species** Cutaneous leishmaniasis is transmitted at the bite of its vector, the female sandfly, in endemic areas of tropical Asia, Africa, and Latin America. *Leishmania* organisms hide within the phagolysosomal system of macrophages. An infected eyelid ulcer may become granulomatous. Scrapings or biopsy material can show intracellular parasites by Giemsa or immunofluorescent stains. The parasites can sometimes be isolated on blood agar or insect tissue culture medium.

Helminths

Onchocerca volvulus Onchocercal filariae are transmitted by the bite of the blackfly of the genus *Simulium*. This fly lays its eggs on trailing vegetation in fast-flowing rivers (hence the common name *river blindness*) and is endemic in parts of sub-Saharan Africa, the Middle East, and Latin America. Microfilariae penetrate the skin and mature in nodules at the site of the fly bite. Maturation to the point of mating and microfilariae production takes approximately 1 year, and worms can live as long as 15 years in the human host. The adult female worm may grow to 100 cm long and liberates as many as 1500 microfilariae each day. Skin snips examined microscopically may demonstrate microfilariae of approximately 300 μm in length.

Migration of microfilariae to the skin and eye results in clinical onchocerciasis, and subsequent blackfly bites can carry the organism to others. Microfilariae may enter the peripheral cornea and reach the inner eye. Keratitis (including punctate keratitis and "snowflake" and sclerosing peripheral corneal opacities), anterior uveitis, and chorioretinitis occur upon death of the microfilariae. Onchocerciasis is cumulative; the severity of disease depends on the degree of exposure to blackfly bites and the density of microfilariae in the tissues. Treatment by nodulectomy, oral ivermectin, and control of local blackfly populations has been successful in selected areas. See *International Ophthalmology*, a BCSC companion book, for fuller discussion and illustrations.

Loa loa larvae enter the skin at the bite of an infected *Chrysops* (mango horsefly). Adult worms may grow to 6 cm in length and migrate through the connective tissues, causing transient hypersensitivity reactions. *Loa loa* may appear beneath the conjunctiva.

***Toxocara* species** Visceral larval migrans is a multisystem disease in young children caused by migrating larvae of *T canis* and *T cati*, natural residents of dogs and cats, respectively. *Toxocara* larvae develop and mate in the intestines of their natural host; human ingestion of fertilized eggs in pet feces results in infection. *Toxocara* larvae in the human intestine do not receive the proper environmental signals and migrate throughout the body, invading and destroying tissues as they go. Ocular larval migrans occurs in older children, and the viscera are typically spared.

Taenia solium, the pork tapeworm, is transmitted to humans from ingestion of undercooked pork containing the cysticercus stage. In the stomach, proteolytic enzymes dissolve the cysticercus capsule. Adult worms attach to the intestinal wall by means of suckers at the head (scolex) and release eggs that then disseminate. A hydatid cyst can subsequently form in various tissues, including the eye and orbit, to cause cysticercosis.

Arthropods

Phthirus pubis Phthiriasis is a venereally acquired crab louse infestation of coarse hair in the pubic, axillary, chest, and facial regions. Adult female crab lice (Fig 6-8) and immature nits on the eyelashes cause blepharoconjunctivitis.

***Demodex* species** *D folliculorum* and *D brevis* inhabit normal superficial hair and eyelash follicles and deeper sebaceous and meibomian glands, respectively. Eyelash colonization increases with age. The organism may be apparent as cylindrical sleeves around eyelash bases and is associated with blepharitis symptoms.

Fly larvae *Myiasis* occurs when maggots invade and feed on the living or dead tissues of humans or animals. *Ophthalmomyiasis* (maggot infestation of the eye) can refer to external or internal infestation and involve almost any ocular tissue. Most myiasis occurs when a female fly lands on the host and deposits eggs or larvae. The larvae of some fly species can penetrate through healthy skin and migrate long distances to infest the eye. Extensive larval infestation of a compromised external eye can result in total destruction of orbital contents.

Collier L, Balows A, Sussman M, eds. *Topley & Wilson's Microbiology and Microbial Infections.* Volume 5, *Parasitology,* edited by Cox FEG, Kreier JP, Wakelin D. London: Arnold; 1998.

Prions

Prions are altered proteins that cause transmissible lethal encephalopathies, including Creutzfeldt-Jakob disease, scrapie in sheep, bovine spongiform encephalitis, and kuru.

Prusiner SB. Shattuck Lecture—Neurodegenerative diseases and prions. *N Engl J Med.* 2001;344:1516–1526.

Diagnostic Laboratory Techniques

The decision to procure clinical specimens for culture, antigen detection, or special chemical stains is based on the likelihood of benefit to the patient's condition. Interpretation of diagnostic specimens requires an understanding of the normal flora and cytology of the ocular surface. Appropriate materials should be available for optimal specimen collection (Table 6-3). The reader is encouraged to also review the discussion of specimen collection and handling in BCSC Section 4, *Ophthalmic Pathology and Intraocular Tumors.*

Specimen Collection and Culturing

See also Chapter 4, Table 4-2, in this volume.

Eyelid specimens

Eyelid vesicles or pustules may be opened with a sharp-pointed surgical blade or small-gauge needle. Material for cytology is smeared onto a glass slide and fixed in methanol or acetone for immunofluorescent staining. Collected vesicular fluid can be inoculated

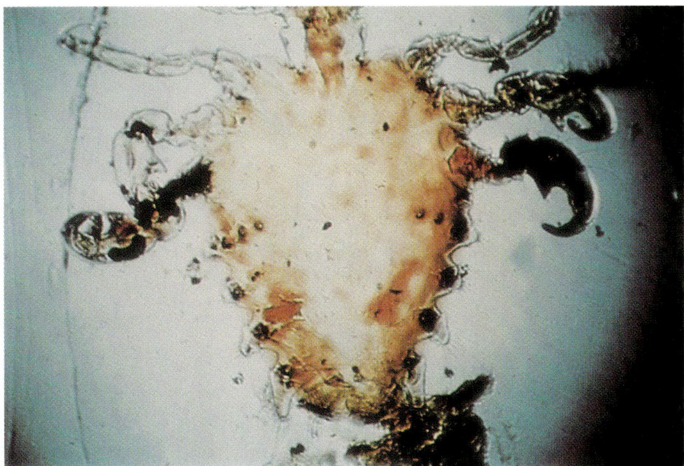

Figure 6-8 Crab louse (*Phthirus pubis.* Wet mount ×200).

Table 6-3 Materials for Collecting Eyelid, Conjunctival, and Corneal Specimens for Ocular Microbiology

Viral Infections	Chlamydial Infections	Microbial Infections
Topical anesthetic	Topical anesthetic	Topical anesthetic
Dacron swabs	Dacron swabs	Calcium alginate or Dacron swabs
Spatula	Saptula	Spatula
Glass slides	Glass slides	Glass slides
Acetone fixative	Methanol or acetone fixative	Methanol fixative
Viral transport medium	Chlamydial transport medium	Blood agar plate
Ice	Ice	Chocolate agar plate
		Thioglycollate or chopped-meat broth
		Sabouraud's dextrose agar plate
		Special media:
		Anaerobic plate
		Brain–heart infusion broth
		Mycobacterial medium
		Nonnutrient agar plate

into chilled viral transport medium for culture isolation in the laboratory. Microbial cultures are obtained by swabbing the abnormal area with a thioglycollate-moistened swab followed by direct inoculation of culture media.

Conjunctival specimens

Specimen collection must debride enough surface conjunctival epithelial cells so that intracellular microbes can be visualized on chemical stains. Sterile Dacron swabs slightly moistened with thioglycollate broth may be used to optimize recovery of microbial specimens. The swabbed material should initially be plated directly onto warmed solid media (blood, chocolate, and Sabouraud's). Then, the "nonhandled" distal end of the swab may be broken off and placed directly into the remaining thioglycollate broth tube. If these media are not available, then specimens should be harvested with any standard Culterette tube system that contains appropriate transport media. The specimen should be sent immediately to any qualified microbiology laboratory for processing.

Conjunctival biopsy can also be performed to assist in the diagnosis of conditions such as Parinaud oculoglandular syndrome or cicatricial pemphigoid. See also Chapter 4.

Corneal specimens

A microbial specimen can be collected from a corneal ulcer by scraping the lesion with a platinum Kimura spatula, sterile needle, surgical blade, or thioglycollate-moistened calcium alginate or Dacron swab. A blade or spatula is preferable for preparation of smears for chemical staining, but either a spatula or swab is acceptable for inoculation of culture media; a combination of techniques may provide added benefit when a paucity of microorganisms is present. Furthermore, because growth patterns on culture media vary among different bacterial species, the material obtained from the corneal ulcer should be used to inoculate microscope slides for stained smears and several different culture media.

Specimens are best inoculated immediately onto microbiologic media that has been warmed to room temperature in anticipation of the culture procedure. To avoid contamination and false positives, care must be taken to avoid touching the blade or swab to the eyelids, and a sterile instrument or swab should be used for each row of C-shaped streaks on each agar plate (Fig 6-9) and for each type of broth culture. For viral culture, a Dacron swab used to obtain viral-infected corneal or conjunctival cells is agitated in chilled viral transport media and discarded. Calcium alginate and cotton swabs should be avoided as the calcium alginate and the wooden shaft of cotton swabs both may inhibit viral recovery.

Corneal biopsy may be necessary in cases of apparent and significant microbial infection when repeated corneal scrapings are negative. A small 2–3 mm trephine (disposable dermatologic skin punch) can be used to create a partial-thickness incision, and

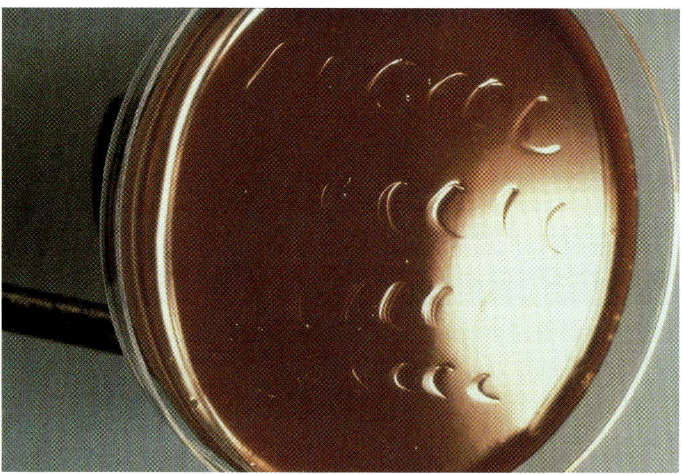

Figure 6-9 "C" streaks on a chocolate blood agar plate. *(Photograph courtesy of James Chodosh, MD.)*

forceps and scissors are used to excise a lamellar flap of cornea. The specimen is generally split in two pieces or separate biopsies taken so that tissue can be evaluated by both histopathology and microbiology.

Isolation techniques

For viral and chlamydial infections, an appropriate tissue-culture cell line is selected for inoculation and examined for the development of cytopathic effects (CPE) and cellular inclusions. For bacterial and fungal infections, directly inoculated blood, chocolate, and Sabouraud's agar and thioglycollate broth are examined daily to detect visible growth. Microorganisms are studied by chemical staining, chemical reactions, and antimicrobial sensitivity testing. *Acanthamoebae* may be identified by trophozoite trails on blood agar, but nonnutrient agar with an overlay of killed *E coli* is the optimal isolation media.

Alexandrakis G, Haimovici R, Miller D, et al. Corneal biopsy in the management of progressive microbial keratitis. *Am J Ophthalmol.* 2000;129:571–576.

Staining Methods

Chapter 4, Diagnostic Approach to Ocular Surface Disease, gives step-by-step procedures for commonly used stains (Table 4-2). See Table 6-4 for recommended stains and media in the setting of suspected microbial keratitis.

Wilhelmus KR, Liesegang TJ, Osato MS, et al. *Laboratory Diagnosis of Ocular Infections.* Washington, DC: American Society for Microbiology; 1994.

Table 6-4 Recommended Stains and Culture Media for Microbial Keratitis

Suspected Organism	Stain	Media
Aerobic bacteria	Gram Acridine orange	Blood agar Chocolate agar Thioglycollate broth
Anaerobic bacteria	Gram Acridine orange	Anaerobic blood agar Phenylethyl alcohol agar in anaerobic chamber Thioglycollate broth
Mycobacteria	Gram Acid-fast Lectin	Blood agar Lowenstein-Jensen agar
Fungi	Gram Acridine orange Calcofluor white	Blood agar (25°C) Sabouraud's agar (25°C) Brain–heart infusion (25°C)
Acanthamoeba	Acridine orange Calcofluor white	Nonnutrient agar with *E coli* overlay Blood agar Buffered charcoal–yeast extract agar

Infectious Diseases of the External Eye: Clinical Aspects

A detailed history and physical examination are essential to proper diagnosis of external eye infections. The patient's chief complaint and a complete systemic and ocular history, including the presence of risk factors for infections of the external eye, should be noted. A complete eye examination should include special attention to the skin of the face and eyelids, the preauricular lymph nodes, the globe-orbit relationship, ocular discharge, and conjunctival and corneal morphology. Diagnostic tests are chosen to differentiate between likely diagnostic entities and to assist in therapy (eg, antimicrobial sensitivity testing in microbial keratitis).

Viral Infections

Molluscum Contagiosum

PATHOGENESIS Molluscum contagiosum virus is spread by direct contact with infected individuals. Infection produces one or more umbilicated nodules on the skin and eyelid margin and, less commonly, on the conjunctiva. Eyelid nodules release viral particles into the tear film.

CLINICAL PRESENTATION A molluscum nodule is smooth with an umbilicated central core. It is smaller and associated with less inflammation than a keratoacanthoma. Punctate epithelial erosions and, rarely, a corneal pannus may occur. Any chronic follicular conjunctivitis should instigate a careful search for lid margin molluscum lesions (Fig 7-1).

LABORATORY EVALUATION AND MANAGEMENT Molluscum contagiosum virus cannot be cultured using standard techniques. Diagnosis is based on the detection of the characteristic eyelid lesions in the presence of a follicular conjunctivitis. Spontaneous resolution occurs but can take months to years. Treatment options include complete excision, cryotherapy, or incision of the central portion of the lesion. Extensive facial and eyelid molluscum lesions occur in association with AIDS (Fig 7-2).

Other Virus-Associated Neoplasms of the Eyelid and Conjunctiva

Verrucae and *papillomas* are caused by papillomavirus infection of the skin and conjunctival epithelium. Venereally acquired conjunctival papillomas resemble those on the lar-

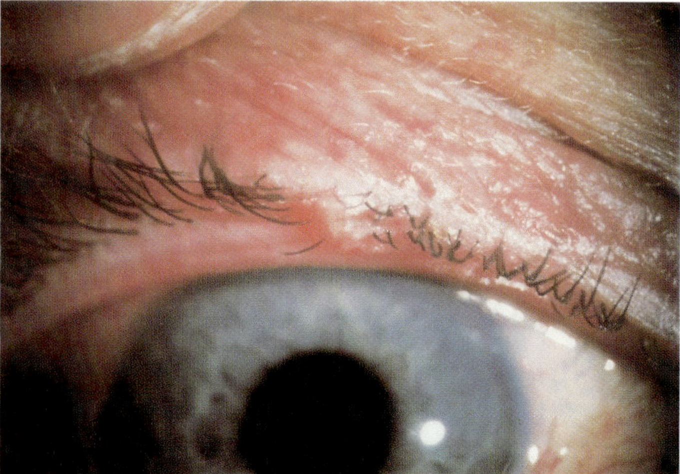

Figure 7-1 Single nodule of molluscum contagiosum at the upper eyelid margin.

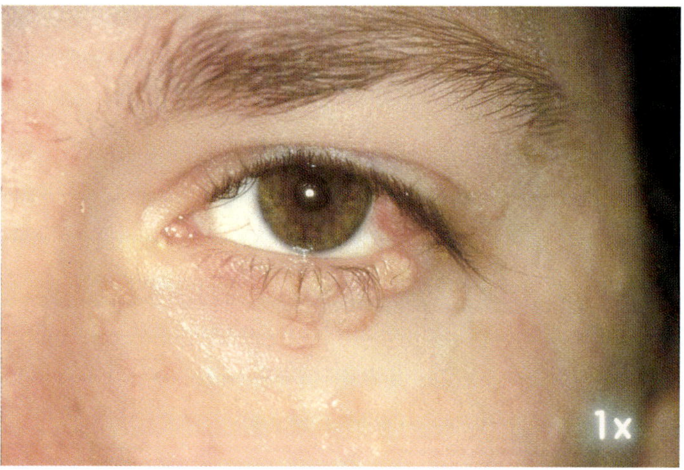

Figure 7-2 Multiple molluscum contagiosum lesions on the eyelid of a patient with AIDS. *(Photograph courtesy of James Chodosh, MD.)*

ynx and urogenital tract. Papillomavirus-associated conjunctival intraepithelial neoplasia and squamous cell carcinoma share many histologic features with similar lesions in the uterine cervix. Another neoplasm, *Kaposi sarcoma* of the skin or conjunctiva, is associated with infection by human herpesvirus type 8. These entities are discussed in greater detail in Chapter 10.

Adenoviral Keratoconjunctivitis

PATHOGENESIS Originally isolated in 1953 from surgically removed human adenoids, adenoviruses cause a broad spectrum of disease including infections of the upper respiratory tract and ocular surface, meningoencephalitis, acute hemorrhagic cystitis of young boys, diarrhea of children, acute respiratory disease of children and military recruits, and respiratory and hepatic failure in the immunocompromised host. Adenoviruses are transmitted by close contact with ocular or respiratory secretions, fomites, or contaminated swimming pools. Transmission occurs more readily in populations living in close quarters, such as schools, nursing homes, military housing, and summer camps. Transmission of adenoviruses by contaminated instruments or eyedrops in physicians' offices is a major source of infectious outbreaks.

CLINICAL PRESENTATION Each subgroup (A–F) and, to a lesser degree, each serotype possesses unique tissue tropisms that reveal the association of specific adenoviruses with distinct clinical syndromes. Most adenoviral eye disease presents clinically as one of three classic syndromes:

- Simple follicular conjunctivitis (multiple serotypes)
- Pharyngoconjunctival fever (most commonly serotypes 3 or 7)
- Epidemic keratoconjunctivitis (EKC; usually serotypes 8, 19, or 37, subgroup D)

Different adenoviral syndromes are indistinguishable early in infection and may be unilateral or bilateral.

Adenoviral follicular conjunctivitis is self-limited, not associated with systemic disease, and often so transient that patients do not seek care. Epithelial keratitis, if present, is mild and fleeting. *Pharyngoconjunctival fever* is characterized by fever, headache, pharyngitis, follicular conjunctivitis, and preauricular adenopathy. The systemic signs and symptoms may mimic influenza. Any associated epithelial keratitis is mild.

Epidemic keratoconjunctivitis is the only adenoviral syndrome with significant corneal involvement. The infection is bilateral in a majority of patients and may be preceded by an upper respiratory infection. One week to 10 days after inoculation, severe follicular conjunctivitis develops, associated with a punctate epithelial keratitis. The conjunctival morphology is follicular but may be obscured by chemosis. Petechial hemorrhages and, occasionally, larger subconjunctival hemorrhages can occur. Preauricular adenopathy is prominent. Pseudomembranes or frank membranes (Fig 7-3) occur predominantly on the tarsal conjunctiva and may be missed on cursory exam. Patients complain of tearing, light sensitivity, and foreign body sensation. Large central geographic corneal erosions can develop and may persist for several days despite patching and lubrication. Within 7–14 days after onset of eye symptoms, multifocal subepithelial (stromal) corneal infiltrates become apparent on slit-lamp examination (Fig 7-4). Photophobia and reduced vision from adenoviral subepithelial infiltrates may persist for months to years.

Epithelial keratitis occurs due to adenovirus replication within the corneal epithelium. Subepithelial infiltrates are likely caused by an immunopathologic response to viral infection of keratocytes in the superficial corneal stroma. The evolution of keratitis in EKC is summarized in Figure 7-5. Chronic complications of conjunctival membranes include subepithelial conjunctival scarring, symblepharon formation, and dry eye due to alterations within the lacrimal glands or lacrimal ducts.

LABORATORY EVALUATION Diagnosis of EKC is suggested in the setting of bilateral follicular conjunctivitis associated with petechial conjunctival hemorrhages, conjunctival pseu-

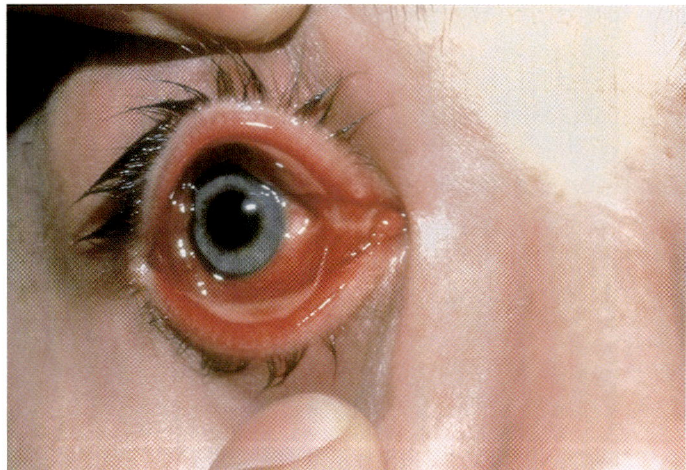

Figure 7-3 Conjunctival membranes in a patient with EKC. *(Photograph courtesy of James Chodosh, MD.)*

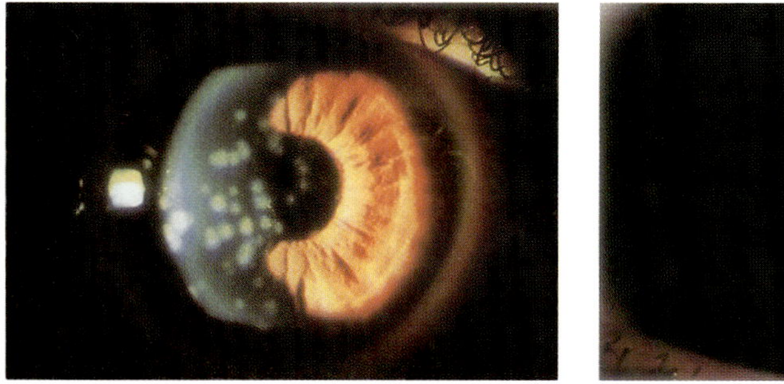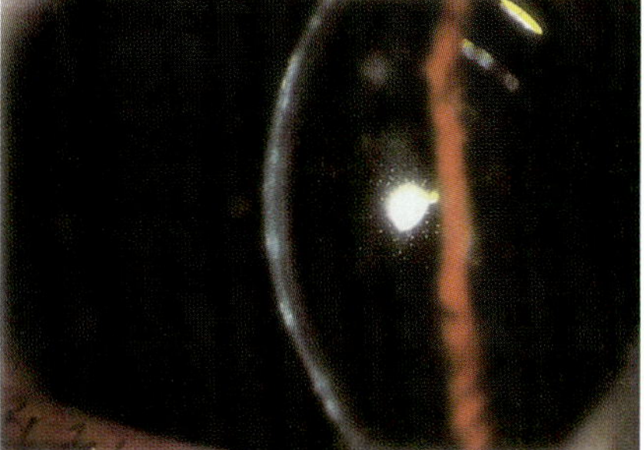

Figure 7-4 Subepithelial corneal infiltrates in a patient with EKC. *(Photographs courtesy of Vincent P. deLuise, MD.)*

domembrane or frank membrane formation, or later on in the clinical course, the presence of bilateral subepithelial infiltrates. Other adenoviral ocular syndromes have less specific signs, but laboratory diagnosis is only rarely indicated. Although viral cultures readily differentiate adenovirus from herpes simplex virus infection, the clinical disease typically subsides or resolves before results become available. Rapid immunodetection assays to detect adenovirus antigens in clinical ocular specimens are under development. Paired serologic titers 2–3 weeks apart allow confirmation of acute adenovirus infection, but this test is rarely performed.

MANAGEMENT Therapy for adenoviral ocular infection is primarily supportive. Cool compresses and artificial tears may provide symptomatic relief. Topical antibiotics may be indicated only when the clinical signs, such as mucopurulent discharge, suggest an associated bacterial infection or when a viral cause is less certain. The antiviral drug ci-

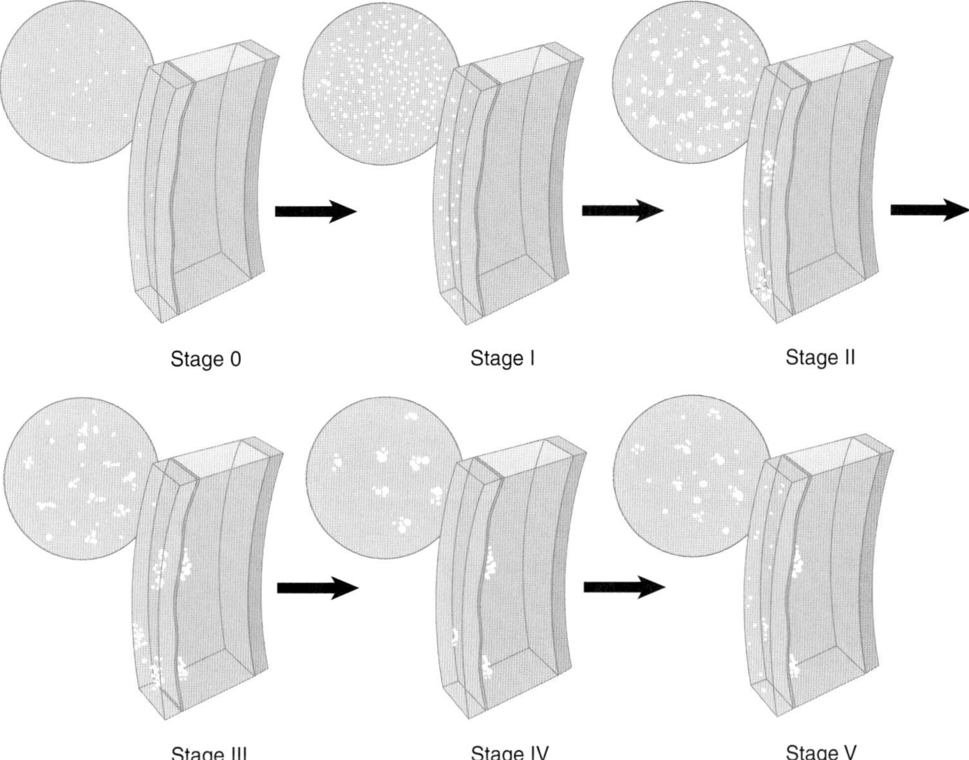

Figure 7-5 Schematic drawing illustrating the natural progression of specific corneal epithelial and stromal pathology in EKC. Epithelial changes proceed from fine punctate epithelial keratitis to coarse punctate epithelial keratitis that stains brightly with rose bengal (first week of infection). Epithelial keratitis resolves soon after the development of subepithelial stromal infiltrates (second week of infection), but late punctate epithelial granularity can occur both adjacent to and distinct from the subepithelial infiltrates. The stages demonstrated are as follows: *Stage 0* (dubium): Poorly staining, minute punctate opacities within the corneal epithelium. *Stage I,* Fine punctate epithelial keratitis (PEK). *Stage II,* Fine and coarse PEK. Stains brightly with rose bengal. *Stage III,* Coarse granular infiltrates within deep epithelium, early subepithelial infiltrates, diminished PEK. *Stage IV,* Classic subepithelial infiltrates without PEK. *Stage V,* Punctate epithelial granularity adjacent to and distinct from the subepithelial infiltrates. *(Adapted from Jones DB, Matoba AY, Wilhelmus KR. Problem solving in corneal and external diseases. Course 626, presented at the American Academy of Ophthalmology. Atlanta, GA; 1995.)*

dofovir blocks replication of adenoviruses but has substantial toxicity and is not FDA approved.

For patients with conjunctival membranes due to EKC, manual removal by the physician with a forceps or cotton swab every 2–3 days, combined with judicious use of topical corticosteroids, may speed resolution and prevent scarring. Topical corticosteroids also reduce photophobia and improve vision impaired by adenoviral subepithelial infiltrates. Because corticosteroids may prolong viral shedding from adenovirus-infected patients and can lead to worsening of herpes simplex infections, their use should be reserved for patients with specific clinical signs of adenovirus infection who present with specific indications for treatment, including conjunctival membranes or photophobia and reduced vision due to bilateral subepithelial infiltrates. Nonsteroidal anti-inflammatory agents are ineffective therapy for adenoviral subepithelial infiltrates, but they may be helpful in preventing recurrence following tapering of steroids.

Actively infected persons readily transmit adenoviruses. Viral shedding may persist for 10–14 days after onset of clinical signs and symptoms. Transmission can be prevented by personal hygiene measures including frequent handwashing; cleaning of towels, pillowcases, and handkerchiefs; and disposal of contaminated facial tissues. Individuals who work with the public, in schools, or in health care facilities in particular should consider a temporary leave of absence from work to prevent infection of others, especially those who are already ill.

Enterovirus and Coxsackievirus Conjunctivitis

Acute hemorrhagic conjunctivitis (AHC), caused by enterovirus type 70 and coxsackievirus A24 variant, and less commonly adenovirus type 11, is one of the most dramatic ocular viral syndromes. Sudden onset of follicular conjunctivitis associated with multiple petechial hemorrhages of bulbar and tarsal conjunctiva characterizes AHC. The hemorrhages may become confluent and appear posttraumatic. Eyelid edema, preauricular adenopathy, chemosis, and punctate epithelial keratitis may be associated with infection. AHC is highly contagious and occurs in large and rapidly spreading epidemics. In approximately 1 out of 10,000 cases due to enterovirus type 70, a polio-like paralysis follows; neurologic deficits are permanent in up to one third of affected individuals.

Herpes Simplex Eye Diseases

PATHOGENESIS Herpes simplex virus (HSV) infection is ubiquitous in humans; almost the entire human population shows serologic evidence of infection by middle age, and nearly 100% of those older than 60 years of age harbor HSV in their trigeminal ganglia at autopsy. It has been estimated that one third of the world population suffers from recurrent infection. Therefore, HSV infections represent a large and worldwide public health problem.

HSV type 1 (HSV-1) and type 2 (HSV-2) are antigenically related and may coinfect the same nerve ganglia. HSV-1 more commonly causes infection above the waist (orofacial and ocular infection), and HSV-2 below the waist (genital infection), but either virus can cause disease in either location. In industrialized societies, 50%–90% of adults have serum antibodies to HSV-1, but the age of serologic conversion is increasing. HSV infection is spread by direct contact with infected lesions or their secretions but most commonly occurs as a result of exposure to viruses shed asymptomatically. HSV can be transmitted to neonates as they pass through the birth canal of a mother with genital infection and, in the newborn, can cause disease confined to the skin and mucous membranes or systemic infection including encephalitis. BCSC Section 6 , *Pediatric Ophthalmology and Strabismus,* discusses neonatal herpes infection in greater detail.

Primary HSV-1 infection in humans occurs most commonly on skin and mucosal surfaces innervated by the cranial nerve V (trigeminal nerve). Primary infection frequently manifests as a nonspecific upper respiratory tract infection and is recognized as

HSV less than 5% of the time. HSV spreads from infected skin and mucosal epithelium via sensory nerve axons to establish latent infection in associated sensory nerve ganglia, including the trigeminal ganglion. Latent infection of the trigeminal ganglion occurs in the absence of recognized primary infection, and reactivation of virus may follow in any of the three branches of CN V despite primary disease in the area of innervation of one particular branch. Approximately 0.15% of the U.S. population has a history of external ocular HSV infection, and of these approximately one fifth develop stromal keratitis, the most common blinding manifestation of infection.

Liesegang TJ. Herpes simplex virus epidemiology and ocular importance. *Cornea.* 2001; 20:1–13.

Primary ocular infections

CLINICAL PRESENTATION Primary ocular HSV infection typically manifests as a unilateral blepharoconjunctivitis. The conjunctival inflammatory response is follicular and accompanied by a palpable preauricular lymph node. Vesicles on the skin (Fig 7-6) or eyelid margin (Fig 7-7) are important for diagnosis. Patients with primary ocular HSV infection can develop epithelial keratitis (see below), but stromal keratitis and uveitis are uncommon.

Signs that can be used to distinguish acute HSV ocular infection from that associated with adenovirus include:

- Cutaneous or eyelid margin vesicles, or ulcers on the bulbar conjunctiva (HSV)
- Dendritic epithelial keratitis (HSV)
- Conjunctival membranes or pseudomembranes (adenovirus)

Laterality is not a reliable distinguishing feature. Although adenoviral infections are more commonly bilateral, they can be unilateral, asymmetric, or bilateral with delayed involvement of the second eye. HSV ocular infection is typically unilateral but can be bilateral in up to 10% of cases, most commonly in patients with underlying atopic disease.

LABORATORY EVALUATION Demonstration of HSV is possible in productive epithelial infection with viral culture or antigen- or DNA-detection methodologies. Serologic tests for neutralizing or complement-fixing immunoglobulins may show a rising antibody titer

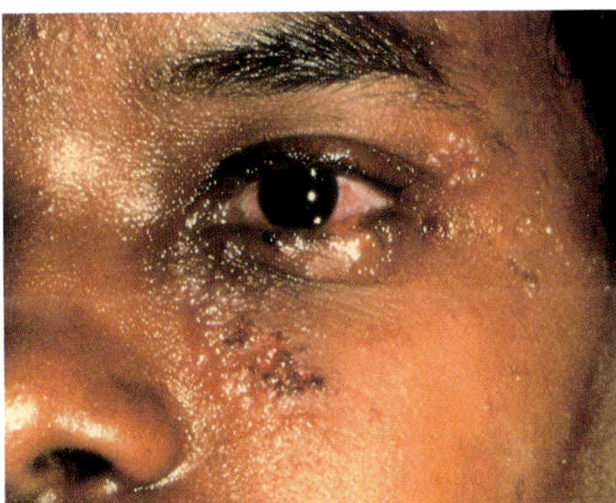

Figure 7-6 Skin vesicles of HSV dermatoblepharitis. *(Photograph courtesy of James Chodosh, MD.)*

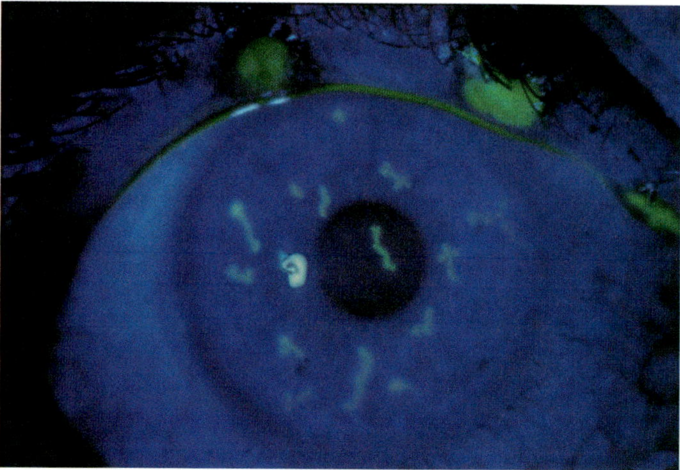

Figure 7-7 Fluorescein staining of eye with primary HSV infection demonstrates characteristic lid margin ulcers and a coarse dendritic epithelial keratitis. *(Photograph courtesy of James Chodosh, MD.)*

during primary infection but are of no diagnostic assistance during recurrent episodes. The vast majority of adults are latently infected with HSV and therefore antibody-positive. Therefore, serologic testing generally is helpful only when negative.

Laboratory tests are indicated in complicated cases when the clinical diagnosis is uncertain, and in all cases of suspected neonatal herpes infection. Vesicles can be opened with a needle, and vesicular fluid cultured. Scrapings from the vesicle base can be tested by cytology or for the presence of HSV antigen. Conjunctival scrapings or impression cytology specimens can be similarly analyzed by culture, antigen detection, or polymerase chain reaction (PCR).

MANAGEMENT (See Table 7-1 for summary of antiviral agents effective against HSV infections.) Primary ocular HSV infection is a self-limited condition. Oral antiviral therapy speeds resolution of signs and symptoms. Topical antiviral therapy with vidarabine ointment is sufficient for infection limited to the conjunctiva.

Recurrent ocular infection

PATHOGENESIS Recurrent lytic HSV infection is caused by reactivation of the virus in latently infected sensory ganglion, transport of virus down the nerve axon to sensory nerve endings, and subsequent infection of ocular surface epithelia. HSV latency in the cornea as a cause of recurrent disease remains a controversial concept.

Anecdotal reports that environmental factors act as triggers for recurrence of HSV ocular disease were not confirmed by a recent prospective multicenter trial. Neither psychologic stress, systemic infection, sunlight exposure, menstrual cycle, nor contact lens wear was demonstrated to induce recurrent ocular HSV infection. An increased rate of recurrence for HSV keratitis was associated with HIV infection in a retrospective study. Interestingly, no difference in the severity of HSV keratitis was found comparing HIV-infected to uninfected persons, despite the observed discrepancy in recurrence rate.

Table 7-1 Antiviral Agents in External/Corneal Infections With Herpes Simplex Virus

Agent	Mechanism of Action	Administration	Dosage for Acute Disease
Vidarabine	Purine analogue Inhibits DNA polymerase	3% ophthalmic ointment[1]	5×/day for 10 days
Trifluridine	Pyrimidine analogue Blocks DNA synthesis	1% ophthalmic solution	8×/day for 10 days
Acyclovir	Activated by HSV thymidine kinase to inhibit viral DNA polymerase	3% ophthalmic ointment[2] 200, 400, 800 mg; 200 mg/5 mL suspension 5% dermatologic ointment[3]	5×/day for 10 days 400 mg 5×/day for 10 days 6×/day for 7 days
Famciclovir[4]	Pro-drug of penciclovir	125, 250, 500 mg	250 mg 3×/day for 10 days
Valacyclovir[4]	L-valyl ester of acyclovir	500, 1000 mg	1000 mg 2×/day for 10 days
Penciclovir	Inhibits viral DNA polymerase	1% dermatologic cream[3]	8×/day for 4 days

[1] No longer manufactured; can be obtained through compounding pharmacies.
[2] Not commercially available in the United States.
[3] Not for ophthalmic use.
[4] Optimal dose for ocular disease not determined.

> Herpetic Eye Disease Study Group. Psychological stress and other potential triggers for recurrences of herpes simplex virus eye infections. *Arch Ophthalmol.* 2000;118:1617–1625.
> Hodge WG, Margolis TP. Herpes simplex virus keratitis among patients who are positive or negative for human immunodeficiency virus: an epidemiologic study. *Ophthalmology.* 1997;104:120–124.

CLINICAL PRESENTATION Recurrent HSV can affect almost any ocular tissue including the eyelid, conjunctiva, cornea, iris, trabecular meshwork, and retina. The most common presentations of clinically recognizable recurrent ocular HSV infection include:

- Blepharoconjunctivitis
- Epithelial keratitis
- Stromal keratitis
- Iridocyclitis

Blepharoconjunctivitis

Eyelid and/or conjunctival involvement can occur in patients with recurrent ocular HSV infection and is clinically indistinguishable from primary infection. The condition is self-limited but can be treated with antivirals to shorten the course of illness.

Epithelial keratitis

CLINICAL PRESENTATION Patients with epithelial keratitis complain of foreign body sensation, light sensitivity, redness, and blurred vision. HSV infection of human corneal epithelium manifests as areas of punctate epithelial keratitis that may coalesce into one or more arborizing dendritic epithelial ulcers with terminal bulbs at the end of each branch. The cytopathic swollen corneal epithelium at the edge of a herpetic ulcer stains with rose bengal (Fig 7-8) due to loss of cell membrane glycoproteins and subsequent lack of mucin binding by the cells. The bed of the ulcer stains with fluorescein (Fig 7-9) due to loss of cellular integrity and absence of intercellular tight junctions. Particularly with use of topical corticosteroids, areas of dendritic keratitis may coalesce further and enlarge into a more expansive *geographic epithelial ulcer* (Fig 7-10). The swollen epithelium at the ulcer's edge will stain with rose bengal, and frequently, dendritic morphology can be seen at the periphery of the ulcer.

Patients with HSV epithelial keratitis exhibit a ciliary flush and mild conjunctival injection. Mild stromal edema and subepithelial white blood cell infiltration may develop beneath epithelial keratitis. Following resolution of dendritic epithelial keratitis, nonsuppurative subepithelial infiltration and scarring may be seen just beneath the area of prior epithelial ulceration, resulting in a ghost image, or *ghost dendrite* (Fig 7-11), reflecting the position and shape of the prior epithelial involvement. Resolution typically occurs without additional therapy.

Focal or diffuse reduction in corneal sensation develops following HSV epithelial keratitis. The distribution of corneal hypoesthesia is related to the extent, duration, severity, and number of recurrences of herpetic keratitis. Sectoral corneal anesthesia may be difficult to detect clinically and is not a reliable sign of herpetic disease.

Other conditions that may produce dendritiform epithelial lesions include:

- Varicella-zoster virus (see below)
- Adenovirus (uncommon)
- Epstein-Barr virus (rare)
- Epithelial regeneration line
- Neurotrophic keratopathy (postherpetic, diabetes mellitus)

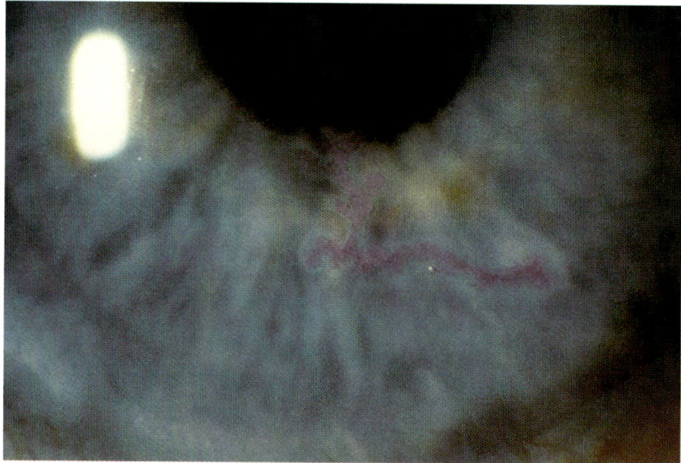

Figure 7-8 Rose bengal staining of herpetic epithelial keratitis outlines a typical dendrite. *(Photograph courtesy of James Chodosh, MD.)*

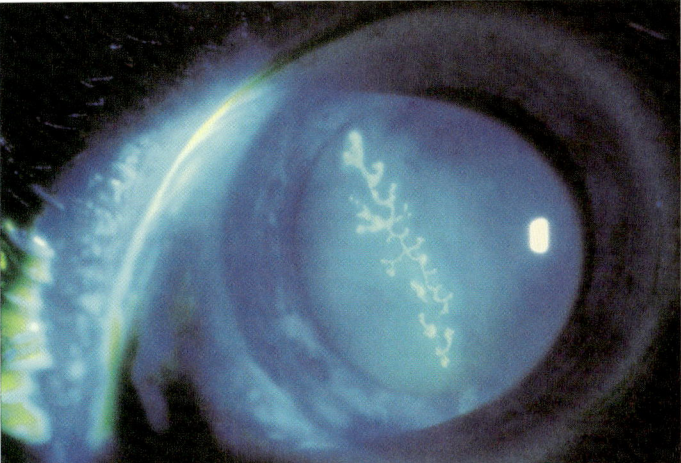

Figure 7-9 Fluorescein staining of herpetic dendritic keratitis. *(Photograph courtesy of James Chodosh, MD.)*

- Soft contact lens wear (thimerosal)
- Topical medications (antivirals, beta blockers)
- *Acanthamoeba*
- Thygeson's superficial punctate keratitis (atypical)
- Epithelial deposits (iron lines, Fabry disease, tyrosinemia type II, systemic drugs)

LABORATORY EVALUATION A specific clinical diagnosis of HSV as the cause of dendritic keratitis can usually be made on the presence of characteristic clinical features. Tissue culture and/or antigen detection techniques may be helpful in establishing the diagnosis in atypical cases.

MANAGEMENT Most cases of HSV epithelial keratitis resolve spontaneously, and there is no evidence to suggest that the form of antiviral therapy influences the subsequent development of stromal keratitis or recurrent epithelial disease. However, treatment shortens the clinical course and might conceivably reduce associated herpetic neuropathy. Minimal wiping debridement of HSV epithelial keratitis with a dry cotton-tipped applicator or cellulose sponge speeds resolution. Antiviral therapy can be used by itself or in combination with epithelial debridement. Topical trifluridine 1% solution eight times daily is efficacious for both dendritic and geographic epithelial keratitis. Vidarabine 3% ointment, previously used for dendritic epithelial keratitis, is no longer manufactured but can still be obtained through some compounding pharmacies. Treatment of HSV epithelial keratitis with topical antivirals generally should be discontinued within 10–14 days to avoid unnecessary toxicity to the ocular surface. Acyclovir 3% ophthalmic ointment has been reported to be as effective as and less toxic than trifluridine and vidarabine for treatment of epithelial keratitis, but the ophthalmic form is not available in the United States. Oral acyclovir has been reported to be as effective as topical antivirals for treatment of epithelial keratitis and, although more expensive, has the advantage of no ocular toxicity. Valacyclovir, a pro-drug of acyclovir likely to be just as effective for ocular disease,

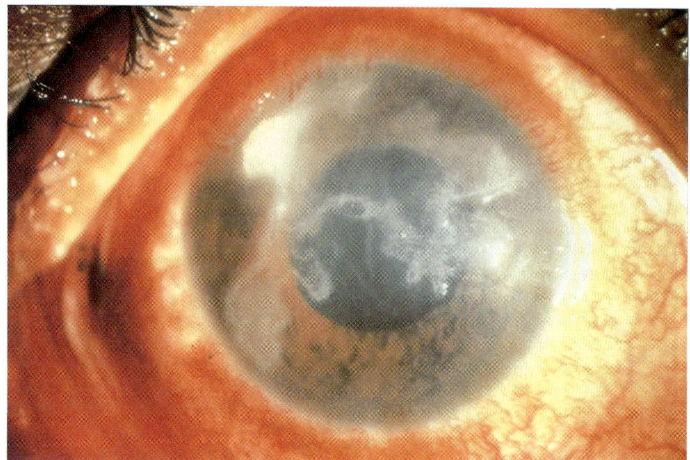

Figure 7-10 Herpetic geographic epithelial keratitis. *(Reprinted with permission from: Chodosh J. Viral keratitis. In: Parrish RK, ed.* The University of Miami Bascom Palmer Eye Institute Atlas of Ophthalmology. *Boston: Current Medicine; 1999.)*

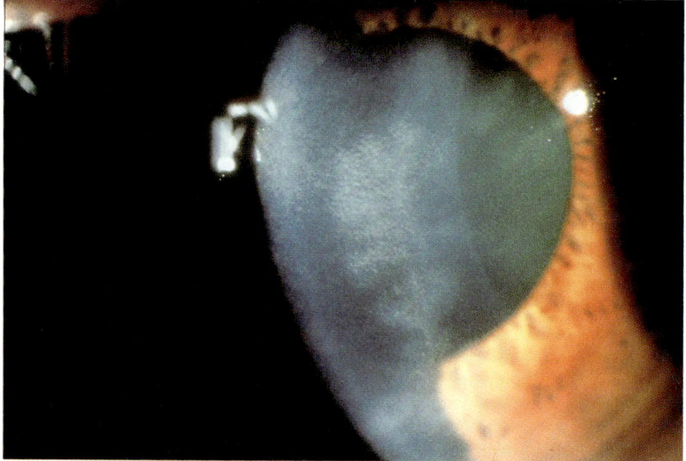

Figure 7-11 Residual stromal inflammation following dendritic epithelial keratitis may leave the impression of a ghost image of the dendrite. *(Reprinted with permission from: Chodosh J. Viral keratitis. In: Parrish RK, ed.* The University of Miami Bascom Palmer Eye Institute Atlas of Ophthalmology. *Boston: Current Medicine; 1999.)*

can cause thrombotic thrombocytopenic purpura/hemolytic uremia syndrome in severely immunocompromised patients such as those with AIDS; thus, it must be used with caution if the immune status is unknown. Topical corticosteroids are contraindicated in the presence of active herpetic epithelial keratitis. Patients with herpetic epithelial keratitis who are using systemic corticosteroids for other indications should be treated aggressively with systemic antiviral therapy.

Stromal keratitis

HSV stromal keratitis is the most common cause of infectious corneal blindness in the United States, and it is the form of recurrent herpetic external disease associated with the greatest visual morbidity. Each episode of stromal keratitis increases the risk of future episodes.

CLINICAL PRESENTATION Herpetic stromal keratitis can be nonnecrotizing (interstitial or disciform) or necrotizing. Different forms of herpetic keratitis may present simultaneously. *Herpetic interstitial keratitis* presents as unifocal or multifocal interstitial haze or whitening of the stroma in the absence of epithelial ulceration (Fig 7-12). Mild stromal edema may accompany the haze, but epithelial edema is not typical. In the absence of significant extracorneal inflammatory signs such as conjunctival injection or anterior chamber cells, it may be difficult to identify active disease in an area of previous scar and thinning. Long-standing or multiply recurrent HSV interstitial keratitis may be associated with corneal vascularization. The differential diagnosis of herpetic interstitial keratitis includes:

- Varicella-zoster virus keratitis
- *Acanthamoeba* keratitis
- Syphilis
- Epstein-Barr virus keratitis
- Mumps keratitis
- Lyme disease
- Sarcoidosis
- Cogan syndrome

Herpetic disciform keratitis presents as corneal stromal and epithelial edema in a round or oval distribution, associated with keratic precipitates underlying the zone of

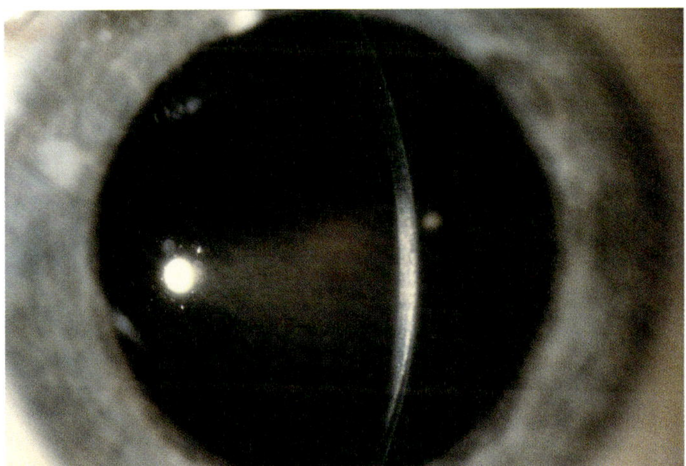

Figure 7-12 Herpetic interstitial keratitis (nonnecrotizing). *(Reprinted with permission from: Chodosh J. Viral keratitis. In: Parrish RK, ed.* The University of Miami Bascom Palmer Eye Institute Atlas of Ophthalmology. *Boston: Current Medicine; 1999.)*

edema (Fig 7-13). Disciform keratitis has also been termed *endotheliitis.* Iridocyclitis can be associated, and the disciform keratitis may be confused with uveitis with secondary corneal endothelial decompensation. However, in disciform keratitis, disc-shaped stromal edema and keratic precipitates appear out of proportion to the degree of anterior chamber reaction. Disciform keratitis due to HSV and VZV are clinically indistinguishable.

Herpetic necrotizing keratitis appears as suppurative corneal inflammation (Fig 7-14). It may be severe, progress rapidly, and appear clinically indistinguishable from fulminant bacterial or fungal keratitis. Overlying epithelial ulceration is common, but the epithelial defect may occur somewhat eccentric to the infiltrate, and the edges of the epithelial ulcer do not stain with rose bengal dye. Corneal stromal vascularization is common. The differential diagnosis of herpetic necrotizing keratitis includes microbial keratitis due to bacteria, fungi, or acanthamoebae, retained foreign body, and topical anesthetic abuse.

PATHOGENESIS The pathogenesis of herpetic stromal keratitis in humans remains unknown. Pathogenesis of herpetic stromal inflammation probably differs depending on the types of stromal inflammation (see above), and animal models of herpetic eye disease do not precisely replicate the human situation. Studies of HSV stromal keratitis in mouse models have variously implicated HSV-specific CD4 and CD8 T lymphocytes and anti-HSV antibodies in keratitis pathogenesis. Recent studies also implicate cell-mediated immunity to corneal antigens up-regulated by HSV infection, and bystander effects of proinflammatory cytokine secretion by infected corneal cells.

Streilein JW, Dana MR, Ksander BR. Immunity causing blindness: five different paths to herpes stromal keratitis. *Immunol Today.* 1997;18:443–449.

MANAGEMENT Many past controversies regarding the optimal management of HSV stromal keratitis have been resolved by the Herpetic Eye Disease Study (HEDS), a prospective multicenter clinical trial funded by the National Eye Institute in the 1990s. Most important, HEDS studies demonstrated that topical corticosteroids given together with a prophylactic antiviral reduce persistence or progression of stromal inflammation and shorten the duration of herpes simplex stromal keratitis; in addition, long-term suppressive oral acyclovir therapy reduces the rate of recurrent HSV keratitis and helps to preserve vision. Long-term antiviral prophylaxis is now recommended for patients with multiple recurrences of HSV stromal keratitis. HEDS studies showed no additional benefit of oral acyclovir in treating active HSV stromal keratitis in those patients also receiving concomitant topical corticosteroids and trifluridine. When given briefly along with trifluridine during an episode of epithelial keratitis, acyclovir also did not appear to prevent subsequent HSV stromal keratitis or iritis.

The experimental protocol applied by HEDS investigators for patients with herpetic stromal keratitis is a useful starting point for a treatment algorithm. Visually significant herpetic interstitial keratitis is treated initially with 1% prednisolone drops every 2 hours accompanied by a prophylactic antiviral drug, either topical trifluridine qid or an oral agent such as acyclovir 400 mg bid or valacyclovir 500 mg once a day. The prednisolone drops are tapered every 1–2 weeks depending on the degree of clinical improvement. The antiviral is used to prevent severe epithelial keratitis should the patient shed HSV while on corticosteroid drops, and it is generally continued until the patient is completely off

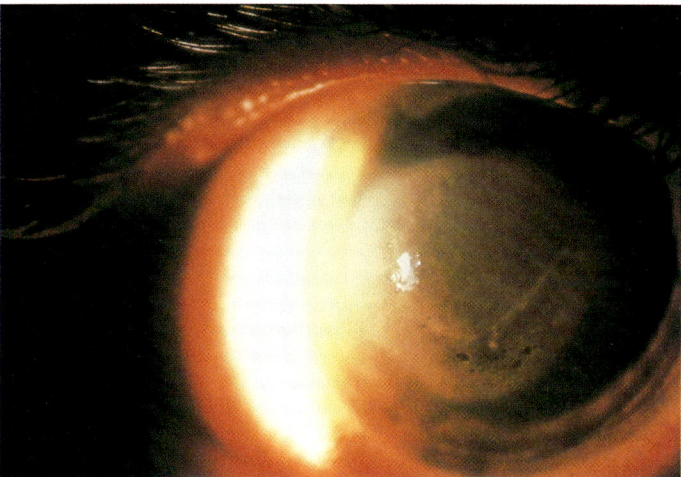

Figure 7-13 Herpetic disciform keratitis (nonnecrotizing). *(Reprinted with permission from: Chodosh J. Viral keratitis. In: Parrish RK, ed.* The University of Miami Bascom Palmer Eye Institute Atlas of Ophthalmology. *Boston: Current Medicine; 1999.)*

corticosteroids or using less than 1 drop of 1% prednisolone per day. Patients should be tapered to the lowest possible corticosteroid dosage that controls their inflammation.

Available topical antiviral medications are not absorbed by the cornea through an intact epithelium, but orally administered acyclovir penetrates an intact cornea and anterior chamber. In this context, anecdotal evidence suggests that oral acyclovir might benefit the deep corneal inflammation of disciform keratitis. The HEDS study showed no additional benefit when acyclovir was added to trifluridine and prednisolone for the treatment of herpetic stromal keratitis, but disciform keratitis was not analyzed as a separate group. Some corneal specialists routinely substitute oral acyclovir for topical trifluridine in treatment of disciform keratitis.

Necrotizing herpetic stromal keratitis is probably the least common form of herpetic keratitis. The diagnosis is frequently one of exclusion following negative cultures for fungal and bacterial pathogens, but it is suggested by a history of HSV facial, conjunctival, and/or corneal infection. The toxicity of topical antiviral agents may be undesirable in the setting of necrotizing inflammation and can confuse the clinical picture. Therefore, an oral antiviral such as acyclovir is preferred for necrotizing herpetic stromal keratitis. Fortunately, necrotizing herpetic keratitis appears to be very sensitive to topical corticosteroids, and twice a day dosing may be sufficient to control inflammation in many patients.

Barron BA, Gee L, Hauck WW, et al. Herpetic Eye Disease Study. A controlled trial of oral acyclovir for herpes simplex stromal keratitis. *Ophthalmology.* 1994;101:1871–1882.

Herpetic Eye Disease Study Group. A controlled trial of oral acyclovir for the prevention of stromal keratitis or iritis in patients with herpes simplex virus epithelial keratitis. The Epithelial Keratitis Trial. *Arch Ophthalmol.* 1997;115:703–712.

Herpetic Eye Disease Study Group. Acyclovir for the prevention of recurrent herpes simplex virus eye disease. *N Engl J Med.* 1998;339:300–306.

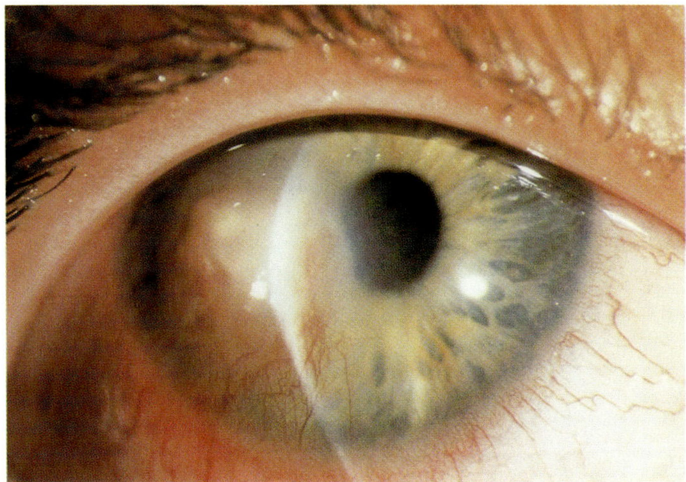

Figure 7-14 Necrotizing herpetic stromal keratitis.

Herpetic Eye Disease Study Group. Oral acyclovir for herpes simplex virus eye disease: effect on prevention of epithelial keratitis and stromal keratitis. *Arch Ophthalmol.* 2000;118:1030–1036.

Wilhelmus KR, Gee L, Hauck WW, et al. Herpetic Eye Disease Study. A controlled trial of topical corticosteroids for herpes simplex stromal keratitis. *Ophthalmology.* 1994;101:1883–1895.

Herpetic iridocyclitis. Granulomatous or nongranulomatous iridocyclitis may accompany necrotizing stromal keratitis or occur independently of corneal disease. Elevated intraocular pressure caused by trabeculitis and/or patchy iris transillumination defects may be found in patients with HSV iridocyclitis. Infectious virus has been cultured from the anterior chamber of such patients, and its presence positively correlated with ocular hypertension. Therefore, the diagnosis of HSV iridocyclitis is suggested by a unilateral presentation associated with an elevated intraocular pressure with or without focal iris transillumination defects. A history or clinical evidence of prior HSV ocular disease is suggestive. One HEDS trial suggested a statistical trend toward benefit of oral acyclovir in the treatment of HSV iridocyclitis in patients also receiving topical corticosteroids, but the number of patients recruited was too small to achieve statistically conclusive results.

Herpetic Eye Disease Study Group. A controlled trial of oral acyclovir for iridocyclitis caused by herpes simplex virus. *Arch Ophthalmol.* 1996;114:1065–1072.

Complications of herpetic eye disease

Complications affect all layers of the cornea. *Epitheliopathy* is common when topical antiviral treatment is prolonged, and its severity and duration are directly related to the duration of antiviral use. Topical antiviral toxicity presents most commonly as diffuse punctate corneal epithelial erosions with conjunctival injection. *Neurotrophic keratopathy* may develop in those patients with reduced corneal sensation secondary to past herpetic infection. Punctate epithelial erosions, sometimes with a vortex pattern of punctate fluorescein staining, chronic epithelial regeneration lines, and frank *neurotrophic ulcers* characterize neurotrophic keratopathy. These ulcers can be distinguished from herpetic epithelial keratitis by a relative absence of rose bengal staining. Neurotrophic ulcers are typically round or oval and located in the central or inferior cornea. Corneal epithelium at the edges of a neurotrophic ulcer may appear to roll under itself and typically has a gray elevated appearance. Liberal use of nonpreserved lubricating drops, gels, and ointments combined with punctal occlusion are the mainstays of therapy. Tarsorrhaphy is indicated for neurotrophic ulcers that fail to respond to conservative therapy in order to prevent progressive stromal thinning and perforation. On occasion, active or resolving interstitial stromal keratitis due to HSV is associated with a chronic epithelial defect that does not stain with rose bengal. This so-called *metaherpetic ulcer* probably results from neurotrophic mechanisms or a devitalized corneal stroma.

Severe or long-standing disciform keratitis can result in persistent bullous keratopathy. Stromal inflammation in general, whether interstitial or necrotizing, commonly leads to permanent corneal scarring and irregular astigmatism. Both scarring and astigmatism may improve with time in some patients. Fitting with a gas-permeable contact lens usually improves visual acuity beyond physician expectations based on spectacle refraction. In patients with deep corneal stromal vascularization due to prior necrotizing herpetic inflammation, secondary lipid keratopathy may further impair the vision. Topical corticosteroids may suppress new vessel growth and halt additional lipid deposition.

SURGICAL TREATMENT *Penetrating keratoplasty* is indicated in selected patients with visually significant stromal scarring and astigmatism not correctable by spectacle or contact lens. Oral antiviral therapy may improve graft survival by reducing the risk of HSV recurrence and allow more liberal use of topical corticosteroids. Oral antivirals lack epithelial toxicity and are therefore generally preferable to topical antivirals in patients after penetrating keratoplasty. *Tectonic penetrating keratoplasty* is indicated in impending or frank corneal perforation due to necrotizing or neurotrophic ulcers. Stromal inflammation, ulceration, and graft failure may develop in inflamed herpetic eyes undergoing tectonic penetrating keratoplasty. Therefore, small descemetoceles and perforations in inflamed eyes may best be treated with application of therapeutic tissue adhesive and a bandage contact lens, with penetrating keratoplasty delayed until inflammation can be controlled. The prognosis for successful optical penetrating keratoplasty approaches 80% in eyes without signs of active inflammation for at least 6 months prior to surgery. Occasionally, lamellar keratoplasty is indicated to remove corneal pannus and allow patients to wear rigid gas-permeable contact lenses.

Varicella-Zoster Virus Dermatoblepharitis, Conjunctivitis, and Keratitis

PATHOGENESIS As with other herpesviruses, varicella-zoster virus (VZV) causes a primary infection (varicella, or chickenpox) and subsequent latency, occasionally followed later by recurrent disease (zoster, or shingles). Primary VZV infection occurs upon direct contact with VZV skin lesions or respiratory secretions via airborne droplets and is highly contagious for naive individuals. VZV infection is usually a self-limited infection of childhood rarely associated with long-term sequelae. Infection of adults or immunosuppressed individuals can be fatal. In children, VZV infection manifests with fever, malaise, and a vesicular dermatitis that lasts 7–10 days. Except for eyelid vesicles and follicular conjunctivitis, ocular involvement is uncommon during primary infection. Like HSV, VZV latency occurs in neural ganglia and, in approximately 20% of infected individuals, reactivates later. Of all cases with zoster, 15% involve the ophthalmic division of cranial nerve V (trigeminal). VZV infection, whether primary or recurrent, can usually be distinguished from infection with HSV by careful history and examination. Distinguishing features of the each infection are listed in Table 7-2.

LABORATORY EVALUATION Laboratory confirmation of acute or recurrent VZV infection is possible by immunodiagnostic methods, viral culture, and PCR. Serologic testing is used primarily to identify varicella-naive adults who might benefit from prophylactic vaccination. As with HSV, scrapings from a vesicle base can be tested by cytology, PCR, or culture, or for the presence of VZV antigen. Conjunctival scrapings or corneal impression cytology specimens can be similarly analyzed by culture, antigen detection, or PCR.

CLINICAL PRESENTATION The rash of chickenpox begins as macules and progresses to papules, vesicles, and then pustules that dry, crust over, and may leave individual scars. Ocular involvement may include follicular conjunctivitis, occasionally associated with a vesicular lesion on the bulbar conjunctiva or eyelid margins. Punctate or dendritic epithelial keratitis is uncommon. Although subepithelial infiltrates, stromal keratitis, disciform keratitis, uveitis, and elevated intraocular pressure are rare, recurrent varicella keratouveitis may cause significant morbidity in some patients.

MANAGEMENT Because infected persons shed the virus in respiratory secretions before the onset of the characteristic rash, avoidance of infected individuals is not always possible. Vaccination against varicella is recommended for anyone older than 12 years of age without a history of chickenpox or with a negative serology. The severity of signs and symptoms may be reduced in clinically ill patients by the administration of oral acyclovir. Significant keratitis or uveitis can be treated with topical corticosteroids.

Table 7-2 Differentiating Features of Eye Disease Caused by Herpes Simplex Virus and Reactivation of Varicella-Zoster Virus

	Herpes Simplex Virus	Varicella-Zoster Virus
Dermatomal distribution	Incomplete	Complete
Pain	Moderate	Severe
Dendrite morphology	Central ulceration with terminal bulbs; geographic in presence of corticosteroids	Smaller without central ulceration or terminal bulbs; dendritiform mucous plaques occur later
Skin scarring	No	Common
Postherpetic neuralgia	No	Common
Iris atrophy	Patchy	Sectoral
Bilateral involvemet	Uncommon	No
Recurrent epithelial keratitis	Common	Rare
Corneal hypoesthesia	Sectoral or diffuse	May be severe

Herpes Zoster Ophthalmicus

PATHOGENESIS Following primary infection, varicella-zoster virus establishes latency in sensory neural ganglia. Zoster (shingles) represents endogenous reactivation of latent virus in persons with a waxing level of immunity to infection. Most patients are in their sixth to ninth decades, and the majority are healthy with no specific predisposing factors. However, zoster is more common in patients on immunosuppressive therapy; in those with a systemic malignancy, a debilitating disease, or HIV infection; and after major surgery, trauma, or radiation.

CLINICAL PRESENTATION Zoster manifests as a painful vesicular dermatitis typically localized to a single dermatome on the thorax or face. Patients may complain initially of fever and malaise, and warmth, redness, and increased sensation in the affected dermatome. The most commonly affected dermatomes are on the thorax (T3 through L3) and those supplied by CN V (trigeminal nerve). The ophthalmic division of the trigeminal nerve is affected more often than the maxillary and mandibular branches, and its involvement is referred to as *herpes zoster ophthalmicus* (HZO) (Fig 7-15). A maculopapular rash, followed by vesicles and then pustules, is characteristic. Zoster dermatitis may result in large scabs that resolve slowly and leave significant scarring. Neurotrophic keratopathy and sectoral iris atrophy are characteristic. Inflammation of almost any ocular tissue can occur and recur in HZO.

Zoster dermatitis is accompanied by pain and dysesthesia. The pain usually decreases as lesions resolve; however, neuralgia in the affected dermatome can continue from months to years. The severity of pain ranges from mild to incapacitating. Ocular involvement occurs in more than 70% of patients with zoster of the first division of CN V and may appear in association with any branch, including the nasociliary, frontal, or lacrimal branches. Ophthalmic complications also may occur with zoster of the second division (maxillary) of CN V. In immunosuppressed patients, zoster may involve more than one

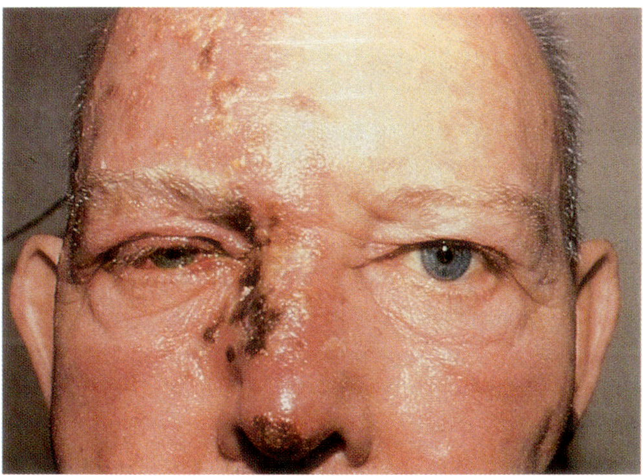

Figure 7-15 Herpes zoster ophthalmicus. *(Photograph courtesy of Vincent P. deLuise, MD.)*

branch of the trigeminal nerve at the same time, can chronically reactivate, and may be multiply recurrent.

Eyelid vesicular eruption can lead to secondary bacterial infection, eyelid scarring, marginal notching, loss of cilia, trichiasis, and cicatricial entropion or ectropion. Scarring and occlusion of the lacrimal puncta or canaliculi may occur. Episcleritis or scleritis associated with zoster may be either nodular, zonal, or diffuse.

Punctate or dendritic epithelial keratitis caused by viral replication in corneal epithelium are common manifestations of ophthalmic zoster. Dendrites may persist and remain chronically culture positive for VZV in AIDS patients. Elevated dendritiform mucous plaques may occur weeks to months after resolution of skin lesions. Diminished corneal sensation develops in up to 50% of patients. Nummular corneal infiltrates are said to be characteristic of zoster stromal keratitis (Fig 7-16), but the interstitial keratitis, disciform keratitis, and anterior uveitis with increased intraocular pressure in HZO are clinically indistinguishable from those caused by herpes simplex virus infection. Chronic corneal stromal inflammation can lead to corneal vascularization, lipid keratopathy (Fig 7-17), and corneal opacity. Corneal anesthesia may be profound, and neurotrophic keratopathy due to HZO can be extremely difficult to manage.

Focal choroiditis, occlusive retinal vasculitis, and retinal detachment have been reported. Ipsilateral acute retinal necrosis (ARN) temporally associated with HZO is uncommon.

Orbital or central nervous system involvement as a result of an occlusive arteritis may lead to eyelid ptosis, orbital edema, and proptosis. Papillitis or retrobulbar optic neuritis may also develop. Cranial nerve palsies have been reported to occur in up to one third of cases of HZO, with CN III (oculomotor) most commonly affected. Cranial nerve involvement may occur within the orbit or the cavernous sinus. Systemic dissemination is unusual in immunocompetent patients but can occur in up to 25% of those who are immunocompromised.

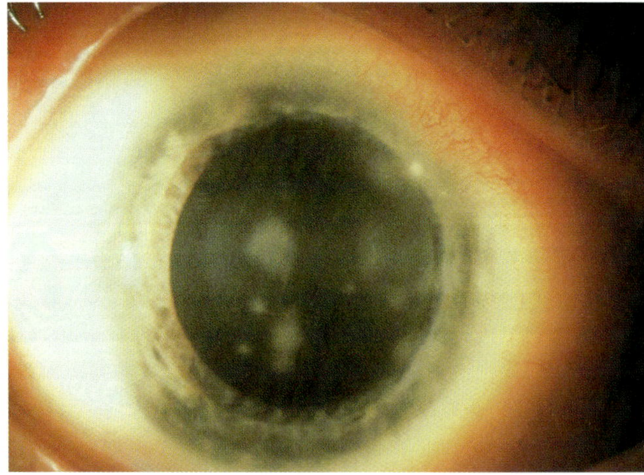

Figure 7-16 Nummular keratitis of herpes zoster ophthalmicus. *(Photograph courtesy of Rhea L. Siatkowski, MD.)*

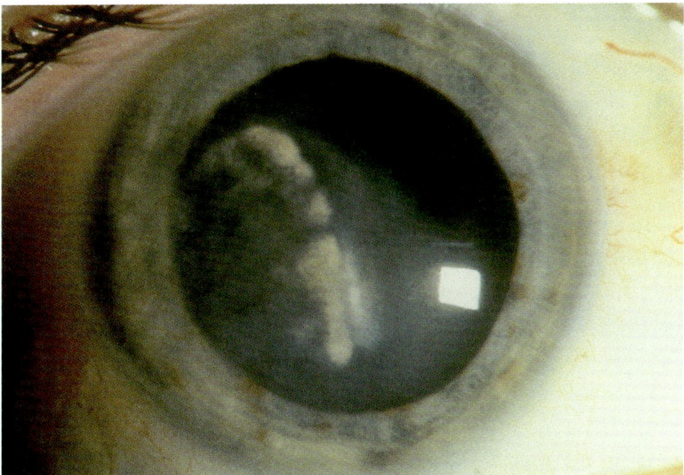

Figure 7-17 Lipid keratopathy following herpes zoster ophthalmicus. *(Reprinted with permission from: Chodosh J. Viral keratitis. In: Parrish RK, ed. The University of Miami Bascom Palmer Eye Institute Atlas of Ophthalmology. Boston: Current Medicine; 1999.)*

MANAGEMENT Oral antiviral therapy for HZO was found in randomized clinical trials to reduce viral shedding from vesicular skin lesions, reduce the chance of systemic dissemination of the virus, and decrease the incidence and severity of the most common ocular complications. Oral antiviral therapy, in particular famciclovir and valacyclovir, may reduce the duration if not the incidence of postherpetic neuralgia if begun within 72 hours of onset of symptoms. Amitriptyline has also been reported to decrease the duration of postherpetic neuralgia if given early on and continued until pain symptoms remit.

The current recommendation for HZO is oral famciclovir 500 mg three time per day, valacyclovir 1 gm three times per day, or acyclovir 800 mg five times per day for 7–10 days, best if started within 72 hours of the onset of skin lesions. Topical antiviral medications are not effective. Intravenous acyclovir therapy is indicated in patients at risk for disseminated zoster due to immunosuppression. Cutaneous lesions may be treated with moist warm compresses and topical antibiotic ointment. Topical corticosteroids and cycloplegics are indicated for keratouveitis. Oral corticosteroids on a tapering dosage over 3 weeks are recommended by some for treatment of patients with HZO over age 60 to reduce early zoster pain and facilitate a rapid return to a normal quality of life.

Postherpetic neuralgia may respond to capsaicin cream applied to the involved skin, but low doses of amitriptyline, desipramine, clomipramine, or carbamazepine may be necessary to control severe symptoms. Aggressive lubrication with nonpreserved tears, gels, and ointments, combined with punctal occlusion and tarsorrhaphy as necessary, may be indicated for neurotrophic keratopathy. Severe recalcitrant pain due to HZO may require referral to a pain management specialist.

Epstein-Barr Virus Dacryoadenitis, Conjunctivitis, and Keratitis

PATHOGENESIS Epstein-Barr virus (EBV) is a ubiquitous herpesvirus that infects the majority of humans by early adulthood. Spread of EBV occurs by the sharing of saliva and results in subclinical infection in the first decade of life; if acquired later in life, it causes infectious mononucleosis. The virus remains latent in B lymphocytes and pharyngeal mucosal epithelial cells throughout life. Ocular disease is uncommon.

CLINICAL PRESENTATION EBV is the most common cause of acute *dacryoadenitis,* characterized by inflammatory enlargement of one or both lacrimal glands. Acute follicular conjunctivitis, Parinaud oculoglandular syndrome, and bulbar conjunctival nodules have been reported in patients with acute infectious mononucleosis and may be the result of EBV infection. Multiple corneal epithelial dendrites involving the central and peripheral cornea were reported in a patient with infectious mononucleosis, but any causal association of EBV with stromal keratitis remains unproved. The three principal forms of EBV stromal keratitis were associated with EBV on the basis of a history of recent infectious mononucleosis and/or persistently high EBV serologic titers:

- Type 1: Multifocal subepithelial infiltrates that resemble adenoviral keratitis
- Type 2: Multifocal, blotchy, pleomorphic infiltrates with active inflammation (Fig 7-18) or granular ring-shaped opacities (inactive form) in anterior to mid-stroma
- Type 3: Multifocal deep or full-thickness peripheral infiltrates, with or without vascularization, that resemble interstitial keratitis due to syphilis

EBV-associated keratitis may be unilateral or bilateral and may, in select cases, appear similar to that induced by herpes simplex virus, varicella-zoster virus, adenovirus, or syphilis.

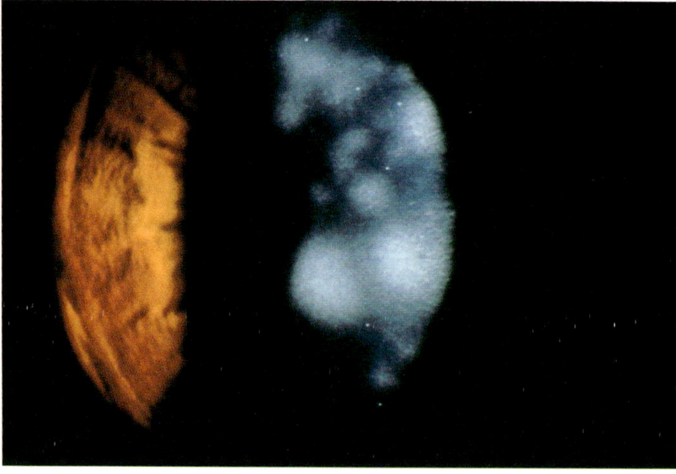

Figure 7-18 Epstein-Barr virus stromal keratitis. *(Reprinted with permission from: Chodosh J. Viral keratitis. In: Parrish RK, ed. The University of Miami Bascom Palmer Eye Institute Atlas of Ophthalmology. Boston: Current Medicine; 1999.)*

MANAGEMENT Because of difficulty in viral isolation, diagnosis of EBV infection depends on the detection of antibodies to various viral components. During acute infection, first IgM and then IgG antibodies to viral capsid antigens (VCA) appear. Anti-VCA IgG may persist for the life of the patient. Antibodies to early antigens (EA) also rise during the acute phases of the disease and subsequently decrease to low or undetectable levels in most individuals. Antibodies to EBV nuclear antigens (EBNA) appear weeks to months later, providing serologic evidence of past infection. Acyclovir is not effective treatment for the clinical signs and symptoms of infectious mononucleosis, but the impact of antiviral therapy on the corneal manifestations of EBV infection remains unknown. Corticosteroids may be effective in patients with reduced vision due to apparent EBV stromal keratitis, but they should not be administered without a prophylactic antiviral if herpes simplex infection is a possibility.

> Chodosh J. Epstein-Barr virus stromal keratitis. *Ophthalmol Clin North Am.* 1994;7(4): 549–556.

Other Viral Infections of the Ocular Surface

RNA viruses

Eye infections due to RNA viruses present to the ophthalmologist less often than those due to DNA viruses, and they most commonly manifest as follicular conjunctivitis associated with an upper respiratory infection. However, certain RNA virus infections may cause pathologic changes in virtually any ocular tissue. For example, *influenza virus* can induce inflammation in the lacrimal gland, cornea, iris, retina, the optic nerve, and other cranial nerves.

In *measles (rubeola) virus* infection, the classic triad of postnatally acquired measles—cough, coryza, and follicular conjunctivitis—can be accompanied by Koplik spots on the conjunctiva and a mild epithelial keratitis. Less common are optic neuritis, retinal vascular occlusion, and pigmentary retinopathy. Measles keratopathy, a major source of blindness in the developing world, typically presents as corneal ulceration in malnourished, vitamin A–deficient children. (For further information on the ocular effects of vitamin A deficiency, see Nutritional and Physiologic Disorders, Vitamin A Deficiency, in Chapter 5 and *International Ophthalmology*, a BCSC companion book.) A rare and fatal complication of measles virus infection, subacute sclerosing panencephalitis (SSPE), occurs in about 1 per 100,000 cases, often years after clinically apparent measles.

Mumps virus infection may result in dacryoadenitis, sometimes concurrent with parotid gland involvement. Follicular conjunctivitis, epithelial and stromal keratitis, iritis, trabeculitis, and scleritis have all been reported within the first 2 weeks after onset of parotitis.

Rubella virus, when acquired in utero, may cause microphthalmos, corneal haze, cataracts, iris hypoplasia, iridocyclitis, glaucoma, and salt-and-pepper pigmentary retinopathy. Congenital ocular abnormalities due to rubella are much worse when maternal infection ensues early in pregnancy. Measles, mumps, and rubella are all uncommon in places where childhood immunization is regularly performed.

Corneal biopsy early in *rabies virus* infection may allow early diagnosis of rabies. Rabies virus can be transmitted via corneal transplant.

Microbial and Parasitic Infections of the Eyelid Margin and Conjunctiva

Staphylococcal Blepharitis

PATHOGENESIS Inflammation of the eyelid margins, called *blepharitis,* is one of the most common causes of external ocular irritation. Blepharitis can have an infectious or inflammatory etiology; the most common causes of blepharitis are staphylococcal infection (usually caused by *S aureus* but occasionally other species) and irritation from oily meibomian gland secretions. The symptoms, signs, and treatment of infectious staphylococcal blepharoconjunctivitis and meibomian gland dysfunction overlap considerably. In general, the term *staphylococcal blepharitis* refers to cases in which bacterial infection of the eyelids (and frequently the conjunctiva) is predominant. *Meibomian gland dysfunction* and *seborrheic blepharitis* designate the presence of chronic abnormal oily secretions producing irritative effects in the eyelid margin and conjunctiva (these two latter conditions are discussed in Chapter 5). Clinical features that may aid in the differential diagnosis of these entities are summarized in Table 7-3.

CLINICAL PRESENTATION Staphylococcal blepharitis is seen more commonly in younger individuals. Symptoms include burning, itching, foreign body sensation, and crusting, particularly upon awakening. Symptoms of irritation and burning tend to peak in the morning and improve as the day progresses, presumably as the crusted material that accumulates on the eyelid margin overnight dissipates.

Typical clinical manifestations include hard, brittle fibrinous scales and hard, matted crusts surrounding individual cilia on the anterior eyelid margin (Fig 7-19). Small ulcers of the anterior eyelid margin may be seen when the hard crusts are removed. Injection and telangiectasis of the anterior and posterior eyelid margins, white lashes (poliosis), lash loss (madarosis), and trichiasis may be seen in varying degrees, depending on the severity and duration of the blepharitis.

Aqueous tear deficiency is found in some patients with staphylococcal blepharitis. Excessive secretion of bacterially modified lipid products into the tear film can increase instability and accentuate evaporative losses, thus further compounding any associated dry eye state. (See additional dry eye discussion in Chapter 5.)

Chronic conjunctivitis

A unilateral or bilateral conjunctivitis that persists for 4 or more weeks is considered chronic. When conjunctivitis accompanies blepharitis, as it frequently does, the condition is known as *staphylococcal blepharoconjunctivitis.* This association is marked by a chronic papillary reaction of the tarsal conjunctiva, particularly the inferior tarsal conjunctiva near the eyelid margin, as well as injection of the bulbar and tarsal conjunctiva. Chronic conjunctivitis tends to be associated with mild conjunctival injection and scant mucopurulent discharge.

Specific clinical signs are commonly seen in patients with chronic conjunctivitis caused by certain bacterial species. *S aureus* is often associated with matted golden crusts and ulcers on the anterior eyelid margin, inferior punctate keratopathy, marginal corneal

Table 7-3 Types of Blepharitis

	Staphylococcal	Meibomian Gland Dysfunction	Seborrheic
Location	Anterior eyelid	Posterior eyelid	Anterior eyelid
Loss and whitening of lashes	Frequent	(−)	Rare
Eyelid crusting	Hard, fibrinous scales; hard, matted crusts (often accompany ulcerative form)	+/−	Oily or greasy
Eyelid ulceration	Occasional	(−)	(−)
Conjunctivitis	Papillary (occasionally with mucopurulent discharge)	Mild to moderate injection, papillary tarsal reaction	Mild injection, follicular or papillary tarsal reaction
Keratitis	Inferior PEE,* marginal infiltrates, vascularization, phlyctenulosis	Inferior PEE, marginal infiltrates, vascular pannus	Inferior PEE
Aqueous tear deficiency	Occasional	Occasional	Occasional
Rosacea	(−)	+ +	+

+ : 0%–33%, + + : 34%–66%.
* PEE: punctate epithelial erosions.

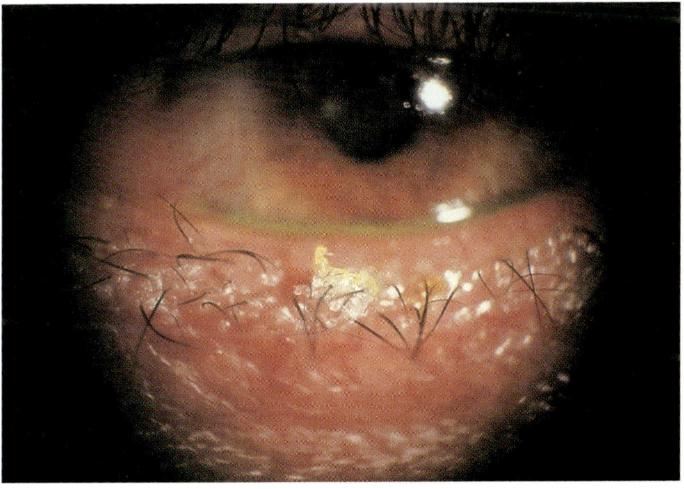

Figure 7-19 Staphylococcal blepharitis with collarettes surrounding eyelashes.

infiltrates, and, rarely, conjunctival or corneal phlyctenules. *Moraxella lacunata* may produce a chronic angular blepharoconjunctivitis with crusting and ulceration of the skin in the lateral canthal angle and papillary or follicular reaction on the tarsal conjunctiva. *Moraxella* angular blepharoconjunctivitis is frequently associated with concomitant *S aureus* blepharoconjunctivitis.

Conjunctival swabbings for culture and sensitivity should be performed in cases that do not respond to initial empiric antibiotic therapy. In cases of persistent chronic unilateral conjunctivitis refractory to therapy, masquerade syndrome (conjunctival malignancy) and factitious illness should be ruled out.

Keratitis

Several forms of keratitis may develop in association with staphylococcal blepharoconjunctivitis.

Punctate epithelial keratopathy manifests as erosions that stain with fluorescein. Frequently, the distribution of the keratopathy is mostly inferior, and it sometimes coincides with the contour of the eyelids across the corneal surface. Occasionally, a diffuse pattern may be observed, and asymmetric or unilateral keratopathy is not uncommon. The degree of corneal involvement can be markedly disproportionate to the severity of the eyelid disease, a circumstance that can lead to diagnostic confusion. Marginal corneal infiltrates may be the most distinctive clinical finding (Fig 7-20).

Phlyctenulosis is a local corneal and/or conjunctival inflammation that is believed to represent a cell-mediated, or delayed, hypersensitivity response induced by microbial antigens such as the cell wall components of staphylococcus. Phlyctenulosis is frequently associated with *S aureus* in developed countries and is classically associated with *Mycobacterium tuberculosis* in malnourished children in areas around the world with endemic tuberculosis. Additional implicated organisms include *Chlamydia lymphogranulomatosis, Candida albicans, Coccidioides immitis, Leishmania* spp, *Ascaris lumbricoides, Ancylostoma duodenale, Hymenolepis nana, Enterobius vermicularis, Entamoeba histolytica,* adenoviruses, and herpes simplex.

Phlyctenules typically present unilaterally at or near the limbus, on the bulbar conjunctiva or cornea, as one or more small, rounded, elevated, gray or yellow, hyperemic, focal inflammatory nodules accompanied by a zone of engorged hyperemic vessels (Fig 7-21). They typically become necrotic and ulcerate centrally, then spontaneously involute over a period of 2–3 weeks. With resolution of corneal phlyctenules, wedge-shaped fibrovascular scars form along the limbus. Conjunctival phlyctenules do not lead to scarring. Bilateral limbus-based fibrovascular corneal scarring that tends to be greater inferiorly than superiorly may indicate previous phlyctenulosis. Corneal involvement is recurrent, and centripetal migration of successive inflammatory lesions may develop. Occasionally, such inflammation leads to corneal thinning and, rarely, perforation.

LABORATORY EVALUATION Eyelid and conjunctival cultures can be performed in suspected cases of staphylococcal blepharoconjunctivitis with a doubtful clinical diagnosis or a poor response to empiric treatment. If the infection is chronic or worsening, diagnostic cultures may be essential. If the patient is still on antibiotics or other topical therapeutic measures, then a brief washout period may be advantageous prior to culturing. (Proce-

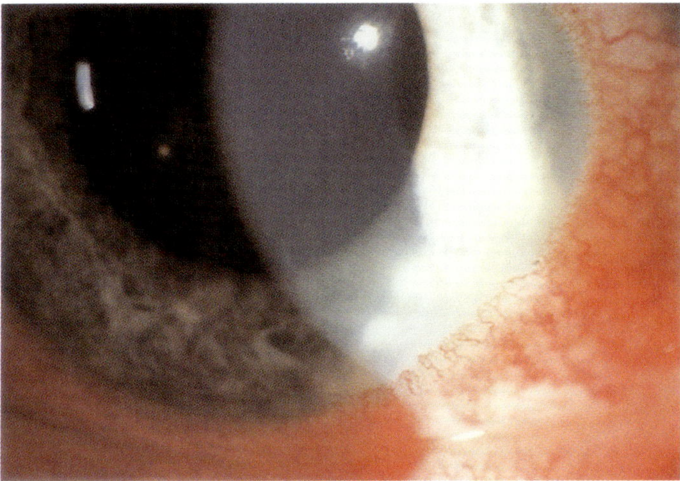

Figure 7-20 Staphylococcal marginal corneal infiltrate.

dures for obtaining, staining, and culturing conjunctival specimens are described in Chapter 4 and Chapter 6.)

The characteristic laboratory finding in staphylococcal blepharoconjunctivitis is a heavy, confluent growth of *S aureus*. Nevertheless, the finding of a light to moderate growth of bacteria and/or the isolation of staphylococcal species other than *S aureus* does not exclude the diagnosis, particularly if a predominant manifestation of the disease is punctate epithelial keratopathy, marginal infiltrates, or phlyctenulosis. Susceptibility testing may be useful in guiding treatment in cases that have been refractory to empiric antibiotic therapy.

MANAGEMENT Treatment consists of antibacterial and anti-inflammatory measures. Eyelid hygiene, using either commercially available lid scrub kits or warm water with diluted baby shampoo, may aid in reducing bacterial colonization and accumulation of sebaceous secretions. Patient education should emphasize treatment directed toward the base of the lashes with a moistened cotton-tipped applicator or a small, soft face cloth sudsed with a dilute concentration of baby shampoo. Following scrubs, a thin film of antibiotic ointment may be applied to the eyelid margins. Further, aqueous tear deficiency and/or lipid-induced tear film instability is frequently present, and the use of artificial tears or other dry eye remedies may be beneficial.

Cases with a prominent conjunctivitis component should be treated with an antibiotic solution. Treatment for staphylococcal blepharitis is frequently prolonged and repeated. This factors into the physician's selection of a topical antibiotic. In order to minimize toxicity and resistance, a well-tolerated, relatively narrow spectrum antimicrobial agent effective against the majority of staphylococci should be selected. When possible, the agents should be demonstrated to be efficacious by susceptibility testing data from the local or regional microbiology laboratory.

Anti-inflammatory therapy consists of limited and judicious use of mild doses of topical corticosteroids in selected cases. Corticosteroids should be reserved for patients

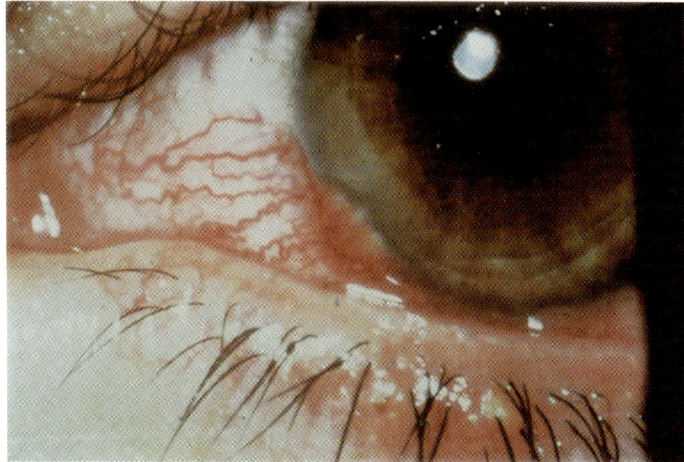

Figure 7-21 Confluent phlyctenules secondary to staphylococcal blepharitis.

who have a strong inflammatory component with little active infection. Patients with routine staphylococcal blepharitis or blepharoconjunctivitis may obtain more rapid symptomatic relief with the use of adjunctive topical corticosteroids, but the potential risks include prolonging or worsening the infection or inducing steroid-related side effects. Therefore, corticosteroid use in routine cases is strongly discouraged.

Corticosteroids provide little therapeutic benefit for toxic-related punctate epithelial keratopathy. In contrast, marginal infiltrates and phlyctenulosis have a strong immunologic component and can thus respond to topical corticosteroid therapy. In these cases, the response to eyelid hygiene and antibiotic therapy alone should first be assessed. If the therapeutic effect is inadequate after a few days (in the case of marginal infiltrates) or weeks (in the case of phlyctenulosis), a time-limited course of low-dose corticosteroid can be prescribed. If epithelial defects are noted over the infiltrates, diagnostic cultures should be obtained before instituting corticosteroid treatment. Chronic or indiscriminate use of corticosteroids should be avoided.

Hordeolum

PATHOGENESIS Hordeola are inflammatory or infectious nodules that develop in the eyelid. Most frequently, they result from inspissation and secondary infection of sebaceous glands. Those occurring on the anterior eyelid in the glands of Zeis or lash follicles are called *external hordeola,* or *styes.* Hordeola occurring at the posterior eyelid from meibomian gland inspissation are termed *internal hordeola.* Either type is associated with a localized purulent abscess, usually caused by *S aureus.*

CLINICAL PRESENTATION Hordeola present as painful, tender, red nodular masses near the eyelid margin. They may rupture, producing a purulent drainage. Hordeola are generally self-limited, improving spontaneously over the course of 1–2 weeks. Internal hordeola occasionally evolve into *chalazia,* which are chronic granulomatous nodules centered around sebaceous glands, usually the meibomian glands. (Chalazia are discussed further in Chapter 5.)

LABORATORY EVALUATION AND MANAGEMENT Cultures are not indicated for isolated, uncomplicated cases of hordeolum. Warm compresses with light massage over the lesion can facilitate drainage. Topically applied antibiotics are generally not effective and, therefore, not indicated unless an accompanying infectious blepharoconjunctivitis is present. Systemic antibiotics are generally indicated only in rare cases of secondary eyelid cellulitis; however, if the patient has a prominent and chronic accompanying meibomitis, oral doxycycline may be necessary. For large or persistent lesions, incision and drainage may be required. In rare cases, a steroid injection may be considered, especially if excision might endanger the lacrimal apparatus. Caution is in order because steroid injection can lead to permanent skin depigmentation.

Fungal and Parasitic Infections of the Eyelid Margin

Demodex is a genus of mites that are normal commensal acarian parasites of humans. The human follicle mites, *Demodex folliculorum* and *Demodex brevis,* are obligate parasites that inhabit hair follicles and sebaceous/meibomian glands respectively. They are commonly seen by slit-lamp biomicroscopy as waxy sleeves around eyelashes or as cylinders extending from sebaceous glands of the eyelid margin. The role of these parasites in the pathogenesis of blepharitis is unclear. Other organisms that survive on lipids of eyelid glands, such as *Malassezia furfur,* have also been incriminated in certain types of blepharitis.

A focal granuloma or dermatitis affecting the eyelid or conjunctiva can be caused by very rare infections, including:

- Blastomycosis
- Sporotrichosis
- Rhinosporidiosis
- Cryptococcosis
- Leishmaniasis
- Ophthalmomyiasis

Lice infestation of the eyelids and eyelashes, also known as *phthiriasis palpebrum,* is an uncommon form of conjunctivitis or blepharitis affecting adolescents and young adults and is caused by the pubic louse and its ova. Rarely, pediculosis involves the ocular region by localized extension of head or body lice (*Pediculus humanus capitis* or *Pediculus humanus corporis,* respectively). Mechanical removal of the lice and nits (eggs) can be performed with jewelers forceps, but pubic hairs are usually treated with a pediculicide. Any ointment can smother the lice and should be applied twice daily for at least 10 days, because the incubation period (of the nits) is 7–10 days. Periodic reexamination is recommended in 10–14 days to detect recurrence and remove any new nits. Bed linen, clothing, and any items of close contact should be washed and dried at the highest temperature setting (at least 50°C).

Bacterial Conjunctivitis in Children and Adults

PATHOGENESIS A bacterial etiology is a less common cause of conjunctivitis in adults. Bacterial conjunctivitis is the result of bacterial overgrowth and infiltration of the conjunctival epithelial layer and sometimes the substantia propria as well. The source of infection is either direct contact with an infected individual's secretions (usually through eye–hand contact) or the spread of infection from the organisms colonizing the patient's own nasal and sinus mucosa.

Although usually self-limited, bacterial conjunctivitis can occasionally be severe and sight-threatening when caused by virulent bacterial species such as *Neisseria gonorrhoeae* or *Streptococcus pyogenes*. In rare cases it may presage life-threatening systemic disease, as with conjunctivitis caused by *N meningitidis*. Direct infection and inflammation of the conjunctival surface, bystander effects on adjacent tissues such as the cornea, and the host's acute inflammatory response and long-term reparative response all contribute to the pathology.

CLINICAL PRESENTATION AND MANAGEMENT Bacterial conjunctivitis should be suspected in patients with conjunctival inflammation and a purulent discharge. The rapidity of onset and severity of conjunctival inflammation and discharge are suggestive of the possible causative organism. Table 7-4 shows the clinical classification of bacterial conjunctivitis based on these parameters.

Acute purulent conjunctivitis

This form of bacterial conjunctivitis is characterized by an acute (less than 3 weeks in duration), self-limited infection of the conjunctival surface that evokes an acute inflammatory response with purulent discharge. Cases may occur spontaneously or in epidemics. The most common etiologic pathogens are *Streptococcus pneumoniae, Staphylococcus aureus*, and *H influenzae*. The relative frequency with which each of these organisms is isolated depends in part on the patient's age and geographic location.

Streptococcus pneumoniae is usually the most common cause of acute purulent bacterial conjunctivitis. Moderate purulent discharge, eyelid edema, chemosis, conjunctival

Table 7-4 Clinical Classification of Bacterial Conjunctivitis

Course of Onset	Severity	Common Organisms
Slow (days to weeks)	Mild–moderate	*Staphylococcus aureus* *Moraxella lacunata* *Proteus* species Enterobacteriaceae *Pseudomonas*
Acute or subacute (hours to days)	Moderate–severe	*Haemophilus influenzae* biotype III* *Haemophilus influenzae* *Streptococcus pneumoniae* *Staphylococcus aureus*
Hyperacute (<24 hours)	Severe	*Neisseria gonorrhoeae* *Neisseria meningitidis*

* Previously referred to as *Haemophilus aegyptius*.

hemorrhages, and occasionally inflammatory membranes on the tarsal conjunctivae are often associated with acute conjunctivitis caused by *S pneumoniae.* Corneal ulceration rarely occurs.

H influenzae conjunctivitis occurs in young children, sometimes in association with otitis media, and in adults, particularly those chronically colonized with *H influenzae* (for example, smokers or patients with chronic bronchopulmonary disease). Acute purulent conjunctivitis caused by *H influenzae* biotype III (previously called *H aegyptius*) resembles that caused by *S pneumoniae;* however, conjunctival membranes do not develop, while peripheral corneal epithelial ulcers and stromal infiltrates occur more commonly.

Staphylococcus aureus may produce an acute blepharoconjunctivitis. The discharge tends to be somewhat less purulent than that seen in pneumococcal conjunctivitis, and the associated signs are generally less severe.

Gram-stained smears and culture of the conjunctiva are not necessary in uncomplicated cases of suspected bacterial conjunctivitis but should be performed in the following situations:

- Certain compromised hosts such as neonates or debilitated or immunocompromised individuals
- Severe cases of purulent conjunctivitis to differentiate it from hyperpurulent conjunctivitis, which generally requires systemic therapy
- Cases unresponsive to initial therapy

MANAGEMENT Most cases of acute purulent conjunctivitis can be managed with empiric antibiotic therapy. Uncomplicated cases that are equivocal or cases likely to represent a viral conjunctivitis should *not* be routinely treated with empiric antibiotics.

Initial medical therapy for acute nonsevere bacterial conjunctivitis includes the following topical agents: erythromycin, bacitracin, or ciprofloxacin ointment; or polymixin combination drops; or aminoglycosides or fluoroquinolone (ciprofloxacin, ofloxacin, levofloxacin, moxifloxacin, or gatifloxacin) drops. The dosing schedule is 4 times daily for approximately 5–7 days unless otherwise indicated. Cases with gram-negative coccobacilli on gram-stained smears are probably caused by *Haemophilus* species and should be treated with polymyxin B–trimethoprim. Furthermore, supplemental oral antibiotics are recommended for patients with acute purulent conjunctivitis associated with pharyngitis, for conjunctivitis-otitis syndrome, and for *Haemophilus* conjunctivitis in children.

When empiric broad-spectrum antibiotic therapy is prescribed in cases of hyperacute conjunctivitis, the initial treatment should be weighted toward the results of the gram-stained morphology of the conjunctival smear, if available. Definitive treatment should be based on the culture results, if available, as smear results may sometimes be inconclusive as to the predominant category of organism responsible for the infection. Cultures of the nose or throat may be performed if an associated sinusitis or pharyngitis is present. Even if no overt sinusitis, rhinitis, or pharyngitis is present, nasal or throat swabs should be considered in cases of relapsing conjunctivitis, because the persistence of organisms colonizing the respiratory mucosa may be the source of infection.

Gonococcal conjunctivitis

This condition presents with explosive onset of severe purulent conjunctivitis: massive exudation; severe chemosis; and, in untreated cases, corneal infiltrates, melting, and perforation. The organism most commonly responsible for hyperpurulent conjunctivitis is *Neisseria gonorrhoeae* (Fig 7-22). Gonococcal conjunctivitis is a sexually transmitted disease resulting from direct genital–eye transmission, genital–hand–ocular contact, or maternal–neonate transmission during vaginal delivery.

The disease is characterized by rapid progression, copious purulent conjunctival discharge, marked conjunctival hyperemia and chemosis, and eyelid edema. Gonococcal conjunctivitis may be associated with preauricular lymphadenopathy and the formation of conjunctival membranes. Keratitis, the principal cause of sight-threatening complications, has been reported to occur in 15%–40% of cases. Corneal involvement may consist of diffuse epithelial haze, epithelial defects, marginal infiltrates, and peripheral ulcerative infectious keratitis that can rapidly progress to perforation.

MANAGEMENT Gonococcal conjunctivitis should be treated with systemic antibiotics. Topical ocular antibiotics can supplement but not replace systemic therapy. Current treatment regimens for gonococcal conjunctivitis reflect the increasing prevalence of *penicillin-resistant N gonorrhoeae (PRNG)* in the United States. Ceftriaxone, a third-generation cephalosporin, is highly effective against PRNG. Gonococcal conjunctivitis without corneal ulceration may be treated on an outpatient basis with one intramuscular ceftriaxone (1 g) injection. Patients with corneal ulceration should be admitted to the hospital and treated with intravenous ceftriaxone (1 g IV every 12 hours) for 3 consecutive days. Patients with penicillin allergy can be given spectinomycin (2 g IM) or oral fluoroquinolones (ciprofloxacin 500 mg or ofloxacin 400 mg orally bid for 5 days).

Erythromycin ointment, bacitracin ointment, gentamicin ointment, and ciprofloxacin solution have been recommended for topical therapy. Just as important as systemic

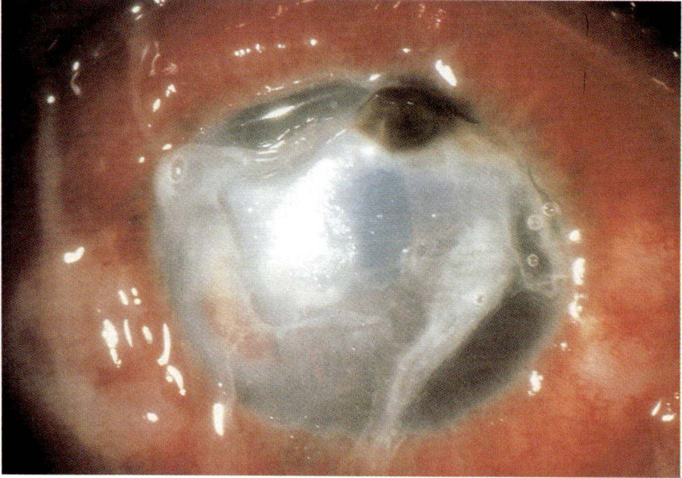

Figure 7-22 Peripheral corneal ulceration and perforation occurring several days after onset of hyperacute conjunctivitis caused by *N gonorrhoeae*.

therapy for the treatment of severe cases is copious, frequent (every 30–60 minutes) irrigation of the conjunctival sac with normal saline. Such lavages help to remove inflammatory cells, proteases, and debris that may be toxic to the ocular surface and contribute to corneal melting.

Up to one third of patients with gonococcal conjunctivitis have been reported to have concurrent chlamydial venereal disease. Because of this frequent association, it is advisable to place patients on supplemental oral antibiotics for treatment of chlamydial infection. These medications include tetracycline 500 mg orally qid for 1 week, doxycycline 100 mg orally bid for 1 week, minocycline 100 mg orally bid for 1 week, erythromycin 250 mg qid for 1 week, or azithromycin 1 g orally once.

Preferred Practice Patterns Committee, Cornea Panel. *Conjunctivitis.* San Francisco: American
Academy of Ophthalmology; 1998.

Bacterial Conjunctivitis in Neonates

Neisseria gonorrhoeae causes the most severe neonatal conjunctivitis. Fortunately, *N gonorrhoeae* is currently responsible for fewer than 1% of all cases of neonatal conjunctivitis in the industrialized countries. In order of decreasing prevalence, the causes of neonatal bacterial conjunctivitis are as follows:

- *Chlamydia trachomatis*
- *Streptococcus viridans*
- *Staphylococcus aureus*
- *Haemophilus influenzae*
- Group D *Streptococcus*
- *Moraxella catarrhalis*
- *Escherichia coli* and other gram-negative rods
- *Neisseria gonorrhoeae*

Ophthalmia neonatorum is discussed in further detail in BCSC Section 6, *Pediatric Ophthalmology and Strabismus;* and *International Ophthalmology,* a BCSC companion book.

Neonatal gonococcal conjunctivitis

The infrequency of neonatal gonococcal conjunctivitis has been attributed to effective prenatal screening for maternal gonococcal genital infection and prophylactic antimicrobial therapy for conjunctivitis in newborns. Infants with gonococcal conjunctivitis typically develop bilateral conjunctival discharge 3–5 days after parturition. The discharge may be serosanguineous during the first several days, and a copious purulent exudate may develop later. Corneal ulceration, corneal perforation, and endophthalmitis have been reported as complications of untreated neonatal gonococcal conjunctivitis. Infected infants may also have other localized gonococcal infections including rhinitis and proctitis. Disseminated gonococcal infection with arthritis, meningitis, pneumonia, and sepsis resulting in death of the infant is a rare complication.

MANAGEMENT Because some strains of *N gonorrhoeae* are developing resistance to various antibiotics, including penicillin, fluoroquinolones (quinolone-resistant *N gonorrhoeae,* or QRNG), and tetracycline, the currently recommended first-line treatment for neonatal gonococcal conjunctivitis is ceftriaxone. For *nondisseminated* infections, a single intramuscular or intravenous ceftriaxone injection (up to 125 mg or a dosage of 25–50 mg/kg) or cefotaxime at a single dose of 100 mg/kg IV or IM is recommended. For *disseminated* infection, treatment should be augmented according to infectious disease consultation. Either of these regimens should be combined with hourly saline irrigation of the conjunctiva until discharge is eliminated. If corneal involvement is suspected, application of topical erythromycin or gentamicin ointment or frequent application of a topical fluoroquinolone should be considered. Topical cycloplegia may also prove beneficial. Systemic treatment is advised for infants born to mothers with active gonorrhea, even in the absence of conjunctivitis.

Centers for Disease Control and Prevention. Sexually Transmitted Diseases Treatment Guidelines 2002. *Morbidity and Mortality Weekly Report.* 2002;51:36–42.

Gonococcal infections. In: Pickering LK, ed. *2000 Red Book: Report of the Committee on Infectious Diseases.* 25th ed. Elk Grove Village, Illinois; American Academy of Pediatrics; 2000:256.

Neonatal chlamydial conjunctivitis

Chlamydial conjunctivitis in neonates differs clinically from adult chlamydial conjunctivitis in the following ways:

- No follicular response appears in newborns
- The amount of mucopurulent discharge is greater in newborns
- Membranes can develop on the tarsal conjunctiva in newborns
- Intracytoplasmic inclusions are seen in a greater percentage of Giemsa-stained conjunctival specimens in newborns
- The infection in newborns is more likely to respond to topical medications

Both Gram and Giemsa stains of conjunctival scrapings are recommended in neonates with conjunctivitis to identify *C trachomatis* and *N gonorrhoeae*, as well as other bacteria as causative agents. Other *Chlamydia*-associated infections such as pneumonitis and otitis media can accompany inclusion conjunctivitis in the newborn. Therefore, systemic erythromycin (12.5 mg/kg oral or IV qid for 14 days) is recommended, even though inclusion conjunctivitis in the newborn usually responds to topical erythromycin or sulfacetamide.

Chlamydial Conjunctivitis

PATHOGENESIS *Chlamydia trachomatis* is an obligate intracellular bacterium that causes several different conjunctivitis syndromes; each is associated with different serotypes of *C trachomatis*:

- Trachoma: serotypes A–C
- Adult and neonatal inclusion conjunctivitis: serotypes D–K
- Lymphogranuloma venereum: serotypes L1, L2, and L3

Rare cases of keratoconjunctivitis in humans have been reported caused by *Chlamydia* species that typically infect animals, such as *C psittaci*, an agent generally associated with disease in parrots, and the feline pneumonitis agent.

CLINICAL PRESENTATION AND MANAGEMENT Trachoma and adult inclusion conjunctivitis are discussed individually below.

Trachoma

Trachoma is an infectious disease that occurs in communities with poor hygiene and inadequate sanitation. It affects approximately 150 million individuals worldwide and is the leading cause of preventable blindness. Trachoma is currently endemic in the Middle East and in developing regions around the world. In the United States it occurs sporadically among American Indians and in mountainous areas of the South. Evidence suggests that the common housefly and other household fomites are important vectors for transmitting *Chlamydia*, and patients with trachoma are repeatedly infected. Other bacteria that cause secondary bacterial infections in patients with trachoma are spread by these fomites as well.

CLINICAL PRESENTATION The initial symptoms of trachoma include foreign body sensation, redness, tearing, and mucopurulent discharge. A severe follicular reaction develops, most prominently in the superior tarsal conjunctiva but sometimes appearing in the superior and inferior fornices, inferior tarsal conjunctiva, semilunar fold, and limbus. In acute trachoma, follicles on the superior tarsus may be obscured by diffuse papillary hypertrophy and inflammatory cell infiltration. Large tarsal follicles in trachoma may become necrotic and eventually heal with significant scarring. Linear or stellate scarring of the superior tarsus *(Arlt's line)* typically occurs (Fig 7-23). Involution and necrosis of follicles may result in limbal depressions known as *Herbert's pits* (Fig 7-24). Corneal findings in trachoma include epithelial keratitis, focal and multifocal peripheral and central stromal infiltrates, and superficial fibrovascular pannus, which is most prominent in the superior third of the cornea but may extend centrally into the visual axis (Fig 7-25).

Clinical diagnosis of trachoma requires at least two of the following clinical features:

- Conjunctival follicles on the upper tarsal conjunctiva
- Limbal follicles and their sequelae (Herbert's pits)
- Typical tarsal conjunctival scarring
- Vascular pannus most marked on the superior limbus

Severe conjunctival and lacrimal gland duct scarring from chronic trachoma can result in aqueous tear deficiency, tear drainage obstruction, trichiasis, and entropion.

The World Health Organization (WHO) has introduced a simple severity grading system for trachoma based on the presence or absence of five key signs:

- Follicular conjunctival inflammation
- Diffuse conjunctival inflammation
- Tarsal conjunctival scarring
- Trichiasis
- Corneal opacification

The WHO grading system was developed for use by trained personnel other than ophthalmologists to assess the prevalence and severity of trachoma in population-based surveys in endemic areas.

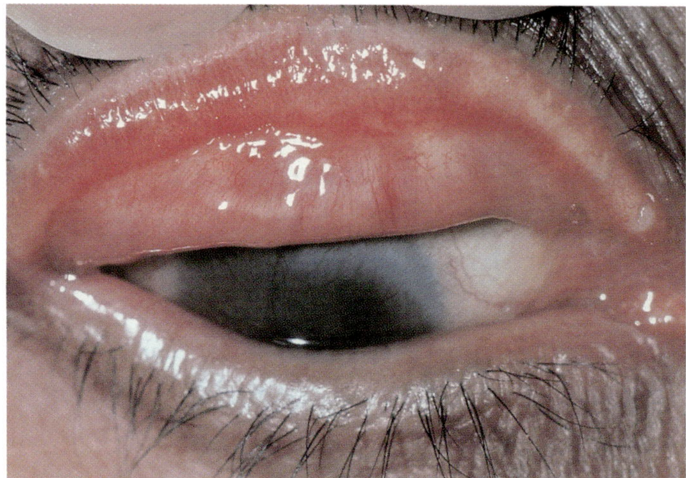

Figure 7-23 Linear scarring of the superior tarsal conjunctiva (Arlt's line) in a patient with old trachoma. *(Photograph courtesy of Vincent P. deLuise, MD.)*

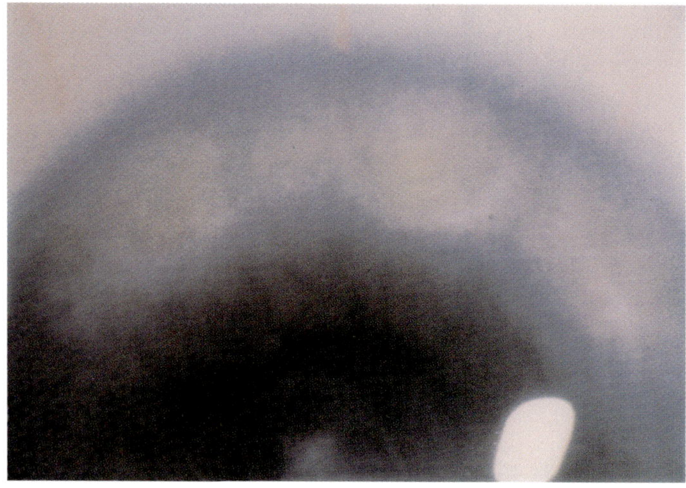

Figure 7-24 Trachoma exhibiting Herbert's pits of the superior limbus (round to oval, relatively lucent areas within pannus).

Thylefors B, Dawson CR, Jones BR, et al. A simple system for the assessment of trachoma and its complications. *Bull World Health Organ.* 1987;65:477–483.

MANAGEMENT Active trachoma is treated with topical and oral tetracycline or erythromycin. Topical tetracycline 1% or erythromycin ointment should be administered twice daily for 2 months. Oral tetracycline in a dosage of 1.5–2.0 g daily in divided doses should be administered for 3 weeks. Oral erythromycin is recommended for treatment of the rare cases of trachoma that are clinically resistant to tetracycline. Azithromycin, a long-acting macrolide, may have utility for mass treatment programs because of the prolonged

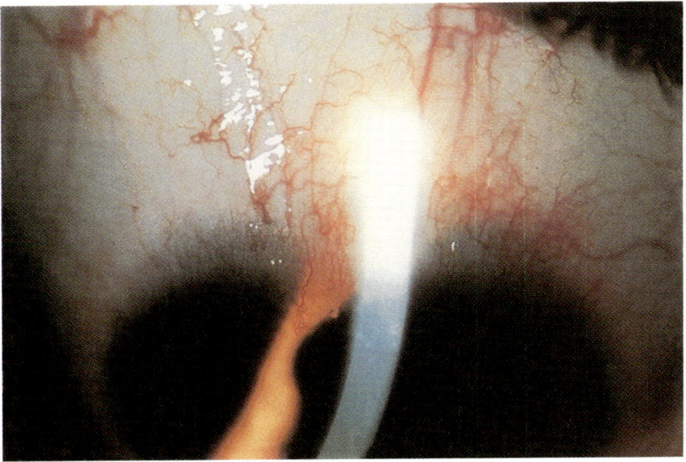

Figure 7-25 Superior corneal micropannus in a patient with adult chlamydial conjunctivitis.

duration of action of single-dose administration. The management of the complications of trachoma may include tear substitutes for dry eye and eyelid surgery for entropion or trichiasis. See further discussion in BCSC Section 13, *International Ophthalmology.*

Adult chlamydial conjunctivitis

This sexually transmitted disease is often found in conjunction with chlamydial urethritis or cervicitis. It is most prevalent in sexually active adolescents and young adults. The eye is usually infected by direct or indirect contact with infected genital secretions, although other modes of transmission may include shared eye cosmetics and inadequately chlorinated swimming pools. Onset of conjunctivitis is typically 1–2 weeks after ocular inoculation and is not as acute as adenoviral keratoconjunctivitis. Often patients may complain of mild symptoms for weeks to months.

CLINICAL PRESENTATION External signs of adult inclusion conjunctivitis include a follicular conjunctival response that is most prominent in the lower palpebral conjunctiva and fornix, scant mucopurulent discharge, and palpable preauricular adenopathy. Follicles in the bulbar conjunctiva and semilunar fold are frequently present, and these are a helpful and specific sign in patients who have not been using topical medications associated with development of bulbar follicles. Inflammatory conjunctival membranes do not develop in chlamydial keratoconjunctivitis.

Corneal involvement may consist of fine or coarse epithelial infiltrates, occasionally associated with subepithelial infiltrates. The keratitis is more likely to be found in the superior cornea but may also occur centrally and resemble adenoviral keratitis. A micropannus, usually extending less than 3 mm from the superior cornea, may develop.

MANAGEMENT Left untreated, adult chlamydial conjunctivitis often resolves spontaneously in 6–18 months. Currently, one of the following antibiotic regimens is recommended:

- Oral tetracycline 250 mg qid for 3 weeks
- Doxycycline 100 mg bid for 3 weeks
- Oral erythromycin 500 mg qid for 3 weeks

A single oral dose of azithromycin 1 g is effective in early active inflammatory stages (Tabbara 1996).

Patients with laboratory-confirmed chlamydial conjunctivitis and their sexual contacts should be evaluated for coinfection with other sexually transmitted diseases such as syphilis or gonorrhea before antibiotic treatment is started. Sexual partners should be concomitantly treated to avoid reinfection.

Tabbara KF, Hyndiuk RA. *Infections of the Eye.* 2nd ed. Boston: Little, Brown; 1996.

Parinaud Oculoglandular Syndrome

Granulomatous conjunctivitis with regional lymphadenopathy is an uncommon condition called *Parinaud oculoglandular syndrome. Cat-scratch disease (CSD),* which causes most cases of the syndrome, is estimated to affect approximately 22,000 persons annually in the United States, with about 10% developing conjunctivitis. The primary causative agent is *Bartonella henselae.* Other infrequent causes of Parinaud oculoglandular syndrome include:

- *Afipia felis*
- *Bartonella clarridgeiae*
- Tularemia
- Lymphogranuloma venereum
- Tuberculosis
- Sporotrichosis
- Syphilis
- Mediterranean spotted fever

PATHOGENESIS *Bartonella henselae* lives on cats and their fleas. Most cases are transmitted by a scratch from a flea-infested kitten. Other modes of transmission include a cat's biting or licking the human skin. Local infection causes a granulomatous reaction.

CLINICAL PRESENTATION Unilateral granulomatous conjunctivitis with one or more raised or flat gelatinous, hyperemic, granulomatous lesions develops on the superior or inferior tarsal conjunctiva, fornix, or bulbar conjunctiva about 3–10 days after inoculation. Either concurrently or 1–2 weeks later, unilateral firm and tender regional preauricular and submandibular lymph nodes, and occasionally cervical nodes, develop. Approximately 10%–40% of the nodes enlarge and become suppurative. Mild systemic symptoms of fever, malaise, headache, and anorexia develop in about 10%–30% of patients with severe, disseminated complications including encephalopathy, encephalitis, thrombocytopenic purpura, osteolysis, hepatitis, and splenitis occurring in approximately 2% of CSD patients. Optic neuritis and neuroretinitis have been reported.

LABORATORY EVALUATION Serologic testing is the most cost-effective means for diagnosing typical CSD. Antibodies to *Bartonella henselae* can be detected by indirect fluorescent antibody testing or by enzyme immunoassay. The enzyme immunoassay for *B henselae* is more sensitive than the indirect fluorescent antibody test and is available from specialty laboratories. The skin test antigen for CSD is neither commercially available nor standardized. Atypical CSD is best approached by combining serologic testing with culture or polymerase chain reaction (PCR).

MANAGEMENT The ideal treatment has not yet been determined. Various antibacterial treatment regimens have reported success. Suggested agents generally include azithromycin, erythromycin, or doxycycline. Rifampin is often used as an adjuvant. Responses to trimethoprim-sulfamethoxazole and fluoroquinolones have also been reported but appear to be inconsistent.

> Jackson LA, Perkins BA, Wenger JD. Cat-scratch disease in the United States: an analysis of three national databases. *Am J Public Health.* 1993;83:1707–1711.

Microsporidial Keratoconjunctivitis

Microsporida are intracellular protozoa that can infect the conjunctival and corneal epithelium in immunosuppressed individuals with AIDS. Patients may also have disseminated microsporidiosis involving the sinuses, respiratory tract, or gastrointestinal tract.

Encephalitozoon hellem and *E cuniculi* cannot be seen within the conjunctiva, although chronic conjunctivitis is typical. Punctate epithelial keratopathy is manifested by a coarse granularity of the corneal epithelium that extends to the limbus. The corneal stroma remains clear, with no or minimal iritis. Scrapings of the ocular surface can be stained to reveal acid-fast spores. Electron microscopy is used to classify the spores and meronts. Medical treatment includes topical fumagillin and oral albendazole. Microsporidial ocular disease is discussed further under the subhead of Microsporidial Keratitis later in this chapter.

Loiasis

Loa loa and other filarial nematodes can cause conjunctivitis as well as dermatologic manifestations. After the bite of an infected vector, such parasites can burrow subcutaneously to reach the eye area. The microfilarial stage is transmitted from human to human by the bite of an infected female deer fly (genus *Chrysops*) indigenous to West and Central Africa. A migrating worm moves under the skin at about 1 cm/min but is most conspicuous when it is seen or felt wriggling under the periocular skin or bulbar conjunctiva. Extraction of the filarial worm cures the conjunctivitis; it is followed by antiparasitic treatment for widespread infestation. Diethylcarbamazine is generally given 2 mg/kg tid for 3 weeks and repeated as necessary. Ivermectin 150 mg/kg may also be effective, but significant side effects have been reported in patients with prominent intravascular loiasis. Concurrent administration of steroids and/or antihistamines may be necessary to minimize allergic reactions.

Microbial and Parasitic Infections of the Cornea and Sclera

Bacterial Keratitis

Bacterial infection is a common sight-threatening condition. Some cases have explosive onset and rapidly progressive stromal inflammation. Untreated, it often leads to progressive tissue destruction with corneal perforation or extension of infection to adjacent tissue. Bacterial keratitis is frequently associated with risk factors that disturb the corneal epithelial integrity. Common predisposing factors include:

- Contact lens wear
- Trauma
- Contaminated ocular medications
- Impaired defense mechanisms
- Altered structure of the corneal surface

The most frequent risk factor for bacterial keratitis in the United States is contact lens wear, which has been identified as such in 19%–42% of patients who develop culture-proven microbial keratitis. Epidemiologic studies have estimated the annual incidence of cosmetic contact lens–related ulcerative keratitis at 0.21% for individuals using extended-wear soft lenses and 0.04% for patients using daily-wear soft lenses. The risk of developing microbial keratitis increases significantly (approximately 15 times) in patients who wear their contact lenses overnight and is positively correlated with the number of consecutive days lenses are worn without removal.

PATHOGENESIS Bacteria have multiple mechanisms of adherence. For example, *S aureus* uses adhesins to bind to collagen and other components of the exposed Bowman's layer and stroma, while *P aeruginosa* can bind to molecular receptors exposed on injured epithelial cells. A clone of bacteria initially proliferates, then—within hours—invades the cornea between stromal lamellae. Corneal inflammation begins with the local production of cytokines and chemokines that enable diapedesis and migration of neutrophils into the peripheral cornea from the limbal vessels. Some microorganisms produce proteases that disrupt the extracellular matrix. Enzymes released by neutrophils and activation of corneal matrix metalloproteinases exacerbate inflammatory necrosis. With antimicrobial control of bacterial replication, wound healing processes begin that may be accompanied by neovascularization and scarring. Progressive inflammation, on the other hand, may lead to corneal perforation.

CLINICAL PRESENTATION Rapid onset of pain is accompanied by conjunctival injection, photophobia, and decreased vision in patients with bacterial corneal ulcers. The rate of progression of these symptoms depends on the virulence of the infecting organism. Bacterial corneal ulcers typically show a sharp epithelial demarcation with underlying dense, suppurative stromal inflammation that has indistinct edges and is surrounded by stromal edema. *P aeruginosa* typically produces stromal necrosis with a shaggy surface and adherent mucopurulent exudate (Fig 7-26). An endothelial inflammatory plaque, marked anterior chamber reaction, and hypopyon frequently occur.

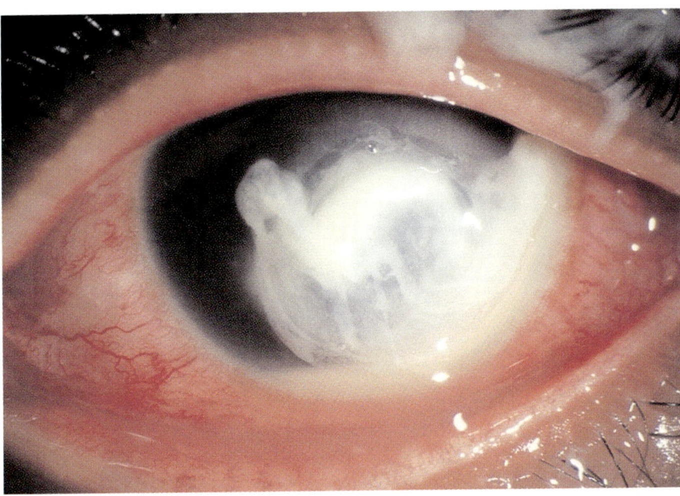

Figure 7-26 Suppurative ulcerative keratitis caused by *P aeruginosa*.

Infections caused by slow-growing, fastidious organisms such as mycobacteria or anaerobes may have a nonsuppurative infiltrate and intact epithelium. *Infectious crystalline keratopathy,* an example of this type of infection, presents as densely packed, white, branching aggregates of organisms in the virtual absence of a host inflammatory response. It is believed to occur when a sequestered colony of slow-growing organisms develops after midstromal implantation in a cornea with compromised inflammatory responses. Corticosteroid use, contact lens wear, and infected corneal grafts can all create a predisposition to this infection. Infectious crystalline keratopathy has been reported with a number of bacterial species, most commonly α-hemolytic *Streptococcus* species (Fig 7-27).

LABORATORY EVALUATION A wide variety of bacterial species can cause microbial keratitis. The prevalence of a particular causative organism depends on the geographic location and risk factors for the infection. Common and uncommon organisms causing bacterial keratitis are listed in Table 7-5.

Because keratitis can be caused by a wide variety of organisms, many of which have unique antimicrobial sensitivity profiles, it can be difficult to determine whether a corneal ulcer has an infectious etiology. Before initiating antimicrobial therapy for cases of suspected bacterial keratitis, the clinician should consider conducting microbiological diagnostic tests. See Chapter 4 and Chapter 6 for specimen collecting, culturing, staining, and interpretation.

If the patient has already been treated with topical antibiotics, the medication should be stopped for 12–24 hours prior to culturing in order to enhance recovery of viable organisms. However, antimicrobial therapy should not be discontinued in severe or rapidly progressive corneal ulcers. An antibiotic removal device, which contains resins to bind antibiotics that might inhibit bacterial growth, may be considered in these cases.

In addition to culturing the cornea, it may be helpful to culture contact lenses, contact lens cases, solutions, and any other potentially contaminating sources such as

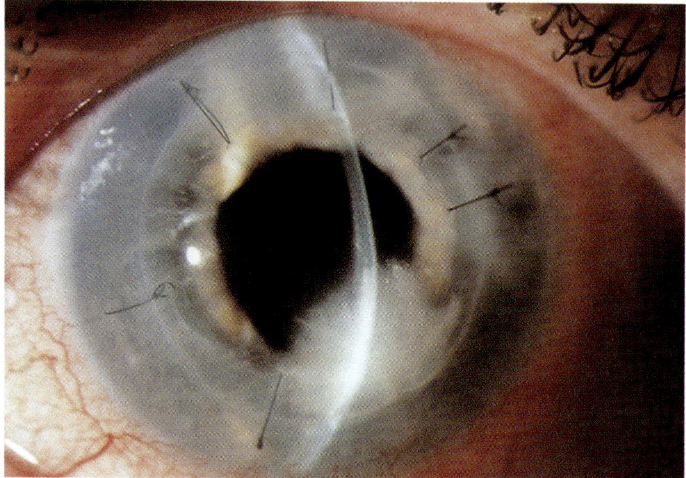

Figure 7-27 Infectious crystalline keratopathy in a corneal graft caused by α-hemolytic *Streptococcus* species.

inflamed eyelids, because any of these might provide a clue to the causative organism in the event that corneal cultures are negative. This approach can also help identify the source of the infection.

MANAGEMENT Currently, no single antibiotic agent is effective against all bacterial species causing microbial keratitis. Initial broad-spectrum therapy is recommended until the offending microorganism is identified in culture. If one type of bacteria is prominently identified on a stained diagnostic smear, therapy may initially be weighted toward that class of microorganism. Broad-spectrum therapy, however, should not be eliminated, as cultures may reveal a different class of microorganism. Once the offending microbe is identified, or the clinical response suggests the change, then appropriate monotherapy may be considered (Table 7-6).

The route of antibiotic administration should be based on the severity of the keratitis. Frequent (every 30–60 minutes) fortified topical antibiotics are now used for bacterial keratitis. Fortified antibiotic solutions produce therapeutic antibiotic concentrations in the corneal stroma, while commercially available antibiotic solutions may result in subtherapeutic concentrations. In severe cases, therapeutic stromal concentrations of antibiotic may be achieved more rapidly by initially administering the antibiotic drop every 5 minutes for 30 minutes as a loading dose. Subconjunctival and IV antibiotics in addition to frequent topical antibiotics are indicated in cases with suspected scleral and/or intraocular extension of infection.

Modification of initial antimicrobial therapy should be based on clinical response, not on the results of antimicrobial sensitivity testing. Determination of antibiotic sensitivity or resistance in traditional antimicrobial sensitivity tests is based on antibiotic concentrations achievable in the serum by oral or parenteral administration. Often, antibiotic concentrations greatly exceeding the mean inhibitory concentrations of bacteria are achieved in the corneal stroma following frequent fortified antibiotic administration.

Table 7-5 Causes of Bacterial Keratitis

Common Organisms	Uncommon Organisms
Staphylococcus aureus	*Neisseria* species
Staphylococcus epidermidis	*Moraxella* species
Streptococcus pneumoniae and other *Streptococcus* species	*Mycobacterium* species
	Nocardia species
Pseudomonas aeruginosa (most common organism in soft contact lens wearers)	Non–spore-forming anaerobes
	Corynebacterium species
Enterobacteriaceae (*Proteus, Enterobacter, Serratia*)	

Table 7-6 Initial Therapy for Bacterial Keratitis

Organism	Antibiotic	Topical Dose	Subconjunctival Dose
Gram-positive cocci	Cefazolin	50 mg/mL	100 mg in 0.5 mL
	Vancomycin*	50 mg/mL	25 mg in 0.5 mL
	Moxifloxacin or gatifloxacin	5 or 3 mg/mL	Not available
Gram-negative rods	Tobramycin	9–14 mg/mL	20 mg in 0.5 mL
	Ceftazidime	50 mg/mL	100 mg in 0.5 mL
	Fluoroquinolones	3 mg/mL	Not available
No organism or multiple types of organisms	Cefazolin with	50 mg/mL	100 mg in 0.5 mL
	Tobramycin or	9–14 mg/mL	20 mg in 0.5 mL
	Fluoroquinolones	3 mg/mL	Not available
Gram-nagative cocci	Ceftriaxone	50 mg/mL	100 mg in 0.5 mL
	Ceftazidime	50 mg/mL	
Mycobacteria	Amikacin	20 mg/mL	20 mg in 0.5 mL

* For resistant *Staphylococcus* species.

Notes for Table 7-6: Preparation of topical antibiotics
Cefazolin 50 mg/mL
1. Add 9.2 mL of Tears Naturale artificial tears to a vial of cefazolin in 1 g (powder for injection).
2. Dissolve. Take 5 mL of this solution and add it to 5 mL of artificial tears.
3. Refrigerate and shake well before instillation.
Vancomycin 50 mg/mL
1. Add 10 mL of 0.9% sodium chloride for injection USP (no preservatives) or artificial tears to a 500-mg vial of vancomycin to produce a solution of 50 mg/mL.
2. Refrigerate and shake well before instillation.
Ceftazidime 50 mg/mL
1. Add 9.2 mL of artificial tears to a vial of ceftazidime 1 g (powder for injection).
2. Dissolve. Take 5 mL of this solution and add it to 5 mL of artificial tears.
3. Refrigerate and shake well before instillation.
Tobramycin 14 mg/mL
1. Withdraw 2 mL of tobramycin injectable vial (40 mg/mL).
2. Add 2 mL to a tobramycin ophthalmic solution (5 mL) to give a 14 mg/mL solution.
3. Refrigerate and shake well before instillation.

An alternate antibiotic regimen should be considered in patients who do not show clinical response or who develop toxicity from the agent(s) used initially. Modification of antibiotic therapy in these cases should be based on antimicrobial sensitivity testing. Several clinical parameters are useful to monitor clinical response to antibiotic therapy:

- Blunting of the perimeter of the stromal infiltrate
- Decreased density of the stromal infiltrate
- Reduction of stromal edema and endothelial inflammatory plaque
- Reduction in anterior chamber inflammation
- Reepithelialization
- Cessation of corneal thinning

The frequency of topical antibiotic administration should slowly be tapered as the stromal inflammation resolves.

Combination therapy with an agent active against gram-positive bacteria (eg, vancomycin, bacitracin, Neosporin, cefuroxime, or cefazolin) and an agent active against gram-negative bacteria (eg, tobramycin, gentamicin, amikacin, ceftazidime, ciprofloxacin, levofloxacin, or ofloxacin) provides good initial broad-spectrum antibiotic coverage. Single-agent therapy with a fluoroquinolone may also be considered. These antibiotics should initially be given every 30–60 minutes and then tapered in frequency according to the clinical response. Fortified antibiotics should generally be continued until substantial infection control has been achieved. Thereafter, a broad-spectrum, nonfortified antibiotic may be given three to eight times daily according to the patient's clinical status.

Disadvantages of fortified antibiotics include ocular irritation, cost, and the inconvenience of extemporaneously preparing a solution that is not commercially available. Their chief advantage is their potential to save vision in aggressive infections. When irritation secondary to epithelial toxicity becomes a concern, lower strength concentrations (eg, 20 mg/mL vancomycin or 20 mg/mL amikacin) may be better tolerated.

An alternative to combination therapy is the use of fluoroquinolone monotherapy, which is most appropriate in compliant patients with less severe ulcers (eg, less than 3 mm in diameter, midperipheral or peripheral, and not associated with significant thinning). Fluoroquinolones (eg, levofloxacin, ciprofloxacin, ofloxacin, moxifloxacin, and gatifloxacin) must be administered at least every hour to maximize therapeutic effect. Because second-generation fluoroquinolones such as ciprofloxacin and ofloxacin typically have variable activity against streptococci, documented streptococcal infections should be treated with a cell wall–active agent (eg, bacitracin, cefazolin, vancomycin, or penicillin G) rather than a second-generation fluoroquinolone, regardless of in vitro testing that may suggest susceptibility.

Corticosteroids

The role of corticosteroid therapy for bacterial keratitis is controversial. It is well recognized that tissue destruction in microbial keratitis results from a combination of the direct effects of lytic enzymes and toxins produced by the infecting organism as well as the damage caused by the inflammatory reaction directed at the microorganisms. An intense suppurative inflammatory reaction consisting predominantly of polymorphonuclear leukocytes is induced by many of the bacteria that cause microbial keratitis. Neutrophils are capable of causing significant tissue destruction by generation of free radicals as well as liberation of proteolytic enzymes, including collagenases and gelatinases that can dissolve the corneal stroma. The rationale for use of corticosteroids is to decrease the tissue destruction caused by these neutrophils.

Several studies using animal models of bacterial keratitis have demonstrated that concurrent use of topical corticosteroids does not impair the killing effect of bactericidal antibiotics against susceptible microorganisms. Clinical series evaluating the effectiveness of corticosteroids for treatment of human bacterial keratitis have reported either no treatment effect or more rapid resolution of stromal inflammation than resulted from antibiotic therapy alone.

However, the use of topical corticosteroids following presumed resolution of gram-negative bacterial keratitis (especially that caused by *P aeruginosa*) has been documented to promote a relapse of the infection. Presumably, virulent organisms that require a low inoculum to establish infection may remain viable in small numbers for some time following clinical resolution of the infection. If the immune system is impaired by administration of topical corticosteroids before complete clearance of these organisms, recurrent infection may result. Topical corticosteroids should therefore be used for treatment of bacterial keratitis with extreme caution and only in qualified circumstances. Following are recommended criteria for instituting corticosteroid therapy for bacterial keratitis:

- Corticosteroids should not be used in the initial phase of the treatment until an etiologic organism has been identified and the organism shows in vitro sensitivity to the antibiotic(s) being used for treatment
- The patient must be able to return for frequent follow-up examinations and demonstrate compliance with appropriate antibiotic therapy
- There is no other associated virulent or difficult-to-eradicate organism

In addition, a favorable clinical response to antibiotic therapy is strongly advised before topical corticosteroids are initiated. Corticosteroid drops may be started in moderate dosages (prednisolone acetate or phosphate 1% every 4–6 hours), and the patient should be monitored at 24 and 48 hours after initiation of therapy. If the patient shows no adverse effects, the frequency of administration may possibly be increased for a short period of time, and then the medication can be tapered based on the clinical response.

Surgery

Penetrating keratoplasty for treatment of bacterial keratitis is indicated if the disease progresses despite therapy, descemetocele formation or perforation occurs, or the keratitis is unresponsive to antimicrobial therapy. The involved area should be identified preoperatively, and an attempt should be made to circumscribe all areas of infection. Peripheral iridectomies are indicated, since patients may develop seclusion of the pupil from inflammatory pupillary membranes. Interrupted sutures are recommended. The patient should be treated with appropriate antibiotics, cycloplegics, and intense topical corticosteroids postoperatively. See Chapters 22–23 for a discussion of penetrating keratoplasty in greater detail.

Preferred Practice Patterns Committee, Cornea Panel. *Bacterial Keratitis.* San Francisco: American Academy of Ophthalmology; 1998.

Schein OD, Glynn RJ, Poggio EC, et al. The relative risk of ulcerative keratitis among users of daily-wear and extended-wear soft contact lenses. A case-control study. Microbial Keratitis Study Group. *N Engl J Med.* 1989;321:773–778.

Fungal Keratitis

PATHOGENESIS Fungal keratitis is less common than bacterial keratitis, generally representing less than 5%–10% of corneal infections in reported clinical series from the United States. Filamentous fungal keratitis occurs more frequently in warmer, more humid parts of the United States than in other regions of the country. Trauma to the cornea with plant or vegetable material is the leading risk factor for fungal keratitis. Especially predisposed are gardeners who use weed trimmers or other similar motorized lawn care equipment without wearing protective eyewear. Trauma related to contact lens wear is another common risk factor for the development of fungal keratitis. Topical corticosteroids are another major risk factor, as they appear to activate and increase the virulence of fungal organisms by reducing the cornea's resistance to infection. The increasing use of topical corticosteroids during the past four decades has been implicated as a major cause for the rising incidence of fungal keratitis during this period. Furthermore, systemic corticosteroid usage may suppress the host's immune response, thereby predisposing to fungal keratitis. Other common risk factors include corneal surgery (eg, penetrating keratoplasty, radial keratotomy) and chronic keratitis (eg, herpes simplex, herpes zoster, or vernal/allergic conjunctivitis).

CLINICAL PRESENTATION Patients with fungal keratitis tend to have fewer inflammatory signs and symptoms during the initial period than those with bacterial keratitis and may have little or no conjunctival injection upon initial presentation. Filamentous fungal keratitis frequently manifests as a gray-white, dry-appearing infiltrate that has irregular feathery or filamentous margins (Fig 7-28). Superficial lesions may appear gray-white,

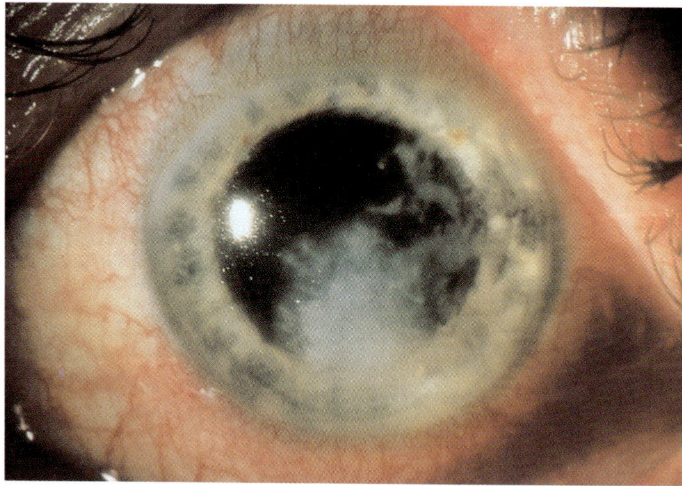

Figure 7-28 Fungal keratitis caused by *Fusarium solani* with characteristic dry white stromal infiltrate with feathery edges.

elevate the surface of the cornea, and have a dry, rough, or gritty texture detectable at the time of diagnostic corneal scraping. Occasionally, multifocal or satellite infiltrates may be present, although these are less common than previously reported. Additionally, a deep stromal infiltrate may occur in the presence of an intact epithelium. An endothelial plaque and/or hypopyon may also occur if the fungal infiltrate(s) are sufficiently deep or large.

As the keratitis progresses, intense suppuration may develop and the lesions may resemble bacterial keratitis. At this point, rapidly progressive hypopyon and anterior chamber inflammatory membranes may develop. Extension of fungal infection into the anterior chamber is often seen in cases with rapidly progressive anterior chamber inflammation. Occasionally, fungus may invade the iris or posterior chamber, and angle-closure glaucoma may develop from inflammatory pupillary block. See also BCSC Section 10, *Glaucoma.*

Yeast keratitis is most frequently caused by *Candida* spp. This form of fungal keratitis frequently presents with superficial white, raised colonies in a structurally altered eye. Although most cases tend to remain superficial, deep invasion may occur with suppuration resembling keratitis induced by gram-positive bacteria.

MANAGEMENT Natamycin 5% suspension is recommended for treatment of most cases of filamentous fungal keratitis, particularly those caused by *Fusarium* spp, which are the most common causative agents for exogenous fungal keratitis occurring in the humid areas of the southern United States. Topical miconazole 1% (10 mg/mL) is the agent of choice to combat *Paecilomyces lilacinus,* an aggressive organism whose conidia are relatively resistant to most sterilization techniques and known to contaminate intraocular lenses. Most clinical and experimental evidence suggests that topical amphotericin B (0.15%–0.3%) is the most efficacious agent available to treat yeast keratitis. An additive effect has been noted when amphotericin B is combined with flucytosine; however, the majority of corneal yeast infections respond readily to amphotericin B. Similarly, amphotericin B is also recommended for filamentous keratitis caused by *Aspergillus* spp. Oral ketoconazole (200–600 mg/day) may be considered for adjunctive therapy in severe filamentous fungal keratitis, and oral fluconazole (200–400 mg/day) for severe yeast keratitis. Oral itraconazole (200 mg/day) has broad-spectrum activity against all *Aspergillus* species and *Candida,* but variable activity against *Fusarium.*

In the presence of a negative smear when fungal infection is suspected, repeated scrapings or biopsy may be necessary to identify fungal material. Furthermore, mechanical debridement may be beneficial for cases of superficial fungal keratitis. Fungal infiltration of the deep corneal stroma may not respond to topical antifungal therapy, because the penetration of these agents is reduced in the presence of an intact epithelium. Penetration of natamycin or amphotericin B has been shown to be significantly enhanced by debridement of the corneal epithelium, and animal experiments indicate that frequent topical application (every 5 minutes) for 1 hour can readily achieve therapeutic levels. Cases with progressive disease despite maximal topical and/or oral antifungal therapy may require therapeutic penetrating keratoplasty to prevent scleral or intraocular extension of the fungal infection. Both of these conditions carry a very poor prognosis for salvaging the eye.

Bron AJ, Seal DV, Hay J. *Ocular Infection: Investigation and Treatment in Practice.* St Louis: Mosby; 1998.

O'Brien TP. Therapy of ocular fungal infections. *Ophthalmol Clin North Am.* 1999;12(1):33–50.

O'Day DM. Fungal keratitis. In: Leibowitz HM, Waring GO III, eds. *Corneal Disorders: Clinical Diagnosis and Management.* 2nd ed. Philadelphia: Saunders; 1998:711–718.

Acanthamoeba Keratitis

PATHOGENESIS Acanthamoebae are free-living ubiquitous protozoa found in freshwater and soil. They are resistant to killing by freezing, desiccation, and the levels of chlorine routinely used in municipal water supplies, swimming pools, and hot tubs. They may exist as motile trophozoites or dormant cysts. The majority (70%) of reported cases of amebic keratitis have been associated with contact lens use. Homemade saline solution prepared by dissolving saline tablets in distilled water appeared to be a significant source of *Acanthamoeba* infection among contact lens wearers until saline tablets were taken off the US market in the 1980s.

CLINICAL PRESENTATION Patients with amebic keratitis commonly have severe ocular pain, photophobia, and a protracted, progressive course. Frequently, they have shown no therapeutic response to a variety of topical antimicrobial agents. *Acanthamoeba* infection is localized to the corneal epithelium in early cases and may manifest as a diffuse punctate epitheliopathy or dendritic epithelial lesion. Cases with epithelial dendrites are often misdiagnosed as herpetic keratitis and treated with antiviral agents and/or corticosteroids. Stromal infection typically occurs in the central cornea, and early cases have a gray-white superficial, nonsuppurative infiltrate. As the disease progresses, a partial or complete ring infiltrate in the paracentral cornea is frequently observed (Fig 7-29). Enlarged corneal nerves, called *radial perineuritis,* may be noted as well as limbitis or focal, nodular, or diffuse scleritis.

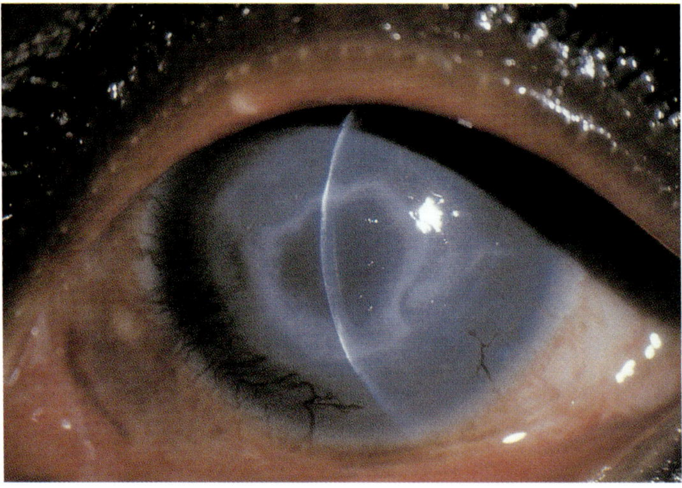

Figure 7-29 Ring infiltrate in *Acanthamoeba* keratitis.

LABORATORY EVALUATION Diagnosis of *Acanthamoeba* keratitis is made by visualizing amoebae in stained smears or by culturing organisms obtained from corneal scrapings. The highest diagnostic yield occurs relatively early in the course of the disease, when the organisms are localized to the epithelium. Later, the organisms penetrate into deeper layers and may be difficult to isolate from superficial scraping. Lamellar corneal biopsy may be required to establish the diagnosis in these cases. In contact lens–associated infections, the contact lenses and contact lens case can be examined.

Amoebae are visualized in smears stained with Giemsa, periodic acid–Schiff (PAS), calcofluor white, or acridine orange stains. Nonnutrient agar with *E coli* or *E aerogenes* overlay is the preferred media for culturing amoebae, although the organisms frequently grow well on blood agar plates and on buffered charcoal–yeast extract agar. Characteristic trails form as the motile trophozoites travel across the surface of the culture plate. Confocal in vivo microscopy can also be used to demonstrate organisms, particularly the cyst forms.

MANAGEMENT Early diagnosis of *Acanthamoeba* keratitis is the most important prognostic indicator of a successful treatment outcome. Unfortunately, many cases are treated initially for herpetic keratitis. Not only is the delay in diagnosis detrimental, but the use of corticosteroids early in the disease may also be correlated with a poor outcome due to compromise of the host's inflammatory response against *Acanthamoeba*. Although controversial, late immunoinflammatory responses after the amoebae have been killed may be reduced by corticosteroids, but this remains an area for further investigation. Clinical features that suggest a diagnosis of *Acanthamoeba* keratitis rather than herpes simplex keratitis include:

- Noncontiguous or multifocal pattern of granular epitheliopathy and subepithelial opacities (unlike the contiguous, dendritic pattern in HSV keratitis)
- Disproportionately severe pain, probably secondary to perineural inflammation (unlike hypoesthesia and disproportionately mild pain secondary to trigeminal nerve involvement in HSV)
- Presence of epidemiologic risk factors such as contact lens use or exposure to possibly contaminated freshwater
- Failure to respond to initial antiviral therapy

Cases diagnosed during the early, epithelial stage of the disease respond well to epithelial debridement, followed by a relatively short (3–4 months) course of antiamebic therapy. The prognosis for visual recovery with only mild residual stromal involvement is very good. Once stromal infiltrates appear, however, eradication of organisms is more difficult, and treatment may be needed for 6–12 months.

A number of antimicrobial agents have been recommended for therapy of *Acanthamoeba* keratitis based on their in vitro amebicidal effects as well as their clinical effectiveness. Agents used for topical administration include:

- Diamidines: propamidine, hexamidine
- Biguanides: polyhexamethylene biguanide (polyhexanide), chlorhexidine
- Aminoglycosides: neomycin, paromomycin
- Imidazoles/triazoles: miconazole, clotrimazole, ketoconazole, itraconazole

Most of these agents are effective against the free-living trophozoite form of the organism but have reduced efficacy in killing cysts. Although there is not yet consensus about the optimal therapeutic agent, successful resolution has been achieved with a biguanide with and without a diamidine. Recent reports favor the use of chlorhexidine 0.02% or polyhexamethylene biguanide (PHMB) 0.02% as initial therapy. Some specialists encourage the combination of chlorhexidine or PHMB in combination with propamidine isethionate 0.1%. Treatment with topical corticosteroids is of uncertain long-term benefit and may contribute to prolonged persistence of viable cysts or potentiate mixed infections when a virus is present.

Penetrating keratoplasty is reserved for cases that are progressing despite maximal medical therapy and showing evidence of severe stromal melting with threatened perforation. The risk for recurrence in this setting is very high. Even in apparently quiet, treated eyes, optical penetrating keratoplasty procedures are associated with a high risk of recurrence if performed within the first year after the onset of infection. The presumed pathogenesis of such recurrences is the persistence of an occasional residual viable cyst in an eye with compromised immunity as the result of the presence of an allograft and the use of topical corticosteroids postoperatively. Therefore, it is advisable to perform any elective penetrating keratoplasty procedure only after a full course of amebicidal therapy has been completed and a minimum of 3–6 months of disease-free follow-up thereafter has been documented.

Corneal Microsporidiosis

In the past decade, the incidence of microsporidial keratitis has risen dramatically in association with AIDS or patients with severe cellular immunodeficiency, usually characterized by an epithelial keratitis caused by *Encephalitozoon*. Of the phylum Microspora, the following genera have been implicated in human infection: *Nosema, Encephalitozoon, Pleistophora, Vittaforma* (formerly *Nosema corneum*), *Trachipleistophora, Enterocytozoon,* and unclassified microsporida. Patients may present with symptoms that include ocular irritation, photophobia, vision decrease, and bilateral conjunctival injection with little or no associated inflammation. Corneal findings include superficial nonstaining opacities described as "mucoid" in appearance along with dense areas of fine punctate fluorescein staining.

In AIDS patients, the greatest number of organisms is found in the superficial conjunctiva; hence, diagnostic swabbing of the inferior cul-de-sac is especially likely to produce positive results. Some authors have discouraged corneal biopsy or scraping because of its potential for promoting additional corneal compromise. Transmission electron microscopy is a sensitive means of identification, and light microscopy using the Brown and Hopps stain may identify small gram-positive spores in the epithelial cells of the conjunctiva. Tissue culture techniques may also be used, but immunofluorescent antibody techniques have greater clinical utility.

Although there is no definitive treatment, topical fumagillin has been used to successfully treat microsporidial keratoconjunctivitis with low toxicity. In severe cases of *Vittaforma corneae,* granulomatous inflammation may lead to necrotic thinning and perforation. Penetrating keratoplasty may then become the only available treatment for severe stromal thinning. In general, medical regimens require long-term use, and recurrence is common after treatment discontinuation. Recent systemic studies with the tumor necrosis factor alpha agent, thalidomide, or highly active antiretroviral treatment strategies show promise.

Bron AJ, Seal DV, Hay J. *Ocular Infection: Investigation and Treatment in Practice.* St Louis: Mosby; 1998.

Murray PR, Baron EJ, Pfaller MA, et al, eds. *Manual of Clinical Microbiology.* 7th ed. Washington, DC: ASM Press; 1999:1413–1420.

Wilkins JH, Joshi N, Margolis TP. Microsporidial keratoconjunctivitis treated successfully with a short course of fumagillin. *Eye.* 1994;8:703–704.

Corneal Stromal Inflammation Associated With Systemic Infections

Nonsuppurative stromal keratitis can be caused by the following:

- Reiter syndrome
- Congenital or acquired syphilis
- Lyme disease
- Tuberculosis
- Hansen disease (leprosy)
- Onchocerciasis

These conditions are discussed in BCSC Section 9, *Intraocular Inflammation and Uveitis.* Additional discussion of onchocerciasis is found in BCSC Section 13, *International Ophthalmology.*

Microbial Scleritis

PATHOGENESIS Bacterial and fungal infections of the sclera are very rare. Most cases result from extension of microbial keratitis involving the peripheral cornea. Trauma and contaminated foreign bodies (including scleral buckles) are possible risk factors. Bacterial scleritis has also occurred in sclerae damaged by previous pterygium surgery, especially when beta irradiation or mitomycin has been used (Fig 7-30). Bacteria and fungi can also invade tissue of the eye wall surrounding a scleral surgical wound, but endophthalmitis is more likely in this setting. Scleral inflammation can also be a feature of syphilis, tuberculosis, nocardia, atypical mycobacteria, and leprosy. Diffuse or nodular scleritis is an occasional complication of varicella-zoster virus eye disease.

LABORATORY EVALUATION Suppurative scleritis is evaluated in a manner similar to microbial keratitis. Smears and cultures are obtained before antimicrobial therapy is begun. The workup of nonsuppurative scleritis is guided by the history and physical examination, as described in Chapter 9.

MANAGEMENT Topical antimicrobial therapy is begun just as for microbial keratitis. Subconjunctival injections and intravenous antibiotics may also be used because of the difficulty in controlling microbial scleritis. In severe cases with threatened eye loss, a subpalpebral lavage system similar to that originally proposed by Hessburg (see Burris et al [1982]) may be the only means of salvaging the eye. In cases of polymicrobial infection,

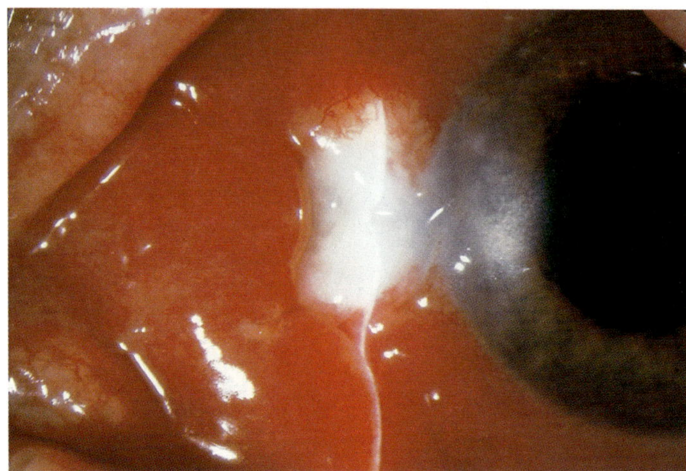

Figure 7-30 Bacterial scleritis occurring 2 weeks after pterygium surgery. *(Photograph courtesy of Kirk R. Wilhelmus, MD.)*

multiple antimicrobial agents may be sequentially administered through a serially connected stop-cock system, employing intervening saline rinses between medications (to prevent precipitation) using a rate of 6–20 drops per minute. The constant irrigation provides gentle continuous debridement, relieves some of the burden on the nursing staff, and is especially helpful with combative elderly or pediatric patients. The role of cryotherapy or debridement remains unclear, and long-term oral therapy shows promise.

Burris TE, Newsom DL, Rowsey JJ. Treatment of *Pseudomonas* corneal and corneoscleral ulcers by Hessburg subpalpebral lavage. *Cornea.* 1982;1:347–355.

PART IV

Immune-Mediated Disorders of the External Eye and Cornea

Ocular Immunology

Immunologic Features of the Cornea and Ocular Surface

For an in-depth discussion of the various features of the innate and adaptive immune system, including the different types of hypersensitivity reactions with relevant ocular examples, see Part I of BCSC Section 9, *Intraocular Inflammation and Uveitis.* The present chapter provides an overview of immune reactivity as it relates to the cornea and ocular surface. The immune system of the ocular surface, cornea, and sclera encompasses features of both the local mucosal immune microenvironment as well as systemic immunity.

The normal, uninflamed conjunctiva contains immunoglobulins, polymorphonuclear leukocytes (neutrophils), lymphocytes, plasma cells, and mast cells within the subepithelial tissue. In addition, the conjunctival stroma has its own endowment of dendritic antigen-presenting cells. The epithelium contains a special subpopulation of dendritic antigen-presenting cells known as *Langerhans cells,* which in many ways function similarly to tissue macrophages found elsewhere in the body. As such, these cells are capable of both antigen uptake and priming (sensitizing) of naive T lymphocytes. Hence, these dendritic cells serve as the sentinel cells of the immune system in the ocular surface. In addition to the presence of immune cells, the conjunctiva has a plentiful supply of lymphatic vessels, which facilitate the trafficking of immune cells and antigens to the draining lymph nodes where the adaptive immune response is largely generated.

The normal, uninflamed cornea also is endowed with dendritic cells. Like those in the conjunctiva, the dendritic cells in the corneal epithelium are also called *Langerhans cells.* In the corneal periphery and limbus, unlike the corneal center, these antigen-presenting cells are in an activated, mature state (expressing class II major histocompatibility complex antigens and costimulatory molecules and hence capable of efficiently stimulating T cells). In addition to these dendritic cells (Fig 8-1), small numbers of lymphocytes are present in the peripheral epithelium and anterior stroma of the cornea. A highly regulated process, mediated by vascular adhesion factors and cytokines, controls the recruitment of the various leukocyte subsets from the intravascular compartment into the limbal matrix. Table 8-1 summarizes the known distribution of certain immune and inflammatory cells in the ocular surface epithelium and substantia propria (stroma).

Unlike the conjunctiva, the normal cornea is considered to be an *immunologically privileged site,* so called because the generation of immune responsiveness to foreign (including transplantation) antigens is relatively suppressed. The cornea's immune privilege is due to a multitude of factors.

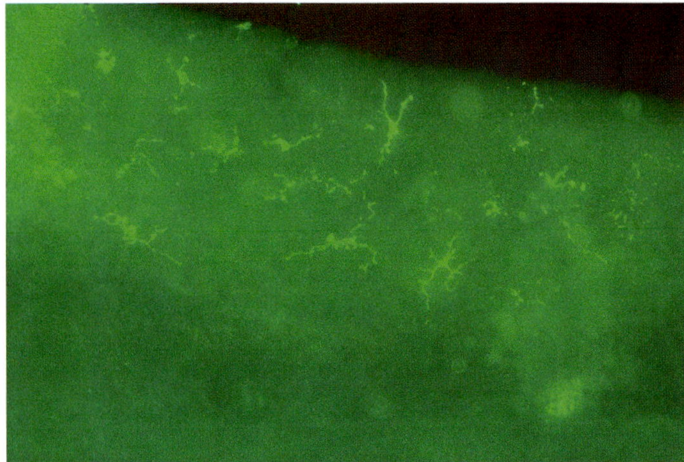

Figure 8-1 Langerhans cells represent a subpopulation of dendritic antigen-presenting cells of the ocular surface epithelium. As the sentinel cells of the immune system, they pick up, process, and present antigens to T cells. This micrograph shows the predominance of MHC class II$^+$ Langerhans cells in the limbus of the uninflamed eye. *(Photograph courtesy of the laboratory of M. Reza Dana, MD.)*

Table 8-1 Immunologic Components of the External Eye

Cell	Epithelium	Substantia Propria
Dendritic cells	+	+
Helper T cells	+	+
Suppressor T cells	+	+
B cells and plasma cells	−	+
Neutrophils	+	+
Eosinophils	−	−
Mast cells	−	+

These include:

- Absence of blood vessels, which impedes delivery of immune effectors
- Absence of lymphatics, which minimizes flow of antigens and antigen-presenting cells to the draining lymph nodes
- Expression of immunosuppressive factors, including transforming growth factor-beta (TGF-β), by the cornea
- Expression of Fas-ligand (CD95 ligand) by corneal cells, which is believed to play a critical part in inducing Fas-mediated apoptosis (programmed cell death) of activated lymphocytes

Hence, it has been postulated that the immune response generated to corneal and anterior chamber antigens may lead to immune unresponsiveness, or even immunological tolerance.

Dana MR, Qian Y, Hamrah P. Twenty-five-year panorama of corneal immunology: emerging concepts in the immunopathogenesis of microbial keratitis, peripheral ulcerative keratitis, and corneal transplant rejection. *Cornea.* 2000;19:625–643.

Dekaris I, Zhu SN, Dana MR. TNF-alpha regulates corneal Langerhans cell migration. *J Immunol.* 1999;162:4235–4239.

Griffith TS, Brunner T, Fletcher SM, Green DR, et al. Fas ligand–induced apoptosis as a mechanism of immune privilege. *Science.* 1995;270:1189–1192.

McClellan KA. Mucosal defense of the outer eye. *Surv Ophthalmol.* 1997;42:233–246.

Soluble Mediators of Inflammation

It is important to recognize that cellular elements of the immune system do not function independently, and up-regulation (or down-modulation) in the expression of many molecules is a critical facet of ocular surface immunoinflammatory responses. For example, many immunoglobulins (primarily dimeric IgA) are normally present in the tear film. However, antibody levels may drop significantly during lacrimal gland atrophy (as protein synthesis in the gland decreases) in severe exocrinopathy in Sjögren syndrome. In contrast, immunoglobulin levels increase in patients with allergic disorders of the external eye or with other disorders that activate the humoral (antibody-dependent) arm of the immune system, such as infections.

The normal tear film also contains components of the complement cascade and a variety of cytokines (see BCSC Section 9, *Intraocular Inflammation and Uveitis* for more in-depth discussion and illustrations of the immune system). These mediators play important roles in various facets of inflammation in the cornea and ocular surface. For example, cytokines such as interleukin-1 (IL-1) and tumor necrosis factor-alpha (TNF-α) are significantly up-regulated in a variety of corneal inflammatory disorders such as corneal graft rejection and dry eye. Similarly, increased expression of growth factors, prostaglandins, neuropeptides, and proteases (including collagenases) has been shown in a wide array of immune disorders of the cornea and ocular surface. Effective immune responses to foreign antigens require cellular effectors in order to traffic through tissues. Although many of the soluble factors (such as cytokines) play important roles in immune cell activation, leukocytes still need to receive directional signaling for effective trafficking. In a condition of inflammation, these signals are provided by soluble mediators called *chemokines* (*chemo*tactic cyto*kines*). To date, a number of chemokines have been identified as playing important roles in corneal inflammation. A brief tabulation of some important soluble mediators involved in corneal and ocular surface immune and inflammatory responses is provided in Table 8-2.

Hendricks RL, Tang Q. Cellular immunity and the eye. In: Pepose JS, Holland GN, Wilhelmus KR, eds. *Ocular Infection and Immunity.* St Louis: Mosby; 1996:71–95.

Luster AD. Chemokines—Chemotactic cytokines that mediate inflammation [review]. *N Engl J Med.* 1998;338:436.

Waldrop JC, Mondino BJ. Humoral immunity and the eye. In: Pepose JS, Holland GN, Wilhelmus KR, eds. *Ocular Infection and Immunity.* St Louis: Mosby; 1996:33–49.

Table 8-2 Soluble Mediators of Ocular Inflammation

Group	Example	Example of Action
Cell adhesion molecules	ICAM-1	Promotes leukocyte recruitment
Chemokines	RANTES	Directs leukocyte traffic
Clotting and fibrinolytic systems	Fibrin	Enhances leukocyte activity
Complement	C5a	Promotes leukocyte recruitment
Corneal proteases	Collagenase	Degrades protein in stromal matrix
Cytokines	Interleukin-1	Promotes leukocyte recruitment
Eicosanoids	Leukotriene B_4	Promotes inflammation and breakdown of blood–ocular barriers
Growth factors	VEGF	Promotes angiogenesis and vascular permeability
Kinin-forming system	Bradykinin	Increases vascular permeability
Leukocyte oxidants	Hydrogen peroxide	Oxidizes free radicals
Neuropeptides	Substance P	Promotes inflammation and pain
Vasoactive amines	Histamine	Dilates blood vessels

Hypersensitivity Reactions of the Conjunctiva, Cornea, and Sclera

Hypersensitivity responses typically involve normal adaptive protective mechanisms that—because of increased antigenic exposure and/or heightened immune status—become so amplified that they lead to tissue pathology. Hypersensitivity reactions are classified into several basic mechanisms grouped as Types I–V (Type V is not discussed in this section; see BCSC Section 9, *Intraocular Inflammation and Uveitis*). Most clinically relevant problems in ophthalmology are probably not due exclusively to a single type of hypersensitivity reaction. Nevertheless, a basic understanding of the mechanisms of hypersensitivity, as shown in Figure 8-2, can be useful in explaining the pathogenesis of several immune-mediated disorders of the cornea and ocular surface (Table 8-3). Below, we will put each type of hypersensitivity response in the context of common corneal and ocular surface inflammatory pathologies. Readers are referred to BCSC Section 9 for a full discussion of basic immunopathogenic mechanisms.

Anaphylactic or Atopic Reactions (Type I)

In *Type I* reactions, antigens combine with IgE antibodies bound to receptors on mast cells, resulting in release of histamine and other preformed (eg, biogenic amine) mediators, as well as new synthesis of prostaglandins and leukotrienes. The pathogenesis of an allergic reaction begins with antigen-presenting cells interacting with $CD4^+$ helper-2 (Th2) cells that release interleukin-4 (IL-4) and other Th2 cytokines.

Atopy is associated with an inherited mutation in the receptor for IL-4 that is associated with enhanced IgE production by B cells and increased numbers of helper T cells. Other features associated with atopy are decreased levels of putative suppressor (or regulatory) T cells that play a role in down-modulating immune responses to common

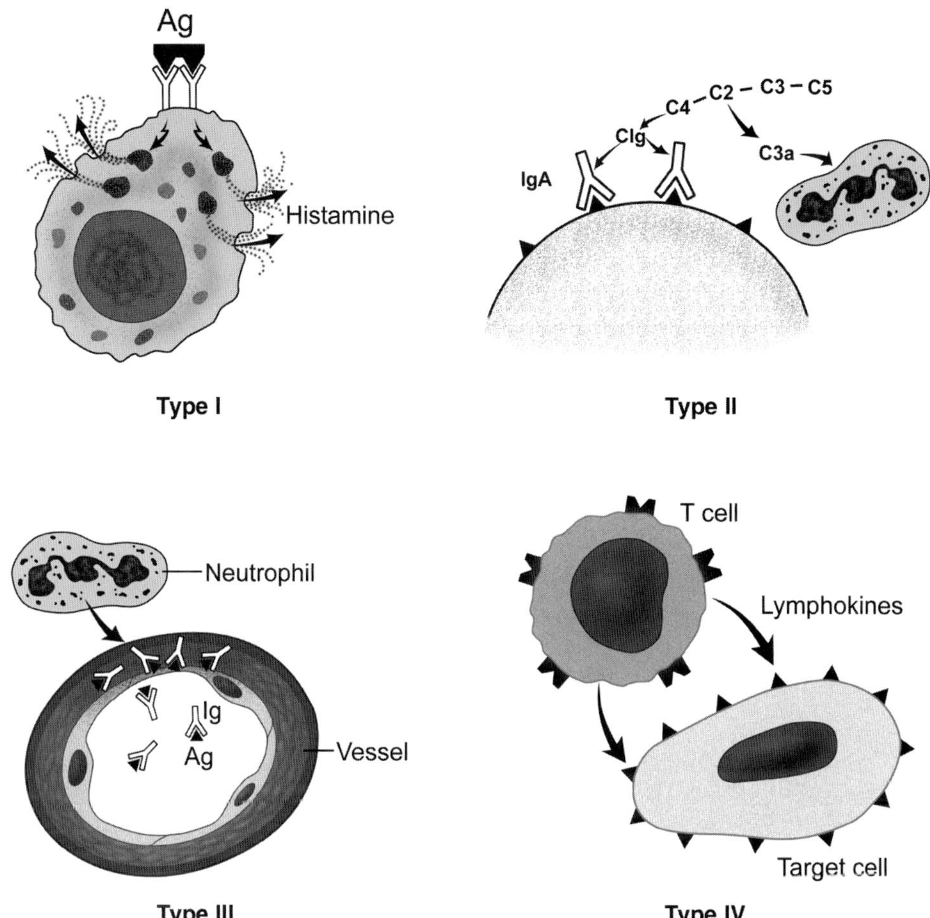

Figure 8-2 Classifications of hypersensitivity reactions. Type I anaphylactic reactions are mediated by IgE antibodies bound to mast cells. Type II cytolytic or cytotoxic reactions are mediated by immunoglobulins against membrane antigens that activate complement. Type III immune-complex reactions occur when antigen-antibody complexes accumulate in a tissue and activate the complement cascade to attract leukocytes. Type IV (delayed hypersensitivity immune reactions) are mediated by T cells that release lymphokines to attract macrophages. *(Illustration by Christine Gralapp.)*

Table 8-3 Hypersensitivity Reactions and Ocular Disease

Type	Ocular Disease
I	Allergic conjunctivitis
II	Ocular cicatricial pemphigoid
III	Scleritis
IV	Contact dermatitis
	Phlyctenulosis
	Corneal graft rejection

antigens in the environment, and the production of autoantibodies to β-adrenergic receptors. Treatment strategies include mast-cell inhibitors, antihistamines, vasoconstrictors, cyclooxygenase inhibitors, and, occasionally, corticosteroids in severe disease. Pharmacological treatment of allergic disease targets a variety of important mediators of atopic disease released by mast cells and eosinophils (Table 8-4).

Cytotoxic Hypersensitivity (Type II)

A *Type II* reaction involves interaction of immunoglobulins with foreign or autoantigens closely associated with cell membranes. Cell lysis may result from complement activation (and development of membrane attack complexes) and from recruitment of leukocytes including neutrophils, lymphocytes, and macrophages. So-called *killer lymphocytes* may be involved in antibody-dependent cell cytotoxicity (ADCC). In general, most investigators maintain that Type II responses do not play a major role in corneal and ocular surface morbidities. However, one disease in which Type II responses are likely relevant is ocular cicatricial pemphigoid (discussed in Chapter 9). In this condition, several antigens along the conjunctival basement membrane zone (BMZ) can react with IgG or IgA antibodies. Treatment of Type II responses usually requires systemic immunosuppression or immune modulation.

Immune-Complex Reactions (Type III)

A *Type III* reaction follows the deposition of antigen-antibody (immune) complexes in tissue with secondary complement and cellular effector activation and recruitment. Immune complexes can fix complement that attracts polymorphonuclear leukocytes. The typical *Arthus reaction* involves vasculitis from immune-complex deposition in small blood vessels. Similarly, the pathophysiology of scleritis and ocular syndromes secondary

Table 8-4 Selected Soluble Mediators Released by Mast Cells and Eosinophils

Substance	Action
Released by mast cells	
Histamine	Vasodilation and increased capillary permeability
Heparin	Anticoagulation
Tryptase	Complement activation
Eosinophil chemotactic factor	Eosinophil chemotaxis
Neutrophil chemotactic factor	Neutrophil chemotaxis
Platelet-activating factor	Vasodilation and increased capillary permeability
Prostaglandins (PGD$_2$)	Vasodilation
Leukotrienes (LTB$_4$)	Leukocyte chemotaxis
Released by eosinophils	
Major basic protein	Mast cell degranulation
Cationic protein	Epithelial cytotoxicity
Peroxidase	Epithelial cytotoxicity
Eotaxin	Eosinophil chemotaxis
Platelet-activating factor	Vasodilation and increased capillary permeability
Leukotrienes (LTC$_4$)	Increased capillary permeability
Slow-reacting substance of anaphylaxis	Increased capillary permeability

to vasculitis (eg, peripheral ulcerative keratitis) has been related to immune-complex deposition. However, a basic understanding of mechanisms is still deficient, since the inciting factors remain largely unknown.

Delayed Hypersensitivity (Type IV)

Type IV, or *cell-mediated, immunity* involves sensitized CD4$^+$ T helper-1 (Th1) lymphocytes. Antigens interact with receptors on the surface of T lymphocytes and result in the release of lymphokines. Contact dermatitis is a common external eye delayed hypersensitivity response caused by lipid-soluble, low-molecular-weight haptens that can penetrate the skin and gain entry into the epidermal layer, where they may be picked up by antigen-presenting cells such as Langerhans cells. These cells can then process the antigen and prime (sensitize) naive T cells in lymphoid organs by coexpressing the processed antigen and major histocompatibility complex (MHC) class II antigens. A similar process is thought to be responsible for corneal graft rejection.

Patterns of Immune-Mediated Ocular Disease

Conjunctiva

The conjunctiva is a mucosa-associated lymphoid tissue (MALT). Humoral immunity in the conjunctiva largely involves IgA, and cellular immunity is dominated by CD4$^+$ T cells. Serosal mast cells that contain neutral proteases are normally present in the conjunctiva, and mucosal mast cells with granules containing only tryptase are increased in the conjunctiva of atopic patients. Mast-cell degranulation produces conjunctival redness, chemosis, mucous discharge, and itching.

Cornea

The normal cornea cannot have either an acute allergic reaction (as it contains no mast cells) or a typical Arthus reaction (as there are no blood vessels). However, the cornea does participate in immune reactions by way of humoral and cellular immune elements that enter the periphery from the limbal blood vessels. These corneal properties may explain why so many immune-mediated disorders occur primarily in the corneal periphery and limbus. Alternatively, ingress of leukocytes through the ciliary body/iris root, and of plasma proteins through breakdown of the blood–ocular barrier (as occurs in uveitis syndromes), provides other pathways of delivery of immune effectors to the cornea.

The cornea can act as an immunologic blotter, soaking up antigens from the ocular surface. This phenomenon was first described by Wessely in 1911, when foreign antigen was injected into the cornea of a previously sensitized animal. A ring-shaped infiltrate formed in the corneal stroma concentric to the limbus, much like an antigen-antibody complex in an immunodiffusion test. Still called a *Wessely immune ring,* this infiltrate contains complement factors and/or neutrophils. Circulating antibodies are not required if sufficient local antibody production is stimulated by antigens deposited in the cornea. The antigen may be a drug, as in the peripheral corneal infiltrates associated with a neomycin reaction, or an unknown substance, as in the corneal infiltrates that occasionally occur in contact lens wearers.

Sclera

Nearly one half of patients with scleritis have an associated systemic immunologic or connective tissue disease. Immune-complex deposition, granulomatous inflammation, and occlusive vasculitis have been implicated in the pathogenesis of scleral inflammation.

Chandler JW. Ocular surface immunology. In: Pepose JS, Holland GN, Wilhelmus KR, eds. *Ocular Infection and Immunity.* St Louis: Mosby; 1996:104–111.

Diagnostic Approach to Immune-Mediated Ocular Disorders

Many, but by no means all, immune-mediated ocular disorders are secondary to a systemic disease. As with most medical problems, diagnostic investigations need to begin with a complete history, including a review of systems, and a general physical examination as indicated. Some of the more common laboratory diagnostic tests that are selected to further narrow the differential diagnosis are listed in Table 8-5. In general, except for rheumatoid arthritis, which has a strong predilection for scleral and ocular surface (and *not* intraocular) involvement, the workup for patients with immune-mediated corneal disease in whom an underlying disease is suspected is quite similar to that for the uveitis patient. Readers are referred to BCSC Section 9 (Chapter 6) for the diagnostic workup of patients with uveitis. Chapter 4 of the present book discusses and illustrates the specific morphological characteristics that can be found on conjunctival or corneal specimens through microscopic examination following standard staining procedures. Table 8-6 shows the clinical interpretation of the findings produced by the procedures described in Chapter 4 for immune-mediated keratoconjunctivitis.

Finally, it should be noted that different corneal and ocular surface morbidities may coexist secondary to an underlying autoimmune or rheumatic disease. For example, many patients with peripheral ulcerative keratitis (PUK) associated with rheumatoid arthritis also have significant lacrimal insufficiency as a manifestation of secondary Sjögren syndrome (see Chapter 5 in this volume for more details). Consequently, in such cases, therapy should be directed at both the PUK and the surface disease due to dry eye. Generally, when a systemic disease is suspected it is also advisable to coordinate care with an internist or rheumatologist, especially if systemic immune suppression is contemplated.

Table 8-5 Common Laboratory Tests for Suspected Systemic Immune-Mediated Disease

Test	Assay
Rheumatoid factor (RF)	Autoantibody (IgG, IgA, or IgM) against epitopes of the Fc portion of IgG
Antinuclear antibody (ANA)	Antibodies against cell nuclear antigens (DNA-histone, double-stranded DNA, single-stranded DNA, histone, RNA, nuclear ribonucleoprotein, etc)
Antineutrophil cytoplasmic antibodies (ANCA)	Autoantibody (IgG) against cytoplasmic antigen (either cytoplasmic proteinase-3 or perinuclear antigens) of neutrophils; positive in Wegener granulomatosis
Urinalysis	Rule out active nephritis by checking for casts, red blood cells, etc
Complete blood count	Abnormally high or low blood counts are indicative of systemic disease
Erythrocyte sedimentation rate or C-reactive protein	High values indicate systemic inflammation

Table 8-6 Clinical Interpretation of Ocular Surface Cytology for Immune-Mediated Keratoconjunctivitis

Finding	Examples
Significant neutrophils	Severe acute/subacute ocular surface inflammation
Predominance of lymphocytes and monocytes	Chronic toxic or allergic conjunctivitis
Eosinophils	Acute allergic conjunctivitis
Basophils or mast cells	Vernal conjunctivitis
Keratinized epithelial cells	Ocular cicatricial pemphigoid Stevens-Johnson syndrome Severe keratoconjunctivitis sicca Graft-versus-host disease

CHAPTER 9

Clinical Approach to Immune-Related Disorders of the External Eye

Immune-Mediated Diseases of the Eyelid

Contact Dermatoblepharitis

PATHOGENESIS Topical application of ophthalmic medications and contact with cosmetics and environmental substances can occasionally trigger allergic reactions. They may occur acutely as anaphylactic reactions or have a delayed onset. Anaphylactic reactions are Type I IgE-mediated hypersensitivity reactions. Contact blepharoconjunctivitis is a Type IV cell-mediated, or delayed hypersensitivity, reaction that may begin 24–72 hours following exposure to the sensitizing agent.

CLINICAL PRESENTATION Type I immediate hypersensitivity reactions typically occur within minutes after application of an allergen. When involving the eyelids, these reactions are associated with itching, eyelid erythema and swelling, and conjunctival redness and chemosis (Fig 9-1). Rarely, patients may develop signs of systemic anaphylaxis. Ocular anaphylactic reactions often resolve spontaneously, without the patient's seeking medical attention, so the true incidence is not easily determined. These reactions have followed instillation of topical anesthetics and antibiotics such as bacitracin, cephalosporins, penicillin, sulfacetamide, and tetracycline.

Delayed Type IV hypersensitivity reactions to medications may begin 24–72 hours following instillation of a topical drug. Patients are often sensitized by previous exposure to the offending drug or preservative. An acute eczema with erythema, leathery thickening, and scaling of the eyelid develops (Fig 9-2). Chronic sequelae of contact blepharoconjunctivitis include hyperpigmentation, dermal scarring, and lower eyelid ectropion. A papillary conjunctivitis and a mucoid or mucopurulent discharge may develop. Punctate epithelial erosions may be noted on the inferior cornea. Medications that are commonly associated with contact blepharoconjunctivitis include:

- Cycloplegics such as atropine and homatropine
- Aminoglycosides such as neomycin, gentamicin, and tobramycin

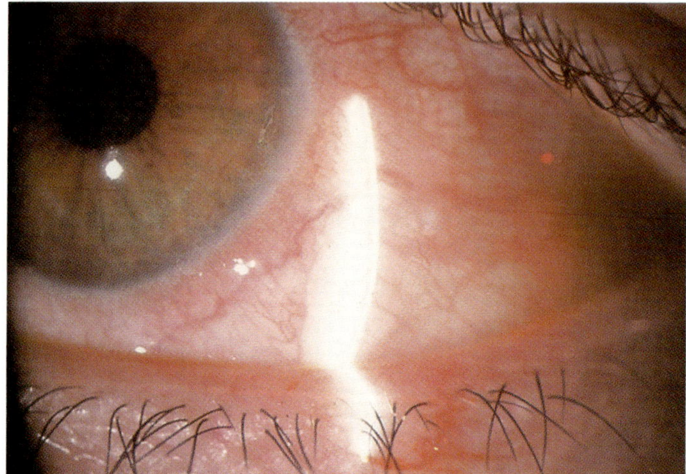

Figure 9-1 Anaphylactic allergic reaction to topical ophthalmic medication with acute conjunctival hyperemia and chemosis.

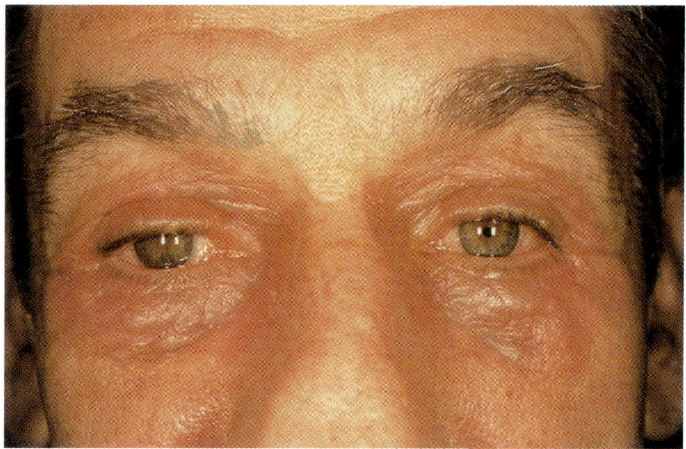

Figure 9-2 Allergic contact dermatitis secondary to topical ophthalmic medication.

- Antiviral agents such as idoxuridine and trifluridine
- Preservatives such as thimerosal and ethylenediaminetetraacetic acid (EDTA)

MANAGEMENT Treatment of hypersensitivity reactions requires identification and discontinuation of the offending agent. Usually, the history provides the necessary clue to determine the offending agent, but sometimes a "rechallenge" is necessary to confirm a suspicion. Rechallenges should never be done in patients with a known systemic allergy to a drug. Type I hypersensitivity reactions are best managed with allergen avoidance or discontinuation. Adjunctive therapy may involve the use of cold compresses, artificial lubricants, topical antihistamines, mast-cell stabilizers, and topical nonsteroidal anti-inflammatory agents in the case of pain. In general, supportive treatment with lubricants and antigen avoidance is adequate in most cases. Topical vasoconstrictors, either alone or in combination with antihistamines, may provide acute symptomatic relief but have been incriminated as causes of chronic blepharoconjunctivitis.

Delayed hypersensitivity reactions are also treated with allergen withdrawal. In severe cases, a brief (several day) course of mild topical corticosteroids applied to the eyelids and periocular skin may speed resolution of eyelid and conjunctival inflammation.

Atopic Dermatitis

PATHOGENESIS Atopic dermatitis is a chronic condition that usually begins in infancy or childhood and may or may not involve the external eye. Environmental irritants, climatic changes, and psychological factors may play a role in genetically susceptible individuals. Immune changes involved in the pathogenesis of atopic dermatitis include increased IgE hypersensitivity, increased histamine release from mast cells and basophils, and impaired cell-mediated immunity.

CLINICAL PRESENTATION Diagnostic criteria for atopic dermatitis include the presence of pruritus, the appearance of lesions on the eyelid and other sites (eg, joint flexures in adolescents and adults; face and extensor surfaces in infants and young children), and a personal or family history of other atopic disorders such as asthma, allergic rhinitis, nasal polyps, and aspirin hypersensitivity. Other ocular findings may include periorbital darkening, exaggerated eyelid folds, ectropion, and chronic conjunctivitis. The appearance of the skin lesions varies depending on the age of the patient. Infants typically have an erythematous rash; children tend to have eczematoid dermatitis with secondary lichenification from scratching; and adults have scaly patches with thickened and wrinkled dry skin.

MANAGEMENT Allergens in the environment and in foods should be minimized whenever possible. In general, the services of an expert allergist should be sought to help identify factors that can exacerbate the patient's condition and to educate the patient. Moisturizing lotions and petrolatum gels can be useful in skin hydration. Acute lesions can be controlled with a topical corticosteroid cream or ointment, but chronic use should be strongly discouraged to avoid skin thinning. Oral antipruritic agents such as antihistamines and mast-cell stabilizers can alleviate itching, but the ophthalmologist should be aware of possible side effects of antihistamines, including dry eye from their anticholinergic activity.

Immune-Mediated Disorders of the Conjunctiva

Hay Fever Conjunctivitis and Perennial Allergic Conjunctivitis

PATHOGENESIS Hay fever (seasonal) and perennial allergic conjunctivitis are largely IgE-mediated immediate hypersensitivity reactions. The allergen is typically airborne. It enters the tear film and comes into contact with conjunctival mast cells that bear allergen-specific IgE antibodies. Degranulation of mast cells releases histamine and a variety of other inflammatory mediators that promote vasodilatation, edema, and recruitment of other inflammatory cells such as eosinophils. The activation and degranulation of mast cells in a presensitized individual can be triggered within minutes of allergen exposure.

CLINICAL PRESENTATION Patients with hay fever conjunctivitis often suffer from other atopic conditions such as allergic rhinitis and asthma. Symptoms develop rapidly after exposure to the allergen and consist of itching, eyelid swelling, conjunctival hyperemia and chemosis, and mucoid discharge. Intense itching is a hallmark symptom. Attacks are usually short-lived and episodic. Contributing factors, including contact lenses and dry eye, should be identified, as these can play an important role in facilitating allergen contact with the ocular surface.

LABORATORY EVALUATION The diagnosis of hay fever conjunctivitis is generally made clinically, although conjunctival scraping can be performed in order to observe the characteristic eosinophils (which are not normally present on the ocular surface—see Chapter 8). Challenge testing with a panel of allergens can be performed using either the conjunctiva or the skin as the responding tissue.

MANAGEMENT Efforts should first be directed at avoidance or abatement of allergen exposure. Thorough cleaning (or changing) of unclean or old carpets, linens, and bedding can be effective in removing accumulated allergens such as animal dander and house dust mites. Simple measures such as wearing glasses or goggles can also serve as physical barriers. Treatment should be based on the severity of patient symptoms and consists of one or more of the following:

- Cold compresses
- Artificial tears
- Topical antihistamines and mast-cell stabilizers
- Topical nonsteroidal anti-inflammatory medications
- Judicious, selective use of topical corticosteroids
- Topical vasoconstrictors

Artificial tears are beneficial in diluting and flushing away allergens and other inflammatory mediators present on the ocular surface. Topical vasoconstrictors, alone or in combination with antihistamines, may provide acute symptomatic relief. However, their use for more than 5–7 consecutive days may predispose to compensatory chronic vascular dilatation and rebound conjunctival hyperemia. Topical mast-cell stabilizing agents such as cromolyn sodium and lodoxamide tromethamine may be useful for treatment of seasonal allergic conjunctivitis, but their primary role is in prophylaxis. Treatment effects usually require continued use over 7 or more days, and hence these agents are generally ineffective in the acute phase of hay fever conjunctivitis. Oral antihistamines may provide symptomatic relief in some patients. Hyposensitization injections (immunotherapy) can be beneficial if the offending allergen has been identified. Certain topical nonsteroidal anti-inflammatory drugs (NSAIDs) have been approved by the Food and Drug Administration for use in ocular atopy, but their efficacy is variable. Topical steroids are very effective in ocular allergy, but they are best avoided except in the very severe cases due to their toxicity.

Vernal Keratoconjunctivitis (VKC)

PATHOGENESIS Usually a seasonally recurring, bilateral inflammation of the conjunctiva, vernal (springtime) keratoconjunctivitis occurs predominantly in male children who frequently, but not invariably, have a personal or family history of atopy. The disease may persist year-round in tropical climates. The immunopathogenesis appears to involve both Type I and Type IV hypersensitivity reactions. The conjunctival inflammatory infiltrate in VKC consists of eosinophils, lymphocytes, plasma cells, and monocytes.

CLINICAL PRESENTATION Symptoms consist of itching, blepharospasm, photophobia, blurred vision, and copious mucoid discharge. Clinically, two forms of VKC may be seen: *palpebral* and *limbal.*

The inflammation in palpebral VKC is located predominantly on the palpebral conjunctiva, where a diffuse papillary hypertrophy develops, usually more prominently on the upper rather than the lower region. Bulbar conjunctival hyperemia and chemosis may occur. In more severe cases giant papillae resembling cobblestones may develop on the upper tarsus (Fig 9-3). Limbal VKC may develop alone or in association with palpebral VKC. It occurs predominantly in patients of African or Asian descent and is also more prevalent in hotter climates. The limbus has a thickened, gelatinous appearance, with scattered opalescent mounds and vascular injection (Fig 9-4). *Horner-Trantas dots,* whitish dots that represent macroaggregates of degenerated eosinophils and epithelial cells, may be observed in the hypertrophied limbus of patients with limbal VKC.

Several different types of corneal changes may also develop in VKC. Punctate epithelial erosions in the superior and central cornea are frequently observed. Pannus occurs most commonly in the superior cornea, but occasionally 360° corneal vascularization may develop. Noninfectious epithelial ulcers with an oval or shield-like shape (the so-called *shield ulcer*) with underlying stromal opacification may develop in the superior or central cornea (Fig 9-5). An association between VKC and keratoconus has been reported.

MANAGEMENT Therapy should be based on the severity of the patient's symptoms and of the ocular surface disease. Mild cases may be successfully managed with topical antihistamines. Climatotherapy such as the use of home air-conditioning or relocation to a cooler environment can promote improvement of the condition. Patients with moderate to severe disease may respond to topical mast-cell stabilizers such as cromolyn sodium or lodoxamide tromethamine. In patients with seasonal exacerbations, these drops should be given four times a day starting at least 1 month prior to the usual time of symptomatic onset. Patients with year-round disease can be maintained chronically on mast-cell stabilizer drops. Topical nonsteroidal anti-inflammatory preparations such as ketorolac 0.5% may offer adjunctive benefit.

Severe cases may require the use of topical corticosteroids or topical immunomodulatory agents such as cyclosporine. Both have been shown to be effective in reducing inflammation and symptoms. Because of the likelihood that patients will develop steroid-related complications from chronic administration, however, corticosteroids should be reserved for exacerbations with moderate to severe discomfort and/or decreased visual acuity. During these exacerbations, intermittent (pulse) therapy is very effective: topical

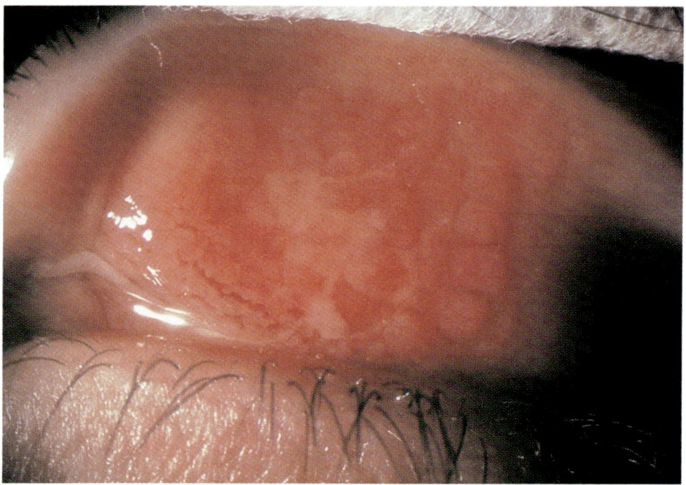

Figure 9-3 Giant papillae of palpebral vernal conjunctivitis.

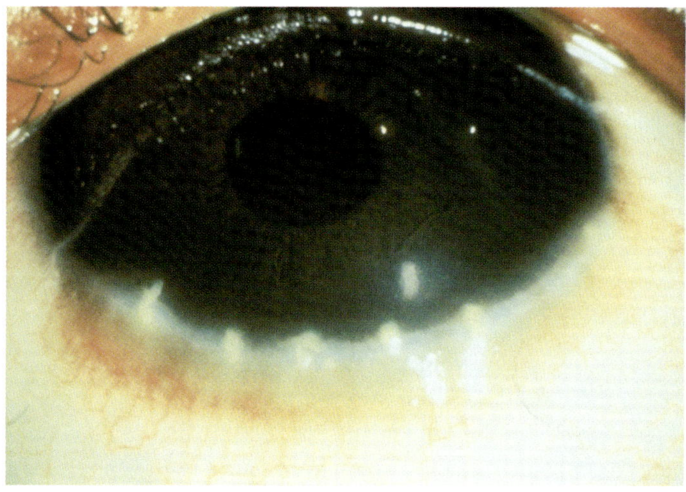

Figure 9-4 Limbal vernal conjunctivitis. *(Photograph courtesy of M. Reza Dana, MD, MPH.)*

corticosteroids are used at relatively high frequency (eg, every 2 hours) for 5–7 days, then rapidly tapered. Because of the propensity of particles of suspended steroid (such as prednisolone acetate) to lodge between papillae, the use of less potent but soluble steroids such as dexamethasone phosphate is preferred. Corticosteroids should be discontinued between attacks. To discourage indiscriminate use for relief of mild symptoms, the patient and family must be thoroughly informed of the potential dangers of chronic topical steroid therapy. Use of systemic anti-inflammatory therapy for severe VKC has been reported, but this should be reserved for very severe cases.

Cooperative patients can be offered an alternative to topical delivery that avoids the problem of continuing self-medication: supratarsal injection of corticosteroid. The su-

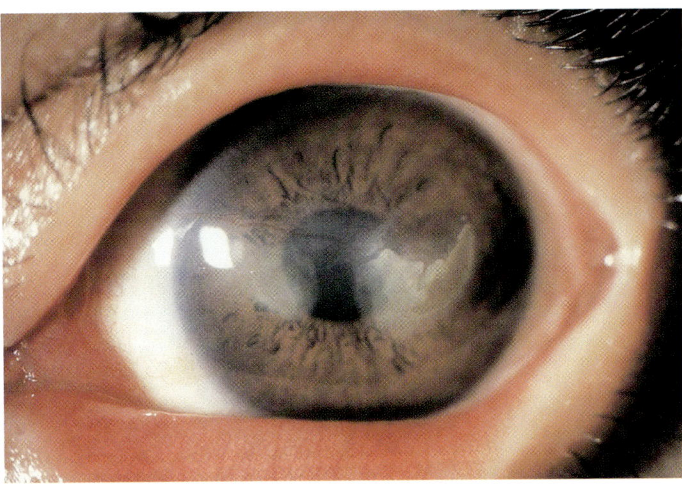

Figure 9-5 Vernal keratoconjunctivitis with focal nonsuppurative keratitis.

pratarsal subconjunctival space is located superior to the upper border of the superior tarsus and is most easily reached by everting the upper eyelid. This space is free of the subepithelial adhesions that bind the superior palpebral conjunctiva to the tarsal plate. After the upper eyelid is everted and the supratarsal conjunctiva has been anesthetized, supratarsal injection of 0.5–1.0 mL of either a relatively short-acting steroid such as dexamethasone phosphate (4 mg/mL) or a longer-acting steroid such as triamcinolone acetonide (40 mg/mL) can be performed. Monitoring of intraocular pressure is mandatory, as steroid-induced pressure spikes are possible.

Topical cyclosporine applied twice daily can also be used for the treatment of refractory cases of VKC. However, this drug is not currently available commercially and must be custom-made by specialized pharmacies. Moreover, there is little data on exact dosing in VKC: although success has been reported with 2% preparations in VKC treatment, significantly lower concentrations have shown efficacy in other ocular surface inflammatory disorders. Reported side effects include punctate epithelial keratopathy and ocular surface irritation. Although systemic absorption after topical instillation is minimal, experience with this agent is limited, and the use of topical cyclosporine in VKC should therefore probably be reserved for the most severe cases.

Atopic Keratoconjunctivitis (AKC)

PATHOGENESIS Keratoconjunctivitis may occur in patients with a history of atopic dermatitis. Approximately one third of patients with atopic dermatitis develop one or more manifestations of atopic keratoconjunctivitis. Atopic individuals demonstrate signs of Type I immediate hypersensitivity responses but also have depressed systemic cell-mediated immunity. As a consequence of this altered immunity, they are susceptible to herpes simplex virus keratitis and to colonization of the eyelids with *Staphylococcus aureus*. Complications related to this predisposition to infection may contribute to, or compound, the primary immunopathogenic manifestations.

CLINICAL PRESENTATION The ocular findings are similar to those of vernal keratoconjunctivitis with the following differences:

- Seasonal exacerbation is minimal. Patients with AKC frequently have disease year-round.
- Patients with AKC are older.
- The papillae are more apt to be small or medium sized, rather than giant.
- The papillae occur in the upper and lower palpebral conjunctiva (Fig 9-6).
- Milky conjunctival edema, with variable subepithelial fibrosis, is often present.
- Extensive corneal vascularization and opacification secondary to chronic epithelial disease (likely due to some degree of limbal stem cell dysfunction) can occur (Fig 9-7).
- Eosinophils seen in conjunctival cytology are less numerous and are less often degranulated.
- Conjunctival scarring often occurs and is sometimes so extensive as to produce symblepharon formation.
- Characteristic posterior subcapsular and/or multifaceted or shield-shaped anterior subcapsular lens opacities may occasionally develop.

MANAGEMENT Treatment of AKC involves allergen avoidance and the use of pharmacotherapeutic agents similar to those used in the treatment of VKC. Additionally, patients should be carefully monitored for infectious disease complications that may warrant specific therapy, such as secondary staphylococcal infections. In the minority of patients in whom the disease takes a very aggressive and destructive course, local pharmacotherapies often fail to control the pathological process. In these severe cases, systemic immune suppression (eg, by oral cyclosporine) may be required.

Abelson MB, Udell IJ. Allergic and toxic reactions. In: Albert DM, Jakobiec FA, eds. *Principles and Practice of Ophthalmology*. Vol 2. 2nd ed. Philadelphia: Saunders; 2000:781–803.

Ligneous Conjunctivitis

PATHOGENESIS Ligneous conjunctivitis is a rare chronic disorder characterized by the formation of firm ("woody"), yellowish fibrinous membranes on the conjunctival surface. These membranes, composed of an admixture of fibrin, epithelial cells, and mixed inflammatory cells, adhere to the conjunctival surface. Although bacteria can be sporadically isolated from cultures of the membranes, they probably represent incidental colonizing microorganisms rather than the etiologic agents, as is the case with infectious membranous conjunctivitis. The cause of ligneous conjunctivitis has recently been linked to severe deficiency in type I plasminogen, and medical therapy by administration of purified plasminogen concentrate to an infant with this condition has been reported.

CLINICAL PRESENTATION Ligneous conjunctivitis can affect all ages. Patients present with symptoms of ocular irritation and foreign body sensation. The cardinal finding consists of yellowish, platelike masses that overlie one or more of the palpebral surfaces and are readily visible with eversion of the eyelid. Ligneous conjunctivitis is generally bilateral and can recur after excision.

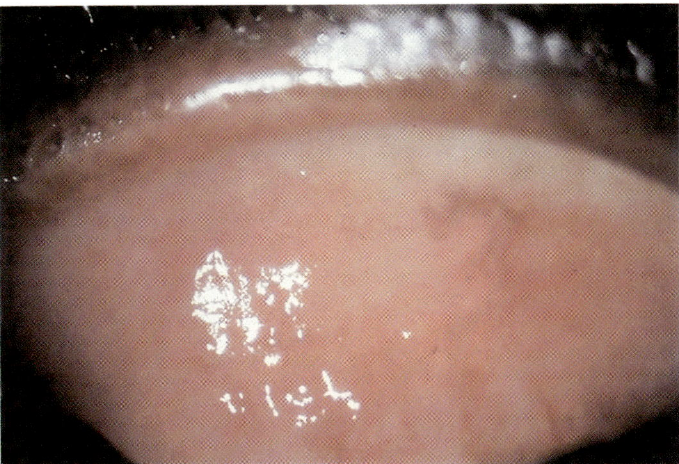

Figure 9-6 Atopic keratoconjunctivitis with small and medium-sized papillae and edema of the tarsal conjunctiva.

MANAGEMENT Cultures can be taken upon initial diagnosis to exclude a bacterial pseudomembranous or membranous conjunctivitis. Surgical excision with or without adjunctive cryotherapy has been advocated. However, recurrences are frequent, and patients and their families should be informed about this possibility. Anecdotal successes have been reported with the use of a variety of pharmacological agents, including topical corticosteroids and cyclosporine, but no single treatment has been shown to be consistently effective or superior. Therapy with purified plasminogen concentrate has also been attempted. Many cases of ligneous conjunctivitis eventually resolve spontaneously after several months to a few years.

> Schott D, Dempfle CE, Beck P, et al. Therapy with purified plasminogen concentrate in an
> infant with ligneous conjunctivitis and homozygous plasminogen deficiency. *N Engl J Med.*
> 1998;339:1679–1686.

Contact Lens–Induced Conjunctivitis

PATHOGENESIS The pathogenesis of contact lens–induced conjunctivitis is not fully understood and may be multifactorial (allergic, dry eye, infectious). Patients with ocular prostheses and exposed monofilament sutures have shown reactions similar to those seen in patients with contact lens–induced conjunctivitis, suggesting that an immune-related response may result from a variety of insults including repeated mechanical trauma of the superior tarsus by the sharp or rough surface of a contact lens, prosthesis, or suture. A hypersensitivity reaction to the contact lens polymer itself (or to antigens or other foreign material adhering to it) has also been postulated but not formally demonstrated. Although most patients who develop contact lens–induced conjunctivitis do not have clinically significant dry eye, the latter condition is present in a significant minority (particularly since contact lenses diminish blinking and hence increase evaporative loss of tears) and may facilitate adhesion of antigens to the surface epithelium.

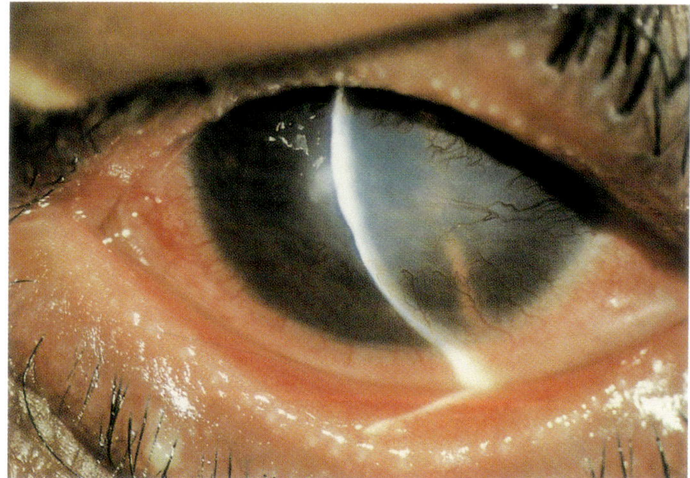

Figure 9-7 Severe corneal vascularization and scarring in a patient with atopic keratoconjunctivitis.

The histologic findings in contact lens–induced conjunctivitis are similar to those observed in vernal keratoconjunctivitis. An abnormal accumulation of mast cells, basophils, and eosinophils is noted in the epithelium and/or the substantia propria of the superior tarsus. Abnormally elevated concentrations of immunoglobulins, specifically IgE, IgG, and IgM, and complement components have been found in the tears of affected patients. These findings suggest a combined mechanical and immune-mediated pathophysiology for contact lens–induced conjunctivitis. It is recognized that surface deposits on worn contact lenses are a risk factor for development and persistence of this condition.

CLINICAL PRESENTATION Some patients who wear contact lenses, in particular extended-wear soft contact lenses, may develop inflammatory symptoms, including redness, itching, and mucoid discharge. One or more of the following signs may be seen during biomicroscopic examination of contact lens wearers with these symptoms:

- Mild papillary reaction (papillae <0.3 mm in diameter) on the superior tarsal conjunctiva
- Punctate epithelial erosions
- Peripheral corneal infiltrates and vascularization

At the more severe end of the spectrum of contact lens–related inflammation is the entity known as *giant papillary conjunctivitis (GPC)*. GPC tends to develop earlier and more frequently in soft contact lens wearers than in hard contact lens wearers and may be recurrent. Symptoms include contact lens intolerance, itching, excessive mucous discharge, blurred vision from mucous coating of the contact lens, contact lens decentration, and conjunctival redness. In rare instances, bloody tears and ptosis secondary to inflammation of the superior tarsal conjunctival may be observed.

The signs of GPC consist of hyperemia, thickening, and abnormally large papillae (diameter >0.3 mm) on the superior tarsal conjunctiva (Fig 9-8). The morphological

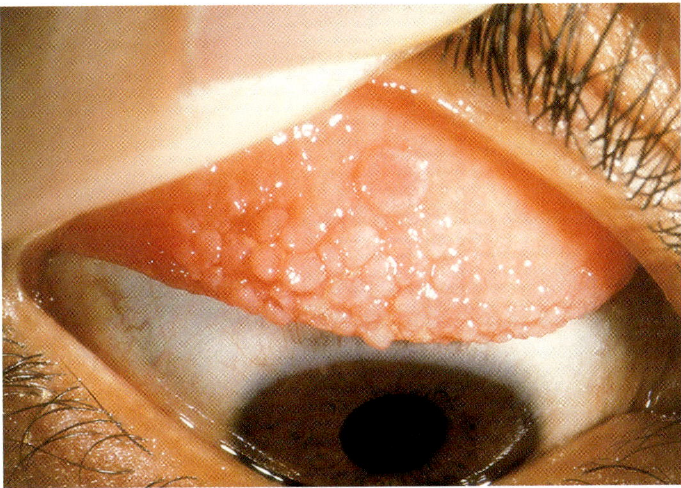

Figure 9-8 Giant papillary conjunctivitis. *(Photograph courtesy of Kirk R. Wilhelmus, MD.)*

appearance of the superior tarsal papillae may be variable in GPC. In some cases the giant papillae cover the entire central tarsus from the posterior eyelid margin to the upper border of the tarsal plate, while involvement in other cases may be less extensive. Occasionally, only a few giant papillae appear, surrounded by smaller papillae. Long-standing or involuted giant papillae on the superior tarsus can resemble follicles.

The symptoms of GPC generally resolve with the discontinuation of contact lens wear. The tarsal conjunctival hyperemia and thickening may resolve in several weeks, but papillae or dome-shaped scars on the superior tarsus can persist for months to years.

MANAGEMENT The goals of GPC treatment are to resolve the symptoms and enable patients to continue wearing contact lenses if possible. Therapeutic strategies include discarding the offending contact lenses and refitting the patient with new ones, improving lens hygiene, and treating conjunctival inflammation with drugs. Simply fitting the patient with new contact lenses frequently resolves GPC. Daily wear rather than extended-wear soft contact lenses should be encouraged, although GPC can also occur with daily wear or even daily disposable contact lenses. Still, periodic planned replacement of soft contact lenses is often beneficial and can easily be accomplished by switching the patient to disposable contact lenses that are used for daily wear and discarded every day or every 2 weeks. Reducing daily wear time or instituting a 1-month contact lens holiday are additional measures that can be helpful in many cases.

Patients should be encouraged to clean their soft contact lenses daily using agents free of preservatives, particularly thimerosal, and to rinse and store lenses in appropriate lens storage solutions. Disinfection of contact lenses with a hydrogen peroxide system appears to be the method best tolerated by the inflamed conjunctiva. Regular enzymatic treatment of contact lenses with papain or subtilisin A may remove inciting contact lens deposits. It is also important to store contact lenses in cases that are routinely cleaned or sterilized; periodic replacement of contact lens cases is encouraged.

If GPC persists, consideration should be given to changing the lens to a different polymer or to daily disposable lenses. Some patients do better with low-water-content lenses. Nevertheless, some patients continue to suffer from GPC as a result of soft contact lens wear despite these measures. In these cases, consideration can be given to fitting the patient with rigid gas-permeable (RGP) contact lenses, which are associated with a lower incidence of GPC. It should be noted that some patients have recurrences of GPC in spite of aggressive lens management and even RGP lens wear; these patients should be counseled about alternatives to contact lens wear.

Pharmacologic therapy can be helpful in the management of patients with GPC. Most practitioners recommend discontinuation of lens wear for several (2–3) weeks while treatment is initiated. Mast-cell stabilizers such as cromolyn sodium have been reported to improve early, mild GPC but have not been successful in advanced, severe cases. However, once advanced cases of GPC have been brought under control, maintenance therapy with topical mast-cell inhibitors may prevent further exacerbations. Topical corticosteroids, though effective in GPC, generally have a limited role because of their potential side effects. If used, they should be discontinued after a short period.

Stevens-Johnson Syndrome (Erythema Multiforme Major) and Toxic Epidermal Necrolysis

PATHOGENESIS Immune-complex deposition in the dermis and conjunctival stroma has been implicated in the pathogenesis of erythema multiforme. The most common inciting agents include drugs such as sulfonamides, anticonvulsants, salicylates, penicillin, ampicillin, and isoniazid; or infectious organisms, such as herpes simplex virus, streptococci, adenovirus, and occasionally mycoplasma.

The distinctive pathologic changes of *Stevens-Johnson syndrome* are subepithelial bullae and subsequent scarring. The most severe form of this condition is referred to as *toxic epidermal necrolysis (TEN)*. TEN, which occurs more commonly in children and people with AIDS, has more superficial (epithelial) inflammation and produces less scarring. It is characterized by interepithelial bullae and extensive sloughing of epidermis, often with conjunctival scarring. See Table 9-1 for a comparison of Stevens-Johnson syndrome, TEN, and other oculocutaneous immune-mediated conditions.

CLINICAL PRESENTATION The term *erythema multiforme* refers to an acute inflammatory vesiculobullous reaction of the skin and mucous membranes. When these hypersensitivity disorders involve only the skin, the term *erythema multiforme minor* is used; when the skin and mucous membranes are involved, the condition is known as *Stevens-Johnson syndrome*, or *erythema multiforme major*, which accounts for 20% of all patients with erythema multiforme. The incidence of Stevens-Johnson syndrome has been shown to be about five cases per million per year. Recent reports have suggested that patients with AIDS are at a higher risk of developing erythema multiforme, particularly patients treated for *Pneumocystis carinii* pneumonia.

Stevens-Johnson syndrome occurs most commonly in children and young adults and in females more often than males, but no age is immune. Fever, arthralgia, malaise, and upper or lower respiratory symptoms are usually sudden in onset. Skin eruption follows within a few days with a classic "target" lesion consisting of a red center surrounded by a pale ring and then a red ring, although maculopapular or bullous lesions are also common. The mucous membranes of the eyes, mouth, and genitalia may be affected by bullous lesions with membrane or pseudomembrane formation. New lesions may appear over 4–6 weeks with approximate 2-week cycles for each crop of lesions. The primary ocular finding is a mucopurulent conjunctivitis and episcleritis. Bullae and extensive areas of necrosis may develop (Fig 9-9). Later ocular complications are caused by cicatrization resulting in conjunctival shrinkage, trichiasis, and tear deficiency. Patients with Stevens-Johnson syndrome are at higher risk of infection due to loss of the epithelial barrier and hence may develop severe ocular infection concurrent with the ocular surface disease.

Table 9-1 Selected Oculocutaneous Immune-Mediated Reactions

Condition	Causes	Eye	Skin	Others
Angioedema	Drugs; foods; insect sting	Eyelid edema	Facial edema; urticaria	Cardiorespiratory distress
Cicatricial pemphigoid	Unknown	Cicatrizing conjunctivitis	Bullous eruptions	Lesions of oropharynx and genitalia
Graft-versus-host disease	Bone-marrow transplant	Dry eye; conjunctivitis	Pigmentary changes	Respiratory and gastrointestinal lesions
Stevens-Johnson syndrome	Drugs; infections	Conjunctival erosion; conjunctivitis; episcleritis	Blisters	Fever; respiratory lesions; sepsis
Toxic epidermal necrolysis	Drugs; infections	Blepharodermatitis; conjunctivitis; corneal exposure	Blisters; necrosis	Fever; respiratory and gastrointestinal lesions

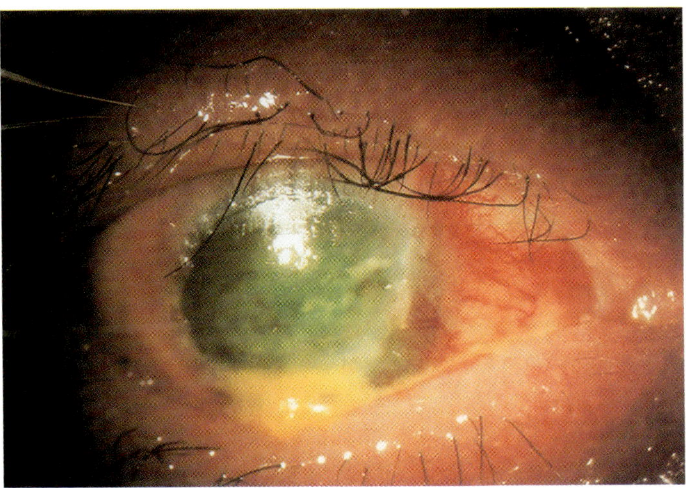

Figure 9-9 Stevens-Johnson syndrome with associated ocular disease.

Cicatricial pemphigoid has also been reported as a rare sequela of Stevens-Johnson syndrome (see below).

MANAGEMENT Management of Stevens-Johnson syndrome is mainly supportive. The mainstay of therapy is ocular lubrication with artificial tears and ointments and vigilant surveillance for the early manifestations of ocular infections. Improved supportive therapy and, in some cases, administration of systemic corticosteroids have reduced the high mortality rate previously associated with this condition. However, the role of corticosteroids remains controversial. Most authorities recommend treating severe cases with oral prednisone, starting with 1 mg/kg/day. Even when used for short periods of time, however, high doses of systemic corticosteroids (primarily when administered intravenously) can be associated with serious complications: gastrointestinal hemorrhage, electrolyte imbalance, and even sudden death. Moreover, they may increase the likelihood of infection. The efficacy of topical corticosteroids for the ocular manifestations of this condition has not been established and remains controversial. On the one hand, steroids may decrease surface inflammation and corneal angiogenesis; on the other hand, they may contribute to corneal thinning and infection. Hence, aggressive lubrication with drops and ointment remains the mainstay of therapy and can prevent nosocomial complications in debilitated patients.

Symblephara may form during the acute phase because the raw, necrotic palpebral and bulbar conjunctival surfaces can adhere to one another (Fig 9-10). Some authors recommend daily lysis of the symblephara and the use of symblepharon rings, but the long-term results of this therapy may be disappointing. In fact, some investigators discourage the use of these strategies, hypothesizing that repeated conjunctival lysis may exacerbate inflammation and surface morbidity.

Late eyelid sequelae, such as entropion, trichiasis, and loss of the fornices, can be surgically corrected after the disease is quiescent. All efforts are aimed at avoiding secondary corneal complications. Because of the altered ocular surface and the corneal neovascularization that frequently develops in these patients, penetrating keratoplasty has an extremely poor prognosis and is generally reserved for progressive thinning or perforation. Favorable results in desperate cases have been achieved with the use of a keratoprosthesis, although its long-term stability may be problematic. Unfortunately, many patients suffering from this condition are young and are left with lifelong ocular morbidity. Ocular surface reconstruction (eg, with amniotic membrane) with limbal grafting has been advocated but controlled prospective data are very limited.

Foster CS. Immunologic disorders of the conjunctiva, cornea, and sclera. In: Albert DM, Jakobiec FA, eds. *Principles and Practice of Ophthalmology*. Vol 2. 2nd ed. Philadelphia: Saunders; 2000:803–829.

Holland EJ, Hardten DR. Stevens-Johnson syndrome. In: Pepose JS, Holland GN, Wilhelmus KR, eds. *Ocular Infection and Immunity*. St Louis: Mosby; 1996:416–425.

Ocular Cicatricial Pemphigoid

PATHOGENESIS The etiology of cicatricial pemphigoid (CP) remains unknown. Antibody activates complement with subsequent breakdown of the conjunctival membrane. Pem-

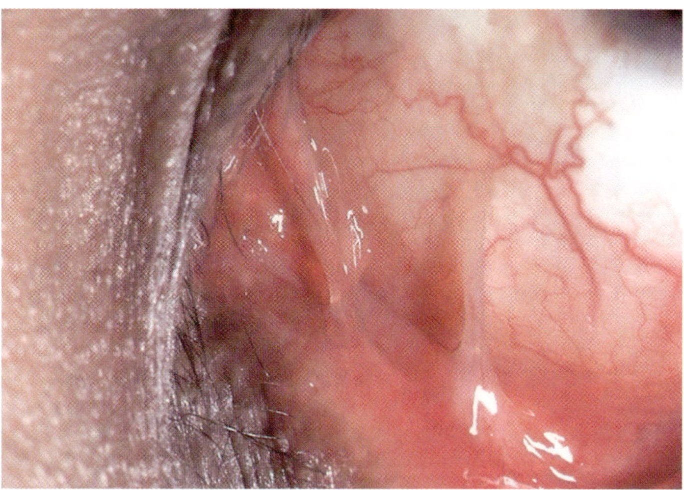

Figure 9-10 Symblepharon formation (adhesion between the globe and palpebral conjunctiva) secondary to conjunctival scarring in Stevens-Johnson syndrome (erythema multiforme major); virtually identical adhesions occur in ocular cicatricial pemphigoid.

phigoid may represent a cytotoxic (Type II) hypersensitivity, in which cell injury results from autoantibodies directed against a cell surface antigen in the basement membrane zone (BMZ). Cellular immunity may also play a role. HLA-DR4, a special genetic locus in the major histocompatibility complex (MHC), has been associated with this condition but by no means are all affected individuals positive for this background; hence HLA typing is not useful.

Pseudopemphigoid, which has a clinical picture similar to pemphigoid, has been associated with the chronic use of certain topical ophthalmic medications. Case reports have implicated pilocarpine, epinephrine, timolol, idoxuridine, echothiophate iodide, and demecarium bromide. The principal difference between pseudopemphigoid and true pemphigoid is that in the former further progression of the disease generally ceases once the offending agent is recognized and removed. The differential diagnosis of cicatrizing conjunctivitis includes four major categories:

- Postinfectious conditions that follow severe episodes of trachoma, adenoviral conjunctivitis, or streptococcal conjunctivitis
- Autoimmune or autoreactive conditions such as sarcoidosis, scleroderma, lichen planus, Stevens-Johnson syndrome, dermatitis herpetiformis, epidermolysis bullosa, atopic blepharoconjunctivitis, and graft-versus-host disease
- Prior conjunctival trauma
- Severe blepharokeratoconjunctivitis caused by rosacea or other disorders (eg, atopic keratoconjunctivitis) that are associated with conjunctival shrinkage

The diagnosis of unilateral CP should be made with caution, since other diseases, including many of those listed above, may masquerade as CP. Finally, linear IgA dermatosis, a rare dermatological condition, can result in an ocular syndrome that is clinically identical to cicatricial pemphigoid and requires similar treatment.

CLINICAL PRESENTATION Cicatricial pemphigoid is a chronic cicatrizing conjunctivitis of autoimmune etiology. Although it is a chronic vesiculobullous disease primarily involving the conjunctiva, it frequently affects other mucous membranes, including the mouth and oropharynx, genitalia, and anus. The skin is involved as well in approximately 15% of the cases. *Pemphigoid* should not be confused with *pemphigus vulgaris,* a skin disease that rarely affects the eyes and with rare exceptions does not cause conjunctival scarring.

Cicatricial pemphigoid affects women more than men by a 2:1 ratio. Patients are usually older than 60 and rarely younger than 30. They frequently present with recurrent attacks of mild and nonspecific conjunctival inflammation with an occasional mucopurulent discharge. In its early phases, CP may present with conjunctival hyperemia, edema, ulceration, and tear dysfunction. Close examination of the conjunctiva in early stages of the disease (stage I) reveals subepithelial fibrosis. Fine gray-white linear opacities, best seen with an intense but thin slit beam, appear in the deep conjunctiva. However, in many cases insidious disease in its early stages produces nonspecific symptoms with minimal overt physical findings such as chronic red eye. Oral mucosal lesions may be a clue that can lead to early diagnosis.

Transient bullae of the conjunctivae rupture, leading to subepithelial fibrosis, particularly of the medial eye. Loss of goblet cells, shortening of the fornices (stage II), symblepharon formation (stage III), and on occasion restricted ocular motility with extensive adhesions between the lid and the globe (stage IV) can follow. Ophthalmologists should attempt to diagnose this condition in its early stages and should therefore watch for an inferior forniceal depth of less than 8 mm, which is abnormal and should prompt further evaluation. Subtle inferior symblephara can be detected when the lower eyelid is pulled down while the patient looks up (Fig 9-11).

Recurrent attacks of conjunctival inflammation can lead to destruction of goblet cells and eventually obstruction of the lacrimal gland ductules. The resultant aqueous and mucous tear deficiency leads to keratinization of the already thickened conjunctiva. En-

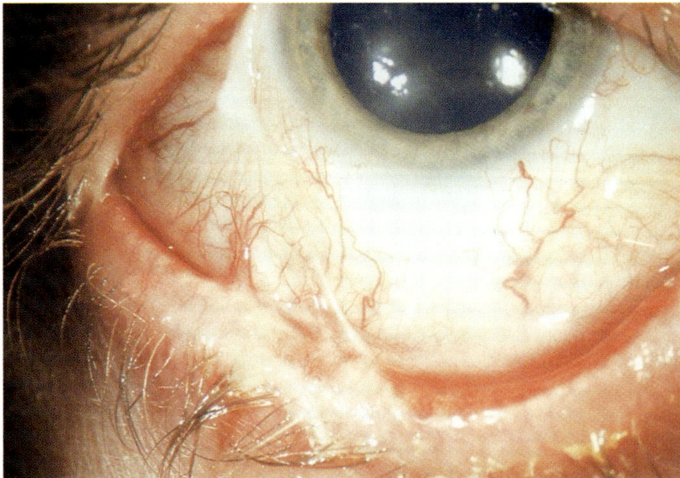

Figure 9-11 Inferior symblepharon as a result of ocular cicatricial pemphigoid.

tropion and trichiasis may develop as scarring progresses, leading to abrasions, corneal vascularization, further scarring, ulceration, and epidermalization of the ocular surface (Fig 9-12). Although the clinical course is variable, progressive deterioration usually occurs in untreated cases. Remissions and exacerbations are common. Surgical intervention can incite to further scarring but may be essential for the management of entropion and trichiasis.

LABORATORY EVALUATION Although cicatricial pemphigoid is a bilateral disease, one eye may be more severely involved than the other. Pathologic support for a diagnosis of pemphigoid can be obtained from a conjunctival biopsy sent for immunofluorescent or immunoperoxidase staining. Biopsy specimens should be obtained from an actively affected area of the conjunctiva or, if diffuse involvement is present, from near the inferior conjunctival fornix. Conjunctival biopsies may or may not be positive for immunoreactants in pseudopemphigoid. Immunohistochemical staining techniques can demonstrate C3, IgG, IgM, and/or IgA localized in the BMZ of the conjunctiva in pemphigoid (Fig 9-13). Circulating anti–basement membrane antibody has been identified in the sera of some patients with pemphigoid.

MANAGEMENT Therapy with systemic corticosteroids alone has limited success in CP. Oral corticosteroids can be used in combination with any of the agents discussed below, although usually for only brief periods of time, measured in months, in severe cases. Because progression is often slow, careful clinical staging of the disease and photo-documentation in differing positions of gaze are generally recommended for evaluation of the disease course and response to therapy. Severity of pemphigoid can be judged by measuring the shortening of the inferior fornix depth (for stage II disease) and the extent of symblepharon along the inferior fornix in quartiles (0%–25%, 25%–50%, 50%–75%, and 75%–100% for stage III–IV disease).

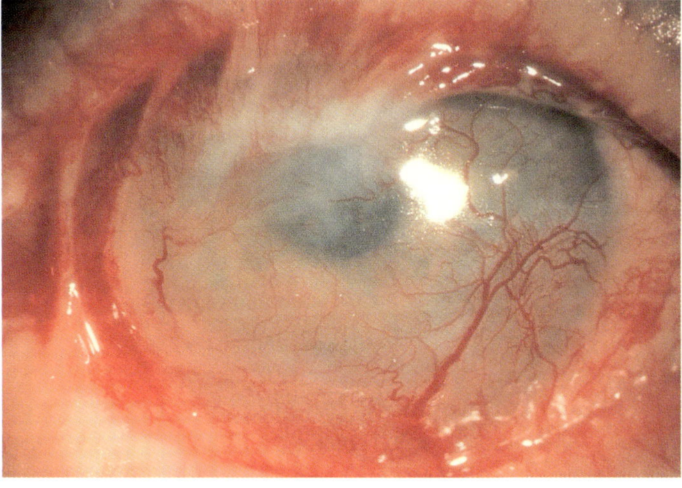

Figure 9-12 Advanced cicatricial pemphigoid.

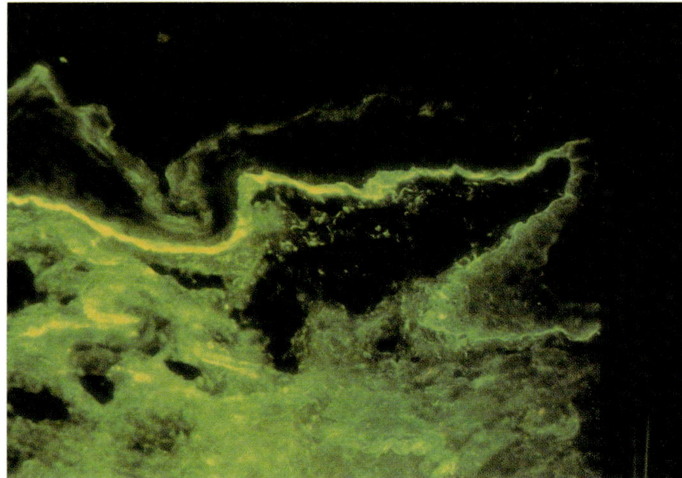

Figure 9-13 Immunofluorescent staining of basement membrane in a patient with cicatricial pemphigoid.

Dapsone, a drug previously used to treat Hansen disease (leprosy) and dermatitis herpetiformis, has been advocated by most authorities as the initial drug of choice in mild cases. It must be used cautiously in patients with glucose-6-phosphate dehydrogenase (G6PD) deficiency or sulfa allergy; therefore, testing for G6PD deficiency is recommended before initiating treatment. However, even those *without* this enzymatic deficiency may develop hemolytic anemia.

Cyclophosphamide (Cytoxan) has been used for treating CP in a manner similar to its use in Wegener granulomatosis. Cyclophosphamide remains a mainstay of therapy in severe disease. The usual therapeutic dose is 1.5–2.0 mg/kg/day in divided doses. The therapeutic target is a reduction in white blood count to the range of 2000–3000 cells per μL. Cytotoxic therapy can bring about disease remission. Consultation with an internist, dermatologist, or oncologist experienced in cytotoxic therapy is recommended for the administration of immunosuppressive agents such as cyclophosphamide. Azathioprine (Imuran) and methotrexate have also been used as alternate agents in moderately severe cases or when cyclophosphamide cannot be tolerated, although the success rate with these agents for severe disease is generally lower.

Topical corticosteroids may suppress the immediate inflammatory response and acute exacerbations. Topical vitamin A has been shown to reverse, to some extent, the keratinization resulting from the squamous metaplasia associated with this condition but is not a standard of care.

Other measures, such as surgical correction of eyelid deformities or lash ablation for trichiasis, are occasionally required to achieve ocular surface quiescence. Intraocular surgery is best delayed until disease activity has been under control for an extended period of time. Hard palate and buccal mucosal grafting can be useful techniques in fornix reconstruction. Punctal occlusion, which may already have resulted from cicatrization, can be useful in the management of any associated dry eye condition. In general, patients with cicatrizing conjunctivitis have a higher rate of spontaneous extrusion of silicone punctal plugs, and thus permanent punctal occlusion with cautery is often required. Standard penetrating keratoplasty generally has a very guarded prognosis in patients who develop severe corneal disease in CP, but keratoprosthesis surgery has been used with some success.

Recently, intravenous immunoglobulin therapy (IVIg) has been reported as adjuvant therapy for several autoimmune disorders including bullous pemphigoid. In some patients, treatment with IVIg has had a steroid-sparing role. However, the optimal dosing strategy and efficacy of this treatment strategy remain to be determined.

Chiou AG, Florakis GJ, Kazim M. Management of conjunctival cicatrizing diseases and severe ocular surface dysfunction. *Surv Ophthalmol.* 1998;43:19–46.

Engineer L, Ahmed AR. Role of intravenous immunoglobulin in the treatment of bullous pemphigoid: analysis of current data. *J Am Acad Dermatol.* 2001;44:83–88.

Foster CS. Immunologic disorders of the conjunctiva, cornea, and sclera. In: Albert DM, Jakobiec FA, eds. *Principles and Practice of Ophthalmology.* Vol 2. 2nd ed. Philadelphia: Saunders; 2000:803–829.

Yaghouti F, Nouri M, Abad JC, et al. Keratoprosthesis: preoperative prognostic categories. *Cornea.* 2001;20:19–23.

Graft-Versus-Host Disease

Graft-versus-host disease (GVHD) is a relatively common complication of allogeneic bone-marrow transplantation, performed most commonly for hematopoietic malignancies. In this condition, the grafted cells can attack the patient's tissues, including the skin, gut, lungs, liver and gastrointestinal system, and eyes. While GVHD can be acute or chronic (developing more than 3 months after bone-marrow transplantation), most ocular complications occur as a manifestation of chronic GVHD. The pathogenesis of ocular surface disease in GVHD is multifactorial but has two main components: (1) conjunctival inflammation with or without subepithelial fibrosis, and (2) severe keratoconjunctivitis sicca from lacrimal gland infiltration by GVHD-effecting T lymphocytes. Conjunctival inflammation in GVHD can be severe and even associated with limbal stem-cell deficiency and secondary corneal scarring, but fortunately, the latter is a rare complication. Typical presentations include conjunctival and corneal epithelial erosions, aqueous tear deficiency, and cicatricial lagophthalmos.

Aggressive lubrication and punctal occlusion are the mainstays of local therapy. Severe filamentary keratitis can be treated further with mucolytic agents (10% acetylcysteine) as needed. Severe ocular surface disease in GVHD may be associated with active nonocular (often skin) GVHD and may require increased systemic immunosuppression by cyclosporine or tacrolimus (FK506).

Kim R, Dana MR. Ocular manifestations of graft-versus-host disease. In: Albert DM, Jakobiec FA, eds. *Principles and Practice of Ophthalmology.* Vol 5. 2nd ed. Philadelphia: Saunders; 2000:4994–5002.

Other Immune-Mediated Diseases of the Skin and Mucous Membranes

Other immune-mediated disorders that can rarely affect the conjunctiva include linear IgA bullous dermatosis, dermatitis herpetiformis, epidermolysis bullosa, lichen planus, paraneoplastic pemphigus, pemphigus vulgaris, and pemphigus foliaceus.

Immune-Mediated Diseases of the Cornea

Thygeson Superficial Punctate Keratitis (SPK)

PATHOGENESIS The etiology of Thygeson superficial punctate keratitis is unknown. Although many of the clinical features resemble a viral infection of the epithelium, attempts to confirm viral particles by electron microscopy or culture have been unsuccessful. The rapid response of the lesions to corticosteroid therapy suggests that Thygeson keratitis is largely immunopathogenically derived.

CLINICAL PRESENTATION This condition, first reported by Thygeson in 1950, is characterized by recurrent episodes of tearing, foreign body sensation, photophobia, and reduced vision. It affects children to older adults and is typically bilateral, although it may develop initially in one eye or may be markedly asymmetrical in some cases. The hallmark finding is multiple (up to 40 but as few as 2–3) slightly elevated corneal epithelial lesions, which are noted during exacerbations. The epithelial lesions are round or oval conglomerates of gray, granular opacities associated with *minimal* conjunctival reaction, in contrast to adenoviral keratoconjunctivitis. High magnification reveals each opacity to be a cluster of multiple smaller pinpoint opacities (Fig 9-14). A characteristic feature is the waxing and waning appearance of individual epithelial opacities, which change in location and number over time. The greatest density of these lesions typically appears in the central cornea. The punctate epithelial lesions stain with fluorescein and rose bengal.

No conjunctival inflammatory reaction is noted during exacerbations, but occasionally patients will have mild bulbar conjunctival injection. Rarely, a mild subepithelial

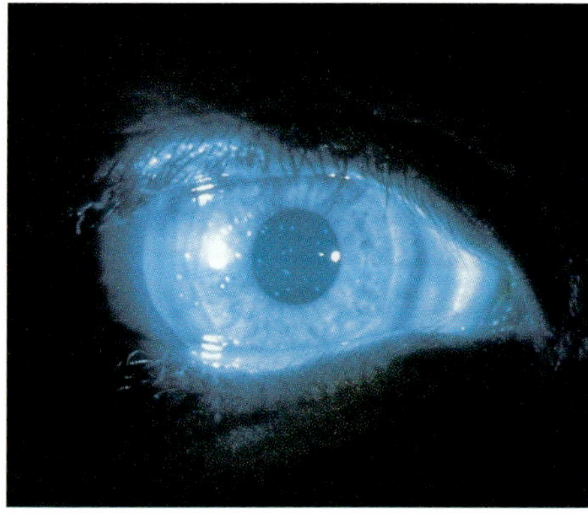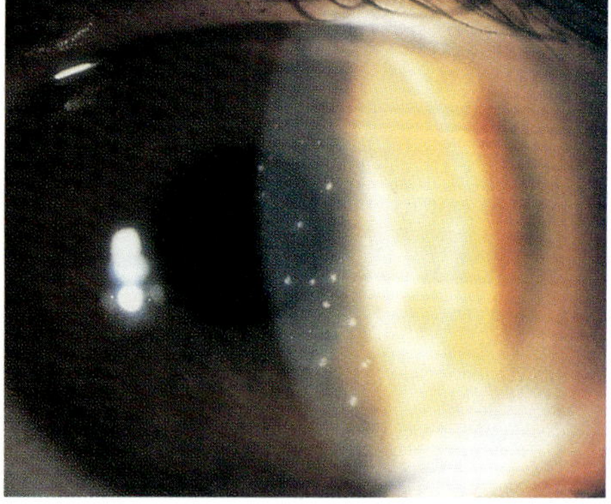

Figure 9-14 Thygeson superficial punctate keratitis; at higher magnification, each lesion is seen to consist of several minute dots.

opacity may develop underlying the epithelial lesion, more commonly in patients who have received topical antiviral therapy. The important facet of this condition is that the patient's symptoms may far exceed the apparent signs; frequently, patients complain bitterly of photophobia and foreign body sensation in the setting of only a few central epithelial lesions.

MANAGEMENT Supportive therapy with artificial tears and bandage soft contact lenses is often adequate in mild cases. Treatment alternatives for persistently symptomatic cases include topical corticosteroids. Antiviral therapy, though recommended by some authors, is not the standard of care at this time, as there are no firm data to associate this condition with an active replicative viral infection.

If a topical corticosteroid is prescribed, only a very mild preparation is needed (eg, fluorometholone 0.1%). Because the lesions are quite responsive to corticosteroids, treatment will hasten their resolution, but they frequently recur in the same or different locations on the cornea after the topical steroids are stopped. Anecdotal reports suggest that use of topical corticosteroids may prolong the disease to more than 15 years, a duration that is uncommon in cases never treated with steroids. Consequently, tapering off of steroids can sometimes be problematic. Topical cyclosporine given twice daily is also effective in causing regression of the lesions, but there is little to suggest that this treatment is superior to steroid therapy.

Schwab IR, Thygeson P. Thygeson superficial punctate keratopathy. In: Pepose JS, Holland GN, Wilhelmus KR, eds. *Ocular Infection and Immunity*. St Louis: Mosby, 1996:403–407.

Interstitial Keratitis Associated With Infectious Diseases

PATHOGENESIS Interstitial keratitis (IK) is a nonsuppurative inflammation of the corneal stroma that features cellular infiltration and usually vascularization without primary involvement of the epithelium or endothelium. Most cases result from a Type IV hypersensitivity response to infectious microorganisms or other antigens in the corneal stroma. The topographic distribution (diffuse versus focal or multifocal) and depth of the stromal infiltration, in addition to associated systemic signs, are helpful in determining the cause of IK.

Congenital syphilis was the first infection to be linked with interstitial keratitis. Herpes simplex virus, which accounts for most cases of stromal keratitis, and varicella-zoster virus keratitis are discussed earlier in this volume. Many other microorganisms are much rarer causes of IK, including:

- *Mycobacterium tuberculosis*
- *M leprae*
- *Borrelia burgdorferi* (Lyme disease)
- Rubeola (measles)
- Epstein-Barr virus (infectious mononucleosis)
- *Chlamydia trachomatis* (lymphogranuloma venereum)
- *Leishmania* species
- *Onchocerca volvulus* (onchocerciasis)

Syphilitic interstitial keratitis

CLINICAL PRESENTATION Syphilitic eye disease is discussed further in BCSC Section 6 *(Pediatric Ophthalmology and Strabismus)* and Section 9 *(Intraocular Inflammation and Uveitis)*. Systemic aspects of syphilis are discussed in BCSC Section 1, *Update on General Medicine.*

Keratitis may be caused by either congenital or acquired syphilis, although most cases are associated with congenital syphilis. Manifestations of congenital syphilis that occur early in life (within the first 2 years) are *infectious.* However, IK is an example of a later, *immune-mediated* manifestation of congenital syphilis. Affected children typically show no evidence of corneal disease in their first years; stromal keratitis lasting for several weeks develops late in the first decade of life (or even later). These patients may also have other nonocular signs of congenital syphilis:

- Dental deformities: notched (Hutchinson) incisors and mulberry molars
- Bone and cartilage abnormalities: saddle nose, palatal perforation, saber shins, and frontal bossing
- Cranial nerve VIII (vestibulocochlear) deafness
- Rhagades (circumoral radiating scars)
- Mental retardation

Congenital syphilitic keratitis is usually bilateral (80%), although both eyes may not be affected simultaneously or to the same degree. Initial symptoms are pain, tearing, photophobia, and perilimbal injection. The inflammation may last for weeks if left untreated. Sectoral superior stromal inflammation and keratic precipitates are typically seen early. As the disease progresses, deep stromal neovascularization develops. Eventually, the inflammation spreads centrally, and corneal opacification and edema may develop (Fig 9-15). In some cases, the deep corneal vascularization becomes so intense that the cornea appears pink, hence the term *salmon patch.* Sequelae of stromal keratitis include corneal

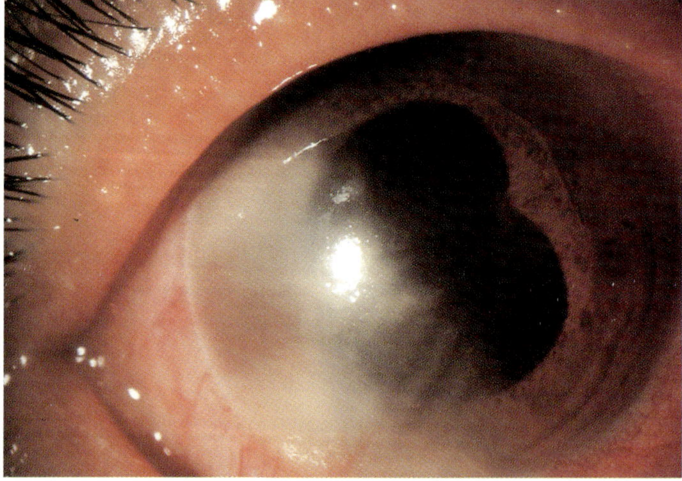

Figure 9-15 Active syphilitic interstitial keratitis.

scarring, thinning, and ghost vessels in the *deep* layers of the stroma. Visual acuity may be reduced because of irregular astigmatism and stromal opacification.

Stromal keratitis only rarely develops in *acquired* (as apposed to congenital) syphilis and, if it does, is typically unilateral (60%). The ocular findings are similar to those seen in congenital syphilitic keratitis. In general, uveitis and retinitis are much more common manifestation of acquired syphilis than keratitis.

LABORATORY EVALUATION AND MANAGEMENT The diagnosis can be confirmed serologically with the rapid plasmin reagin test and a treponeme-specific antibody test (FTA-ABS or MHA-TP). During the acute phase, ocular inflammation should be treated with cycloplegic agents and topical corticosteroids in order to limit stromal inflammation and late scarring. The corneal disease can be suppressed effectively with topical corticosteroids; however, even if left untreated the disease typically burns out after several weeks, though it can lead to severe corneal opacification before doing so. Systemic syphilis (or neuroretinal manifestations) should be treated with penicillin or an appropriate alternative antibiotic according to a protocol appropriate for either congenital or acquired syphilis. The necessity of lumbar puncture in syphilitic interstitial keratitis is uncertain. See BCSC Section 9, *Intraocular Inflammation and Uveitis,* for a more in-depth discussion of noncorneal syphilitic disease.

Reiter Syndrome

Reiter syndrome is a systemic disorder characterized by the classic triad of ocular (conjunctivitis/episcleritis, iridocyclitis, or keratitis), urethral, and joint inflammation. The joint inflammation is often highly asymmetrical and involves a few joints (oligoarticular). These manifestations can appear simultaneously or separately in any sequence. Less common manifestations include keratoderma blennorrhagicum (a scaling skin eruption), balanitis, aphthous stomatitis, fever, lymphadenopathy, pneumonitis, pericarditis, and myocarditis. Attacks are self-limited, lasting from 2 to several months, but they may recur periodically over the course of several years.

Reiter syndrome may occur after gram-negative bacterial dysentery (most frequently associated with *Salmonella, Shigella,* and *Yersinia*) or after nongonococcal urethritis caused by *Chlamydia trachomatis.* More than 75% of patients with Reiter syndrome are HLA-B27 positive. See BCSC Section 9, *Intraocular Inflammation and Uveitis,* for discussion of HLA-B27–related diseases and illustrations of nonocular manifestations of Reiter syndrome.

A bilateral papillary conjunctivitis with mucopurulent discharge is the most common ocular finding in Reiter syndrome; it has been reported in 30%–60% of patients. The conjunctivitis is self-limited, lasting for days to weeks. Some patients present more with episcleritis rather than conjunctivitis. Mild nongranulomatous iritis has been reported to occur in 3%–12% of patients. Various forms of keratitis may rarely occur, including diffuse punctate epithelial erosions, superficial or deep focal infiltrates, and superficial or deep vascularization. Reiter syndrome should be considered in any case of chronic, nonfollicular, mucopurulent conjunctivitis with negative cultures.

Treatment is mainly palliative. Corneal infiltrates and vascularization often respond to topical corticosteroids. Systemic antibiotic treatment of the related infection, if any, may be beneficial. Occasionally, the intraocular (uveitic) component of the disease can be very severe and require systemic immune suppression—see BCSC Section 9, *Intraocular Inflammation and Uveitis.*

Cogan Syndrome

PATHOGENESIS Cogan syndrome is an autoimmune disorder that produces stromal keratitis, vertigo, and hearing loss. The etiology of Cogan syndrome is obscure, but the disease shares some clinicopathologic features with polyarteritis nodosa.

CLINICAL PRESENTATION Cogan syndrome typically occurs in young adults, the majority of whom have had an upper respiratory infection 1–2 weeks prior to the onset of ocular or vestibuloauditory symptoms (vertigo, tinnitus, and hearing loss). The earliest corneal findings are bilateral faint white subepithelial infiltrates similar to those occurring in viral keratoconjunctivitis but located in the peripheral cornea. Multifocal nodular infiltrates may develop in the *posterior* cornea later in the course of this condition. Some patients develop a systemic vasculitis that presents as polyarteritis nodosa.

LABORATORY EVALUATION When the cause of stromal keratitis is not apparent, VDRL or RPR and FTA-ABS or MHA-TP are obtained (VDRL and RPR may become nonreactive in congenital syphilis). Other infectious syndromes should also be considered. Since there are no specific laboratory findings, Cogan syndrome is essentially a diagnosis of exclusion.

MANAGEMENT The acute keratitis of Cogan syndrome is treated with frequent topical corticosteroids. Oral corticosteroids are recommended for the vestibuloauditory symptoms, because this treatment enhances the long-term prognosis and recovery of normal hearing. Cytotoxic agents may also have a therapeutic role but are reserved for severe and unresponsive cases.

Marginal Corneal Infiltrates Associated With Blepharoconjunctivitis

PATHOGENESIS The limbus plays an important role in immune-mediated corneal disorders. As reviewed in Chapter 8, the limbus has a population of antigen-presenting cells that constitutively express class II MHC antigens and are capable of efficient mobilization and induction of T-cell responses. Therefore, immune-related corneal changes often occur in a peripheral location adjacent to the limbus. In addition, because the peripheral cornea is adjacent to the vascularized (posterior) limbus, circulating immune cells, immune complexes, and complement factors tend to deposit adjacent to the terminal capillary loops of the limbal vascular arcades, thereby producing a variety of immune phenomena that manifest in the corneal periphery. Predisposing causes include

- Blepharoconjunctivitis
- Contact lens wear
- Trauma
- Endophthalmitis

CLINICAL PRESENTATION Marginal infiltrates (also referred to as *catarrhal infiltrates*) usually occur where the eyelid margins intersect with the corneal surface: the 10, 2, 4, and

8 o'clock positions. Marginal infiltrates in staphylococcal blepharitis are typically gray-white, well circumscribed, and located approximately 1 mm inside the limbus, with a characteristic clear (intervening) zone of cornea between the infiltrate and the limbus (see Figure 7-20). In chronic disease, superficial blood vessels may cross the clear interval into the area of corneal infiltration. The epithelium overlying marginal infiltrates may be intact, show punctate epithelial erosions, or be ulcerated. Stromal opacification, peripheral corneal thinning, and/or pannus may develop following resolution of the acute marginal infiltrates.

Peripheral Ulcerative Keratitis Associated With Systemic Immune-Mediated Diseases

PATHOGENESIS Autoimmune peripheral keratitis may develop in patients who have systemic immune-mediated and rheumatic diseases. Peripheral ulcerative keratitis (PUK) occurs most often in association with rheumatoid arthritis but may also be seen in Wegener granulomatosis, systemic lupus erythematosus, polyarteritis nodosa, ulcerative colitis, relapsing polychondritis, and other inflammatory diseases such as rosacea (Table 9-2). Biopsy of conjunctival tissue adjacent to marginal corneal disease—although not a standard diagnostic procedure—typically shows evidence of immune-mediated vaso-occlusive disease.

CLINICAL PRESENTATION A history of connective tissue disease is often (but not invariably) present, although in some cases the ocular finding of peripheral corneal infiltration or frank stromal melting may be the first sign of the underlying systemic illness. Autoimmune peripheral ulcerative keratitis generally correlates with exacerbations of systemic disease activity. Follow-up of these patients reveals that, if they are treated inadequately, a high proportion may suffer severe disease-related morbidity. The term *keratolysis* refers to significant (and often rapid) stromal melting seen in some cases of immune-mediated PUK associated with systemic autoimmunity.

Although autoimmune peripheral ulcerative keratitis can sometimes be bilateral and extensive, it is usually unilateral and limited to one sector of the peripheral cornea (Fig 9-16). The initial lesions appear in a zone within 2 mm of the limbus and are accompanied by varying degrees of vaso-occlusion of the adjacent limbal vascular networks. In most cases, the epithelium is absent in the affected area and the underlying stroma thinned; however, if the disease is detected early, the epithelial involvement may be patchy and the stroma still of near-normal thickness. Ulceration may or may not be associated with a significant cellular infiltrate in the corneal stroma, and the adjacent conjunctiva can be minimally or severely inflamed.

MANAGEMENT The goal of therapy is to provide local supportive measures to decrease melting. This is achieved through maneuvers directed at (1) improving wetting, (2) promoting reepithelialization, and (3) suppressing the systemic-mediated inflammation.

Maintaining enhanced lubrication of the surface is very important: first, because many rheumatoid patients have keratoconjunctivitis sicca as a manifestation of their secondary Sjögren syndrome; and second, because lubrication may help in diluting the effect of inflammatory cytokines in the preocular tear film. Melting will stop or slow

Table 9-2 Differential Diagnosis of PUK

Ocular
  Microbial
    Bacterial
      Staphylococcus
      Streptococcus
      Gonococcus
      Moraxella
      Haemophilus
    Viral
      Herpes simplex
      Herpes zoster
      Acanthamoeba
    Fungal
  Mooren ulcer
  Traumatic or postsurgical
  Terrien marginal degeneration
  Exposure keratopathy
  Rosacea
Systemic
  Microbial
    Bacterial
      Tuberculosis
      Syphilis
      Gonorrhea
      Borreliosis
      Bacillary dysentery
    Viral
      Herpes zoster
      AIDS
      Hepatitis C
    Helminthiasis
  Rheumatoid arthritis
  Systemic lupus erythematosus
  Wegener granulomatosis
  Polyarteritis nodosa
  Relapsing polychondritis
  Progressive systemic sclerosis and scleroderma
  Sjögren syndrome
  Behçet syndrome
  Sarcoidosis
  Inflammatory bowel disease
  α_1-antitrypsin deficiency
  Malignancy

(Adapted with permission from Dana MR, Qian Y, Hamrah P. Twenty-five-year panorama of corneal immunology: emerging concepts in the immunopathogenesis of microbial keratitis, peripheral ulcerative keratitis, and corneal transplant rejection. *Cornea.* 2000;19:625–643.)

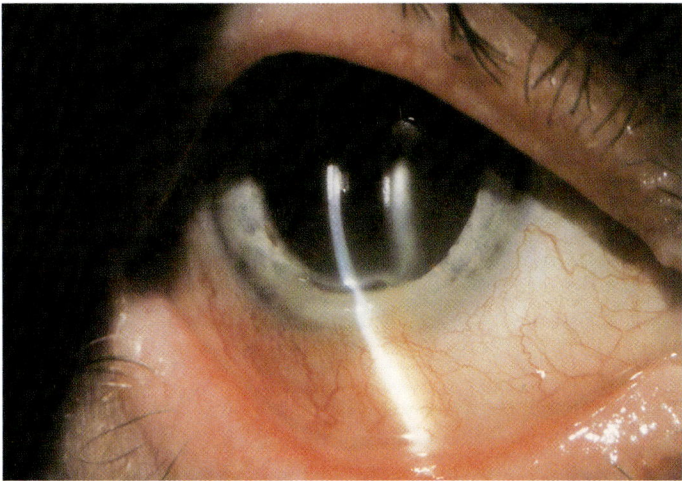

Figure 9-16 Peripheral ulcerative keratitis as a result of rheumatoid disease.

appreciably if the epithelium can be made to heal by means of lubricants, patching, or a bandage soft contact lens. Topical collagenase inhibitors such as sodium citrate 10% or tetracycline and systemic collagenase inhibitors such as tetracyclines (eg, doxycycline) are of possible value.

Topical corticosteroids, which also inhibit collagenase function, often have variable effects. Although they may suppress corneal inflammation when there is profound leukocyte infiltration in the cornea, they also may delay reepithelialization, predispose to superinfection, and even exacerbate melting by suppressing collagen production. In general, if the cornea has become significantly thinned, corticosteroid therapy is not indicated. Excision or recession of adjacent limbal conjunctiva (as has been advocated for Mooren ulcer—see the following section) is often followed by healing of the ulcer, presumably because the procedure eliminates a source of inflammatory cells and collagenolytic enzymes.

Definitive management often cannot be achieved by local measures alone and requires institution or escalation of systemic treatment, including immunosuppressive therapy using cytotoxic agents such as cyclophosphamide or immunomodulatory agents such as methotrexate or cyclosporine. Severe, rapidly melting cases may require intravenous therapy with high-dose cyclophosphamide, with or without corticosteroid therapy. Threatened perforation should be treated with temporizing measures such as cyanoacrylate glue and bandage contact lens placement until systemic therapy has been initiated, since lamellar or penetrating grafts are also susceptible to melting. Sometimes multiple tectonic grafts are required to preserve the globe while the systemic therapy is being adjusted. Once the underlying disease process has been controlled, reconstructive keratoplasty can be performed (see Chapters 22–23). While conjunctival flaps can be very helpful for controlling the stromal melting in difficult-to-manage microbial keratitis, they are probably best avoided in immune-mediated disease. The melting could potentially be accelerated by bringing the conjunctival vasculature in even closer proximity to the area of corneal disease.

Mooren Ulcer

PATHOGENESIS Although the etiology of this peripheral ulcerative keratitis is unknown, evidence is mounting that autoimmunity plays a key role. The following have been found in patients with Mooren ulcer:

- Deficiency of suppressor T cells
- Increased level of IgA
- Increased concentration of plasma cells and lymphocytes in the conjunctiva adjacent to the ulcerated areas
- Tissue-fixed immunoglobulins and complement in the conjunctival epithelium and peripheral cornea

A significant number of resident cells in Mooren ulcer specimens express MHC class II antigens—a reflection of the degree of immune-mediated inflammation in the tissue. It has been suggested that autoreactivity to a cornea-specific antigen may play a role in the pathogenesis of this disorder, and humoral and cell-mediated immune mechanisms may be involved in the initiation and perpetuation of corneal destruction. The proximity of the ulcerative lesion to the limbus probably has pathophysiologic importance (as discussed above in the section on PUK), because resection or recession of the limbal conjunctiva can often have a beneficial therapeutic effect.

Although the cause of Mooren ulcer is unknown, precipitating factors include accidental trauma or surgery and exposure to parasitic infection. The latter is of considerable importance, as the incidence of Mooren ulcer is particularly high in areas where parasitic (eg, helminthic) infections are endemic. The principal hypotheses are that inflammation associated with previous injury or infection may alter the expression of corneal or conjunctival antigens (to which autoantibodies are then produced) or that cross-reactivity occurs between the immune effectors generated in response to infection and corneal autoantigens. By definition, Mooren ulcer is of unknown cause. Cases of peripheral corneal ulceration (PUK) due to known local (eg, rosacea) or systemic (eg, rheumatoid arthritis) diseases should not be called Mooren ulcer.

CLINICAL PRESENTATION Mooren ulcer is a chronic, progressive, painful, idiopathic ulceration of the peripheral corneal stroma and epithelium. Typically, the ulcer starts in the periphery of the cornea and spreads circumferentially and then centripetally, with a leading undermined edge of de-epithelized tissue (Fig 9-17). A slower movement of ulceration proceeds toward the sclera. The eye is inflamed and pain can be intense, with photophobia and tearing. Perforation may occur with minor trauma or during secondary infection. Extensive vascularization and fibrosis of the cornea may occur.

Two clinical types of Mooren ulcer have been described. Unilateral Mooren ulcer typically occurs in an older patient population. Sex distribution is equal in this form, which is slowly progressive. A second type of Mooren ulcer is more common in Africa. This form is usually bilateral, rapidly progressive, and poorly responsive to medical or surgical intervention (Fig 9-18). Corneal ulceration and perforation are frequent. Many of the patients with this form of Mooren ulcer also have coexisting parasitemia. It is possible that in this subgroup of West African males, Mooren ulcer may be triggered by

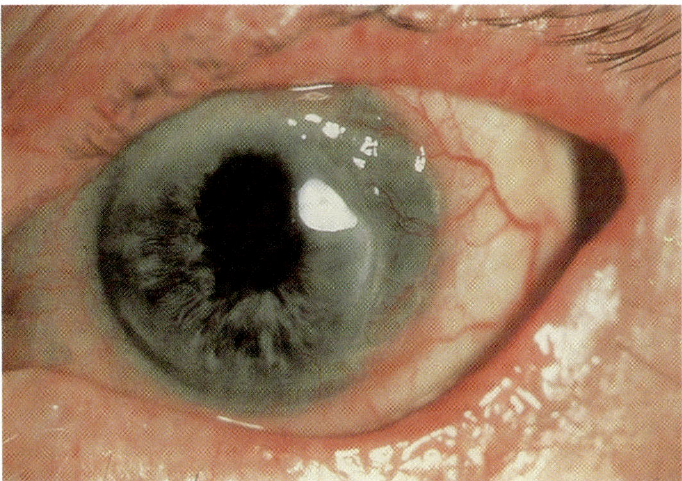

Figure 9-17 Mooren ulcer. *(Photograph courtesy of Vincent P. deLuise, MD.)*

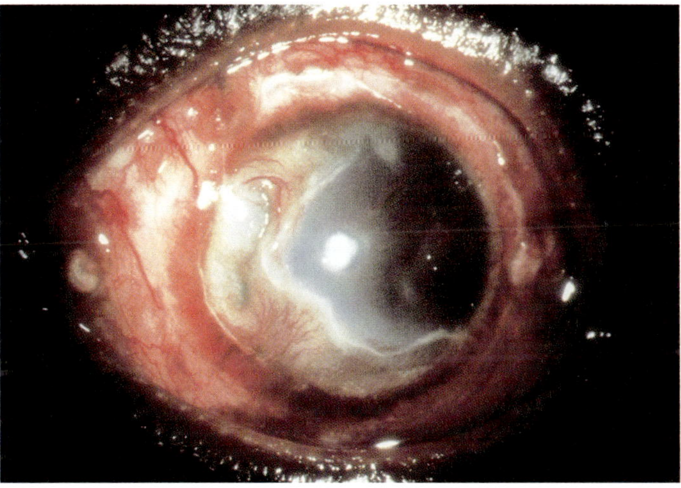

Figure 9-18 Mooren ulcer with severe superior limbal ulceration and thinning.

antigen-antibody reaction to helminthic toxins or antigens deposited in the limbal cornea during the bloodborne phase of parasitic infection.

MANAGEMENT The multitude of therapeutic strategies employed against Mooren ulcer underscores the relative lack of effective treatment. Topical corticosteroids, contact lenses, acetylcysteine (Mucomyst 10%) and L-cysteine (0.2 molar), topical cyclosporine, limbal conjunctival excision, and lamellar keratoplasty have all been described with variable success. In general, severe cases can seldom be controlled by local measures alone. Systemic immunosuppressives such as oral corticosteroids, cyclophosphamide, methotrexate, and cyclosporine have shown promise in these cases. Hepatitis C–associated cases of "Mooren ulcer"–type PUK have responded to interferon therapy.

Gottsch JD, Stark WJ, Liu SH. Cloning and sequence analysis of human and bovine corneal antigen (CO-Ag) cDNA: identification of host-parasite protein calgranulin C. *Trans Am Ophthalmol Soc.* 1997;95:111–125.

Immune-Mediated Diseases of the Episclera and Sclera

Episcleritis

PATHOGENESIS Episcleritis is a self-limited, generally benign inflammation of the episcleral tissues. The pathophysiology of this disorder remains obscure. An underlying systemic cause is found in only a minority of patients.

CLINICAL PRESENTATION Episcleritis is typically a transient (usually days to weeks), self-limited disease of adults, usually 20–50 years of age. The chief complaint is usually ocular redness without irritation, which resolves spontaneously. Slight tenderness may be present. The disease occurs most commonly in the exposure zone of the eye, often in the area of a pinguecula, and it may recur in the same or different locations. About one third of patients have bilateral disease at one time or another.

Episcleritis is diagnosed clinically by localizing the site of inflammation to the episclera. Unlike the deeper inflammation seen in scleritis (often with associated scleral edema clearly discernible on slit-lamp exam), episcleral inflammation is superficial. The characteristic color in episcleritis is bright red or salmon pink color in natural light, unlike the violaceous hue in most forms of scleritis. Additionally, the redness in episcleritis (unlike that associated with scleritis) will blanch with application of topical phenylephrine.

Episcleritis is classified as *simple* (diffuse injection) or *nodular.* In simple episcleritis, the inflammation is localized to a sector of the globe in 70% of cases, and the entire episclera in 30% of cases. A localized mobile nodule develops in nodular episcleritis (Fig 9-19). Small peripheral corneal opacities can be observed adjacent to the area of episcleral inflammation in 10% of patients. Episcleritis generally resolves without producing any lasting destructive effects on tissues of the eye.

MANAGEMENT A workup for underlying causes (eg, autoimmune connective tissue disease such as Sjögren syndrome, rheumatoid arthritis, or other conditions such as gout, herpes zoster, syphilis, tuberculosis, rosacea) is rarely indicated except after multiple recurrences. Episcleritis generally clears without treatment, but topical or oral nonsteroidal anti-inflammatory agents may be prescribed for patients bothered by pain. Most patients simply need reassurance that their condition is not sight-threatening and can be treated with lubricants alone. The use of topical corticosteroids should be kept to a minimum in this benign, self-limited condition. However, in unusual cases of severe disease that does not respond to standard therapy with lubricants and NSAIDs, a short course of corticosteroids may be necessary.

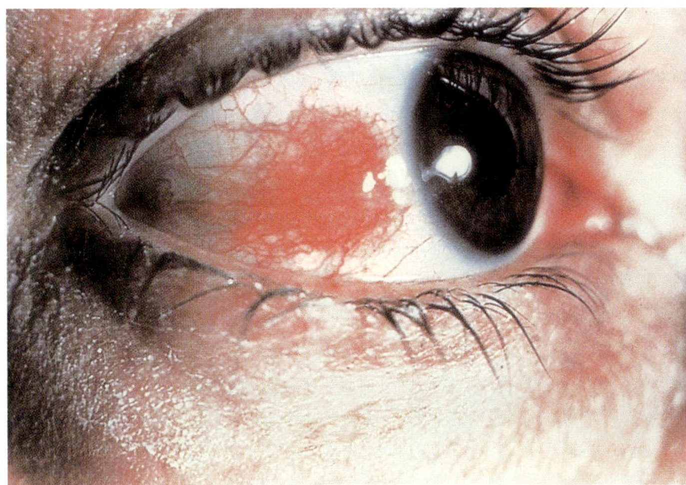

Figure 9-19 Nodular episcleritis.

Scleritis

PATHOGENESIS Scleritis is a much more severe ocular inflammatory condition than episcleritis. It is caused by an immune-mediated (typically immune-complex) vasculitis that frequently leads to destruction of the sclera. Scleritis is frequently associated with an underlying systemic immunologic disease; about one third of patients with diffuse or nodular scleritis and two thirds with necrotizing scleritis have a detectable connective tissue or autoimmune disease. Scleritis causes significant pain and may lead to structural alterations of the globe with attendant visual morbidity. It is exceedingly rare in children, occurs most often in the fourth to sixth decades of life, and is more common in women. About one half of scleritis cases are bilateral at some time in their course.

CLINICAL PRESENTATION The onset of scleritis is usually gradual, extending over several days. Most patients with scleritis develop severe boring or piercing ocular pain, which may worsen at night and occasionally awaken them from sleep. The pain may be referred to other regions of the head or face on the involved side, and the globe is often tender to touch. The inflamed sclera has a violaceous hue best seen in natural sunlight. Inflamed scleral vessels have a crisscross pattern, adhere to the sclera, and cannot be moved with a cotton-tipped applicator. Scleral edema, often with overlying episcleral edema, is noted by slit-lamp examination. Scleritis can be classified clinically based on the anatomical location (anterior versus posterior scleritis) and appearance of scleral inflammation (Table 9-3).

Diffuse versus nodular anterior scleritis

Diffuse anterior scleritis is characterized by a zone of scleral edema and redness. A portion of the anterior sclera (<50%) is involved in 60% of cases, and the entire anterior segment is involved in 40% of cases (Fig 9-20). In *nodular anterior scleritis,* the scleral nodule is a deep red-purple color, immobile, and separated from the overlying episcleral tissue, which is elevated by the nodule (Fig 9-21).

Table 9-3 Subtypes and Prevalence of Scleritis

Location	Subtype	Prevalence
Anterior sclera	Diffuse scleritis	40%
	Nodular scleritis	44%
	Necrotizing scleritis	14%
	with inflammation	(10%)
	without inflammation *(scleromalacia perforans)*	(4%)
Posterior sclera		2%

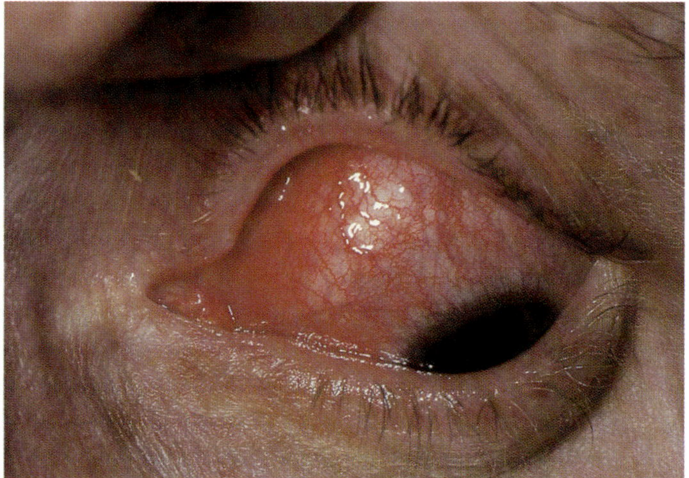

Figure 9-20 Diffuse anterior scleritis.

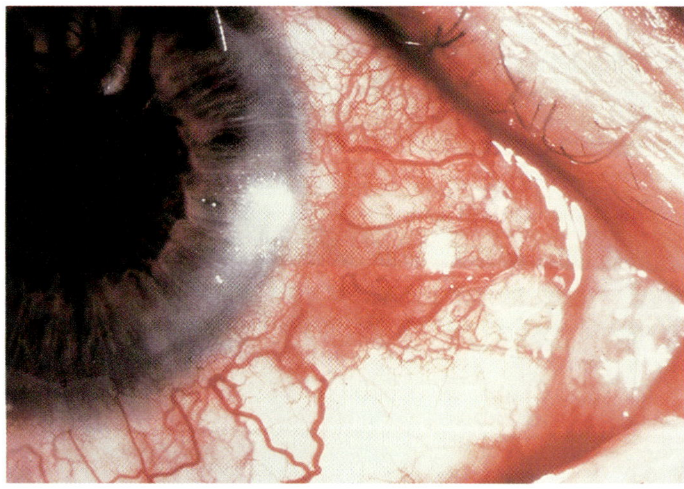

Figure 9-21 Nodular scleritis.

Necrotizing scleritis

Necrotizing scleritis is the most destructive form of scleritis. Of the patients affected 60% develop ocular and systemic complications; 40% suffer loss of vision; and a significant minority may die prematurely as a result of complications of vasculitis. Patients with *necrotizing scleritis with inflammation* typically present with severe pain. Most commonly, a localized patch of inflammation is noted initially, with the edges of the lesion more inflamed than the center. In more advanced disease (25% of cases), an avascular edematous patch of sclera is seen (Fig 9-22). Untreated, necrotizing scleritis may spread posteriorly to the equator and circumferentially until the entire anterior globe is involved. Severe loss of tissue may result if treatment is not intensive and prompt. The sclera may develop a blue-gray appearance (due to thinning, which allows the underlying choroid to show) and reveal an altered deep episcleral blood vessel pattern (large anastomotic blood vessels that may circumscribe the involved area) after the inflammation subsides.

Necrotizing scleritis without inflammation (scleromalacia perforans)

This form of scleritis, though undoubtedly due to inflammation, is said to be "without inflammation" because its clinical presentation is distinct from the other forms of anterior scleritis in which typical signs (redness, edema) and symptoms (pain) of inflammation are readily apparent.

Scleromalacia perforans typically occurs in patients with long-standing rheumatoid arthritis. Signs of inflammation are minimal, and this type of scleritis is generally painless. As the disease progresses, the sclera thins and the underlying dark uveal tissue becomes visible (Fig 9-23). In many cases the uvea is covered with only thin connective tissue and conjunctiva. Large abnormal blood vessels surround and cross the areas of scleral loss. A bulging staphyloma develops if the intraocular pressure is elevated; spontaneous perforation is rare, although these eyes may rupture with minimal trauma.

Posterior scleritis

Posterior scleritis can occur in isolation or concomitant with anterior scleritis. Some investigators include posterior scleritis as an anterior variant of inflammatory pseudotumor. Patients present with pain, tenderness, proptosis, visual loss, and, occasionally, restricted motility. Choroidal folds, exudative retinal detachment, papilledema, and angle-closure glaucoma secondary to choroidal thickening may develop. Retraction of the lower eyelid may occur in upgaze, presumably caused by infiltration of muscles in the region of the posterior scleritis. The pain may be referred to other parts of the head, and the diagnosis can be missed in the absence of associated anterior scleritis. Demonstration of thickened posterior sclera by echography, CT scan, or MRI may be helpful in establishing the diagnosis. Often, no related systemic disease can be found in patients with posterior scleritis.

Complications of scleritis

Complications are frequent and include peripheral keratitis (37%), uveitis (30%), cataract (7%), glaucoma (18%), and scleral thinning (33%). Anterior uveitis may occur as a spillover phenomenon in eyes with anterior scleritis. Some degree of posterior uveitis occurs in all patients with posterior scleritis and may also occur in anterior scleritis when

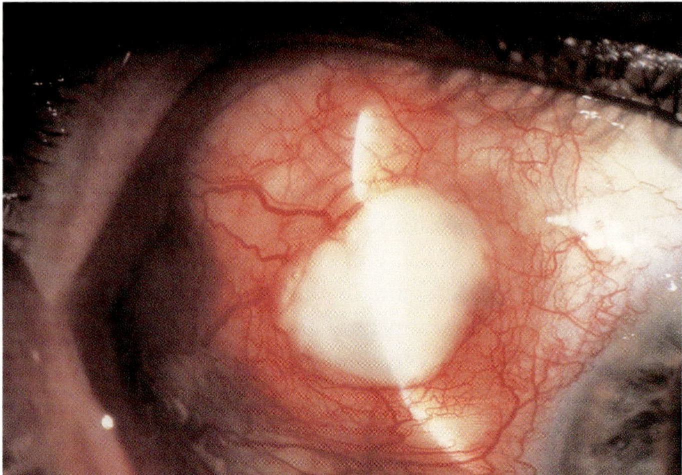

Figure 9-22 Necrotizing scleritis.

the overlying sclera is inflamed. Although one third of patients with scleritis have evidence of scleral translucency and/or thinning, frank scleral defects are seen only in the most severe forms of necrotizing disease and in the late stages of scleromalacia perforans.

A wide variety of corneal findings may coincide with scleritis. Rarely, corneas may develop central stromal keratitis in conjunction with scleritis, associated with heavy vascularization and opacification in the absence of treatment. In nodular or sectoral scleritis, the corneal changes are usually localized to the area of inflammation.

In *sclerokeratitis*, the peripheral cornea becomes opacified by fibrosis and lipid deposition in conjunction with neighboring scleritis (which may be severe or very mild) (Fig 9-24). The area of involvement may gradually move centrally, resulting in opacification of a large segment of cornea. This type of keratitis commonly accompanies herpes zoster scleritis but may also occur in rheumatic diseases.

LABORATORY EVALUATION Scleritis can occur in association with various systemic infectious diseases, including syphilis, tuberculosis, herpes zoster, Lyme disease, cat-scratch disease, and Hansen disease. It is most frequently seen in association with autoimmune connective tissue diseases such as rheumatoid arthritis, systemic lupus erythematosus, and seronegative spondyloarthropathies (eg, ankylosing spondylitis) or secondary to vasculitides such as Wegener granulomatosis, polyarteritis nodosa, or giant cell arteritis. Metabolic diseases such as gout may also rarely be associated with scleritis. More than one half of patients with scleritis have an associated identifiable systemic disease. The differential diagnosis of scleritis is similar to that of PUK (see Table 9-2).

Because patients with certain forms of scleritis, especially necrotizing scleritis, have an increased rate of extraocular morbidity, its presence should be recognized as a manifestation of a potentially serious systemic disease. The workup of scleritis should therefore include a complete physical examination, with attention to the joints, skin, and cardiovascular and respiratory systems. Usually, this is best done in conjunction with a rheumatologist or other internist with experience in the diagnosis and management of

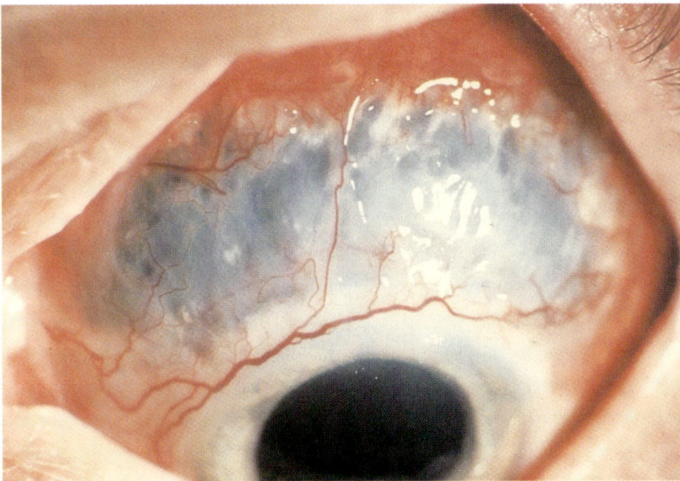

Figure 9-23 Scleromalacia perforans in a patient with long-standing rheumatoid arthritis. *(Photograph courtesy of Vincent P. deLuise, MD.)*

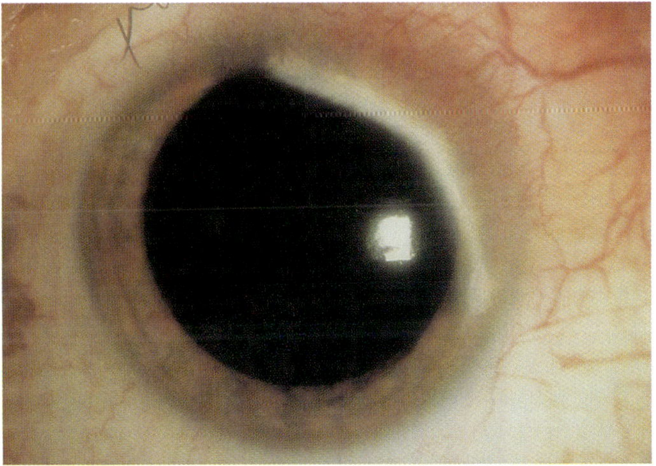

Figure 9-24 Sclerokeratitis.

these conditions. There is no single approach used in the diagnosis of these patients' possible underlying illness, and laboratory studies should always be guided by the history and physical exam. However, the following laboratory tests are generally recommended as an initial screening. Other tests may then be ordered based on a more thorough rheumatological (or infectious disease) examination:

- Complete blood count (CBC) with differential
- Erythrocyte sedimentation rate (ESR) or C-reactive protein (CRP)
- Serum autoantibody screen (antinuclear antibodies [ANA], anti-DNA antibodies, rheumatoid factor [RF], antineutrophil cytoplasmic antibodies [ANCA])

- Urinalysis
- Serum uric acid
- Syphilis serology
- Chest x-ray
- Sarcoidosis screen (serum angiotensin-converting enzyme [ACE] and lysozyme) as appropriate

Additional laboratory tests may be indicated based on the clinical findings.

MANAGEMENT Topical corticosteroids may occasionally reduce ocular inflammation in mild cases of diffuse anterior and nodular scleritis, but in general the treatment of scleritis is systemic. For nonnecrotizing disease, especially diffuse disease, oral NSAIDs may be effective. Severe nodular disease and necrotizing disease almost always require more potent anti-inflammatory therapy. Treatment is usually commenced with oral corticosteroids. Although subconjunctival steroids may be effective in reducing scleral inflammation, they have been reported to cause scleral necrosis and exacerbate epithelial defects; therefore, use of depot steroid injections in these cases is generally contraindicated.

It is important to clearly define treatment goals: treatment failure may be considered as progression of disease to a more severe form (eg, nodular to necrotizing) or failure to achieve response to treatment after 2–3 weeks of therapy, in which case an alternate therapeutic strategy will need to be instituted.

Oral and/or high-dose (pulsed) IV steroids may be effective for some cases of necrotizing scleritis or sclerokeratitis. If no therapeutic response is observed with corticosteroids, however, systemic immunosuppressive therapy with an antimetabolite (methotrexate), an immunomodulator (eg, cyclosporine), or a cytotoxic agent (eg, cyclophosphamide) is recommended. Although there is no consensus, most clinicians place rheumatoid arthritis patients on methotrexate, and reserve more potent cytotoxic therapy for patients with active vasculitic disease such as Wegener granulomatosis. Patients receiving systemic immunosuppressive therapy for scleritis should be monitored closely for systemic complications associated with these drugs. Antituberculosis and anti-*Pneumocystis* coverage may be necessary for at-risk patients. Both the treatment and long-term management of these patients are best done as a collaborative effort between the ophthalmologist and rheumatologist.

Dana MR, Reddy CV, Foster CS. Adult rheumatoid arthritis. In: Albert DM, Jakobiec FA, eds. *Principles and Practice of Ophthalmology.* Vol 5. 2nd ed. Philadelphia: Saunders; 2000:4555–4563.

Dubord PJ, Chalmers A. Scleritis and episcleritis: diagnosis and management. In: *Focal Points: Clinical Modules for Ophthalmologists.* San Francisco: American Academy of Ophthalmology; 1995:vol 13, no 9.

PART V

Neoplastic Disorders of the Eyelids, Conjunctiva, and Cornea

Tumor Cell Biology and Diagnostic Approaches to Ocular Surface Neoplasia

The Eyelid Skin and Ocular Surface

Microanatomy

The anatomy of the eyelids and the ocular surface and the pathologic processes that affect these tissues are reviewed in BCSC Section 2, *Fundamentals and Principles of Ophthalmology*, and Section 4, *Ophthalmic Pathology and Intraocular Tumors*.

The skin of the upper eyelid is the thinnest of the body, and it thins further with aging. Keratinocytes arranged into the basal, prickle, squamous, granular, and keratin layers form the epidermis of the eyelid skin. Basal keratinocytes contain a variable amount of melanin pigment. *Dendritic melanocytes* and *Langerhans cells* are scattered throughout the epidermis. *Nevus cells*, modified melanocytes found in clumps in the epidermis and dermis, have varying degrees of pigmentation, depending on their expression of tyrosinase and melanogenic activity. Basal epidermal cells produce a basement membrane to which they attach by hemidesmosomes. Downward projections of the epidermis into the dermis are called *rete ridges*, and the corresponding upward projections of the dermis are termed *dermal ridges*, or *dermal papillae*(Fig 10-1). The dermis of the eyelid skin lacks well-defined papillae and consists of a thin layer of fibrovascular tissue containing hair follicles, sebaceous glands, and sweat glands but no fat. The dermis is firmly attached to the underlying orbicularis oculi muscle only at the eyelid creases, canthi, and lid margins.

The epithelium of the conjunctiva and cornea includes basal cells, wing cells, and superficial cells but lacks granular and keratin layers. Goblet cells, melanocytes, and Langerhans cells are present in the conjunctival epithelium. Pigmented and nonpigmented nevus cells reside in nests of the conjunctival epithelium and substantia propria. Langerhans cells and occasional melanocytes are present in the peripheral cornea. Basal epithelial cells produce a basement membrane to which they attach by hemidesmosomes. The substantia propria of the conjunctiva and the stroma of the cornea consist of fibrous tissue.

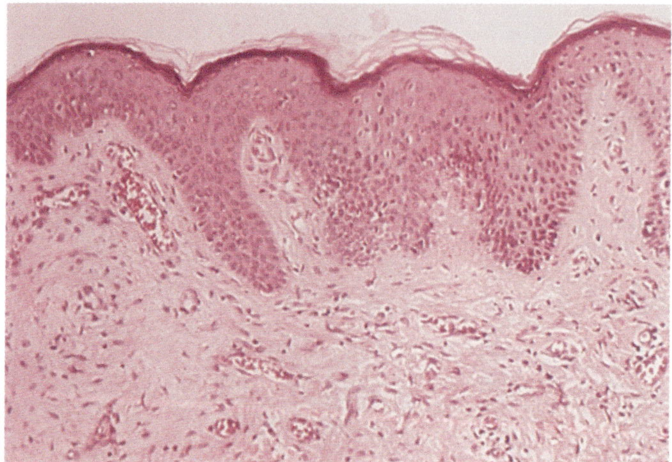

Figure 10-1 Normal eyelid skin, with typical downward projections of epidermis and upward projections of dermis. (Hematoxylin-eosin, ×100.)

Stem Cells and Cell Turnover

Stem cells for skin and mucous membranes reside in basal epithelial layers, in locations relatively sheltered from environmental insults. Epidermal stem cells reside in rete ridges; conjunctival epithelial stem cells in the basal conjunctival epithelium, with concentrations in the fornix and just posterior to the lid margin; and corneal epithelial stem cells at the corneal limbus. The eyelid epidermis is replaced every 2 weeks, and conjunctival and corneal epithelial cells are replaced weekly.

Histopathologic Processes and Conditions

A *tumor* is a tissue mass that may be caused by inflammation, fibrovascular proliferation, cystic enlargement, or malignant transformation. The most common growths of the external eye, such as pterygia and chalazia, are reactive rather than malignant. True malignancies of the eyelids and ocular surface are disturbances of squamous epidermis or epithelium, melanocytes, or altered mesenchymal cells. Neoplastic tumors are associated with specific cellular and tissue changes (Table 10-1).

Neoplasia is the unregulated proliferation of cells. The pattern of growth may be described clinically or histologically. For example, the term *papilloma,* used clinically, refers to any epidermal or epithelial growth that extends outward in a multilobulated pattern and contains a central vascular core in each lobule. A neoplasm may be benign or malignant. Histopathologic criteria that differentiate benign from malignant neoplasms are based on cellular and nuclear morphology and on tissue organization (Table 10-2).

Dysplasia indicates a trend toward malignancy; it is characterized by acanthosis, cellular atypia, and abnormal polarity. *Anaplasia* is severe dysplasia that indicates malignancy. Lesions classified as *precancerous*—for example, intraepithelial neoplasms—are

Table 10-1 Cellular and Tissue Reactions

Histopathologic Term	Definition
Hypertrophy	Increase in size of cells or tissue without increase in number of cells
Hyperplasia	Increase in number of cells in excess of normal but not progressive
Metaplasia	Transformation of one type of tissue into another
Atrophy	Decrease in size of cells or tissue
Necrosis	Secondary death of cells or tissue
Apoptosis	Normal or abnormal programmed death of cells
Dysplasia	Abnormal growth of cells
Neoplasia	Unregulated increase in number of cells

those in which malignant transformation has taken place at a cellular level, but no invasion of the basement membrane or metastasis has occurred.

Carcinoma indicates invasion of dysplastic cells beneath the basement membrane and/or metastatic spread. Malignant neoplasms invade and destroy surrounding tissue and may metastasize to form secondary centers of neoplastic growth.

Overview of Oncogenesis

Cancer results from mutations in cellular genes that regulate proliferation; by definition, it originates in long-lived cells such as stem cells. Dysregulation of cell replication is a necessary component of neoplasia. Oncogenesis is a multistep process. Table 10-3 gives examples of risk factors that can lead to cancer. Tumors may be initiated by inherited genetic mutations and/or exposure to environmental mutagens or carcinogens that irreversibly damage cellular DNA. In one model of oncogenesis, an inherited mutated allele in the germ line is followed by loss of a second allele in a somatic cell. Subsequent carcinogenesis may result from activation of a cellular oncogene or, more commonly, from loss of oncogene suppression. Genes involved in the development of cancer include those that regulate progression through the cell cycle, direct differentiation pathways, resist programmed cell death (apoptosis), or normally prevent replication errors. Abnormal levels of growth factors may result in uncontrolled proliferation with malignant transformation and angiogenesis. Local invasion and metastasis involve additional genetic changes, with unbalanced regulation of extracellular matrix (eg, basement membrane) degradation, adhesion, and motility. In carcinogenesis, irreversible DNA changes in a subpopulation of cells may be partially attenuated by apoptosis of genetically damaged cells. However, frank annulment of apoptotic mechanisms by gene mutations or an ascendancy of cellular proliferation over apoptosis favors neoplastic growth.

Tumor Immunology

The emerging field of tumor immunology holds tremendous but as yet unrealized potential for the treatment of human cancers. Although tumors are antigenic, lymphocytes and immune effector molecules can have positive as well as negative effects on tumor growth. For example, immune system cells can induce tumor growth and angiogenesis.

Table 10-2 Histopathologic Features of Neoplasia

Histopathologic Term	Definition	Implication
Acanthosis	Thickening of the squamous layer as a result of increased mitosis of basal cell layer	Active cell proliferation, whether benign, preinvasive, or malignant
Hyperkeratosis	Increased thickness of the keratin layer of the epidermis (also called *epidermalization* when occurring on mucosal epithelium)	Active cell proliferation, whether benign, preinvasive, or malignant (called *leukoplakia* when a visible white plaque is seen on the conjunctiva)
Parakeratosis	Hyperkeratosis in which nuclei persist in the superficial cells	Active cell proliferation, whether benign, preinvasive, or malignant
Dyskeratosis	Keratinization of individual cells that lie within the epidermis or epithelium, rather than at the surface	Active cell proliferation, whether benign, preinvasive, or malignant
Cellular atypia	Increased nucleus-to-cytoplasm ratio (hyperchromasia); nuclei may be increased in size or number, be abnormally shaped, or have abnormal mitotic figures	Isolated atypical cells may indicate premalignant lesions; abundant atypical cells occur in malignancy
Abnormal polarity	Loss of normal transition from basal cells to superficial cells, and all epidermal or epithelial cells look alike	Mild loss of normal cell maturation may indicate premalignant lesions; disorganized architecture occurs in malignancy

Table 10-3 Examples of Initiating Causes of Neoplasms of the Eyelid and Ocular Surface

Risk Factor	Benign	Preinvasive/Invasive
Physical/chemical exposure (eg, sunlight)	Squamous cell papilloma Nevus	Actinic keratosis Basal cell carcinoma Lentigo maligna melanoma
Virus	Molluscum contagiosum Verruca Conjunctival papilloma	Kaposi sarcoma Conjunctival/corneal intraepithelial neoplasia (CIN) Squamous cell carcinoma
Heredity	Neurofibromatosis Muir-Torre syndrome Gardner syndrome Multiple endocrine neoplasia (MEN) syndromes Lipoid proteinosis Benign hereditary intraepithelial dyskeratosis	Basal cell nevus syndrome Xeroderma pigmentosum

Conversely, the rare spontaneous regression of a tumor in a healthy individual may occur due to immune recognition and tumor cell death; in addition, immunosuppressed patients carry an increased risk of cancer, including lymphomas, sarcomas, and epithelial carcinomas. These latter observations affirm the potential of the immune system to have an antitumor effect. Cell-mediated tumor immunity provides

- Lymphocytes that attack tumor cells
- Activated macrophages that secrete proteolytic enzymes, free radicals, and other factors to cause tumor necrosis
- Neutrophils

In some cases, cancer cells avoid immune-mediated destruction by expressing surface ligands that induce apoptosis of incoming T cells.

Many tumors are antigenic but not immunogenic. Antigens expressed by tumor cells include those normally expressed on the cell of origin as well as those that are tumor specific. Dedifferentiated cells may express antigens associated with an earlier developmental stage of the parent cell line. Examples are carcinoembryonic antigen and α-fetoprotein. Tumor-specific antigens may be particular to a given neoplastic cell type or may cross-react with other neoplasms of the same histogenesis. The presence of such antigens gives hope that immunotherapy utilizing antigen-specific cytotoxic T cells may reduce tumor burden or eliminate tumors completely.

Ksander BR, Murray TG. Immunology of ocular tumors. In: Pepose JS, Holland GN, Wilhelmus KR, eds. *Ocular Infection and Immunity*. St Louis· Mosby; 1996:157–182.

Sogn JA. Tumor immunology: the glass is half full. *Immunity*. 1998;9:757–763.

Diagnostic Approaches

Noninvasive Investigation

The clinician should investigate whether the lesion is congenital or acquired, the time of onset and growth pattern, and if an acquired tumor might have arisen from sun exposure, a previous injury, a preexisting lesion, or systemic disease. Many neoplastic lesions of the eyelid or ocular surface have typical clinical features, and an accurate diagnosis can often be made with a history and careful clinical inspection prior to biopsy and histopathologic confirmation. External inspection, palpation, and slit-lamp biomicroscopy should be used to distinguish epithelial and subepithelial lesions and cystic and solid tumors and to determine the presence of inflammation. Malignancy should be suspected in cases of rapid growth, changing color, chronic inflammation, ulceration, or bleeding. Regional lymph nodes should be checked. Periodic observation and sequential photographs are used to follow presumed benign lesions such as nevi.

Biopsy Decisions and Techniques

History and physical examination are not substitutes for detailed histopathologic examinations of suspicious lesions. Biopsy is considered for any possibly malignant lesion (Fig 10-2). An *excisional biopsy* removes the entire lesion with adjacent normal margins.

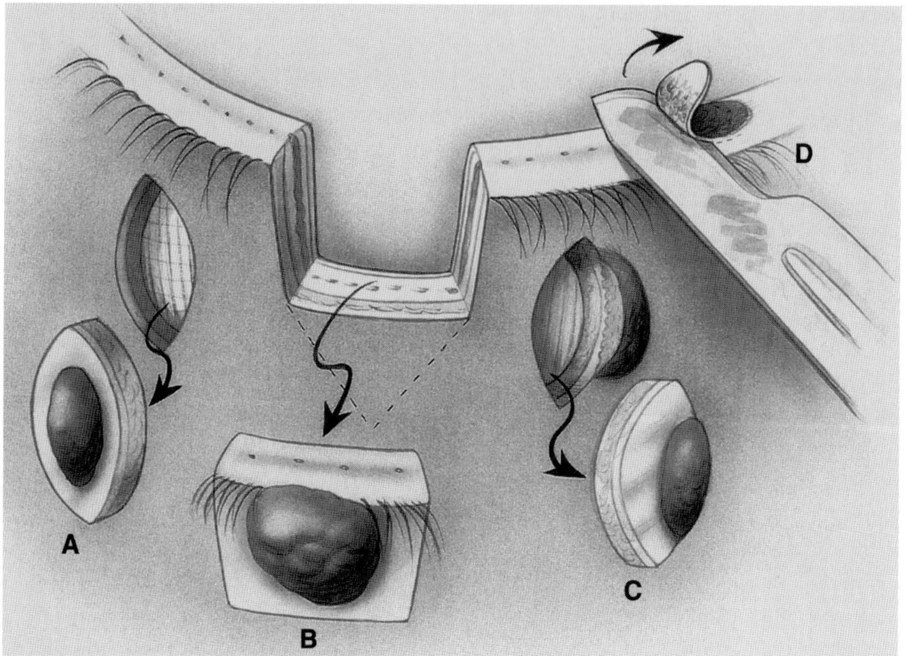

Figure 10-2 Techniques of eyelid biopsy. **A,** Excisional biopsy. **B,** Full-thickness eyelid biopsy. **C,** Incisional or punch biopsy, including normal skin. **D,** Shave biopsy of eyelid margin lesion. *(Illustration by Christine Gralapp.)*

An *incisional biopsy* removes a representative portion of the lesion. A *shave biopsy* is a type of excisional biopsy for removing a superficial lesion of the epidermis or outer dermis. Microscopic control using frozen sections or Mohs' resection technique can ensure completeness of an excisional biopsy (see BCSC Section 4, *Ophthalmic Pathology and Intraocular Tumors*).

Primary excisional biopsy is undertaken for small lesions that are symptomatic or suspected to be malignant. If a biopsy is planned, an excisional biopsy is often preferred to completely remove the lesion. An incisional biopsy is reserved for large lesions where extensive reconstructive surgery would be required if excisional biopsy were performed primarily. The choice of whether to primarily close or to use a skin or mucous membrane graft depends on the extent of the surgery.

The excision should be deep enough to contain the lesion and a small amount of adjacent unaffected tissue. Lesions of the eyelid skin are usually excised, when possible, by a small ellipse aligned along the orbicularis fibers. A lesion of the eyelid margin is often removed with a wedge resection. Frozen sections determine completeness of excision. A limbal lesion can be removed with a lamellar conjunctivosclerectomy (Fig 10-3). Gentle handling to avoid crush injury and distortion of the histopathologic findings is essential. Marking the tissue and making a diagram when cutting appropriate cross sections help to orient the pathologist.

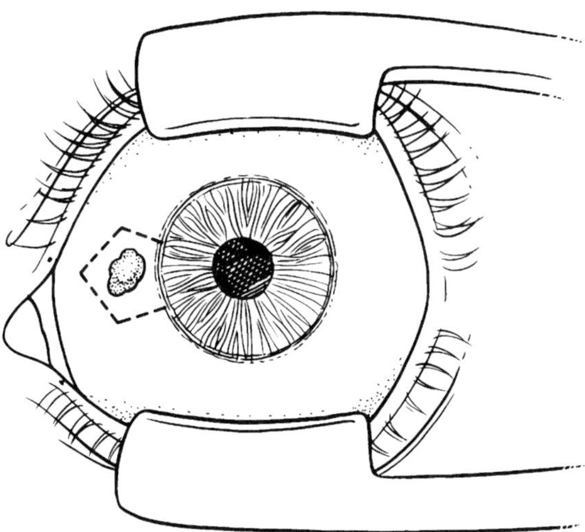

Figure 10-3 Excisional biopsy of conjunctival lesion. *(Illustration by Christine Gralapp.)*

Approximately 80% of cutaneous eyelid lesions are benign. The diagnosis by an experienced ophthalmologist of malignancy or premalignancy is approximately 90% predictive of subsequent histopathologic evaluation. If the initial histopathologic findings do not agree with a clinical impression of malignancy, repeat biopsy should be considered.

Management

Therapeutic approaches include surgery, cryotherapy, radiotherapy, and chemotherapy. Drugs that inhibit replication of oncogenic viruses, kill proliferating cells, block angiogenesis, or clot blood vessels feeding a tumor are under development. Consultation with a tumor board, a multidisciplinary group of physicians that meets to review cancer cases, can aid in the decision-making process of cancer care. See also BCSC Section 7, *Orbit, Eyelids, and Lacrimal System*.

Shields JA, Shields CL, De Potter P. Surgical management of conjunctival tumors. The 1994 Lynn B. McMahan Lecture. *Arch Ophthalmol.* 1997;115:808–815.

Clinical Approach to Neoplastic Disorders of the Conjunctiva and Cornea

Approximately 1 person in 2500 seeks ophthalmic care for a tumor of the eyelid or ocular surface each year, totaling about 100,000 per year in the United States. Benign neoplasms are at least three times more frequent than malignant lesions. Most of these tumors arise from the eyelid skin and are discussed in BCSC Section 4, *Ophthalmic Pathology and Intraocular Tumors*, and Section 7, *Orbit, Eyelids, and Lacrimal System*.

Neoplastic tumors of the conjunctiva and cornea are considered together because the lesions often affect both tissues in a similar fashion. These lesions are classified by the type of cell, such as epithelium, melanocytes and nevus cells, vascular endothelium and mesenchymal cells, and lymphocytes. Many are analogous to lesions affecting the eyelid (Table 11-1). Several infectious and inflammatory lesions of the conjunctiva, limbus, and cornea are associated with exophytic growth. Lesions discussed elsewhere in this

Table 11-1 Comparison Between Some Cutaneous and Mucosal Manifestations of Neoplastic and Pigmentary Conditions

Eyelid	Conjunctiva
Surface lesions	
Epidermal inclusion cyst	Epithelial inclusion cyst
Squamous cell papilloma	Squamous cell papilloma
Actinic keratosis	Mild conjunctival intraepithelial neoplasia
Intraepidermal squamous cell carcinoma	Severe conjunctival intraepithelial neoplasia
Squamous cell carcinoma	Squamous cell carcinoma
Pigmentary lesions	
Freckle	Freckle
Dermal melanocytosis	Ocular melanocytosis
Nevus	Nevus
Junctional	Junctional
Compound	Compound
Intradermal	Subepithelial
Lentigo maligna	Primary acquired melanosis
Melanoma	Melanoma

volume are hordeolum; various granulomatous reactions such as chalazion, sarcoidosis, cat-scratch disease, and lymphogranuloma venereum; and corneal keloid (consult the index). See also BCSC Section 4, *Ophthalmic Pathology and Intraocular Tumors.*

Shields JA, Shields CL. *Atlas of Eyelid and Conjunctival Tumors.* Philadelphia: Lippincott Williams & Wilkins; 1999.

Cysts of the Epithelium

Epithelial Inclusion Cyst

Inclusion cysts of the conjunctival epithelium are commonly found (Fig 11-1). One or more small cysts are often seen in the lower fornix of healthy people.

PATHOGENESIS Like epidermal cysts of the eyelids, cysts of conjunctival epithelium can be congenital or can develop during life. Small cysts are likely formed by apposition of conjunctival folds. Large, single cysts are usually a result of epithelium implanted into the substantia propria by trauma, surgery, or inflammation.

CLINICAL FINDINGS Conjunctival inclusion cysts appear clear and are lined by normal conjunctival epithelium. A corneal epithelial inclusion cyst is rare, but it can occur if trauma or surgery displaces ocular surface epithelium into the stroma. Lymphangiectasia may mimic an inclusion cyst of the bulbar conjunctiva.

MANAGEMENT Epithelial inclusion cysts will re-form after simple incision because the inner epithelial cell wall remains. Marsupialization or complete excision is necessary to prevent recurrence.

Tumors of Epithelial Origin

Table 11-2 lists the epithelial tumors of the conjunctiva and cornea.

Margo CE. Nonpigmented lesions of the ocular surface. In: *Focal Points: Clinical Modules for Ophthalmologists.* San Francisco: American Academy of Ophthalmology; 1996; vol 14, no 9.

Warner MA, Jakobiec FA. Squamous neoplasms of the conjunctiva. In: Krachmer JH, Mannis MJ, Holland EJ, eds. *Cornea.* Vol 2. St Louis: Mosby; 1997:701–714.

Benign Epithelial Tumors

Conjunctival papilloma

The two forms of conjunctival papilloma—sessile and pedunculated—have etiologic, histologic, and clinical differences. Papillomatous growth of conjunctival intraepithelial neoplasia is discussed below.

PATHOGENESIS Human papillomavirus (HPV), subtype 6 or 11, initiates a neoplastic growth of epithelial cells with vascular proliferation that gives rise to a verruca vulgaris (wart) of the eyelid skin or a pedunculated papilloma of the conjunctiva (Fig 11-2). In contrast, a sessile conjunctival lesion is more likely to represent a dysplastic or carcinom-

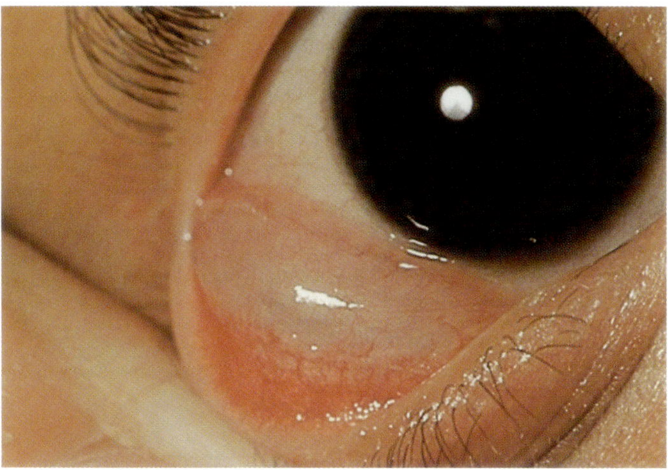

Figure 11-1 Conjunctival epithelial inclusion cyst.

Table 11-2 Neoplastic Tumors of Ocular Surface Epithelium

Benign	Preinvasive	Malignant
Papilloma	Conjunctival and corneal intraepithelial neoplasia	Squamous cell carcinoma
Pseudoepitheliomatous hyperplasia		Mucoepidermoid carcinoma
Benign hereditary intraepithelial dyskeratosis		

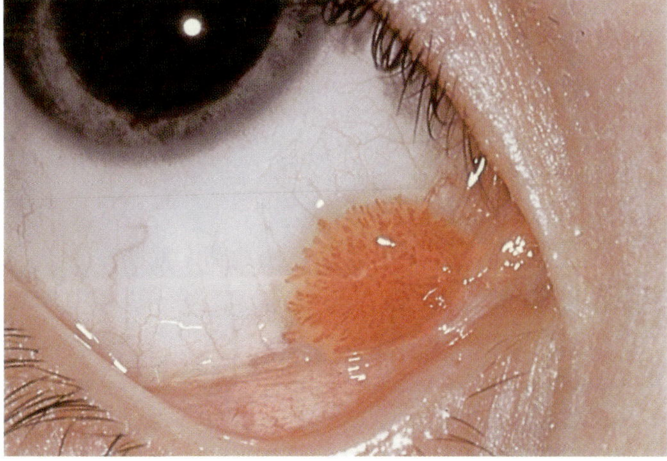

Figure 11-2 Conjunctival squamous papilloma.

atous lesion and is usually caused by HPV-16 or HPV-18 (see Chapter 10 of this volume). These latter oncogenic virus strains, along with HPV-31, are also strongly associated with the pathogenesis of human cervical carcinoma.

CLINICAL FINDINGS A pedunculated conjunctival papilloma is a fleshy, exophytic growth with a fibrovascular core. It often arises in the inferior fornix but can also present on the tarsal or bulbar conjunctiva or along the semilunar fold. The lesion emanates from a stalk and has a multilobulated appearance with smooth, clear epithelium and numerous underlying, small corkscrew blood vessels. Multiple lesions sometimes occur, and the lesion may be extensive in patients with HIV infection.

A sessile papilloma is more typically found at the limbus and has a flat base. The glistening surface and numerous red dots resemble a strawberry. Spread onto the cornea can occur. Signs of dysplasia include keratinization (leukoplakia), inflammation, and invasion. A very rare variant is an inverted papilloma.

MANAGEMENT Many conjunctival papillomas regress spontaneously. A pedunculated papilloma that is small, cosmetically acceptable, and nonirritating may be observed, although spontaneous resolution can take months to years. An incomplete excision, however, can stimulate growth and lead to a worse cosmetic outcome. Cryotherapy, excision with cryotherapy to the base, or excision with adjunctive application of mitomycin-C or α-interferon is sometimes curative, but recurrences are frequent. Surgical manipulation should be minimized to reduce the risk of virus dissemination to uninvolved healthy conjunctiva.

A sessile limbal papilloma must be observed closely or excised. If the lesion enlarges or shows clinical features suggesting dysplastic or carcinomatous growth, then excisional biopsy with adjunctive cryotherapy is indicated.

Pseudoepitheliomatous hyperplasia

Somewhat common on the eyelid, pseudoepitheliomatous hyperplasia and keratoacanthoma occur rarely on the conjunctiva. Pseudoepitheliomatous hyperplasia can be found histologically in the conjunctival epithelium overlying a pterygium or pinguecula.

Preinvasive Epithelial Lesions

Conjunctival intraepithelial neoplasia

Conjunctival intraepithelial neoplasia (CIN) is analogous to actinic keratosis of the eyelid skin. In CIN, the neoplastic process does not invade the underlying basement membrane and is referred to as mild, moderate, or severe CIN, depending on the extent of involvement of the epithelium with atypical cells. Other terms include *squamous dysplasia,* if atypical cells involve only part of the epithelium, and *carcinoma in situ,* when cellular atypia extends throughout the epithelial layer (Fig 11-3).

PATHOGENESIS The relative contributions to this condition of human papillomavirus infection, sunlight exposure, and host factors have not been determined. The lesion most commonly develops on exposed areas of the bulbar conjunctiva, at or near the limbus, in light-complected, older male smokers who may have been exposed to petroleum products or to the sun over long periods of life. Rapid growth may occur when the lesion is present in a person with AIDS. Systemic immunosuppression appears to potentiate squamous neoplasia. In a young adult, CIN should instigate a serologic test for HIV infection.

Karp CL, Scott IU, Chang TS, et al. Conjunctival intraepithelial neoplasia. A possible marker for human immunodeficiency virus infection? *Arch Ophthalmol.* 1996;114:257–261.

CLINICAL FINDINGS Conjunctival intraepithelial neoplasia has three principal clinical variants (Fig 11-4):

- Papilliform, in which a sessile papilloma harbors dysplastic cells
- Gelatinous, as a result of acanthosis and dysplasia
- Leukoplakic, caused by hyperkeratosis, parakeratosis, and dyskeratosis

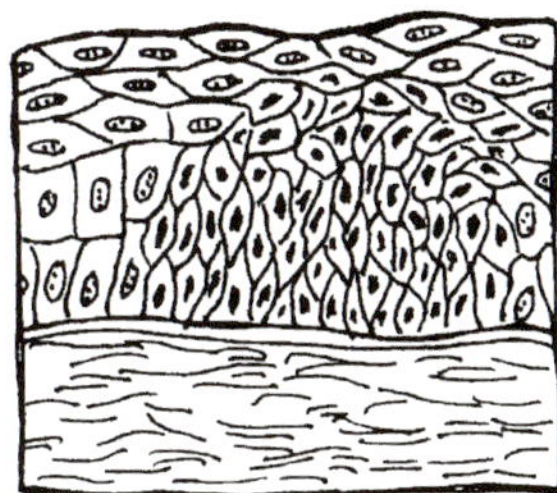
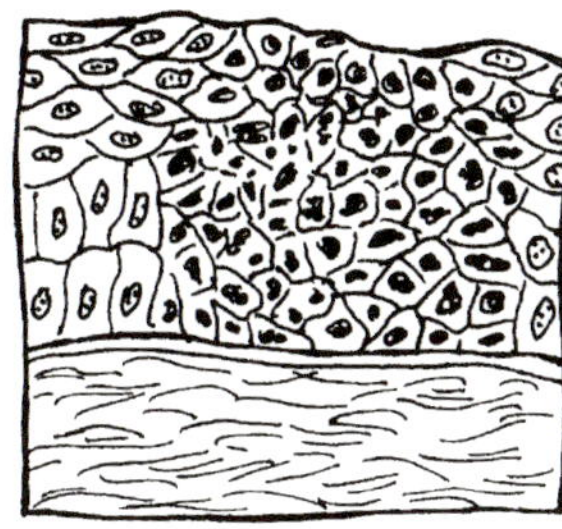
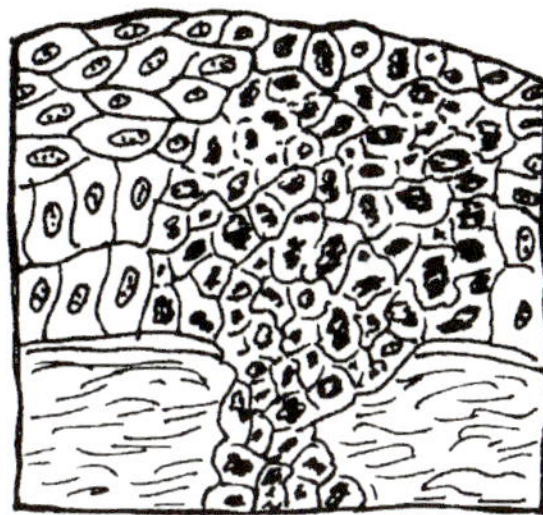

Mild conjunctival intraepithelial neoplasia (squamous dysplasia)

Severe conjunctival intraepithelial neoplasia (carcinoma in situ)

Squamous cell carcinoma

Figure 11-3 Conjunctival epithelial neoplasia.

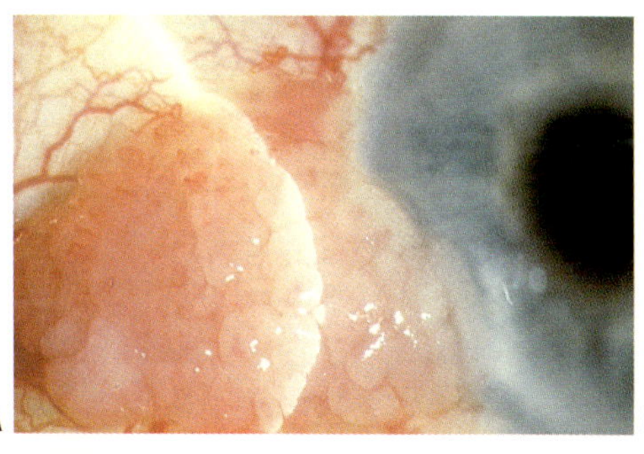
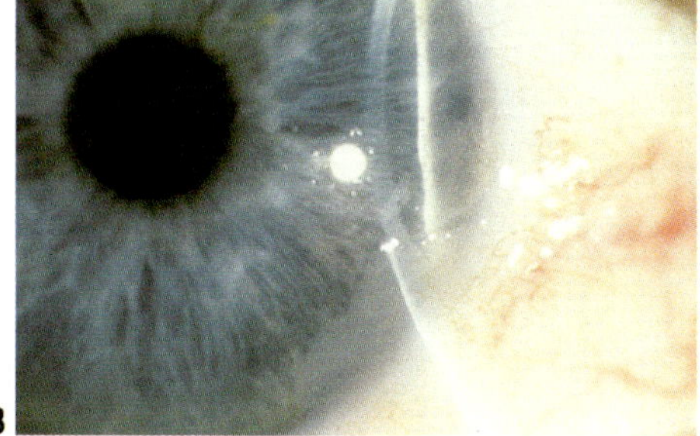
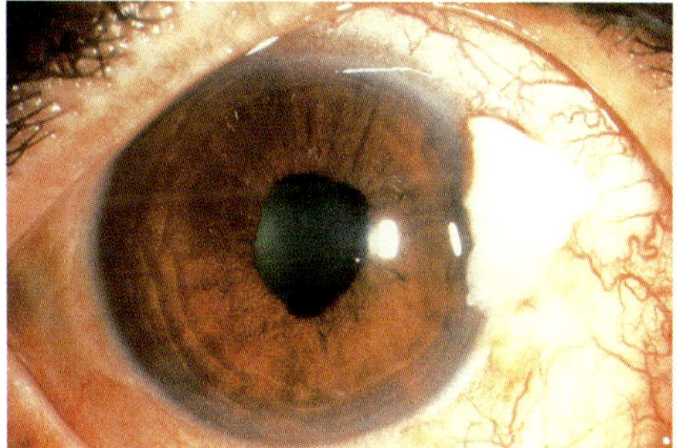

Figure 11-4 Conjunctival intraepithelial neoplasia: **A,** Papilliform. **B,** Gelatinous. **C,** Leukoplakic. *(Photographs courtesy of James Chodosh, MD.)*

Mild inflammation and various degrees of abnormal vascularization may accompany CIN lesions, but large feeder blood vessels indicate a higher probability of invasion beneath the epithelial basement membrane (squamous cell carcinoma; see Fig 11-3). CIN lesions are slow-growing tumors nearly always centered at the limbus but with the potential to spread to other areas of the ocular surface, including the cornea.

MANAGEMENT The surgical management of CIN is the same as for squamous cell carcinoma of the conjunctiva and cornea. By 10 years after surgical excision, CIN has recurred in approximately one third of eyes with negative surgical margins and one half of eyes with positive surgical margins. Lesions with dysplastic cells at the excision edge recur sooner than lesions that have been completely excised. Therefore, although excisional biopsy with adjunctive cryotherapy is still recommended, recent reports have focused on topical chemotherapeutic agents with the potential to treat the entire ocular surface without regard to surgical margins. Interferon, mitomycin-C, and 5-fluorouracil applied topically as eyedrops appear in some cases to completely eradicate CIN lesions. Ten years or more may ensue before clinical recurrence following surgery, and long-term studies of newer therapies have not been performed. Nevertheless, the ability of topical agents to treat microinvasive or frankly invasive disease is doubtful, and the role of topical antitumor agents for the treatment of CIN remains uncertain.

Maskin SL. Regression of limbal epithelial dysplasia with topical interferon. *Arch Ophthalmol.* 1994;112:1145–1146.

Tabin G, Levin S, Snibson G, et al. Late recurrences and the necessity for long-term follow-up in corneal and conjunctival intraepithelial neoplasia. *Ophthalmology.* 1997;104:485–492.

Vann RR, Karp CL. Perilesional and topical interferon alfa-2b for conjunctival and corneal neoplasia. *Ophthalmology.* 1999;106:91–97.

Wilson MW, Hungerford JL, George SM, et al. Topical mitomycin C for the treatment of conjunctival and corneal epithelial dysplasia and neoplasia. *Am J Ophthalmol.* 1997;124:303–311.

Corneal intraepithelial neoplasia

The cornea adjacent to intraepithelial neoplasia of the conjunctiva can also be affected. Sometimes, the conjunctival or limbal component is not clinically apparent, and only a sheet or individual islands of well-demarcated, geographic, epithelial granularity are seen.

PATHOGENESIS Corneal intraepithelial neoplasia is associated with the same risk factors as conjunctival intraepithelial neoplasia and presumably shares the same pathogenesis.

CLINICAL FINDINGS A granular, translucent, gray epithelial sheet broadly based at the limbus extends onto the cornea. Occasionally, free islands of punctate granular epithelium are present on the cornea. The edges of corneal lesions have characteristic fimbriated margins and pseudopodia-like extensions (Fig 11-5). Corneal neovascularization does not typically occur, which helps to differentiate CIN lesions from limbal stem-cell failure.

MANAGEMENT Corneal involvement may be treated by gently scraping away the opalescent epithelium from the underlying Bowman's layer or by observation. Bowman's layer should not be disturbed. Excision of the grossly normal but often histologically abnormal adjacent limbal tissue is important, even if the lesion appears to be primarily corneal.

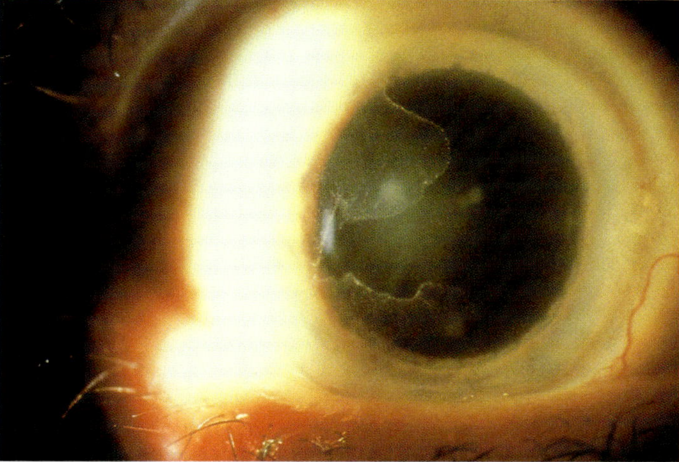

Figure 11-5 Corneal intraepithelial neoplasia. *(Photograph courtesy of James Chodosh, MD.)*

Cryotherapy of the remaining adjacent conjunctiva and absolute alcohol application to the adjacent corneal epithelium and sclera underlying the limbal source can destroy any abnormal cells and possibly reduce the likelihood of recurrence.

Malignant Epithelial Lesions

Squamous cell carcinoma

This plaquelike, gelatinous, or papilliform growth occurs in limbal and bulbar conjunctiva in the interpalpebral fissure zone of older individuals.

PATHOGENESIS Ultraviolet radiation is an important influence on the development of squamous cell carcinoma, but viral and genetic factors probably also play a role. Squamous cell carcinoma is more common and more aggressive in HIV-infected individuals and in those with xeroderma pigmentosum.

CLINICAL FINDINGS A broad base is usually present along the limbus. The lesion tends to grow outward with sharp borders and may appear leukoplakic (Fig 11-6). Although histologic invasion beneath the epithelial basement membrane is present, growth usually remains superficial, infrequently penetrating the sclera or Bowman's layer. Pigmentation can occur in dark-skinned patients. Engorged conjunctival vessels feed the tumor. Adenoid squamous cell carcinoma is a variant that arises in sun-exposed conjunctiva and may be more common in tropical regions. It presents with inflammation, is locally invasive, and can metastasize.

MANAGEMENT When possible, complete local excision of the tumor, accompanied by adjunctive cryotherapy, is suggested. The treatment of choice includes excision of conjunctiva 4 mm beyond the clinically apparent margins of the tumor, along with a thin lamellar scleral flap beneath the tumor; treatment of the remaining sclera with absolute alcohol; and cryotherapy applied to the conjunctival margins. As with CIN, the risk of recurrence depends on the status of the surgical margins. If neglected, squamous cell

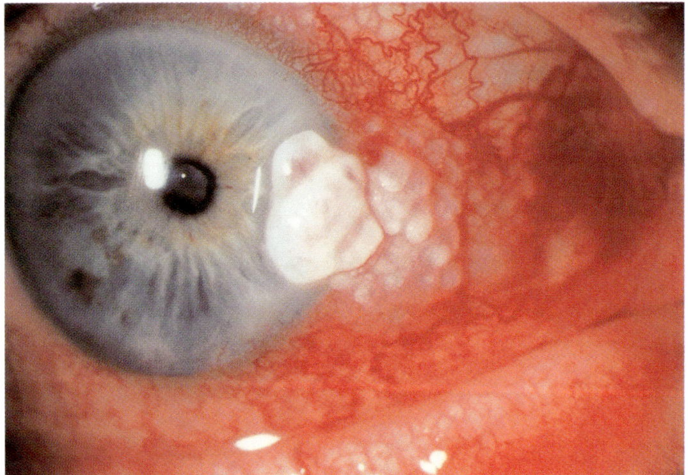

Figure 11-6 Limbal squamous cell carcinoma.

carcinoma can eventually invade the interior of the eye, where the tumor can exhibit vigorous growth. Invasion of the iris or trabecular meshwork provides the tumor with access to the systemic circulation and may be the route by which metastases occur. Extensive external spread can necessitate orbital exenteration. Radiation therapy may be indicated as adjunctive therapy in select cases.

Lee GA, Hirst LW. Ocular surface squamous neoplasia. *Surv Ophthalmol.* 1995;39:429–450.

Shields JA, Shields CL, De Potter P. Surgical management of conjunctival tumors. The 1994 Lynn B. McMahan Lecture. *Arch Ophthalmol.* 1997;115:808–815.

Mucoepidermoid carcinoma

This tumor is a very rare carcinoma of the limbal conjunctiva, fornix, or caruncle that clinically resembles an aggressive variant of squamous cell carcinoma. In addition to neoplastic epithelial cells, malignant goblet cells can be demonstrated with mucin stains. Compared to squamous cell carcinoma, mucoepidermoid carcinoma is more likely to invade the globe or orbit. Treatment is wide surgical excision; adjuvant therapy can include cryotherapy and radiotherapy.

Other carcinomas

Spindle cell carcinoma is a rare tumor of the bulbar or limbal conjunctiva in which the anaplastic cells appear spindle-shaped like fibroblasts. Basal cell carcinoma arising from the conjunctiva is also very unusual.

Glandular Tumors of the Conjunctiva

Oncocytoma

A slow-growing cystadenoma, this tumor arises from ductal and acinar cells of main and accessory lacrimal glands. In elderly individuals, an oncocytoma may present as a reddish brown nodule on the surface of the caruncle.

Dacryoadenoma

This extremely rare conjunctival tumor occurs in children or young adults and may represent a benign proliferation of accessory lacrimal gland cells. The tumor appears as a round pink elevation on the palpebral or bulbar conjunctiva.

Sebaceous Gland Carcinoma

Sebaceous adenocarcinoma

Sebaceous gland carcinomas account for approximately 1% of all eyelid tumors and 5% of eyelid malignancies. They affect elderly individuals but may be seen in younger individuals after radiation therapy. They may masquerade as chalazia or as chronic unilateral blepharoconjunctivitis (Fig 11-7).

PATHOGENESIS Most sebaceous gland carcinomas of the eyelid arise from a meibomian gland, but some develop from the glands of Zeis, from sebaceous glands of the caruncle, or from the pilosebaceous glands of the eyelids and eyebrows. The multifocal nature of sebaceous carcinomas suggests that environmental factors leading to malignant transformation act diffusely on sebaceous gland cells.

CLINICAL FINDINGS Lesions tend to involve the eyelid margin and are more common on the upper eyelid than the lower, possibly because of the greater number of meibomian glands along the upper eyelid margin. The clinical appearance is variable, as the tumor tends to spread beneath the surface. It may be associated with inflammation and be

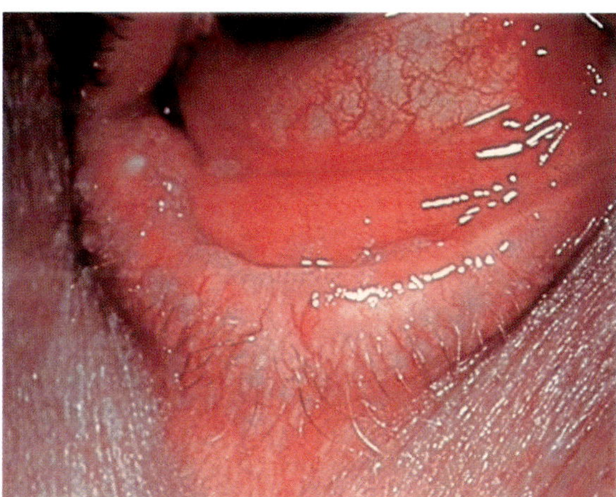

Figure 11-7 Sebaceous gland carcinoma.

multicentric. A painless, slow-growing, firm, nonmobile, yellowish nodule would be a typical presentation. When the tumor arises from a meibomian gland or a gland of Zeis at the eyelid margin, intraepithelial pagetoid spread into the conjunctiva with inflammation may mask the site of origin, produce chronic papillary conjunctivitis, and significantly delay the diagnosis. Any chronic unilateral conjunctivitis in an elderly patient should raise suspicion for a sebaceous cell carcinoma. An enlarged preauricular lymph node may indicate metastatic spread.

MANAGEMENT A full-thickness biopsy is performed for histopathologic confirmation. Mapping biopsies may be needed because of skip areas. Wide excision with tumor-free margins is necessary. Multifocal or spreading tumors may require exenteration. Adjunctive radiotherapy can be given. Complications of the disease include orbital invasion, recurrence, and metastases. Local recurrence occurs in 10%–20% of patients, and distant metastases affect 15%–25% of cases. Tumor-related mortality is about 10%. A poor prognosis is associated with a duration longer than 6 months, extensive tumor dedifferentiation and invasion, and incomplete excision.

Tumors of Neuroectodermal Origin

Table 11-3 lists the ocular surface tumors that arise from melanocytes, nevus cells, and other neuroectodermal cells. Some pigmented lesions of the globe are normal. For example, a *pigment spot of the sclera* is a collection of melanocytes associated with an intrascleral nerve loop or perforating anterior ciliary vessel. The term *melanosis* refers to excessive pigmentation without an elevated mass that may be congenital (whether epithelial or subepithelial) or acquired (whether primary or secondary). Conjunctival pigmentation can also occur from epinephrine, silver, and mascara.

> Helm CJ. Melanoma and other pigmented lesions of the ocular surface. In: *Focal Points: Clinical Modules for Ophthalmologists.* San Francisco: American Academy of Ophthalmology; 1996: vol 14, no 11.

Table 11-3 Neoplastic Tumors and Related Conditions of Neuroectodermal Cells of the Ocular Surface

Cell of Origin	Benign	Preinvasive/Malignant
Epithelial melanocytes	Freckle Benign acquired melanosis	Primary acquired melanosis Melanoma
Subepithelial melanocytes	Ocular melanocytosis Blue nevus Melanocytoma	Melanoma
Nevus cells	Intraepithelial nevus Compound nevus Subepithelial nevus	Melanoma
Neural and other cells	Neurofibroma	Leiomyosarcoma

McLean IW. Melanocytic neoplasms of the conjunctiva. In: Krachmer JH, Mannis MJ, Holland EJ, eds. *Cornea*. Vol 2. St Louis: Mosby; 1997:715–722.

Benign Pigmented Lesions

Congenital epithelial melanosis (freckle or ephelis)

A conjunctival freckle is a flat brown patch, usually of the bulbar conjunctiva near the limbus. It is more common in darkly pigmented individuals and is present at an early age.

Benign acquired melanosis

Increasing pigmentation of the conjunctiva of both eyes is a common occurrence in middle-aged individuals with dark skin. This pigmentation, which affects predominantly darkly pigmented indivduals, is often most apparent in the bulbar conjunctiva. The stimulus to melanocytic hyperplasia is unknown but may be related to sunlight exposure. Benign acquired melanosis is characterized by light brown pigmentation of the perilimbal (Fig 11-8) and interpalpebral bulbar conjunctiva. Streaks and whorls called *striate melanokeratosis* sometimes extend into the peripheral corneal epithelium.

Ocular melanocytosis

Congenital melanosis of the episclera occurs in about 1 in every 2500 individuals and is more common in the black, Hispanic, and Asian populations.

PATHOGENESIS Ocular melanocytosis consists of focal proliferation of subepithelial melanocytes (blue nevus).

CLINICAL FINDINGS Patches of episcleral pigmentation appear slate gray through the normal conjunctiva (Fig 11-9) and are nonmobile. Affected patients may have a diffuse nevus of the uvea evident as increased pigmentation of the iris and choroid. About one half of

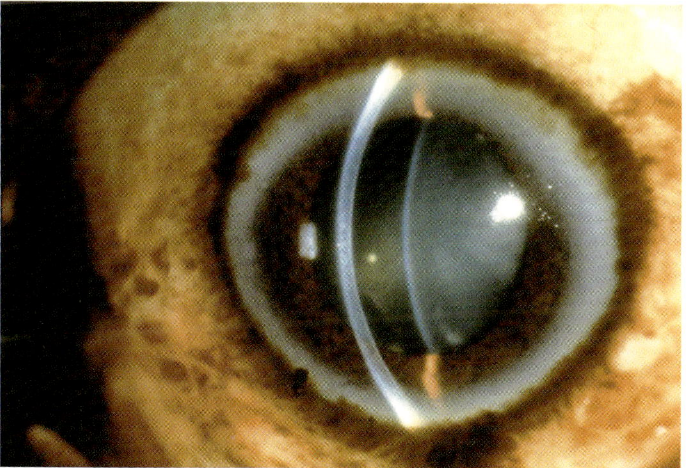

Figure 11-8 Benign acquired melanosis in a patient with corneal arcus. *(Photograph courtesy of James Chodosh, MD.)*

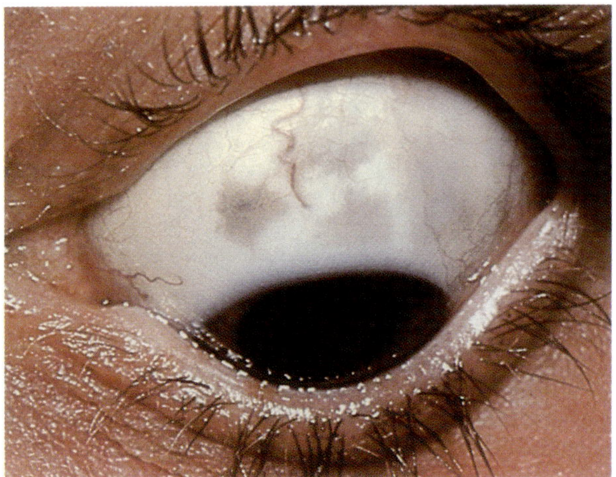

Figure 11-9 Congenital ocular melanocytosis.

patients with ocular melanocytosis have ipsilateral dermal melanocytosis (nevus of Ota), a proliferation of dermal melanocytes in the periocular skin of the first and second dermatomes of cranial nerve V. The combined ocular and cutaneous pigmentations are referred to as *oculodermal melanocytosis.* Approximately 5% of cases are bilateral.

MANAGEMENT Secondary glaucoma occurs in the affected eye in 10% of patients. Malignant transformation is possible but rare and seems to occur only in patients with a fair complexion. Malignant melanoma can develop in the skin, conjunctiva, uvea, or orbit. The lifetime risk of uveal melanoma in a patient with ocular melanocytosis is about 1 in 400, significantly greater than the 1 in 13,000 risk of the general population.

Nevus

Nevocellular nevi of the conjunctiva are hamartia that arise during childhood and adolescence. A nevus can be junctional, compound, or subepithelial.

PATHOGENESIS Pure intraepithelial nevi are rare except in children, and these junctional nevi may be difficult to distinguish histopathologically from primary acquired melanosis. The subepithelial nevus of the conjunctiva is the equivalent of the intradermal nevus of the skin.

CLINICAL FINDINGS A nevus near the limbus is usually almost flat. Those appearing elsewhere on the bulbar conjunctiva, semilunar fold, caruncle, or eyelid margin tend to be elevated. Pigmentation of conjunctival nevi is variable; they may be light tan in color or amelanotic (Fig 11-10). A subepithelial nevus often has a cobblestone appearance.

Small epithelial inclusion cysts occur within about half of all conjunctival nevi, particularly the compound or subepithelial varieties. Secretion of mucin by goblet cells in the inclusion cysts can cause a nevus to enlarge, producing a false impression of malignant change. Cellular proliferation may induce secondary lymphocytic inflammation. Rapid enlargement can occur at puberty, giving rise to a clinical impression of conjunctival melanoma. When inflamed, an amelanotic, vascularized nevus may resemble an angioma.

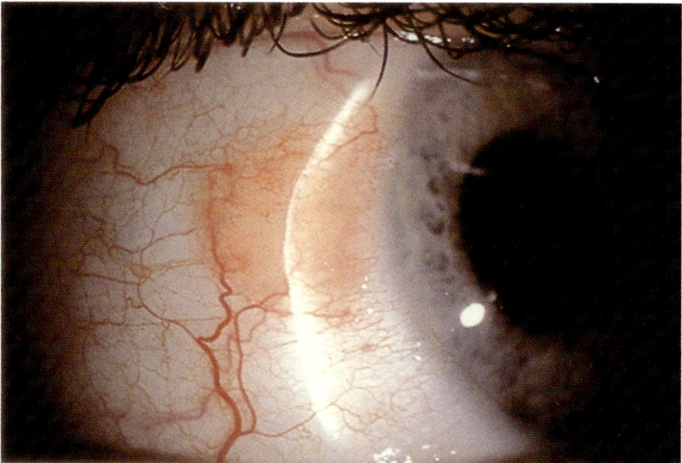

Figure 11-10 Amelanotic conjunctival nevus.

MANAGEMENT Conjunctival nevi have a high prevalence of junctional activity. Even so, they rarely become malignant. Nevertheless, excision of suspicious lesions may be preferred to prolonged observation or sequential photography. Because nevi are rare on the palpebral conjunctiva, pigmented lesions on the tarsus or in the fornix should be excised rather than observed.

Preinvasive Pigmented Lesions

Primary acquired melanosis

This acquired pigmentation of the conjunctival epithelium may be analogous to lentigo maligna of the skin (Hutchinson's freckle), a preinvasive intraepidermal lesion of sun-exposed skin. The term *primary acquired melanosis (PAM)* refers to flat, brown lesions of the conjunctival epithelium that are commonly encountered in clinical practice (Fig 11-11). By definition, the condition differs from congenital pigmented lesions and from secondary acquired melanosis, such as that caused by Addison disease, radiation, or pregnancy. Table 11-4 compares the various pigmentary lesions of the conjunctiva. Most types of acquired melanosis remain benign, but in one study, PAM associated with cellular atypia progressed to conjunctival melanoma in 46% of cases (see BCSC Section 4, *Ophthalmic Pathology and Intraocular Tumors*).

> Folberg R, McLean IW, Zimmerman LE. Primary acquired melanosis of the conjunctiva. *Hum Pathol.* 1985;16:129–135.

PATHOGENESIS Abnormal melanocytes proliferate in the basal conjunctival epithelium of middle-aged, light-skinned individuals for reasons that are unknown. Pigmentation in an individual with dark skin is called benign acquired melanosis rather than PAM, but the two conditions may be related.

CLINICAL FINDINGS Multiple flat brown patches of noncystic pigmentation appear within the superficial conjunctiva of one eye. Changes in size may be associated with inflam-

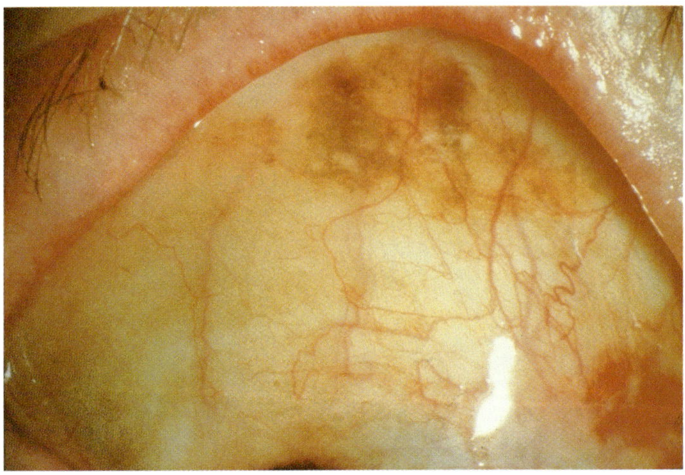

Figure 11-11 Primary acquired melanosis. *(Photograph courtesy of James Chodosh, MD.)*

Table 11-4 Clinical Comparison of Conjunctival Pigmentary Lesions

Lesion	Onset	Area	Location	Malignant Potential
Freckle	Youth	Small	Conjunctiva	No
Benign acquired melanosis	Adulthood	Patchy or diffuse	Conjunctiva	No
Conjunctival nevus	Youth	Small, cystic	Conjunctiva	Low (conjunctival melanoma)
Ocular and oculodermal melanocytosis	Congenital	Patchy or diffuse	Episcleral	Yes (skin, conjunctival, uveal, orbital melanoma)
Primary acquired melanosis	Middle age	Patchy or diffuse	Conjunctiva	Yes (conjunctival melanoma)

mation or may be the result of hormonal influences. Malignant transformation should be suspected when a lesion shows nodularity, enlargement, or increased vascularity. Small typical areas of PAM can be observed and biopsy delayed until progression is observed.

MANAGEMENT The best treatment for this condition remains undetermined. An excisional biopsy utilizing the same techniques as for squamous neoplasia of the conjunctiva (see the section "Squamous cell carcinoma") should be performed for large, progressive, or dark lesions, when melanoma is considered. All pigmented palpebral conjunctival lesions should be excised. When lesions show atypia on histopathologic examination, the clinician should check the margins carefully and perform additional resection until the lesion is completely removed. For lesions that show atypia or malignancy, cryotherapy can be a useful adjunct; topical mitomycin-C may also be useful. Regional lymph nodes should be checked regularly.

McLean IW. Melanocytic neoplasms of the conjunctiva. In: Krachmer JH, Mannis MJ, Holland EJ, eds. *Cornea.* Vol 2. St Louis: Mosby; 1997:715–722.

Malignant Pigmented Lesions

Melanoma

With a prevalence of approximately 1 per 2 million in the population of European ancestry, conjunctival melanomas make up less than 1% of ocular malignancies. Conjunctival melanomas are rare in black and Asian populations. Although malignant melanoma of the conjunctiva can metastasize, it has a better prognosis than cutaneous melanoma.

PATHOGENESIS Conjunctival melanomas may arise from acquired nevi, from PAM, or from clinically normal conjunctiva. Malignant transformation of a congenital conjunctival nevus is very rare. Intralymphatic spread increases the risk of metastasis. In rare cases, an underlying ciliary body melanoma can extend through the sclera. Cutaneous melanoma can, in very rare instances, metastasize to the conjunctiva.

CLINICAL FINDINGS Although conjunctival melanomas can arise in palpebral conjunctiva, they are most commonly found in bulbar conjunctiva or at the limbus (Fig 11-12). The degree of pigmentation is variable. Because heavy vascularization is common, these tumors may bleed easily. They grow in a nodular fashion and can invade the globe or orbit. Outcome is partly determined by the site involved: bulbar conjunctival melanomas have a better prognosis than melanomas of the palpebral conjunctiva, fornix, or caruncle. Conjunctival melanomas may metastasize to regional lymph nodes, the brain, and other sites. Cytologic risk factors for metastasis are large size, multicentricity, epithelioid cell type, and lymphatic invasion.

MANAGEMENT An excisional biopsy should be considered for any suspicious pigmented epibulbar lesions; biopsy seems not to increase the risk of metastasis. The recommended treatment comprises excision of conjunctiva 4 mm beyond the clinically apparent mar-

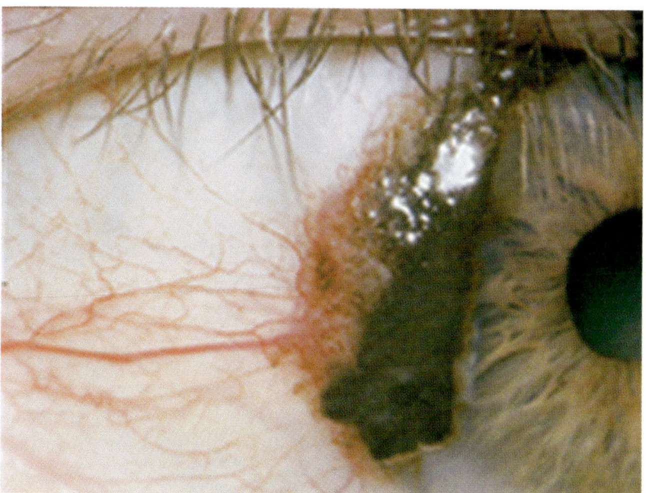

Figure 11-12 Malignant melanoma of the limbal conjunctiva. *(Reproduced with permission from Helm CJ. Melanoma and other pigmented lesions of the ocular surface. In: Focal Points: Clinical Modules for Ophthalmologists. San Francisco: American Academy of Ophthalmology; 1996; vol 14, no 11. Photograph courtesy of Thomas Pettit, MD.)*

gins of the tumor, along with a thin lamellar scleral flap beneath the tumor; treatment of the remaining sclera with absolute alcohol; and cryotherapy applied to the conjunctival margins. Primary closure is performed when feasible, but conjunctival or amniotic membrane grafts are necessary for large excisions. Topical mitomycin-C has been used after excision and cryotherapy to treat residual disease. Orbital exenteration is performed for advanced disease when local excision or enucleation would be insufficient to completely excise the tumor (when metastases have been excluded) or as palliative treatment for advanced, aggressive tumors. Fatal metastases are more likely with thick tumors, multifocal tumors, and melanomas arising in the caruncle or palpebral conjunctiva.

Conjunctival malignant melanomas are potentially deadly tumors. In a recently reported study, metastasis was detected in 26% of patients, and death occurred in 13% of patients 10 years after surgical excision. Melanomas arising de novo (not in preexisting nevi or from PAM), tumors not involving the limbus, and residual involvement at the surgical margins were especially poor prognostic factors. The role of radiotherapy or excision of regional lymph nodes has not been determined.

Seregard S. Conjunctival melanoma. *Surv Ophthalmol.* 1998;42:321–350.

Shields CL, Shields JA, Gunduz K, et al. Conjunctival melanoma: risk factors for recurrence, exenteration, metastasis, and death in 150 consecutive patients. *Arch Ophthalmol.* 2000;118:1497–1507.

Singh AD, Campos OE, Rhatigan RM, et al. Conjunctival melanoma in the black population. *Surv Ophthalmol.* 1998;43:127–133.

Neurogenic and Smooth Muscle Tumors

Subconjunctival peripheral nerve sheath tumors such as *neurofibromas, schwannomas,* and *neuromas* have been reported, especially in multiple endocrine neoplasia (MEN). A neurofibroma of the conjunctiva or eyelid is almost always a manifestation of neurofibromatosis, an autosomal dominant phakomatosis (see BCSC Section 6, *Pediatric Ophthalmology and Strabismus*). A *neurilemoma* is a very rare tumor of the conjunctiva that originates from Schwann cells of a peripheral nerve sheath (Fig 11-13). A *leiomyosarcoma* is a very rare limbal lesion with the potential for orbital invasion.

Vascular and Mesenchymal Tumors

Vascular lesions of the eyelid margin or conjunctiva generally are benign hamartomas or secondary reactions to infection or other stimuli (Table 11-5).

Benign Tumors

Hemangioma

Isolated capillary and cavernous hemangiomas of the bulbar conjunctiva are rare and are more likely to represent extension from adjacent structures. The palpebral conjunctiva is frequently involved with an eyelid capillary hemangioma. Diffuse hemangiomatosis of the palpebral or forniceal conjunctiva indicates an orbital capillary hemangioma. A cavernous hemangioma of the orbit may present initially under the conjunctiva.

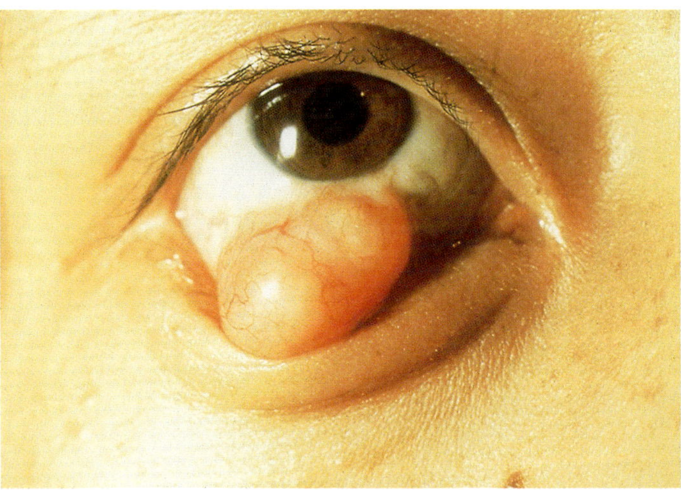

Figure 11-13 Conjunctival neurilemoma. *(Reproduced with permission from Charles NC, Fox DM, Avendano JA, et al. Conjunctival neurilemoma. Report of 3 cases. Arch Ophthalmol. 1997; 115:547–549. Photograph courtesy of Norman Charles, MD.)*

Table 11-5 Neoplastic Tumors of Blood Vessels of the Eyelid and Conjunctiva*

Hamartoma	Reactive	Malignant
Nevus flammeus	Pyogenic granuloma	Kaposi sarcoma
Capillary hemangioma	Glomus tumor	Angiosarcoma
Cavernous hemangioma	Intravascular papillary endothelial hyperplasia	

* Tumors are not listed in a particular order, and lesions in one column do not necessarily correspond to those in parallel columns.

Nevus flammeus, a congenital lesion described as a port-wine stain, may occur alone or as part of Sturge-Weber syndrome, associated with vascular hamartomas, secondary glaucoma, and/or leptomeningeal angiomatosis. Some cases result from a genetic mutation coding for the vascular endothelial protein receptor for angiopoietin-1, which controls the assembly of perivascular smooth muscle. *Ataxia-telangiectasia* is a syndrome of epibulbar telangiectasis, cerebellar abnormalities, and immune alterations.

Inflammatory vascular tumors

Inflammatory conjunctival lesions often show vascular proliferation. *Pyogenic granuloma,* a common type of reactive hemangioma, is misnamed because it is not suppurative and does not contain giant cells. The lesion may occur over a chalazion or when minor trauma or surgery stimulates exuberant healing tissue with fibroblasts (granulation tissue) and proliferating capillaries that grow in a radiating pattern. This rapidly growing lesion is red, pedunculated, and smooth (Fig 11-14), bleeds easily, and stains with fluorescein dye. Topical or intralesional corticosteroids may be curative. Excision with cauterization to

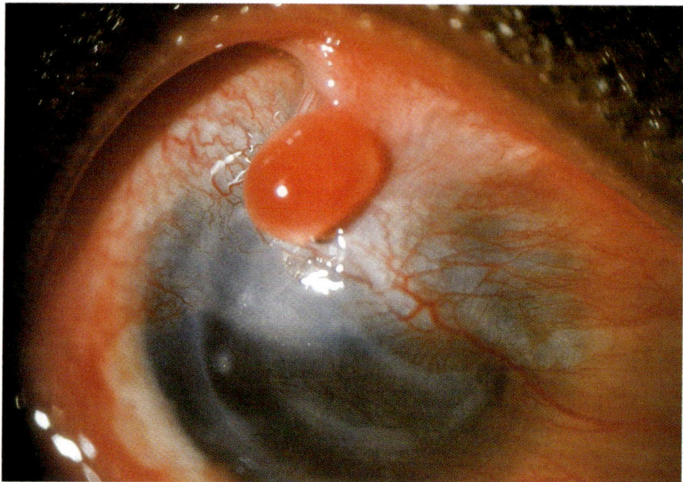

Figure 11-14 Pyogenic granuloma.

the base, primary closure of the wound, and generous postoperative topical corticosteroids may minimize recurrences.

Subconjunctival granulomas may form around parasitic and mycotic infectious foci. They have also occurred with connective tissue diseases such as rheumatoid arthritis. Sarcoid nodules appear as tan-yellow elevations that can resemble follicles. *Juvenile xanthogranuloma* is a histiocytic disorder that can present as a conjunctival mass. A *fibrous histiocytoma*, composed of fibroblasts and histiocytes with lipid vacuoles, arises on rare occasions on the conjunctiva or limbus. *Nodular fasciitis* is a very rare benign tumor of fibrovascular tissue in the eyelid or under the conjunctiva; it may originate at the insertion site of a rectus muscle.

Malignant Tumors

Kaposi sarcoma

This malignant neoplasm of vascular endothelium involves the skin and mucous membranes. Internal organs are occasionally involved as well.

PATHOGENESIS Infection with Kaposi sarcoma–associated herpesvirus/human herpesvirus 8 (KSHV) is responsible for this disease; in young patients, it occurs most often in the setting of AIDS.

CLINICAL FINDINGS On the eyelid skin, Kaposi sarcoma presents as a purplish nodule. Orbital involvement may produce eyelid and conjunctival edema. In the conjunctiva, Kaposi sarcoma presents as a reddish, highly vascular subconjunctival lesion that may simulate a subconjunctival hemorrhage. Lesions are most often found in the inferior fornix and may be nodular or diffuse (Fig 11-15). Nodular lesions may be relatively less responsive to therapy.

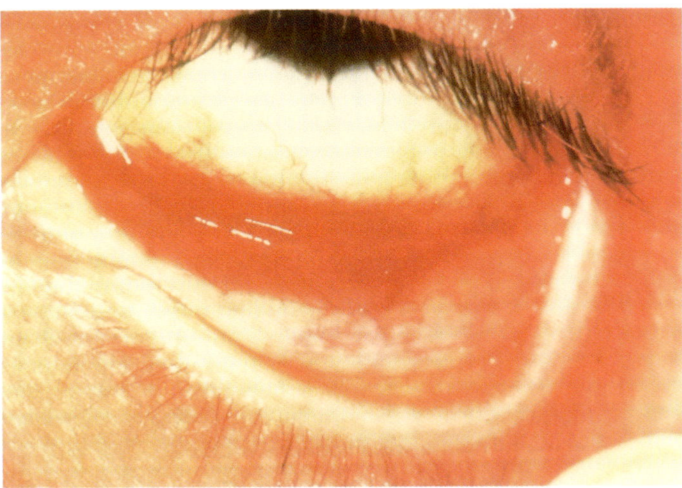

Figure 11-15 Kaposi sarcoma of the conjunctiva. *(Reproduced with permission from Holland GN, Pepose JS, Pettit TH. Acquired immune deficiency. Ocular manifestations.* Ophthalmology. *1983;90:859–873. Photograph courtesy of Gary N. Holland, MD.)*

MANAGEMENT Treatment may not be curative. Options for controlling symptoms include surgical debulking, cryotherapy, and radiotherapy. Local or systemic chemotherapy may be required. Intralesional interferon alfa-2a has been reported to be effective.

Other malignant tumors

Malignant mesenchymal lesions that rarely involve the conjunctiva are malignant fibrous histiocytomas, liposarcomas, leiomyosarcomas, and rhabdomyosarcomas.

Lymphatic and Lymphocytic Tumors

Lymphoid tumors of the conjunctiva may be benign, malignant, or indeterminate. Many of these lesions have overlapping clinical and pathologic features. About 20% of patients with a conjunctival lymphoid tumor have detectable extraocular lymphoma.

Lymphangiectasia and Lymphangioma

Lymphangiectasia appears on the eye as irregularly dilated lymphatic channels in the bulbar conjunctiva. It may be a developmental anomaly or can follow trauma or inflammation. Anomalous communication with a venule can lead to spontaneous filling of the lymphatic vessels with blood. *Lymphangiomas* are proliferations of lymphatic channel elements. Like a capillary hemangioma, lymphanigomas are usually present at birth and may enlarge slowly. The lesion appears as a patch of vesicles with edema. Intralesional hemorrhage, producing a "chocolate cyst," makes differentiation from a hemangioma difficult.

Lymphoid Hyperplasia

PATHOGENESIS Formerly called *reactive hyperplasia*, this benign-appearing accumulation of lymphocytes and other leukocytes may represent a low-grade B-cell lymphoma. Most patients are older than 40 years although, in rare instances, extranodal lymphoid hyperplasia has occurred in children.

CLINICAL FINDINGS This mass presents as a minimally elevated salmon-colored subepithelial tumor with a pebbly appearance corresponding to follicle formation (Fig 11-16); it is clinically indistinguishable from conjunctival lymphoma. It is often moderately or highly vascularized. Primary localized amyloidosis can have a similar appearance.

MANAGEMENT Lymphoid hyperplasia may resolve spontaneously, but it has been treated with local excision, topical corticosteroids, or radiation. Biopsy specimens require special handling to complete many of the unusual histochemical and immunologic studies. Because a patient with an apparently benign polyclonal lymphoid lesion has the potential to develop a systemic lymphoma, general medical consultation is advisable.

Lymphoma

A neoplastic lymphoid lesion of the conjunctiva is generally a monoclonal proliferation of B lymphocytes.

PATHOGENESIS A lymphoma can arise in the conjunctival lymphoid follicles. Some lymphomas are limited to the conjunctiva; others occur in conjunction with systemic malignant lymphoma. Some are polyclonal, but most conjunctival lymphomas are monoclonal B-cell lymphomas. Conjunctival plasmacytoma, Hodgkin lymphoma, and T-cell lymphomas are less common.

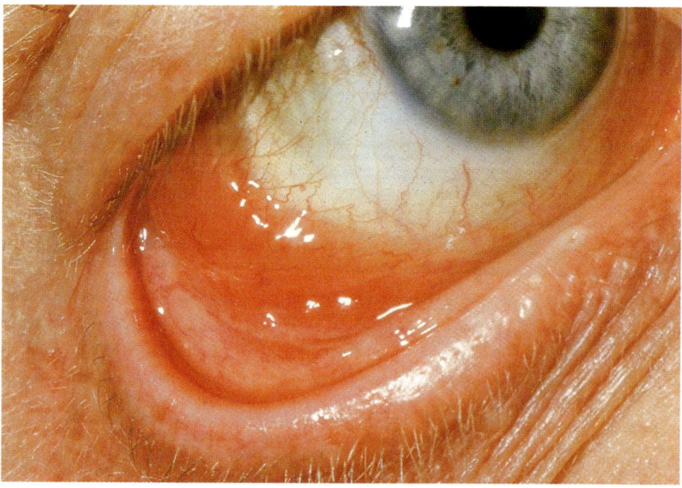

Figure 11-16 Conjunctival lymphoid hyperplasia.

CLINICAL FINDINGS Non–Hodgkin B-cell lymphoma has essentially the same clinical appearance as benign lymphoid hyperplasia. It appears as a salmon pink, mobile mass on the conjunctiva (Fig 11-17). A diffuse lesion may masquerade as chronic conjunctivitis. An epibulbar mass fixed to the underlying sclera may be a sign of extrascleral extension of uveal lymphoid neoplasia. Most patients with conjunctival lymphoma are either over 50 years of age or immunosuppressed. Patients with AIDS are at increased risk.

LABORATORY EVALUATION AND MANAGEMENT Patients should be referred to an oncologist for systemic evaluation. Unless a tumor is small enough to be removed completely, incisional biopsy is indicated for histopathologic diagnosis. Local external beam radiation therapy is usually curative for lesions confined to the conjunctiva, but systemic chemotherapy is required for the treatment of systemic lymphoma.

Metastatic Tumors

Metastatic tumors to the conjunctiva are much less common than those from the uveal tract and orbit, but such tumors have arisen from cancer of the breast, lung, kidney, and elsewhere, including cutaneous melanoma. Metastatic lesions to the uveal tract, orbit, or paranasal sinuses can extend into the conjunctiva. Metastases or leukemic infiltrates to the limbus or cornea also occur.

Epibulbar Choristomas

A *hamartoma* is a congenital tumor resulting from abnormal tissue residing at its normal site. Nevi and hemangiomas, which were discussed previously, are hamartomas. A *choristoma* is a heterotopic congenital lesion that results from normal tissue being placed in an abnormal location during embryogenesis. The most common episcleral choristoma is a *dermoid*. Although present at birth, a choristoma in the eyelid or orbit may

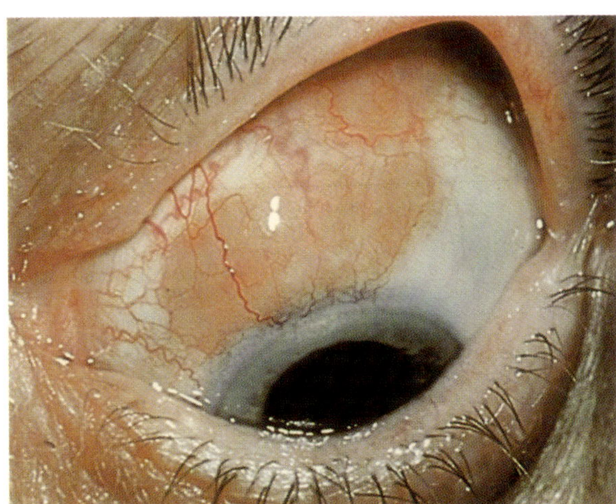

Figure 11-17 Conjunctival lymphoma.

not be apparent until later in life. Intraocular lacrimal gland tissue is an extremely rare choristoma.

Epidermoid and Dermoid Cyst

A congenital *epidermoid cyst* is a somewhat rare choristomatous anomaly caused by displacement of normal embryonic tissue. An epidermoid cyst containing accessory skin structures in its wall is called a *dermoid cyst.* Epidermoid and dermoid cysts most commonly occur near the frontozygomatic suture and, less often, near the nasofrontal suture. Excision is recommended when an epidermoid or dermoid cyst threatens to cause amblyopia or a cosmetic deformity.

Epibulbar Dermoid Tumor

The congenital *epibulbar dermoid tumor* typically occurs on the inferotemporal globe or temporal limbus as a smooth, elevated, solid mass embedded in the superficial sclera or cornea (Fig 11-18). About 1 in 10,000 individuals is affected.

PATHOGENESIS A dermoid tumor results from faulty development of the eyelid folds and consists of displaced embryonic tissue that was destined to become skin. Dermoids are composed of fibrous tissue and occasionally hair with sebaceous glands; they are covered by conjunctival epithelium. Epibulbar dermoids are solid rather than cystic and are not fully entrapped beneath the surface, unlike dermoid cysts.

CLINICAL FINDINGS Dermoids are well-circumscribed, porcelain white, round to oval lesions that occur most often at the inferotemporal limbus, but they can also be found on the central cornea, in the subconjunctival space, or in the orbit. Fine hairs may protrude from some dermoids. A limbal dermoid often has an arcuslike deposition of lipid along its anterior corneal border. Corneal astigmatism caused by a dermoid can

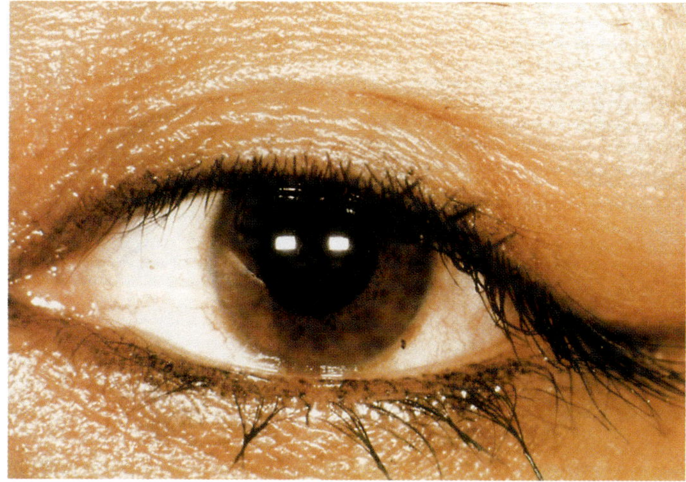

Figure 11-18 Limbal dermoid. *(Reproduced with permission from Marines HM, Patrinely JR. Benign eyelid tumors. Ophthalmol Clin North Am. 1992;5:243–260.)*

lead to anisometropic amblyopia. The flattest meridian of the cornea is adjacent to the limbal dermoid.

Dermoids are often associated with a congenital malformation known as *Goldenhar syndrome* (oculoauriculovertebral dysplasia), a sporadic or autosomal dominant syndrome of the first branchial arch, characterized by the presence of epibulbar dermoid, coloboma of the upper eyelid, preauricular skin tags and aural fistulae, and vertebral anomalies. BCSC Section 6, *Pediatric Ophthalmology and Strabismus*, discusses and illustrates Goldenhar syndrome in greater detail.

MANAGEMENT Dermoids grow along with the child and the eye and have virtually no malignant potential. The elevated portion of a dermoid may be excised, but the lesion often extends deep into underlying tissues. Some corneal astigmatism often remains after a shaving dissection of a limbal dermoid. A relaxing incision or other corrective measure may be considered. Lamellar keratoplasty can improve the cosmetic appearance.

Dermolipoma

A dermolipoma is a pale yellow dermoid containing adipose tissue that should be distinguished from herniation of orbital fat. It typically occurs superotemporally and may extend posteriorly.

Ectopic Lacrimal Gland

Lacrimal gland tissue occurring outside of the lacrimal fossa may be associated with a complex choristoma (see below), or it may occur alone as a round, pink, vascularized mass at the limbus.

Other Choristomas

A *complex choristoma*, usually on the superotemporal globe, consists of multiple tissues, including cartilage, bone, lacrimal gland lobules, hair follicles, hair, sebaceous glands, and adipose tissue (Fig 11-19). An *osseous choristoma* is a solitary nodule of bone surrounded by fibrous tissue that is also located superotemporally. A *neuroglial choristoma* is more diffuse. A *phakomatous choristoma* is a subcutaneous nodule in the inferomedial eyelid composed of disorganized lens cells.

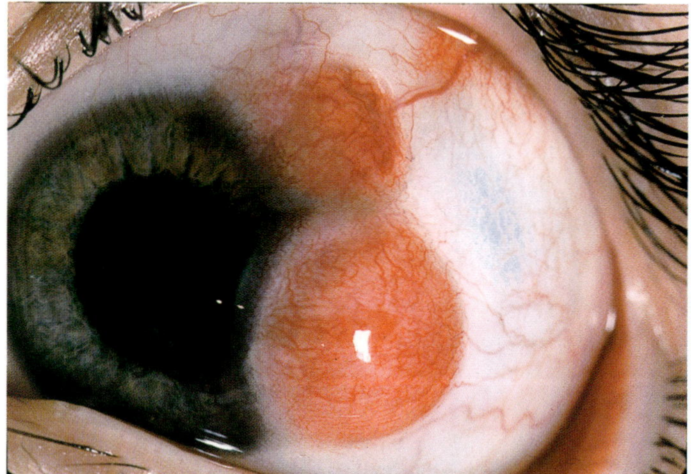

Figure 11-19 Complex choristomas showing rose coloring caused by presence of richly vascularized ectopic lacrimal gland tissue. *(Reproduced with permission from Margo CE. Nonpigmented lesions of the ocular surface. In: Focal Points: Clinical Modules for Ophthalmologists. San Francisco: American Academy of Ophthalmology; 1996; vol 14, no 9.)*

PART VI

Congenital Anomalies of the Cornea and Sclera

Basic Concepts of Congenital Anomalies of the Cornea and Sclera

Normal Prenatal Development of the Eyelids, Conjunctiva, and Cornea

Just as with the eye as a whole, three parts of the primitive embryo contribute to the development of the external eye: *neuroectoderm, neural crest cells,* and *surface ectoderm.* Mesoderm provides only the endothelium of the vasculature, the orbicularis muscles of the eyelids, and the temporal portion of the sclera. The optic primordium appears at day 24 of gestation in the neural folds (Table 12-1). The optic vesicle evaginates at day 25, and neural crest cells migrate to surround it. The vesicle induces development of the lens placode from the surface ectoderm at day 28.

In the second month of gestation, the optic and lens vesicles invaginate, and two layers of corneal epithelium originating from the surface ectoderm form over the lens vesicle. The first wave of neural crest cells migrates centrally, separating the lens vesicle from the surface ectoderm and forming the primitive corneal endothelium and acellular corneal stroma (Figs 12-1, 12-2). In the sixth week, the eyelid folds appear. At the seventh week, a second wave of neural crest mesenchyme invades the corneal stroma posteriorly, then anteriorly. This wave condenses as sclera, which then begins posterior migration. In the eighth week, the third wave of neural crest mesenchyme advances to form the primitive anterior chamber, iris stroma, and pupillary membrane. In the twelfth week, the eyelid folds meet and fuse, allowing the conjunctiva and corneal epithelium to develop away from amniotic fluid.

In the third month of gestation, iris and ciliary body, cilia, goblet cells, and meibomian glands become evident. Endothelium thins to one layer. Descemet's membrane has become a continuous structure by 12 weeks. In the fourth month, characteristic banding of Descemet's membrane begins, and the keratocytes realign and assume a spindle shape. Collagen lamellae are laid down in a spiral, orthogonal pattern proceeding from posterior to anterior. The corneal epithelium develops wing cells and appears more orderly than the conjunctiva. Aqueous humor forms and moves anteriorly. Iris sphincter muscle develops from the neuroectoderm, and the Zeis and Moll glands form in the eyelids.

Table 12-1 Human Anterior Segment Development

Mo	Week	Day	Length of Embryo (MM)	Event
1	3	22	2–3.5	Optic sulci present in forebrain
	4	24	2.4–4.5	Optic vesicles form
				Lens placode thickens
		26	3.0–5.0	Neural crest mesenchyme surrounds optic vesicle
2	5	28		Optic cup and lens pit form invaginations
				Surface ectoderm formed
				Lens and corneal epithelial basement membranes are fused
	6	40	11–14	*First wave of neural crest cells forms corneal endothelium*
		41		Eyelid folds develop
	7	44	13–17	Anterior chamber forming
		49	24	*Second wave forms stromal keratocytes and sclera*
	8	54	25	Lacrimal gland buds from conjunctiva
				Acellular corneal stroma present
				Episclera (Tenon's layer) becoming evident
			35–40	*Third wave forms iris and pupillary membrane*
3	10		43–48	Conjunctiva forming from eyelid and cornea
				Anterior banded Descemet's membrane forms
				Sclera condenses from anterior to posterior
	12		48–52	Cilia form
			50–55	Krause, Wolfring glands form from conjunctival recess
			52	Goblet cells formed
			80	Meibomian glands form
4			87	Sclera forms lamina cribosa
				Collagen fibrils appear as lamellae and take on adult form
				Aqueous is formed
			80–100	Glands of Moll and Zeis form
			170	Eyelids keratinized
5			320	Anterior eyelid border opens
6			385	Posterior eyelid opens

In the fifth month, scleral fibrils have formed around the axonal bundles of the optic nerve. Keratinization of the eyelid margin from within the pilosebaceous complex causes the eyelids to begin to separate anteriorly. Full separation is present in the sixth month, when the dilator muscle of the iris also becomes apparent. In the seventh month, the fibrous lamina cribrosa is fully formed, and the pupillary membrane begins to atrophy. At birth, the pupillary membrane has regressed, and the cornea has grown from 2 mm in diameter at 3 months to 9.5–10.5 mm and has assumed its typical lenticular shape, although it will not reach adult size for 1–2 years. The lacrimal gland is present but reflex tearing is absent until about 3 weeks after birth; the gland continues to grow for 3–4 years. Lacrimal drainage does not begin until near or shortly after birth and can be delayed for several months.

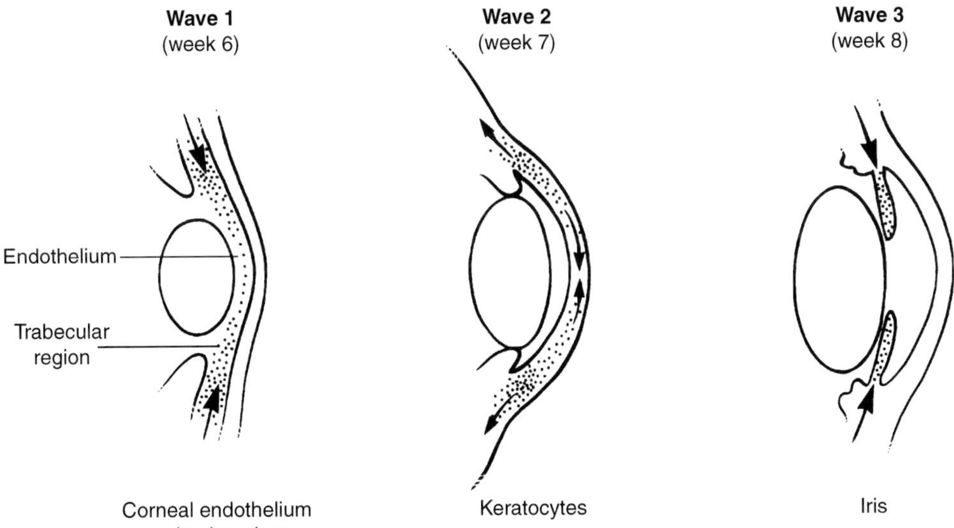

Figure 12-1 The three waves of neural crest cell migration during embryogenesis: Wave 1, trabecular meshwork and corneal endothelium; wave 2, corneal stroma and keratocytes; wave 3, iris. *(Illustration by Christine Gralapp, modified from Bahn CF, Falls HF, Varley GA, et al. Classification of corneal endothelial disorders based on neural crest origin.* Ophthalmology. *1984;91:559.)*

Causes of Congenital Corneal Anomalies

Congenital anomalies manifest as alterations in gross morphology evident at the time of birth. They may be sporadic or familial and unilateral or bilateral and may or may not be heritable. They are the result of abnormal development during embryonic or fetal life caused by various genetic influences and local or environmental effects.

Ocular anomalies can occur along with a constellation of cranial, facial, or somatic abnormalities, making it difficult to incriminate a specific chromosomal abnormality, intrauterine infection, or maternal toxin as the cause. Ocular structures are most at risk in the period of organogenesis, from 18 to 60 days. Anomalies occur when either intrinsic or extrinsic factors disrupt the intricate sequencing of embryonic events. *Intrinsic factors* include

- Altered, defective, or imperfect genes
- Impaired cellular induction and proliferation
- Defective cell migration
- Cell death
- Abnormal extracellular substrates
- Inadequate differentiation
- Physical constraint

Extrinsic factors include health of the mother and exposure to a teratogen, which can vary in its nature, timing, and degree.

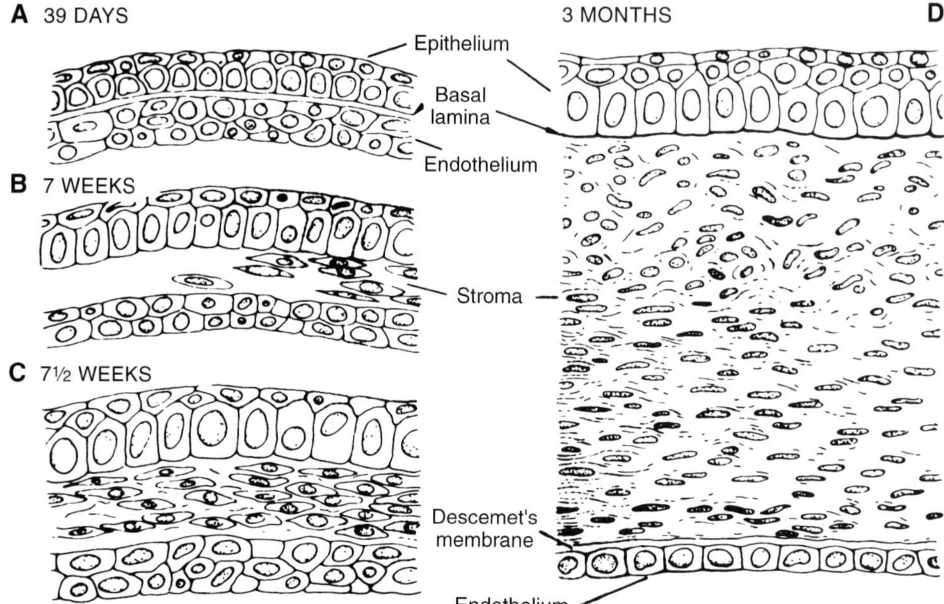

Figure 12-2 Development of cornea in central region. **A,** At day 39, two-layered epithelium rests on basal lamina and is separated from endothelium (two to three layers) by narrow acellular space. **B,** At week 7, mesenchymal cells from periphery migrate into space between epithelium and endothelium. **C,** Mesenchymal cells (future keratocytes) are arranged in four to five incomplete layers by 7½ weeks, and a few collagen fibrils are present among cells. **D,** By 3 months, epithelium has two to three layers of cells, and stroma has about 25–30 layers of keratocytes that are arranged more regularly in the posterior half. Thin, uneven Descemet's membrane lies between the most posterior keratocytes and the now single layer of endothelium. *(Reproduced with permission from Cook CS, Ozanics V, Jakobiec FA. Prenatal development of the eye and its adnexa. In: Tasman W, Jaeger EA, eds.* Duane's Foundations of Clinical Ophthalmology. *Philadelphia: Lippincott; 1991.)*

Teratogens are infectious, pharmacologic, chemical, or physical agents that lead to defects in the developing embryo or fetus. The term means, literally, "induce a monster." Confirmed ocular teratogens with effects on the anterior segment other than cataract include the following:

- Radiation
- Fetal alcohol syndrome
- Rubella
- Cytomegalovirus
- Syphilis
- Herpes simplex virus
- Maternal diabetes
- Maternal ingestion of thalidomide, antiseizure medications, coumarin anticoagulants, lysergic acid diethylamide (LSD), and retinoic acid

Many other chemicals and environmental factors are suspected but not confirmed teratogens. No topical administration of ophthalmic medication is suspected or confirmed to produce a teratogenic effect. *Mutagens* are chemical or physical agents that induce a heritable change in offspring as opposed to acting directly on the developing embryo. BCSC Section 2, *Fundamentals and Principles of Ophthalmology*, discusses in depth in Part II, Embryology, the issues covered in this chapter and the next. A helpful glossary and numerous illustrations are included. Part III, Genetics, in the same volume discusses mutations in detail.

Diagnostic Approach

The prevalence of childhood blindness in Western countries has been estimated to be 1–3 per 10,000 live births. When further analyzed by cause, malformations of the cornea and anterior segment (excluding congenital cataract) are responsible for roughly 1%–3% of all blindness in childhood. Approximately one half of all blind children have one or more associated nonocular defects. Diagnosis of congenital anomalies requires careful ophthalmic and general examination. The infant should be sedated if required. The examination should include the following:

- Documentation of eyelid and orbit orientation, formation, and anatomy
- Measurement of corneal diameter horizontally and vertically
- Biomicroscopy of the cornea, with attention to the limbus, Bowman's membrane, stromal clarity, and Descemet's membrane
- Gonioscopy, if corneal clarity allows
- Assessment of iris and pupil shape
- Investigation of lens anomalies and posterior segment
- Documentation of intraocular pressure
- Echography of the posterior segment if no view of the anterior chamber or fundus is possible
- Ultrasound biomicroscopy of the anterior segment structures, which can be very helpful in cases where opacified media prevent direct observation

See also BCSC Section 6, *Pediatric Ophthalmology and Strabismus*.

Once an anomaly is identified, thorough family and prenatal histories should be explored with the parents to separate familial from sporadic causes. The presence of antimongoloid or pronounced mongoloid slant of the palpebral fissures, colobomas, epicanthal folds, hypertelorism, multiple systemic malformations, ptosis, strabismus, or mental retardation should prompt consultation with an ocular geneticist to identify familial syndromes or chromosomal abnormalities and to provide genetic counseling and prognostic information to patients or parents. The preliminary findings dictate which tests should subsequently be used: biochemical and chromosomal analysis, CT and MRI, tissue biopsies, and echography are the common choices. Prenatal diagnosis is an emerging field that may hold promise for the identification of ocular anomalies present in the parents or siblings.

Kim T, Palay DA. Developmental abnormalities of the cornea. In: Krachmer JH, Mannis MJ, Holland EJ, eds. *Cornea*. Vol 2. St Louis: Mosby; 1997:871–884.

McKusick VA. *Mendelian Inheritance in Man: A Catalog of Human Genes and Genetic Disorders.* 12th ed. Baltimore: The Johns Hopkins University Press; 1998. See also, under OMIM Allied Resources, the Online Mendelian Inheritance in Man website, updated daily (www.ncbi.nlm.nih.gov/omim). Site developed by the National Center for Biotechnology Information, National Library of Medicine, Bethesda, MD.

Wilson FM. Congenital anomalies of the cornea and conjunctiva. In: Smolin G, Thoft RA, eds. *The Cornea: Scientific Foundations and Clinical Practice.* 3rd ed. Boston: Little, Brown; 1994:535–533.

Clinical Aspects of Congenital Anomalies of the Cornea and Sclera

Congenital anomalies are also discussed in depth in BCSC Section 6, *Pediatric Ophthalmology and Strabismus*. Chapter 19 of that volume covers diseases of the cornea and anterior segment. See also BCSC Section 2, *Fundamentals and Principles of Ophthalmology*, which discusses these anomalies in Part II, Embryology.

Abnormalities of the Globe and Sclera

Cryptophthalmos

"Hidden eye" is a very rare condition with fewer than 150 reported cases. It is usually bilateral. The eyelids and associated structures of the brows and lashes fail to form *(ablepharon)*. The cornea is merged with the epidermis, and the anterior chamber, iris, and lens are variably formed or are absent (Fig 13-1). The conjunctiva is typically absent. *Pseudocryptophthalmos* occurs when the eyelids and associated structures form but fail to separate *(ankyloblepharon)*.

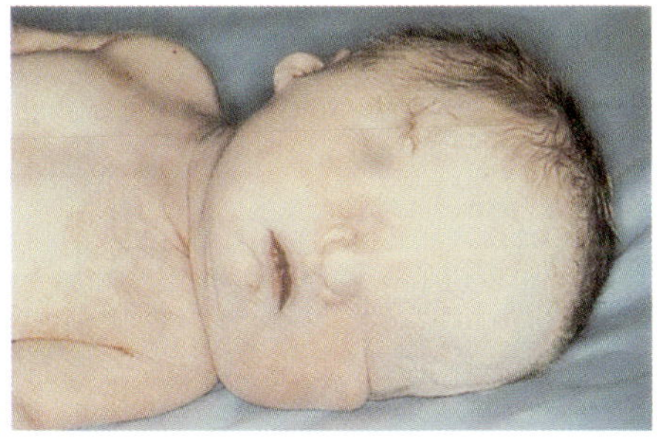

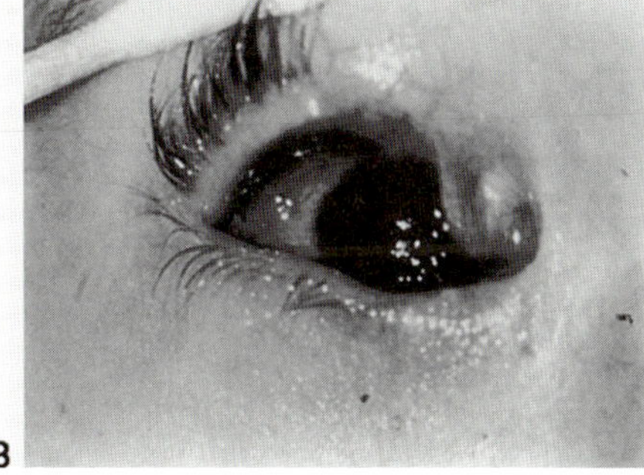

Figure 13-1 **A,** Complete cryptophthalmos, both eyes. **B,** Incomplete cryptophthalmos of the right eye, with eyelid fused to cornea superonasally.

PATHOGENESIS The pathogenesis of this syndrome is unknown. The inward migration of all three waves of neural crest cells fails to occur. Similarities with maternal hypovitaminosis A in animal models suggest that pathogenesis may be related to retinoic acid metabolism.

CLINICAL FINDINGS Cryptophthalmos demonstrates equal sex distribution and equal occurrence in male and female siblings, consanguinity in families with more than one affected child, and lack of vertical transmission—strongly suggesting autosomal recessive inheritance. Ocular findings include the following:

- Dermoid transformation of the cornea and conjunctiva into skin
- Absence of the eyelid structures, lacrimal glands, and canaliculi
- Absence or transformation into connective tissue of the iris, Schlemm's canal, trabecular meshwork, anterior chamber, and lens

Cryptophthalmos syndrome includes any nonocular malformation associated with cryptophthalmos. Fraser syndrome (cryptophthalmos-syndactyly) may occur with anophthalmos and normal eyelids and, frequently, renal agenesis.

MANAGEMENT Cryptophthalmos requires surgical intervention only for cosmesis or relief of pain from absolute glaucoma. Pseudocryptophthalmos may benefit from eyelid separation, but ongoing management of the reconstructed eyelids to prevent secondary complications is necessary.

Microphthalmos

Microphthalmos is a small disorganized globe (Fig 13-2). There is often an associated cystic outpouching of the posteroinferior sclera. This condition has been associated with failure of the fetal fissure to close properly, and colobomatous defects of the iris, ciliary body, uvea, and optic nerve are often present.

PATHOGENESIS Normal embryonic development proceeds through at least the formation of the optic vesicle. Multiple associations have been made with microphthalmos, including trisomies of almost every chromosome (typically trisomy 13), maternal infections, and exposure to toxins and radiation. Autosomal dominant, recessive, and X-linked modes of inheritance have been observed. Terminal deletion with a breakpoint at Xp22.2 is lethal for males. One family is confirmed to have a translocation of the short arm of chromosome 16 [t(2;16)(p22.3;p13.3)].

CLINICAL FINDINGS Associated ocular abnormalities may include leukomas, anterior segment disorders, retinal dysplasia, colobomas, cysts, marked internal dysgenesis, persistent fetal vasculature (PFV), small orbit, ptosis, and blepharophimosis. Systemic associations are numerous, including mental retardation and dwarfism among many others.

MANAGEMENT Associated conditions should be sought and managed appropriately, and genetic counseling should be considered. A cosmetic shell or contact lens may be indicated in selected patients.

Goldberg MF. Persistent fetal vasculature (PFV): an integrated interpretation of signs and symptoms associated with persistent hyperplastic primary vitreous (PHPV). LIV Edward Jackson Memorial Lecture. *Am J Ophthalmol.* 1997;124:587–626.

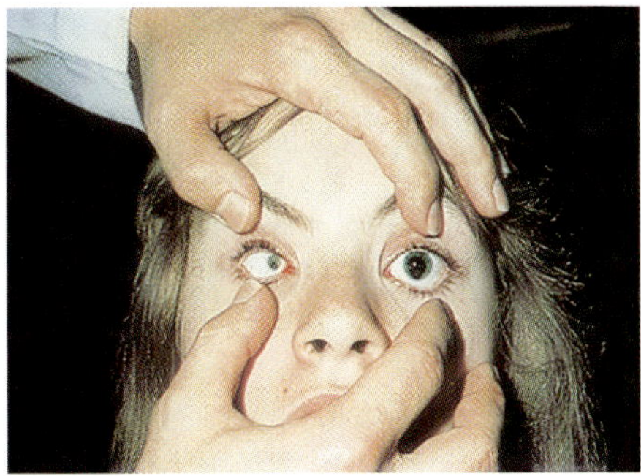

Figure 13-2 Severe microcornea and microphthalmos OD. Both irides are colobomatous.

Nanophthalmos

Nanophthalmos is characterized by a small, functional eye with relatively normal internal organization and proportions. Patients have a high degree of hyperopia (7–15 diopters) due to a short axial length (15–20 mm). Patients also have a high lens-to-eye volume ratio that can lead to crowding of the anterior segment and angle-closure glaucoma.

PATHOGENESIS The cause of this condition is unknown, and both autosomal dominant (nanophthalmos 1) and autosomal recessive (nanophthalmos 2) inheritance patterns have been reported. One gene locus for the autosomal dominant form has been mapped to chromosome arm 11p. The recessive form of the disease has been mapped to chromosome arm 15q.

CLINICAL FINDINGS Patients have high axial hyperopia, narrow palpebral fissures, thickened sclera, and crowded anterior segments associated with angle-closure glaucoma. Peripheral choroidal effusion can occur spontaneously. Large choroidal effusions or hemorrhage have been frequently encountered during anterior segment surgery, possibly secondary to impaired venous outflow through the vortex veins as a result of scleral inelasticity.

MANAGEMENT Hyperopia and glaucoma are managed medically. Peripheral laser iridotomy sometimes combined with peripheral laser iridoplasty may be effective treatment of the angle-closure component. Cataract surgery may be complicated by uveal effusion or hemorrhage and exudative retinal detachment unless full-thickness sclerectomies are carried out in all four quadrants. Extremely high intraocular lens powers are required to achieve emmetropia.

Yamani A, Wood I, Sugino I, et al. Abnormal collagen fibrils in nanophthalmos: a clinical and histologic study. *Am J Ophthalmol.* 1999;127:106–108.

Blue Sclera

The striking clinical picture of blue sclera is related to generalized scleral thinning, with increased visibility of underlying uvea. This anomaly must be distinguished from the slate gray appearance of ocular melanosis bulbi and from acquired causes of scleral thinning such as rheumatoid arthritis or staining from minocycline treatment.

PATHOGENESIS Genetic mutations and altered proteins have been identified for two syndromes associated with blue sclera:

- *Osteogenesis imperfecta type I* is a somewhat common, dominantly inherited, generalized connective tissue disorder characterized mainly by bone fragility and blue sclerae. "Functional null" alleles of *COL1A1* on chromosome 17 or *COL1A2* on chromosome 7 lead to reduced amounts of normal type I collagen in most cases.
- *Ehlers-Danlos syndrome type VI (EDS VI)* is a somewhat rare syndrome with autosomal recessive inheritance characterized by joint hyperextensibility, moderate to severe kyphoscoliosis, cardiac anomalies, and skin abnormalities of easy bruisability, abnormal scarring, and soft distensibility. EDS VI is associated with molecular defects in the gene for lysyl hydroxylase *(PLOD)* on 1p36.3–p36.2 in some patients.
- A third syndrome of brittle cornea, blue sclera, keratoglobus, and joint hyperextensibility may be the same as EDS VI with a normal level of lysyl hydroxylase.

CLINICAL FINDINGS All three syndromes may share similar manifestations of fractures from minor trauma in childhood, kyphoscoliosis, joint extensibility, and elastic skin. Decreased hearing and tinnitus may also occur.

MANAGEMENT Regular hearing evaluations after adolescence are recommended. Postmenopausal women should engage in a long-term physical therapy program to strengthen the paraspinal muscles. Estrogen and progesterone replacement, adequate calcium intake, and perhaps calcitonin or fluoride may be specifically indicated for these patients. Fractures are treated with standard methods. See also Chapter 15.

Abnormalities of Size and Shape of the Cornea

Microcornea

Microcornea is a somewhat common condition that refers to a clear cornea of normal thickness whose diameter is less than 10 mm (or 9 mm in a newborn). If the whole anterior segment is small, the term *anterior microphthalmos* applies. If the entire eye is small and malformed, the term *microphthalmos* is used in contrast to *nanophthalmos*, in which the eye is small but otherwise normal.

PATHOGENESIS Cause is unknown and may be related to fetal arrest of growth of the cornea in the fifth month. Alternatively, it may be related to overgrowth of the anterior tips of the optic cup, which leaves less space for the cornea to develop.

CLINICAL FINDINGS Microcornea may be transmitted as an autosomal dominant or recessive trait with equal sex predilection. Dominant transmission is more common. Because their corneas are relatively flat, patients with microcornea are usually hyperopic and have a higher incidence of angle-closure glaucoma. Of patients who avoid angle-closure glaucoma, 20% develop open-angle glaucoma later in life. Important ocular anomalies often associated with microcornea include persistent fetal vasculature, congenital cataracts, anterior segment dysgenesis, and optic nerve hypoplasia. Significant systemic associations include myotonic dystrophy, fetal alcohol syndrome, achondroplasia, and Ehlers-Danlos syndrome.

MANAGEMENT If microcornea occurs as an isolated finding, the patient has an excellent visual prognosis with spectacles to treat the hyperopia resulting from the flat cornea. Concurrent ocular pathology such as cataract, persistent fetal vasculature, and glaucoma may require treatment following the usual procedures for those conditions.

Megalocornea

This rare, X-linked condition is a nonprogressive corneal enlargement. Affected subjects have histologically normal corneas measuring 13.0–16.5 mm in diameter (Fig 13-3). Males are more typically affected, but heterozygous women may demonstrate a slight increase in corneal diameter.

PATHOGENESIS The cornea has normal thickness, endothelial cell count, and clarity but may be steeper keratometrically. The etiology may be related to failure of the optic cup to grow and of its anterior tips to close, leaving a larger space for the cornea to fill. Alternatively, megalocornea may represent arrested buphthalmos and exaggerated growth of the cornea in relation to the rest of the eye. An abnormality in collagen production is suggested by the association of megalocornea with systemic disorders of collagen synthesis. The gene locus has been identified at Xq21.3–q22.

CLINICAL FINDINGS Megalocornea may be associated with iris translucency (diaphany), miosis, microcoria, goniodysgenesis, cataract, ectopia lentis, arcus juvenilis, mosaic corneal dystrophy (central cloudy dystrophy of François) (Fig 13-4), and glaucoma (but not congenital glaucoma). It is usually bilateral and X-linked recessive. Sporadic, autosomal recessive, and autosomal dominant cases have also been reported.

Systemic associations include craniosynostosis, frontal bossing, hypertelorism, facial anomalies, dwarfism, facial hemiatrophy, mental retardation, hypotonia, Down syndrome, Marfan syndrome, Alport syndrome, osteogenesis imperfecta, mucolipidosis type II, or occasionally other genetic syndromes. Anterior megalophthalmos is the most common familial form of megalocornea, which includes bilateral megalocornea; ciliary ring enlargement; and secondary effects of iridodonesis, miosis, atrophy of iris stroma, and, frequently, cataractous lens.

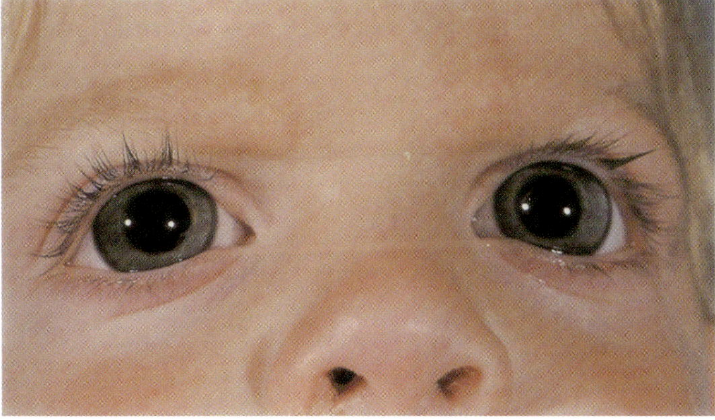

Figure 13-3 Megalocornea.

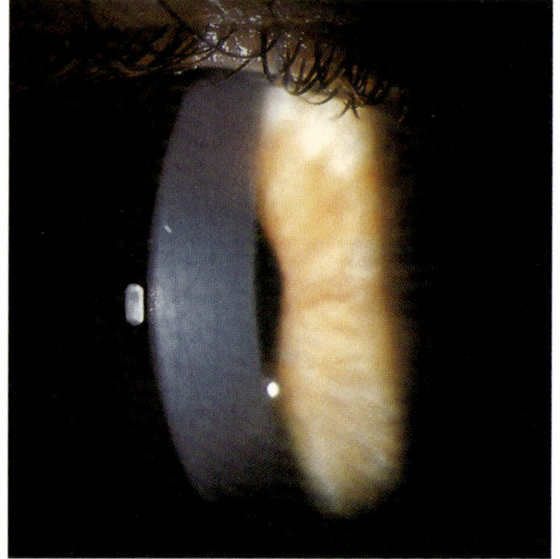

Figure 13-4 Central cloudy dystrophy of François in megalocornea.

MANAGEMENT Congenital glaucoma must be ruled out by intraocular pressure testing and careful biomicroscopy. Ultrasonography may be of value in determining the short vitreous length, deep lens and iris position, and normal axial length that distinguish megalocornea from buphthalmos caused by congenital glaucoma. Myopia and with-the-rule astigmatism are managed as in unaffected patients. Care must be taken during cataract surgery to implant the intraocular lens into the lens capsular bag. Standard-sized posterior chamber lenses are typically too short to be fixated in the ciliary sulcus, and anterior chamber lenses are similarly problematic in the enlarged anterior chamber.

Mackey DA, Buttery RG, Wise GM, et al. Description of X-linked megalocornea with identification of the gene locus. *Arch Ophthalmol.* 1991;109:829–833.

Cornea Plana

Cornea plana is a rare condition that refers to a flat cornea, where the radius of curvature is less than 43 diopters (D), and readings of 20–30 D are common. Corneal curvature that is the same as the adjacent sclera is pathognomonic. Sclerocornea also features flat corneas, but it is distinguished by the loss of transparency as well (see Figure 13-10).

PATHOGENESIS Similar to sclerocornea, the second wave of neural crest cells between weeks 7 and 10 fails to form the limbal anlage and differentiates into tissue resembling sclera instead of corneal stroma. The absence of the limbus is associated with failure of the corneal curve to develop.

CLINICAL FINDINGS Cornea plana is often seen in association with sclerocornea or microcornea. Other associated ocular or systemic abnormalities include cataracts, anterior and posterior colobomas, or Ehlers-Danlos syndrome. Cornea plana usually produces hyperopia, but any type of refractive error may be present because of variations in globe size. Angle-closure glaucoma occurs because of a morphologically shallow anterior chamber, and open-angle glaucoma occurs because of angle abnormalities. Both dominant and the more severe recessive forms exist. Three fourths of isolated cases appear in

Finnish patients, with both the autosomal recessive and dominant forms linked to chromosome arm 12q21 (*CNA2* locus).

MANAGEMENT Refractive errors are neutralized and glaucoma must be considered. Loss of central clarity may indicate penetrating keratoplasty, but cornea plana increases the risk of graft rejection and postkeratoplasty glaucoma.

Keratectasia and Congenital Anterior Staphyloma

Keratectasia and congenital anterior staphyloma are very rare unilateral conditions that are both characterized by protrusion of the opaque cornea between the eyelids at birth. They differ only in the presence of a uveal lining of the cornea in congenital anterior staphyloma.

PATHOGENESIS Intrauterine perforation from an infection or from thinning following secondary failure of neural crest cell migration results in dermoid transformation of the cornea to stratified squamous epithelium, sparing the eyelids and conjunctiva. Keratectasia is probably not the result of abnormal development but rather intrauterine keratitis or vitamin deficiency and subsequent corneal perforation. Histopathologically, Descemet's membrane and endothelium are absent, and a uveal lining is present (except in keratectasia). The cornea is variably thinned and scarred and the anterior segment disorganized, with the lens occasionally adherent to the posterior cornea, resembling unilateral Peters anomaly.

CLINICAL FINDINGS An opaque, bulging cornea is accompanied by a deep anterior segment. These cases are typically unilateral, and all are sporadic, with no familial or systemic association.

MANAGEMENT Except in very mild cases, visual prognosis is poor because of associated severe damage to the anterior segment. Penetrating keratoplasty is rarely warranted, and enucleation may be required for a blind, glaucomatous, painful eye.

Dysgenesis of the Anterior Segment

Abnormalities of Corneal Structure and/or Clarity

Posterior embryotoxon

This condition involves a thickened and centrally displaced anterior border ring of Schwalbe. Schwalbe's ring represents the junction of the trabecular meshwork with the termination of Descemet's membrane, and it is visible in 8%–30% of normal eyes as an irregular, opaque ridge 0.5–2.0 mm central to the limbus. The term *posterior embryotoxon* is used when Schwalbe's ring is visible by external examination (Fig 13-5). Posterior embryotoxon is usually inherited as a dominant trait. The eye is usually normal but can manifest a number of other anterior segment anomalies that are part of ocular or systemic syndromes, such as Alagille syndrome (arteriohepatic dysplasia), X-linked ichthyosis, and familial aniridia.

Axenfeld-Rieger syndrome

The conditions previously referred to as *Axenfeld anomaly* and *syndrome* and *Rieger anomaly* and *syndrome* have overlapping findings and have now been grouped into a single entity known as *Axenfeld-Rieger syndrome*. This syndrome represents a spectrum of disorders characterized by an anteriorly displaced Schwalbe's ring (posterior embryotoxon) with attached iris strands, iris hypoplasia, and glaucoma in 50% of the cases occurring in late childhood or in adulthood (Fig 13-6). Associated skeletal, cranial, facial, and dental abnormalities are often present.

Transmission is usually dominant (75%) for the Axenfeld-Rieger group, but it can be sporadic. Evidence suggests that a spectrum of mutations of transcription factors located in chromosome region 6p25, known as forkhead genes, are responsible for many developmental defects of the anterior chamber of the eye. (See BCSC Section 2, *Fundamentals and Principles of Ophthalmology*, Part III, Genetics.)

Nishimura DY, Searby CC, Alward WL, et al. A spectrum of FOXC1 mutations suggests gene dosage as a mechanism for developmental defects of the anterior chamber of the eye. *Am J Hum Genet.* 2001;68:364–372.

Peters anomaly

Peters anomaly is a central corneal opacity present at birth that is often associated with focal areas of iridocorneal adhesion extending from the region of the iris collarette to the border of the opacity (Fig 13-7). Approximately 60% of cases are bilateral. Associated ocular abnormalities are present in approximately 50% of cases. Ocular abnormalities include keratolenticular touch, cataract, congenital glaucoma, microcornea, aniridia, and persistent fetal vasculature. Characteristic histopathologic findings in Peters anomaly include a localized absence of the corneal endothelium and Descemet's membrane beneath the area of opacity.

Peters anomaly has been associated with systemic malformations in up to 60% of patients. These abnormalities include developmental delay, heart defects, external ear abnormalities, hearing loss, CNS deficits, spinal defects, gastrointestinal and genitourinary defects, facial clefts, and skeletal anomalies. Although systemic malformations may be associated with genetically transmitted syndromes (trisomy 13–15, Peters-plus syndrome, Kivlin syndrome, Pfeiffer syndrome), these associations are the exception rather than the rule.

Most cases of Peters anomaly occur sporadically; however, both autosomal recessive and dominant modes of inheritance have been reported. Mutations at the *PAX6* gene on chromosome 11 are found in heterogeneous anterior segment malformations, including Peters anomaly.

Kivlin JD, Apple DJ, Olson RJ, et al. Dominantly inherited keratitis. *Arch Ophthalmol.* 1986;104:1621–1623.

Traboulsi EI, Maumenee IH. Peters' anomaly and associated congenital malformations. *Arch Ophthalmol.* 1992;110:1739–1742.

Circumscribed posterior keratoconus

The presence of a localized central or paracentral indentation of the posterior cornea without any protrusion of the anterior surface, as is seen in typical keratoconus, char-

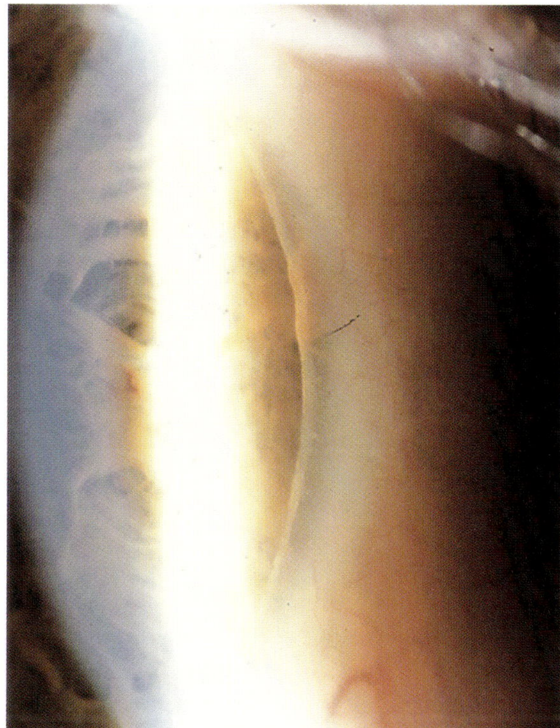

Figure 13-5 Posterior embryotoxon displaying a prominent and anteriorly displaced Schwalbe's ring.

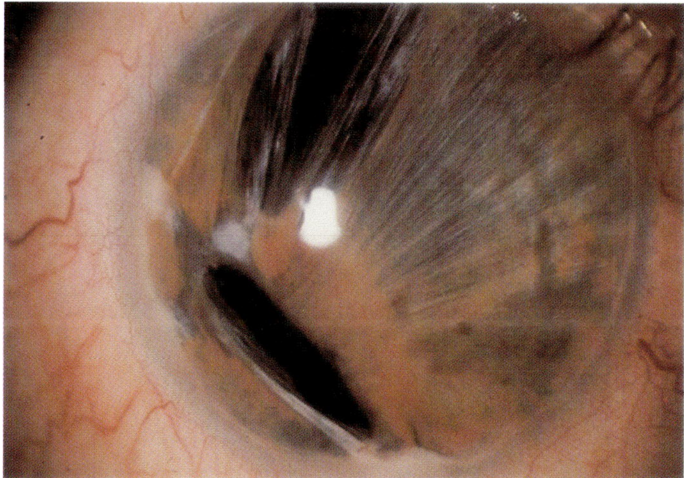

Figure 13-6 Axenfeld-Rieger syndrome exhibiting iris atrophy, corectopia, and pseudopolycoria. *(Photograph courtesy of Vincent P. deLuise, MD.)*

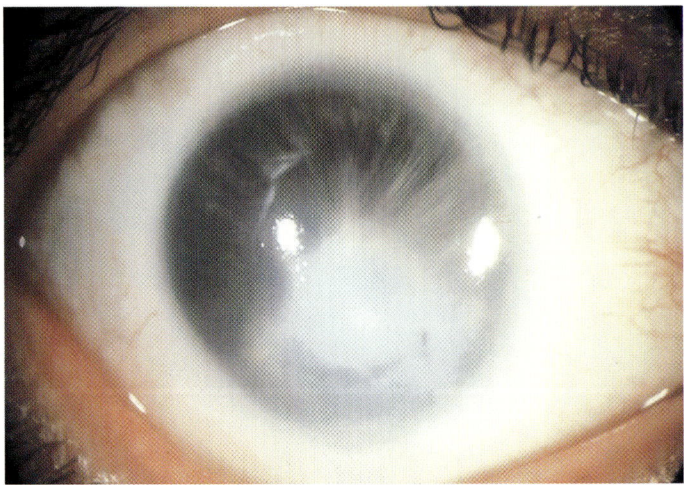

Figure 13-7 Peters anomaly.

acterizes circumscribed posterior keratoconus. A variable amount of overlying stromal haze is also usually present. Loss of stromal substance can lead to corneal thinning approaching one third of normal (Figs 13-8, 13-9) Descemet's membrane and endothelium are usually present in the area of defect. Focal deposits of pigmentation and guttae are often present at the margins of the opacity. Most cases are unilateral, nonprogressive, and sporadic. Astigmatism and/or amblyopia may occur.

Arcus juvenilis

This deposition of lipid in the peripheral corneal stroma occasionally occurs as a congenital anomaly. Usually the condition involves only a sector of the peripheral cornea and is not associated with abnormalities of serum lipid.

Sclerocornea

This nonprogressive, noninflammatory scleralization of the cornea may be limited to the corneal periphery, or the entire cornea may be involved. The limbus is usually ill-defined, and superficial vessels that are extensions of normal scleral, episcleral, and conjunctival vessels cross the cornea (Fig 13-10). The most common associated ocular finding is cornea plana, which occurs in 80% of cases. Angle structures are also commonly malformed. No sex predilection is evident, and 90% of cases are bilateral. Multiple systemic anomalies have been reported in association with sclerocornea.

Sclerocornea is usually sporadic, but both autosomal dominant and recessive patterns of inheritance have been reported.

Congenital hereditary stromal dystrophy (CHSD)

This extremely rare dominant stationary dystrophy presents at birth with bilateral central superficial corneal clouding. The anterior corneal stroma exhibits an ill-defined flaky or feathery appearance. The cornea is clear peripherally. No edema, photophobia, or tearing occurs, but the opacities can be sufficiently dense to cause a reduction in vision.

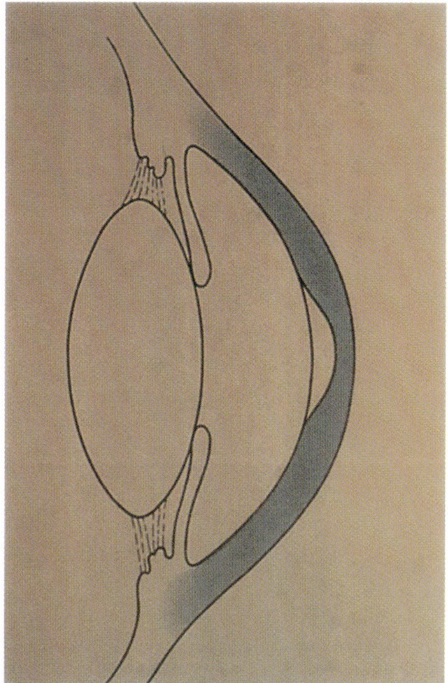

Figure 13-8 Circumscribed posterior keratoconus. Schematic diagram shows loss of central stromal thickness, normal anterior corneal curvature, and a central posterior corneal crater.

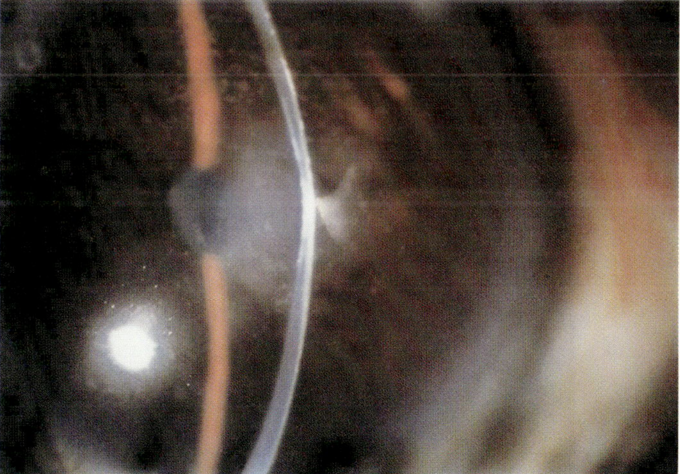

Figure 13-9 Circumscribed posterior keratoconus. A slit-lamp photograph shows loss of stromal thickness, stromal haze, and posterior corneal crater.

Posterior amorphous corneal dystrophy

This very rare autosomal dominant stromal dystrophy is bilaterally symmetrical. It appears early in life and may be congenital. Examination reveals diffuse gray-white, sheetlike stromal opacities concentrated in the posterior stroma. Although the central cornea is

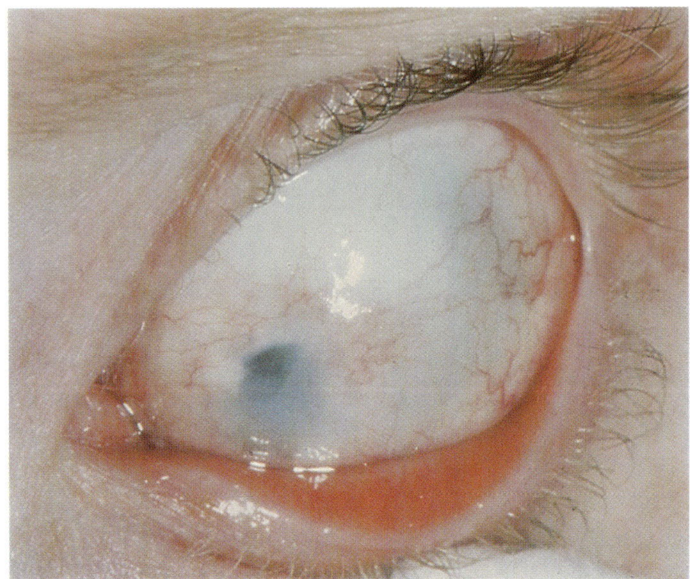

Figure 13-10 Sclerocornea.

most heavily involved, the lesions extend to the limbus. The epithelium appears normal, but Descemet's membrane shows involvement, with focal areas of endothelial disruption. Other findings include central corneal thinning, hyperopia, flattened corneal topography, anterior iris abnormalities, and fine iris processes extending to Schwalbe's line for 360°. A peripheral variant features a clear central cornea, but these patients do not show the iris processes. The dystrophy is either nonprogressive or slowly progressive. The corneal thinning produces little irregular astigmatism, and visual acuity remains good.

Dunn SP, Krachmer JH, Ching SS. New findings in posterior amorphous corneal dystrophy. *Arch Ophthalmol.* 1984;102:236–239.

Congenital hereditary endothelial dystrophy (CHED)

CHED is a cause of bilateral congenital corneal edema, but more common causes such as birth trauma and congenital glaucoma must be ruled out. Two forms of CHED are recognized. The more common autosomal recessive type (CHED 2) presents at birth, remains stationary, and is accompanied by nystagmus. The bluish white cornea may be two to three times normal thickness and have a ground-glass appearance, but this finding is not associated with tearing or photophobia. There may be diffuse nonbullous epithelial edema. A uniform thickening of Descemet's membrane may be seen, but no guttate changes are present.

The dominant form (CHED 1) presents in the first or second year of life, although expressivity is variable. It is slowly progressive and accompanied by pain, photophobia, and tearing, but nystagmus is not present. The cornea exhibits a diffuse, blue-gray, ground-glass appearance (Fig 13-11). The primary abnormality is thought to be a degeneration of endothelial cells during or after the fifth month of gestation.

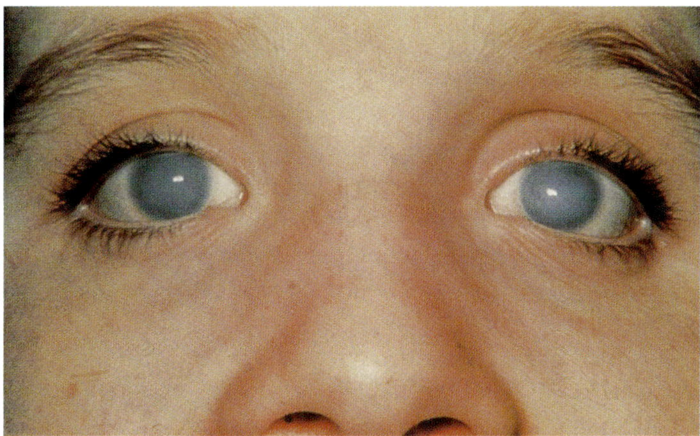

Figure 13-11 Congenital hereditary endothelial dystrophy.

Both forms of CHED are thought to be examples of anterior segment dysgenesis, probably caused by abnormal differentiation of neural crest ectoderm that forms corneal endothelium. CHED has no consistent associations with other systemic abnormalities, although axial myopia is common in these patients. Its gene locus is mapped to the pericentric region of chromosome 20 (20p11.2–q11.2).

Congenital Corneal Opacities in Hereditary Syndromes and Chromosomal Aberrations

Mucopolysaccharidoses (MPS) and *mucolipidoses* are disorders caused by abnormal carbohydrate metabolism. Corneal clouding and haziness may be present in early life in varying degrees in many of these entities, including Scheie syndrome (MPS IS) and Hurler syndrome (MPS IH). A more detailed discussion of these conditions appears in Chapter 15.

Secondary Abnormalities Affecting the Fetal Cornea

Intrauterine Keratitis: Bacterial and Syphilitic

Maternally transmitted congenital infections can cause ocular damage in several different ways:

- Through direct action of the infecting agent, which damages tissue
- Through a teratogenic effect resulting in malformation
- Through a delayed reactivation of the agent after birth, with inflammation that damages developed tissue

A posterior corneal defect called *von Hippel internal corneal ulcer* may follow intrauterine inflammation. Often, signs of inflammation may still be present after birth, including corneal infiltrates and vascularization, keratic precipitates, and uveitis. The iris adhesions are extensive and may arise from areas apart from the collarette; the lens is usually involved. Corneal ulcers and endophthalmitis were common complications of gonococcal ophthalmia neonatorum before the widespread use of silver nitrate prophylaxis and antibiotics. Neonatal conjunctivitis is discussed in Chapter 7.

Congenitally acquired syphilis infections caused by the *Treponema pallidum* spirochete can lead to fetal death or premature delivery. A variety of systemic manifestations have been described. *Interstitial keratitis* can develop in the first decade of life in children with untreated congenital syphilis. It presents as a rapidly progressive corneal edema followed by abnormal vascularization in the deep stroma adjacent to Descemet's membrane. The cornea may assume a salmon pink color because of intense vascularization, giving rise to the term *salmon patch*. Over several weeks to months, blood flow through these vessels gradually ceases, leaving empty "ghost" vessels in the corneal stroma. (See Chapter 9 for a more complete discussion of interstitial keratitis.)

Congenital Corneal Keloid

Corneal keloids are relatively rare lesions most commonly described following corneal perforation or trauma. Congenital corneal keloids, often bilateral, have been described in Lowe disease (oculocerebrorenal syndrome) and the ACL syndrome (acromegaly, cutis gyrata, cornea leukoma syndrome). They can be seen in association with cataracts, aniridia, and glaucoma and may represent a developmental anomaly with failure of normal differentiation of corneal tissue. Histopathologic examination reveals thick collagenase bundles haphazardly arranged, with focal areas of myofibroblastic proliferation. Autosomal dominant inheritance has been observed in the ACL syndrome. Acquired corneal keloid is discussed in Chapter 17.

Congenital Corneal Anesthesia

Congenital corneal anesthesia is a rare condition that is difficult to diagnose. Most cases are bilateral and present with painless corneal opacities and sterile epithelial ulcerations during infancy and childhood. A thorough systemic examination, including neuroradiologic studies, should be carried out in order to rule out associated systemic conditions. Congenital cornea anesthesia has been associated with congenital mesenchymal anomalies, congenital trigeminal hypoplasia, and diffuse brain stem anomalies. Treatment should include frequent topical lubrication, nighttime lid splinting, and, in some cases, lateral tarsorrhaphy.

Mathen MM, Vishnu S, Prajna NV, et al. Congenital corneal anesthesia: a series of four case reports. *Cornea.* 2001;20:194–196.

Congenital Glaucoma

Primary congenital glaucoma is evident either at birth or within the first few years of life. It is believed to be caused by dysplasia of the anterior chamber angle without other ocular or systemic abnormalities. Characteristic findings in the newborn include the triad of epiphora, photophobia, and blepharospasm. External eye examination may reveal buphthalmos, with corneal enlargement greater than 12 mm in diameter during the first year of life. (The normal horizontal corneal diameter is 9.5–10.5 in full-term infants.)

Corneal edema is present in 25% of affected infants at birth and in more than 60% by the sixth month. It may range from mild haze to dense opacification in the corneal stroma because of elevated IOP. Tears in Descemet's membrane called *Haab's striae* may occur acutely as a result of corneal stretching. They are typically oriented horizontally or concentric to the limbus. BCSC Section 6, *Pediatric Ophthalmology and Strabismus*, also discusses pediatric glaucoma.

Birth Trauma

Progressive corneal edema developing during the first few postnatal days, accompanied by vertical or oblique posterior striae, may be caused by birth trauma (Fig 13-12). Ruptures occur in Descemet's membrane and the endothelium. Healing usually takes place, leaving a hypertrophic ridge of Descemet's membrane. The edema may or may not clear; if it does clear, the cornea can again become edematous at any time later in life. High astigmatism and amblyopia may be associated. Congenital glaucoma can present with similar findings and should be considered in the differential diagnosis.

Iridocorneal Endothelial Syndrome (ICE)

Iridocorneal endothelial syndrome is a spectrum of disorders characterized by varying degrees of corneal edema, glaucoma, and iris abnormalities (Fig 13-13).

PATHOGENESIS The pathogenesis of ICE syndrome is unknown but appears to involve an abnormal clone of endothelial cells that takes on the ultrastructural characteristics of epithelial cells. The condition appears to represent an acquired maldifferentiation of a group of endothelial cells, although the abnormal clone could originate at birth or before. Varying degrees of endothelialization take place in the anterior chamber angle and on the iris surface. Herpesvirus DNA has been identified in some corneal specimens following keratoplasty and in the aqueous humor of some patients. This raises the intriguing possibility that a herpes simplex virus infection may induce these changes.

CLINICAL FINDINGS When the pathology is confined to the inner corneal surface, corneal edema may result from subnormal endothelial pump function, producing the Chandler variant of ICE syndrome. Frequently, the border between the abnormal and normal endothelium can be seen at the slit lamp using specular reflection. When the abnormal endothelium migrates over the anterior chamber angle, the resultant peripheral anterior synechiae and outflow obstruction produce glaucoma. When the abnormal endothelium spreads onto the surface of the iris, the resulting contractile membrane may produce iris atrophy, corectopia, and polycoria, hallmarks of the essential iris atrophy variant of ICE syndrome. The Cogan–Reese (or iris nevus) variant shows multiple pigmented iris nodules, also produced by the contracting endothelial membrane.

This congenital syndrome becomes apparent most commonly in middle-aged females and is almost always unilateral. Asymmetric posterior polymorphous dystrophy, as well as other causes of unilateral corneal edema, must be included in the differential diagnosis of ICE syndrome.

MANAGEMENT Penetrating keratoplasty is an effective treatment for the corneal component of this syndrome. Glaucoma is an important feature of the ICE syndrome. Long-

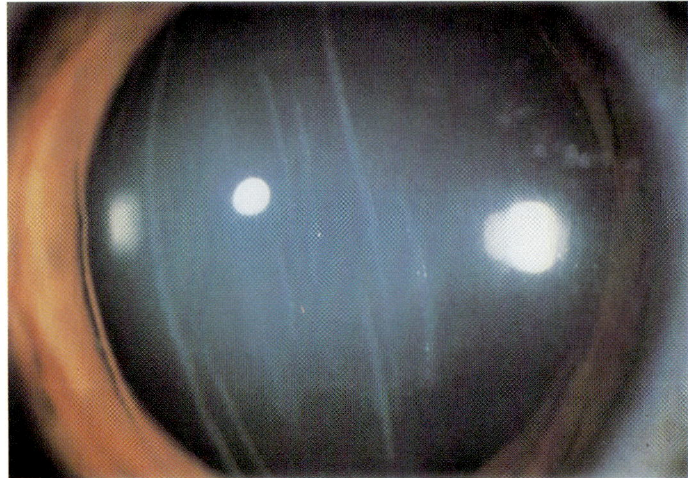

Figure 13-12 Birth trauma demonstrating vertical ruptures of Descemet's membrane secondary to traumatic delivery. *(Photograph courtesy of Vincent P. deLuise, MD.)*

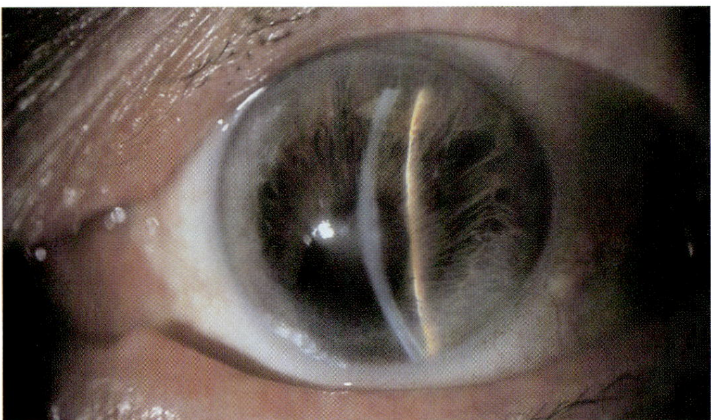

Figure 13-13 Iridocorneal endothelial syndrome with corectopia.

term graft clarity depends on the successful control of IOP, which can be difficult (see BCSC Section 10, *Glaucoma*).

Alvarado JA, Underwood JL, Green WR, et al. Detection of herpes simplex viral DNA in the iridocorneal endothelial syndrome. *Arch Ophthalmol.* 1994;112:1601–1609.

Patel A, Kenyon KR, Hirst LW, et al. Clinicopathologic features of Chandler's syndrome. *Surv Ophthalmol.* 1983;27:327–344.

Corneal Dystrophies and Metabolic Disorders Involving the Conjunctiva, Cornea, and Sclera

CHAPTER 14

Molecular Genetics of Corneal Dystrophies and Metabolic Disorders

This chapter includes an introduction to the genetic basis of disease and its role in diagnosis. See BCSC Section 2, *Fundamentals and Principles of Ophthalmology*, Part III, for a more extensive review of genetics.

Principles of Genetics

Linkage means that a known biochemical (eg, blood type) or genetic marker (eg, polymorphic DNA marker) and phenotype are coinherited and therefore located closely together on the same physical piece of DNA. The mapping of different phenotypes to specific genetic loci (regions of DNA in the genome) has enhanced our understanding of the pathogenesis of many corneal dystrophies and diseases with complex, multifactorial origins. Many diseases have been mapped to specific areas of the genome, and linkages can be used to establish the potential carrier status of parents or siblings. This allows more specific genetic counseling than just assessing risks based on the inheritance patterns of the diseases.

Structure of Chromosomes and Genes

The nuclear material of human cells condenses into chromosomes during cell division. *Chromosomes* are composed primarily of proteins and *deoxyribonucleic acid (DNA)*. DNA is a giant, highly ordered molecule in a double-helical configuration consisting of deoxyribose (5-carbon sugar) molecules linked by phosphates and carrying one nitrogenous base each. The nitrogenous base is either a *purine* (adenine or guanosine) or a *pyrimidine* (thymine or cytosine). An individual sugar-phosphate unit with its nitrogen base is called a *nucleotide (nt)*.

In double-stranded helical DNA, each nitrogen base can form a hydrogen bond only with a specific counterpart: thymine (T) always pairs with adenine (A) and guanine (G) always pairs with cytosine (C), so TA, AT, GC, and CG are the possible combinations. These combinations are known as *base pairs (bp)*. Three billion base pairs make up human DNA. The nucleotides are arranged on each strand in a complementary manner, with a polarity from the 5′ to 3′ ends. A full, double-stranded 7-bp fragment of DNA is written

5′–C T G G C A T–3′
| | | | | | |
3′–G A C C G T A–5′

The genetic code determines the composition of cellular proteins in an elegant manner. The 20 amino acids are the building blocks of proteins, and each amino acid is specified by a grouping of 3 nucleotides (a *codon*) on the chromosome. There are 64 possible combinations of nucleotides, so some amino acids have more than one *codon* (ie, the codon is degenerate).

Ribonucleic acid (RNA) is a second type of nucleic acid found primarily in the cytoplasm. It contains the sugar ribose instead of deoxyribose and substitutes uracil (U) for the thymine nitrogenous base. Single-stranded RNA is formed by the process of *transcription* from double-stranded DNA in the nucleus. The DNA strand has some regions that do not code for protein and some that regulate the coding.

A region of the DNA that is ultimately translated into protein consists of *exons* and *introns*, which are spliced out of the RNA before it leaves the nucleus. Removal of the introns creates *messenger RNA (mRNA)*, the functional blueprint of the genetic code, which leaves the nucleus and goes to the ribosomes. *Transfer RNA (tRNA)* binds to the mRNA in a complementary fashion, aligning the specific amino acids in the correct sequence for protein synthesis.

Genes are the smallest segments of DNA. They contain individual units of information that code for a single trait or a single polypeptide chain. (See BCSC Section 2, *Fundamentals and Principles of Ophthalmology,* Part III.)

Clinical Genetics

More than 8800 human diseases are known to be inherited, and 10%–15% of these are confined to the eye. Another 15% have ocular manifestations. As of this writing, the Human Genome Project has completed the first draft of sequencing the 3.2 billion base pairs in about 30,000 genes that make up the human genome. Not all of the functions of these genes are understood, but knowing the location has significant value both for diagnosis and for possible future linkage to a specific protein or biochemical cause of disease.

Hereditary diseases can be classified by their inheritance patterns:

- Autosomal dominant
- Autosomal recessive
- X-linked
- Y-linked
- Mitochondrial

This classification is based on the chromosomal location and phenotypic behavior of the gene. The *genotype* of an individual refers to the biologic state of that person's genes. The *phenotype* refers to the observable physical, biochemical, molecular, or physiologic characteristics of the individual. These characteristics are determined by the genotype but may be modified by environment, maternal exposures, and other factors. Individuals can have the same phenotype but have very different genotypes (genetic heterogeneity). For example, tyrosinase-positive and tyrosinase-negative albinism have a similar phenotype, but they are not the result of mutations of the same gene. Conversely, different phenotypes may result from mutations in a single gene through a process called *pleiotropism* (phenotypic diversity). For example, mutations in the *BIGH3* (also known as *TGFBI* [transforming growth factor beta–induced]) gene can lead to Reis-Bücklers dystrophy, Thiel-Behnke dystrophy, granular dystrophy, or lattice dystrophy. A *trait* is typically a physical characteristic that distinguishes one individual from another. A *phenocopy* is a clinical picture similar to a given phenotype but is actually the result of environmental causes without the same genotype. For example, congenital rubella retinopathy is a phenocopy of retinitis pigmentosa.

Alleles are alternate forms of a gene at the same locus on each of an identical pair of chromosomes. If the alleles are the same, the individual is *homozygous* for the gene at that locus. If the alleles are distinct from each other, the individual is *heterozygous*. If there is only one allele at a locus, the gene is termed *hemizygous*. *Polymorphisms* are genetic variations that occur at a specific locus with an appreciable frequency in the general population. These sequence variants may not have any appreciable effect on gene function, but they can be useful for mapping the gene through linkage. During meiosis, genes may "cross over" from one chromosome to the other. The likelihood that two genes, two markers of a gene, and a gene and a marker will be separated from one another during such a recombination event is proportional to the distance between them in the genome. Thus, linkage is exploited to create maps of genes and markers by observing the inheritance patterns of markers and disease phenotypes in large numbers of individuals.

A trait is *dominant* if the responsible gene is expressed when only a single copy exists in the chromosomal pair. A trait is *recessive* if the responsible gene can be masked by a normal allele and expressed only when homozygous. A gene is either *penetrant* or *nonpenetrant* depending on whether any phenotypic effect appears in an individual. The fraction of a population with a gene that shows effect is the gene's penetrance.

Online Mendelian Inheritance in Man (OMIM). McKusick-Nathans Institute for Genetic Medicine, Johns Hopkins University (Baltimore, MD) and National Center for Biotechnology Information, National Library of Medicine (Bethesda, MD), 2000. Website updated daily: www.ncbi.nlm.nih.gov/omim.

Diagnostic Approach

Diagnosis of corneal dystrophies and metabolic abnormalities requires suspicion based on symmetry, progression of the disease, and careful family history. Confirmation may come from the typical appearance and clinical course of the disorder or from molecular techniques.

Pedigree Analysis

The family history for ocular and nonocular conditions can be summarized in a pedigree chart that carefully illustrates the *proband* (first person with the recognized disease) and all the relatives available through history and by examination. In the United States in 1990, 28% of babies were born outside legal marriage, and the nonpaternity rate is currently 5%–15%, so delicate questioning may be necessary in obtaining answers about family history. The information obtained is used to determine type of inheritance and to aid in linkage analysis, and it is essential in genetic counseling.

Molecular Biologic Techniques

See BCSC Section 2, *Fundamentals and Principles of Ophthalmology,* Part III, for a more extensive review of molecular biologic techniques.

Several methods are used to determine linkage of a disease to a specific area of a chromosome:

- *Somatic cell hybrid technique* is used to map known human DNA fragments and genes with a known product to a specific locus.
- *In situ hybridization* can also be used to identify the chromosomal location of a gene for which a cloned complementary DNA (cDNA) or a genomic clone is available (rhodopsin was mapped to 3q21 by this method).
- *Deletion* or *duplication mapping* correlates reduced or excess gene product with deficiency or duplication of specific segments of a chromosome (esterase D was assigned to 13q14 because of its association with retinoblastoma patients with this deletion).
- *Linkage disequilibrium* refers to the tendency of specific alleles to occur with specific alleles of another locus on the same chromosome. Polymorphic DNA markers are used as a tool to search for linkage disequilibrium.

Once established, linkage can be useful in predicting candidate genes for a specific defect. When specific genes are known, the point mutation or the resulting protein can be used for diagnosis and for genetic counseling of the family. Linkage can be valuable in diagnosis, even without knowledge of the specific gene or its function.

Determination of point mutations through molecular genetics has dramatically increased with polymerase chain reaction (PCR)–based methods such as single-stranded conformation polymorphism assay, heteroduplex analysis, oligonucleotide ligation assay, and allele-specific priming, just to mention a few.

The first linkage of disease to a human chromosome was the observation that protanopia was linked to the X chromosome. In 1937, hemophilia was observed to be linked to congenital color deficiency, and in 1963, the Coppock cataract was the first autosomal gene to be linked (to the Duffy blood group locus on chromosome 1). Table 14-1 lists corneal dystrophies and conditions with known linkages. Normal keratocytes also acquire various aneuploid cytogenetic abnormalities.

Multiple genes are involved in the morphogenesis and health of the cornea and outer eye. For example, the *PAX6* gene codes for a transcription factor that targets other genes. *PAX6* mutations can thus have multiple effects, including aniridia, Peters anomaly, and

Table 14-1 Linkages of Inherited Corneal Conditions

Condition	Inheritance*	Chromosome (Gene)	Protein Affected
Congenital syndromes, often diagnosed in infants and children			
Alkaptonuria	AR	3q21 (H or O gene)	Homogentisate 1,2-dioxygenase
Aniridia	AD	11p13 *(PAX6)*	PAX6 homeoprotein
Astigmatism	AD	Unknown	Unknown
Autosomal dominant keratitis	AD	11p13 *(PAX6)*	PAX6 homeoprotein
Benign hereditary intraepithelial dyskeratosis	AD	4q35	Unknown
Congenital hereditary corneal dystrophy (CHED1)	AD	20p13	Unknown
Congenital hereditary corneal dystrophy (CHED2)	AR	20	Unknown
Congenital pterygium	AD	Unknown	Unknown
Corneal dermoid	X, AR, AD	x24–1ter	Unknown
Cornea plana	AD	12q *(CNA1)*	Keratocan; mimecan
	AR	12q22 *(CNA2)*	
Cystinosis	AR	17p13 *(CTNS)*	Cystinosin
Darier disease	AD	12q23–q24.1 *(ATP2A2)*	Calcium-ATPase type 2
Ectodermal dysplasia 1	X	Xq12 *(EDA1)*–q13.1	Ectodysplasin-A
Ectodermal dysplasia 2	AD	13q12	Gap junction
Ectodermal dysplasia 3	AD	2q11–q13	Ectodysplasin-A
Ehlers-Danlos syndrome type VIA	AR	1p36.3–p36.2	Unknown, possibly lysyl hydroxylase
Ehlers-Danlos syndrome type VIB	AR	1p36.3–p36.2 . . .	Unknown
Fish eye disease	AR	16q22.1	Apolipoprotein A-I; lecithin-cholesterol acyltransferase
Ichthyosis, X-linked	X	Xp22.32	Steroid sulfatase
Megalocornea	X, AR	Xq21.3–q22	Unknown
Mucopolysaccharidosis type I	AR	4p16 *(IDUA)*	Alpha-L-iduronidase
Multiple endocrine neoplasia type IIB	AD	10q11	Unknown
Pachyonychia congenita type 2	AD	17q	Keratin-17
Peters anomaly	AR, AD	11p13 *(PAX6)*	PAX6 homeoprotein
		4q25–q26	PTX2
		2p22–p21	CYP1B1
		6p25	FOXC1
Sclerocornea	AD, AR	14q32	Unknown
Tyrosinemia type 2	AR	16q22 *(TAT)*	Tyrosine aminotransferase
Xeroderma pigmentosum	AR	3p25 *(XPC)*	Unknown
Corneal dystrophies, usually diagnosed in adolescents and adults			
Corneal epithelial basement membrane dystrophy	AD	Unknown	Unknown
Meesman corneal dystrophy	AD	12q12	Keratin-3 or -12
Reis-Bücklers corneal dystrophy	AD	5q31 *(BIGH3)*†	Keratoepithelin
Thiel-Behnke corneal dystrophy	AD	10q24	Unknown

(Continued)

* *AD = autosomal dominant; AR = autosomal recessive; X = X-linked.*
† *BIGH3 also known as TGFBI.*

Table 14-1 Linkages of Inherited Corneal Conditions (Continued)

Condition	Inheritance*	Chromosome (Gene)	Protein Affected
Granular corneal dystrophy	AD	5q31 *(BIGH3)*	Keratoepithelin
Avellino corneal dystrophy	AD	5q31 *(BIGH3)*	Keratoepithelin
Lattice corneal dystrophy type I	AD	5q31 *(BIGH3)*	Keratoepithelin
Lattice corneal dystrophy type II	AD	9q32–34 *(GSN)*	Gelsolin
Lattice corneal dystrophy type III	AR	5q31 *(BIGH3)*	Keratoepithelin
Lattice corneal dystrophy type IIIA	AD	5q31 *(BIGH3)*	Keratoepithelin
Macular corneal dystrophy type I	AR	16q22	CHST6
Macular corneal dystrophy type II	AR	16q22	CHST6
Gelatinous droplike corneal dystrophy	AR	1p32	M1S1
Schnyder central crystalline dystrophy	AD	1p36	Unknown
Fleck corneal dystrophy	AD	Unknown	Unknown
Central cloudy corneal dystrophy	AD	Unknown	Unknown
Fuchs corneal dystrophy	AD	1p34–p32	COL8A2
Posterior polymorphous corneal dystrophy	AD	20p11.2–q11.2	VSX1
		1p34	COL8A2
Keratoconus (majority of cases are sporadic)	AD	20p11.2	VSX1

* AD = autosomal dominant; AR = autosomal recessive; X = X-linked.
† *BIGH3* also known as *TGFBI.*

congenital cataract. Knowledge of specific mutations enables prenatal counseling and testing and should soon lead to new ways to replace or to correct genetic deficiencies.

Bron AJ. Genetics of the corneal dystrophies: what we have learned in the past twenty-five years. *Cornea.* 2000;19:699–711.

Klintworth GK. Advances in the molecular genetics of corneal dystrophies. *Am J Ophthalmol.* 1999;128:747–754.

Taylor GR, ed. *Laboratory Methods for the Detection of Mutations and Polymorphisms in DNA.* Boca Raton, FL: CRC Press; 1997.

Vincent AL, Rootman D, Munier FL, et al. A molecular perspective on corneal dystrophies. *Dev Ophthalmol.* 2003;37:50–66.

CHAPTER 15

Clinical Approach to Corneal Dystrophies and Metabolic Disorders

A *dystrophy* is a bilateral, symmetric, inherited condition that appears to have little or no relationship to environmental or systemic factors. Dystrophies begin early in life but may not become clinically apparent until later. They tend to be slowly progressive. Corneal dystrophies can be classified according to genetic pattern, severity, histopathologic features, biochemical characteristics, or anatomic location. The anatomic scheme that classifies the dystrophies according to the levels of the cornea that are involved is the one used most often.

> Klintworth GK. Advances in the molecular genetics of corneal dystrophies. *Am J Ophthalmol.* 1999;128:747–754.

Anterior Corneal Dystrophies

Corneal Basement Membrane Dystrophies

Corneal epithelial basement membrane dystrophy (EBMD)

Also known as *map-dot-fingerprint* or *Cogan microcystic dystrophy*, EBMD is the most common anterior corneal dystrophy. It is bilateral and may have dominant inheritance (often with incomplete penetrance) but is more often sporadic. EBMD occurs in 6%–18% of the population, more commonly in women, with increasing frequency over the age of 50 years.

PATHOGENESIS EBMD is an abnormality of epithelial turnover, maturation, and production of basement membrane. Histopathologic findings include the following:

- A thickened basement membrane with extension into the epithelium
- Abnormal epithelial cells with microcysts (often with absent or abnormal hemidesmosomes)
- Fibrillar material between the basement membrane and Bowman's layer

CLINICAL FINDINGS Gray patches, microcysts, and/or fine lines in the central epithelial layer are seen on examination. These are usually best seen with sclerotic scatter, retroillumination, or a broad tangential beam. The findings are quite variable and may change with time. Three kinds of lesions are seen with the epithelium and its immediately subjacent basement membrane:

- Fingerprint lines
- Map lines
- Dots or microcysts

These abnormalities occur in varying combinations and change in number and distribution from time to time. Fingerprint lines are thin, relucent, hairlike lines; several of them are often arranged in a concentric pattern so they resemble fingerprints. Map lines are the same as fingerprint lines except thicker, more irregular, and surrounded by a faint haze; they resemble irregular coastlines or geographic borders on maps (Fig 15-1). Maps and fingerprints consist of thickened or multilaminar strips of epithelial basement membrane. Dots are intraepithelial spaces containing the debris of epithelial cells that have collapsed and degenerated before having reached the epithelial surface (Fig 15-2). The gray-white dots have discrete edges. When they are very prominent, the term *Cogan microcystic dystrophy* may be used.

Symptoms that are related to recurrent epithelial erosions and to transient blurred vision are more common in patients older than 30 but can be seen at any age. It is estimated that 10% of patients with EBMD will have corneal erosions and that 50% of patients with recurrent epithelial erosions have evidence of this anterior dystrophy. Both eyes must be examined because evidence of the dystrophy may be found in the uninvolved eye. In some circumstances, clinical findings may mimic corneal intraepithelial dysplasia, and removed material should be submitted for histopathology.

MANAGEMENT Treatment may need to be extended for months. It consists of varying combinations of the following (see also discussion of recurrent corneal erosions in Chapter 5):

- 5% sodium chloride drops or ointment
- Lubricating drops or ointment
- Epithelial debridement
- Patching
- Fitting of a thin, loose bandage (soft contact) lens

Recalcitrant cases of recurrent corneal erosion may require anterior stromal puncture of the epithelium using a 20- to 25-gauge needle (0.1 mm is sufficient depth). Multiple small punctures disturb Bowman's layer, thereby promoting a tighter adhesion and stimulating the cornea to produce functional basement membrane complexes. The Nd:YAG laser and 5 mm diamond burr have also been reported to be effective in creating anterior stromal disturbance as treatment of recurrent erosion. Removal of damaged epithelium alone may be very effective. Phototherapeutic keratectomy (PTK) with excimer laser into the anterior 2–4 µm of Bowman's membrane after removal of the epithelium may be used for central or recurrent erosions. Recurrence of erosive symptoms after PTK occurs in 13%–44% of patients and may require repetition of PTK.

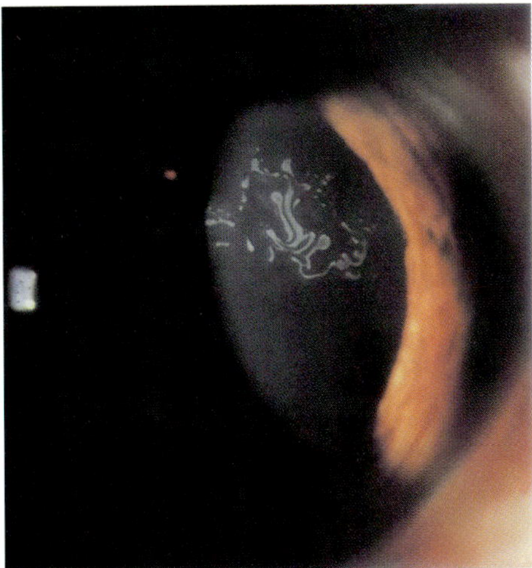

Figure 15-1 Epithelial basement membrane dystrophy, showing thick geographic map lines, or "putty marks." *(Photograph courtesy of Vincent P. deLuise, MD.)*

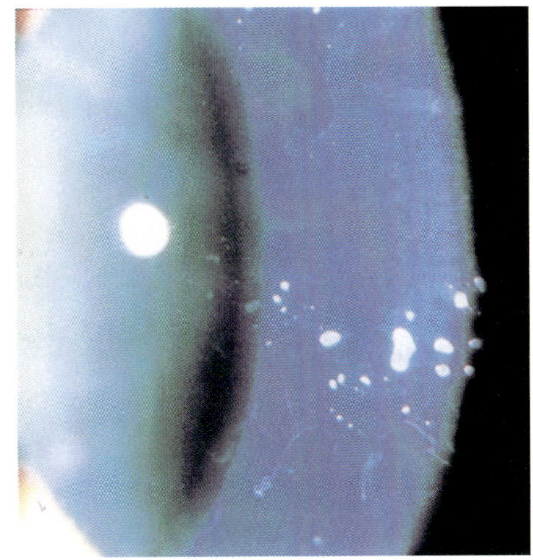

Figure 15-2 EBMD dystrophy, showing microcysts and geographic map line areas. *(Photograph courtesy of Vincent P. deLuise, MD.)*

Dinh R, Rapuano CJ, Cohen EJ, et al. Recurrence of corneal dystrophy after excimer laser phototherapeutic keratectomy. *Ophthalmology.* 1999;106:1490–1497.

Meesmann (juvenile epithelial) dystrophy

This rare bilateral autosomal dominant epithelial dystrophy appears very early in life.

PATHOGENESIS Thickened epithelium and a multilaminar, thickened basement membrane with projections into the basal epithelium are seen. The epithelial cells contain an electron-dense accumulation of "peculiar substance," a fibrillogranular material of unknown composition.

CLINICAL FINDINGS Tiny epithelial vesicles are seen—most easily with retroillumination—extending out to the limbus. They appear as tiny, bubblelike blebs and are most numerous in the interpalpebral area (Fig 15-3). The surrounding epithelium is clear. Whorled and wedge-shaped epithelial patterns have been reported. The cornea may be slightly thinned and corneal sensation may be reduced. Symptoms are limited to mild irritation and a slight decrease in visual acuity.

MANAGEMENT Most patients require no treatment, but soft contact lens wear may be helpful if patients show frequent symptoms. Superficial PTK is useful for reducing symptoms but is rarely required.

Reis-Bücklers dystrophy

This progressive autosomal dominant dystrophy appears in the first few years of life and mainly affects Bowman's layer. Reis-Bücklers dystrophy has been linked to chromosome 5q31 in the same region as granular, lattice, and Avellino (granular-lattice) dystrophies (see the following sections).

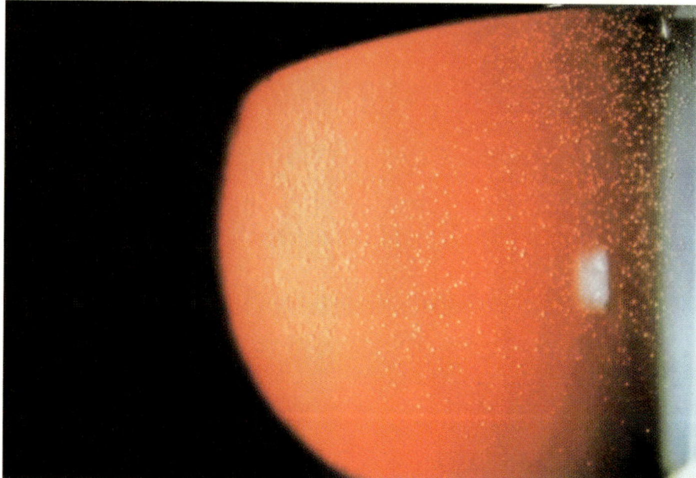

Figure 15-3 Meesmann dystrophy, appearing as tiny, bubblelike blebs against the red reflex. *(Photograph courtesy of Vincent P. deLuise, MD.)*

PATHOGENESIS A mutation occurs in the BIGH3 (human transforming growth factor beta–induced) gene responsible for formation of keratoepithelin, but the exact material accumulating is unknown. Degenerative changes occur in the deep epithelium, but basement membrane is not thickened. Bowman's layer is disrupted or absent and replaced by fibrocellular tissue in an undulating, or "sawtooth," fashion that corresponds clinically to areas of subepithelial opacification.

CLINICAL FINDINGS Biomicroscopy reveals a superficial geographic, or honeycomb, gray-white reticular opacification that is greatest in the central cornea. The posterior cornea appears normal, but in advanced cases the anterior scarring can lead to surface irregularity. Symptoms often begin in the first or second decade with painful recurrent epithelial erosions. Vision is reduced by both anterior scarring with surface irregularity and anterior stromal edema.

LABORATORY EVALUATION Some authors divide corneal dystrophy of Bowman's membrane (CDB) into two types based on the transmission electron microscopic appearance. CDB type I (geographic, or true Reis-Bücklers, dystrophy) has rod-shaped bodies similar to granular dystrophy. CDB type II (honeycomb-shaped, or Thiel-Behnke, dystrophy) has "curly fibers" (see discussion below).

MANAGEMENT Initial treatment is aimed at the recurrent erosions. Superficial keratectomy, lamellar keratoplasty (LK), PTK, or, in rare instances, penetrating keratoplasty (PK) may be performed. Recurrence in the graft is common (Fig 15-4).

Laibson PR. Anterior corneal dystrophies. In: Krachmer JH, Mannis MJ, Holland EJ, eds. *Cornea.* Vol 2. St Louis: Mosby; 1997:1033–1042.

Munier FL, Korvatska E, Djemai A, et al. Kerato-epithelin mutations in four 5q31-linked corneal dystrophies. *Nat Genet.* 1997;15:247–251.

Yee RW, Sullivan LS, Lai HT, et al. Linkage mapping of Thiel-Behnke corneal dystrophy (CDB2) to chromosome 10q23-q24. *Genomics.* 1997;46:152–154.

Thiel-Behnke dystrophy

Thiel-Behnke dystrophy was previously classified as Reis-Bücklers dystrophy type II, with autosomal dominant inheritance and honeycomb opacification of the superficial central cornea. Unlike Reis-Bücklers (CDB type I), Thiel-Behnke dystrophy demonstrates curly fibers on electron microscopy and is linked to chromosome 10q24. Thiel-Behnke may be the more prevalent form of Bowman's layer dystrophy.

Stromal Corneal Dystrophies

Posterior amorphous corneal dystrophy and congenital hereditary stromal dystrophy are discussed in Chapter 13. Conditions related to those discussed in the following section are also described later in this chapter under the heading "Disorders of Protein Metabolism." Table 15-1 provides information on the histopathologic identification of stromal corneal dystrophies.

Granular dystrophy and Avellino dystrophy

Granular dystrophy is one of the three most common stromal dystrophies. Transmission is autosomal dominant and the gene has been linked to chromosome 5q31, along with lattice, Avellino, and Reis-Bücklers dystrophies.

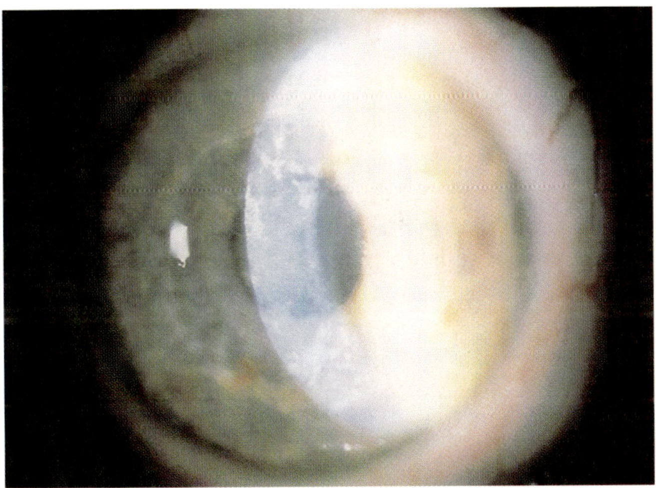

Figure 15-4   Reis-Bücklers corneal dystrophy: recurrence in graft.

Table 15-1 Histopathologic Differentiation of Granular, Macular, and Lattice Dystrophies

Dystrophy	Masson	Alcian Blue	PAS	Amyloid*	Birefringence
Granular	+	−	−	−	−
Macular	−	+	−	−	−
Lattice	+	−	+	+	+

* Stains for amyloid: Congo red, crystal violet, and thioflavine T.

PATHOGENESIS Microscopically, the granular material is hyaline and stains bright red with Masson trichrome stain. An electron-dense material made up of rod-shaped bodies immersed in an amorphous matrix is seen ultrastructurally. Histochemically, the deposits are noncollagenous protein that may derive from the corneal epithelium and/or keratocytes. Although the exact cause is unknown, a mutation different from that in Reis-Bücklers, lattice, and Avellino dystrophies has been identified in the *BIGH3* gene responsible for formation of keratoepithelin. Homozygous cases of R124H mutation found in Avellino dystrophy may develop juvenile corneal opacities significant enough to require keratoplasty.

CLINICAL FINDINGS Three clinical forms are identified, but all have the same electron microscopic features. *Type I* is most frequent and corresponds to Groenouw dystrophy type I. Onset occurs early in life with crumblike opacities that broaden into a disciform appearance as the patient reaches the teens. The lesions do not extend to the limbus but can extend anteriorly through focal breaks in Bowman's layer (Fig 15-5). The dystrophy is slowly progressive, with vision only rarely dropping to 20/200 after age 40. *Type II* presents in the second decade, with fewer, larger ring- or disc-shaped granular deposits in the anterior stroma, sharply defined by intervening clear areas. The deposits can be found progressively deeper as the patient ages. Erosions are infrequent and vision is usually better than 20/70. *Type III* is more superficial and presents in infancy with erosions. Fine granular deposits are confined to Bowman's layer or anterior stroma. This form clinically resembles Reis-Bücklers dystrophy and has a distinct mutation of the *BIGH3* gene.

Avellino corneal dystrophy, a variant of granular dystrophy, was originally described in a small number of families who traced their roots to Avellino, Italy. The affected patients have a granular dystrophy both histologically and clinically. Lattice lesions are also present in some patients. Older patients have anterior stromal haze between deposits, which reduces visual acuity. Pathologically, both the hyaline deposits typical of granular

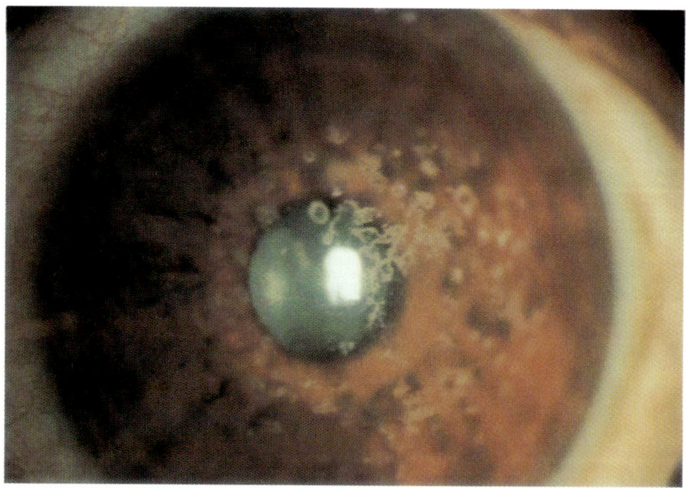

Figure 15-5 Granular dystrophy.

dystrophy and the amyloid deposits typical of lattice dystrophy (see the following section) are seen, and Avellino dystrophy is also known as *granular-lattice dystrophy.*

The relationship among these four different phenotypes of stromal dystrophy (granular, Avellino, lattice, and Reis-Bücklers) is not fully understood, and different mutations in the *BIGH3* gene result in differences in the phenotypic expression.

MANAGEMENT Early in the disease process, no treatment is needed. Recurrent erosions in superficial granular dystrophy may be treated with therapeutic contact lenses, superficial keratectomy, or PTK. When visual acuity is affected, penetrating keratoplasty has a good prognosis. Recurrence in the graft (anteriorly and peripherally) may occur after many years as fine subepithelial opacities varying from original presentation.

Fujiki K, Hotta Y, Nakayasu K, et al. Six different mutations of TGFBI (betaig-h3, keratoepithelin) gene found in Japanese corneal dystrophies. *Cornea.* 2000;19:842–845.

Lattice dystrophy

This autosomal dominant dystrophy is very common. Variable expression is characterized by typical glasslike branching lines in the stroma.

PATHOGENESIS Light microscopy of lattice dystrophy demonstrates amyloid deposits concentrated most heavily in the anterior stroma. Amyloid may also accumulate in the subepithelial area, giving rise to poor epithelial–stromal adhesions. Amyloid stains rose to orange-red with Congo red dye and metachromatically with crystal violet dye, and it exhibits dichroism and birefringence. The specific genetic defect is in the *BIGH3* gene responsible for formation of keratoepithelin. This mutation is not in one of the 128 known amyloid-associated genes.

LABORATORY EVALUATION In vivo confocal microscopy reveals characteristic linear images that should be differentiated from those seen in infection with fungal hyphae.

CLINICAL FINDINGS The spectrum of corneal changes is broad, and the classic branching lattice figures may not be present in all cases. Refractile lines, central and subepithelial ovoid white dots, and diffuse anterior stromal haze appear early in life. Initially, the white dots resemble granular dystrophy. The refractile lines, so-called *lattice lines,* are best seen against a red reflex or with retroillumination (Fig 15-6). The stroma can take on a ground-glass appearance, but the peripheral cornea remains clear. Recurrent epithelial erosions occur often. In addition, stromal haze and epithelial surface irregularity may decrease vision.

This disorder is a primary localized corneal amyloidosis, in which the amyloid deposits may result from corneal epithelial cells and keratocytes. At least three types of lattice dystrophy have been identified.

Type I (Biber-Haab-Dimmer) This form is classic lattice dystrophy, with onset of erosions or visual symptoms at the end of the first decade. There is no systemic amyloid deposition (see primary localized amyloidosis later in this chapter). Type I is linked to chromosome 5q31.

Type II (Meretoja syndrome) This form combines lattice dystrophy with coexisting systemic amyloidosis and manifests around age 20 years. In addition to lattice corneal

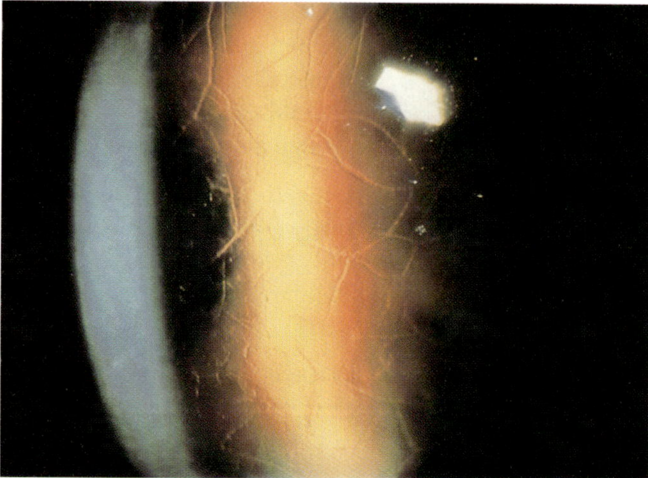

Figure 15-6 Lattice corneal dystrophy. *(Photograph courtesy of Vincent P. deLuise, MD.)*

changes, patients with Meretoja syndrome (Finnish type) have a characteristic facial mask; blepharochalasis; pendulous ears; cranial and peripheral nerve palsies; and dry, lax skin with amyloid deposition. The classic corneal lattice lines are less numerous and more peripherally located in this form. The amyloid in this condition is related to gelsolin and does not stain for type AA or AP. A mutation in chromosome 9q34 has been found in Meretoja syndrome.

Type III These deposits are midstromal and larger than the deposits in age-matched individuals with type I. Type III deposits are type AP amyloid, in contrast to the type AA seen in type I lattice dystrophy. The inheritance pattern of type III appears to be autosomal recessive, with symptoms delayed until the fifth to seventh decade. A variant described as type IIIA differs in some respects: Recurrent erosions are common, inheritance is autosomal dominant, and this form is reported only in white patients. These patients appear to have a distinct mutation in the *BIGH3* gene.

MANAGEMENT Recurrent erosions are managed with therapeutic contact lenses, superficial keratectomy, or PTK. Severe cases of lattice dystrophy with visual loss are treated with penetrating keratoplasty. Recurrence of this dystrophy in the corneal graft, usually in 2–12 years, occurs more frequently than after grafting for granular or macular dystrophy.

Chiou AG, Beuerman RW, Kaufman SC, et al. Confocal microscopy in lattice corneal dystrophy. *Graefes Arch Clin Exp Ophthalmol.* 1999;237:697–701.

Dighiero P, Drunat S, Ellies P, et al. A new mutation (A546T) of the betaig-h3 gene responsible for a French lattice corneal dystrophy type IIIA. *Am J Ophthalmol.* 2000;129:248–251.

Macular dystrophy

This least common of the three classic stromal dystrophies differs from both lattice and granular dystrophies: It has an autosomal recessive inheritance, involves the corneal periphery, may involve the corneal endothelium, and features a decrease in vision at an earlier age. Two types are described here.

PATHOGENESIS The deposits in macular dystrophy are glycosaminoglycans (GAGs; acid mucopolysaccharide), and they stain with colloidal iron and Alcian blue. They accumulate in the endoplasmic reticulum and not in lysosomal vacuoles as seen in systemic mucopolysaccharidoses. Both types I and II have been linked to chromosome 16q22, suggesting different mutations of the same allele.

CLINICAL FINDINGS Corneas are clear at birth and begin to cloud at ages 3–9. Patients with macular dystrophy show focal, gray-white, superficial stromal opacities that progress to involve full stromal thickness and extend to the corneal periphery. Macular spots have indefinite edges, and the stroma between the opacities is diffusely cloudy (Fig 15-7). Involvement of Descemet's membrane and the endothelium is indicated by the presence of cornea guttata. Epithelial erosions are possible, but symptoms usually involve decrease in vision. Central corneal thinning has been noted. The two types of macular dystrophy are based on biochemical differences.

Type I Patients with this more prevalent form of macular dystrophy lack antigenic keratan sulfate in their cornea, serum, and cartilage. These patients have a normal synthesis of dermatan sulfate–proteoglycan. An error occurs in the synthesis of keratan sulfate and in the activity of specific sulfotransferases involved in the sulfation of the keratan sulfate lactose aminoglycan side chain.

Type II Patients with this form synthesize a normal ratio of keratan sulfate and dermatan sulfate–proteoglycans, but synthesis is 30% below normal. Moreover, the dermatan sulfate–proteoglycan chains are 40% shorter than normal. Clinical presentation is similar to type I.

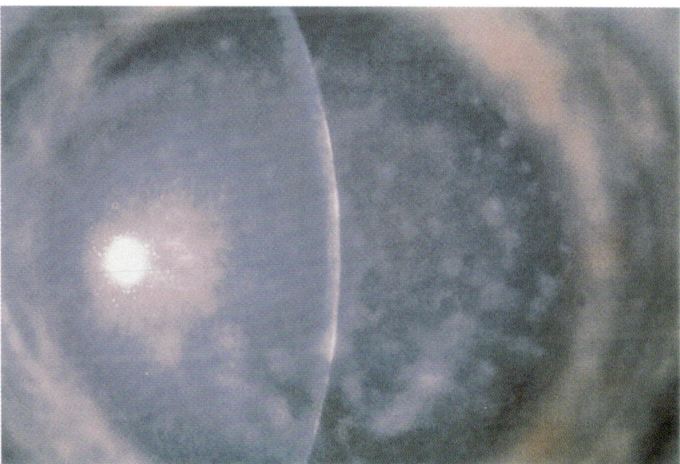

Figure 15-7 Macular dystrophy, showing involvement to the limbus with diffuse haze. *(Photograph courtesy of Vincent P. deLuise, MD.)*

LABORATORY EVALUATION An enzyme-linked immunosorbent assay (ELISA) can measure sulfated keratan sulfate. This test can help in the diagnosis of macular dystrophy, even in preclinical forms and carriers.

MANAGEMENT Recurrent erosions are treated as for other stromal dystrophies, and photophobia may be relieved with tinted contact lenses. PTK can be used for symptomatic anterior macular dystrophy. Definitive treatment is by penetrating corneal transplantation, although recurrences may be seen with both LK and PK.

Comparison of granular dystrophy, lattice dystrophy, and macular dystrophy shows that the frequency of regraft is highest in lattice dystrophy, followed by granular dystrophy and then macular dystrophy. However, the age of presentation of clinical findings is youngest in macular dystrophy, followed by lattice dystrophy and then granular dystrophy.

Gelatinous droplike dystrophy (primary familial amyloidosis)

This uncommon autosomal recessive corneal dystrophy maps to chromosome 1p. It features typical amyloid occurring as subepithelial deposits (see also the subsection Disorders of Protein Metabolism later in this chapter). Electron microscopy suggests the source of the amyloid is the basal epithelial layer. Most reports are in the Japanese literature. Onset occurs in the first decade and may resemble band keratopathy, but advancing disease develops protruding, mulberrylike subepithelial deposits (Fig 15-8). Management is similar to lattice dystrophy, and the recurrence rate is very high following keratoplasty.

Schnyder crystalline corneal dystrophy

This rare, slowly progressive autosomal dominant stromal dystrophy may become apparent as early as the first year of life, with the deposition of subepithelial corneal crystals (Fig 15-9A). However, diagnosis is usually made by the second or third decade, although it may be further delayed in patients who have the acrystalline form of the disease (Fig 15-9B). It has been linked to chromosome 1p36.

PATHOGENESIS This condition is thought to be a local disorder of corneal lipid metabolism. Pathologically, the opacities are accumulations of unesterified and esterified cho-

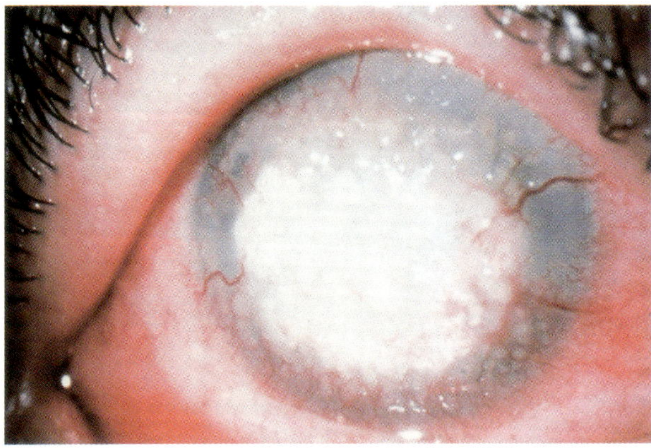

Figure 15-8 Gelatinous droplike dystrophy.

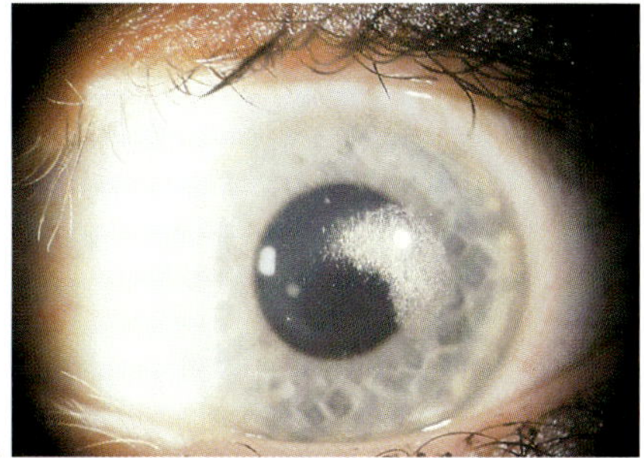

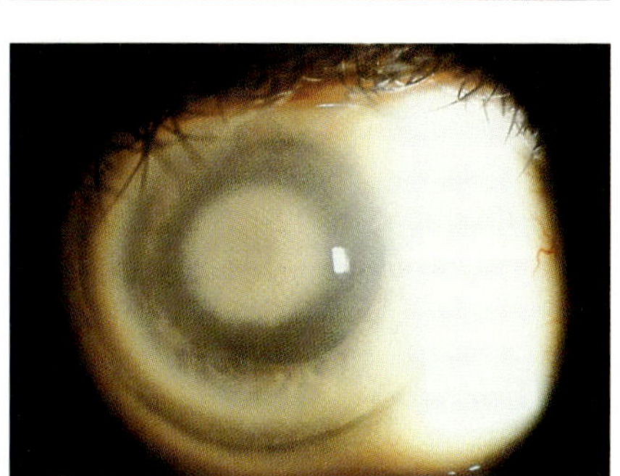

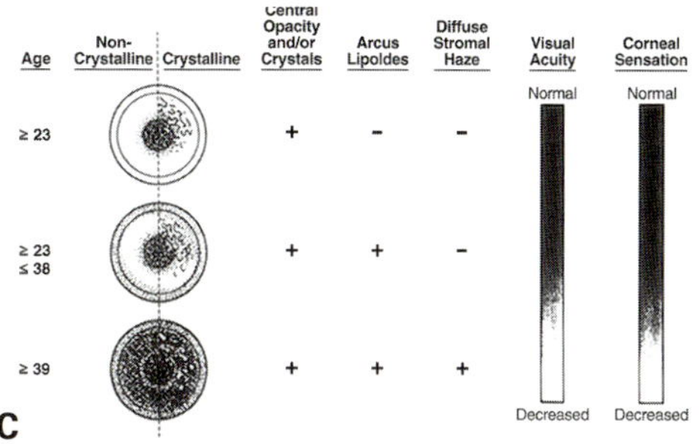

Figure 15-9 **A,** Schnyder crystalline dystrophy with central subepithelial crystalline deposition. **B,** Schnyder crystalline dystrophy with central panstromal corneal opacity and arcus lipoides. No crystals are present. **C,** Natural history of Schnyder's with age. *(Parts A and B courtesy of Jayne S Weiss, MD. Part C from Weiss JS. Schnyder's crystalline dystrophy: A Swede-Finn connection.* Cornea. *1992;11:93–101.)*

lesterol and phospholipids. Oil red O stains the phospholipids red. In the normal process of embedding tissue in paraffin, cholesterol and other fatty substances are dissolved; therefore, the pathologist must be made aware of the requirements for special stains. Electron microscopy will demonstrate abnormal accumulation of lipid and dissolved cholesterol in the epithelium, Bowman's layer, and throughout the stroma.

CLINICAL FINDINGS Affected patients show predictable changes on the basis of age (Fig 15-9C):

- Central subepithelial crystals (seen in only 50% of patients)
- Central corneal opacification
- Dense corneal arcus lipoides
- Midperipheral corneal opacification
- Decreased corneal sensation

Only 50% of patients develop subepithelial corneal crystal deposition. The central and midperipheral corneal opacification can be panstromal, thereby affecting the entire stromal thickness. Initially, the central opacification may take on a doughnutlike shape, sparing the visual axis. The epithelium is usually uninvolved clinically and remains smooth, and the cornea does not vascularize. Dense corneal arcus begins to develop in the third decade. Finally, in the fourth decade, lipid deposition in the midperipheral cornea results in a diffuse corneal opacification. These changes are accompanied by progressive loss of corneal sensation and decrease in photopic vision. Many patients are reported to have Swede-Finn ethnicity, but the disease has been reported in other groups.

LABORATORY EVALUATION Fasting lipid profile should be done for possible hyperlipoproteinemia (type II-a, III, or IV) or hyperlipidemia. Approximately 50% of affected patients have elevated serum cholesterol, which responds to diet or medication. Unaffected family members may also have an abnormal lipid profile. Confocal microscopy demonstrates intracellular and extracellular highly reflective deposits leading to eventual disruption of the subepithelial nerve plexus.

MANAGEMENT Despite maintenance of excellent scotopic vision, Schnyder crystalline dystrophy can disproportionately reduce photopic vision, leading to corneal transplantation in a minority of those affected. After penetrating keratoplasty (PK), recurrences can occur. PTK has been used to treat decreased vision from subepithelial crystals, but it does not treat panstromal haze. Abnormal serum lipids are managed by diet and/or medication but do not affect the progression of the corneal dystrophy.

> Weiss JS. Schnyder's dystrophy of the cornea. A Swede-Finn connection. *Cornea.* 1992;11:93–101.
>
> Weiss JS. Schnyder crystalline dystrophy sine crystals. Recommendation for a revision in nomenclature. *Ophthalmology.* 1996;103:465–473.

Fleck dystrophy

This uncommon nonprogressive stromal dystrophy begins very early in life and may be congenital. It can show extreme asymmetry (unilateral only) and is probably autosomal dominant.

PATHOGENESIS Affected keratocytes contain two abnormal substances: excess glycosaminoglycan, which stains with Alcian blue and colloidal iron; and lipids, demonstrated by Sudan black B and oil red O.

LABORATORY INVESTIGATION In vivo confocal microscopy demonstrates accumulation of pathologic material in stromal cells and inclusions in the basal nerves.

CLINICAL FINDINGS Discrete, flat, gray-white, dandrufflike (sometimes ring-shaped) opacities appear throughout the stroma to its periphery. The epithelium, Bowman's layer, Descemet's membrane, and the endothelium are not involved. Symptoms are minimal, and vision is usually not reduced. However, fleck dystrophy may be associated with decreased corneal sensation, limbal dermoid, keratoconus, central cloudy dystrophy, punctate cortical lens changes, pseudoxanthoma elasticum, or atopy.

Central cloudy dystrophy of François

This bilateral, symmetrical stromal dystrophy is nonprogressive or only very slowly progressive. It is autosomal dominant. No management is required.

PATHOGENESIS Cause is unknown. Pathologically, the collagen of the deep stroma is thrown into sawtooth folds. Extracellular deposition of mucopolysaccharide and lipidlike material has been reported.

CLINICAL FINDINGS The opacity is densest centrally and posteriorly and fades both anteriorly and peripherally (Fig 15-10). Opacities consist of multiple nebulous, polygonal, gray areas separated by cracklike intervening clear zones. The epithelium, Bowman's layer, stromal thickness, Descemet's membrane, and endothelium are normal. Vision is usually not reduced. This condition differs from posterior crocodile shagreen principally in

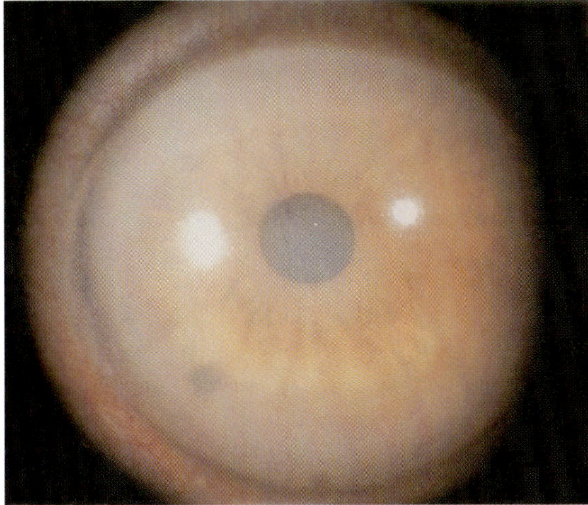

Figure 15-10 Central cloudy dystrophy (François), showing mild stromal haze and peripheral clearing.

showing a strong autosomal dominant inheritance pattern and having haze extend anteriorly into the cornea.

Mannis MJ, DeSousa LB, Gross RH. The stromal dystrophies. In: Krachmer JH, Mannis MJ, Holland EJ, eds. *Cornea*. Vol 2. St Louis: Mosby; 1997:1043–1062.

Endothelial Dystrophies

Fuchs endothelial dystrophy

This very common condition ranges from asymptomatic cornea guttata to a decompensated cornea with stromal edema, subepithelial fibrosis, and epithelial bullae. The condition shows variable autosomal dominant transmission and may be sporadic. Onset occurs after 50 years, with a female preponderance.

PATHOGENESIS Primary dysfunction of the endothelial cells manifests as increased corneal swelling and deposition of collagen and extracellular matrix in Descemet's membrane. The cause of the abnormal function is unknown, but there is a reduction in the number of Na^+,K^+-ATPase pump sites or in pump function. It is not clear whether the reduction in the posterior nonbanded zone and the increase in thickness of the posterior banded zone (posterior collagenous layer) is a primary effect of endothelial dysfunction or is secondary to chronic corneal edema.

CLINICAL FINDINGS Findings vary with the severity of the disease. Cornea guttata are first evident centrally and spread toward the periphery. Descemet's membrane becomes thickened, and folds develop secondary to stromal edema (Fig 15-11).

Increased endothelial pigmentation is also seen. As the endothelium further decompensates, the central corneal thickness may approach 1 mm (0.52–0.56 mm is normal). Epithelial edema develops (Fig 15-12), leading to microcystic edema; this later progresses to epithelial bullae, which may rupture.

Microscopically, the endothelial cells are noted to be larger and more polymorphic than normal and are disrupted by excrescences of excess collagen, a product of the

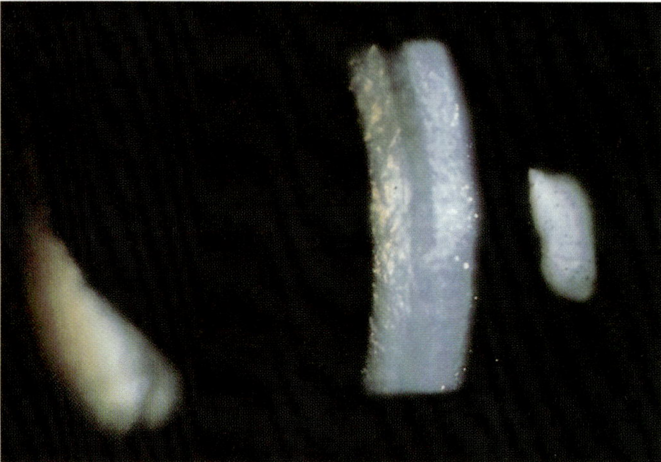

Figure 15-11 Fuchs endothelial dystrophy showing stromal edema, Descemet's folds, and endothelial guttata. *(Photograph courtesy of Vincent P. deLuise, MD.)*

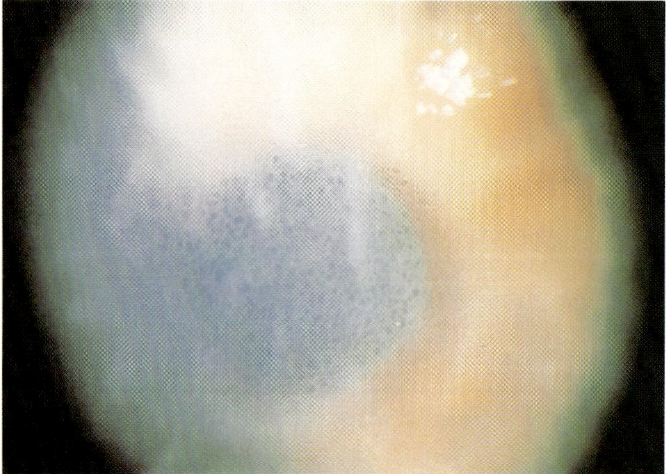

Figure 15-12 Fuchs endothelial dystrophy showing microcystic epithelial edema.

stressed endothelial cells (Fig 15-13). Descemet's membrane is thickened. Long-standing cases lead to subepithelial fibrosis.

Symptoms are rare before age 50 and are related to the edema, which causes a decrease in vision and pain secondary to ruptured bullae. Symptoms are worse upon awakening because of decreased surface evaporation during sleep. Painful episodes may subside once subepithelial fibrosis occurs.

LABORATORY EVALUATION Specular microscopy may be helpful in diagnosing Fuchs and following the clinical course for loss of endothelial cells. Corneal pachymetry may indicate relative endothelial function and change with progression of the disease. Both are useful in determining the relative safety of cataract or other intraocular surgery. Endothelial cell

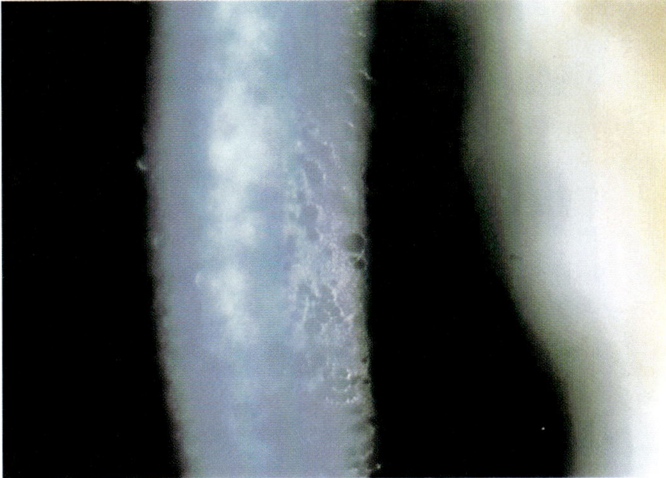

Figure 15-13 Fuchs endothelial dystrophy. Endothelial cells are large and disrupted by numerous guttata (specular reflection photomicrograph).

count less than 1000/mm^2 or corneal thickness greater than 0.65 mm suggests caution and the possibility that the cornea may decompensate with surgery (see Chapter 2).

MANAGEMENT Treatment is first aimed at reducing corneal edema and relieving pain. Use of sodium chloride drops and ointment (5%) and measures to lower intraocular pressure (IOP) may temporarily help the edema. Lubricating drops and a soft bandage lens are useful in the treatment of ruptured bullae. In advanced cases, a conjunctival flap may be considered, but restoration of vision requires corneal transplantation. Surgery should be performed before vascularization, and most authorities would recommend surgery before the entire cornea becomes edematous. Prognosis for graft survival is good. Alternatives to traditional full-thickness keratoplasty are being explored. Preliminary results of posterior lamellar keratoplasty (PLK) through a sclerocorneal pocket incision appear promising.

> Melles GR, Lander F, van Dooren BT, et al. Preliminary clinical results of posterior lamellar keratoplasty through sclerocorneal pocket incision. *Ophthalmology.* 2000;107:1850–1856.

Posterior polymorphous dystrophy (PPMD)

This uncommon, slowly progressive autosomal dominant or recessive dystrophy presents early in life. It has a variable clinical spectrum and can often be asymmetric and overlooked. PPMD has been mapped to chromosome 20q11 (congenital hereditary endothelial dystrophy links to 20p13).

PATHOGENESIS The most distinctive microscopic finding is the appearance of abnormal, multilayered endothelial cells that look and behave like epithelial cells or fibroblasts. These cells

- Show microvilli
- Stain positive for keratin

- Show rapid and easy growth in cell culture
- Have intercellular desmosomes
- Manifest proliferative tendencies

Similar changes that are not limited to the cornea are seen in iridocorneal endothelial (ICE) syndrome (see Chapter 13). A diffuse abnormality of Descemet's membrane is common, including thickening, a multilaminated appearance, and polymorphous alterations.

CLINICAL FINDINGS Careful examination of the posterior corneal surface will show any or all of the following:

- Isolated grouped vesicles
- Geographic-shaped discrete gray lesions
- Broad bands with scalloped edges (Fig 15-14)

Variable amounts of stromal edema, corectopia, or broad iridocorneal adhesions are also seen (Fig 15-15). Fine, glasslike adhesions may be seen gonioscopically. Both angle-closure and open-angle glaucoma can occur, and 14% of patients have elevated IOP.

LABORATORY EVALUATION Specular microscopy may show typical vesicles and bands, in contrast to the involved cells in ICE syndrome, which appear as dark areas with central highlights and light peripheral borders. Opinion is divided on the value of relying on specular microscopy alone in making the diagnosis. Confocal microscopy reveals alterations in Descemet's membrane. This may be a useful adjunct in the presence of corneal edema when slit-lamp examination and specular microscopy may not be able to demonstrate changes in Descemet's membrane.

MANAGEMENT Most patients are stable and asymptomatic. Mild corneal edema may be managed as with early Fuchs dystrophy. Stromal micropuncture to induce subepithelial pannus can be used to manage localized swelling. With more severe disease, glaucoma

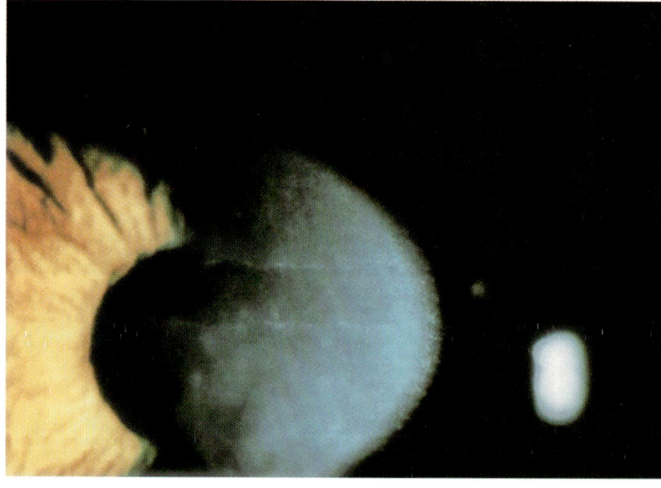

Figure 15-14 Posterior polymorphous dystrophy showing scallop-edged endothelial band.

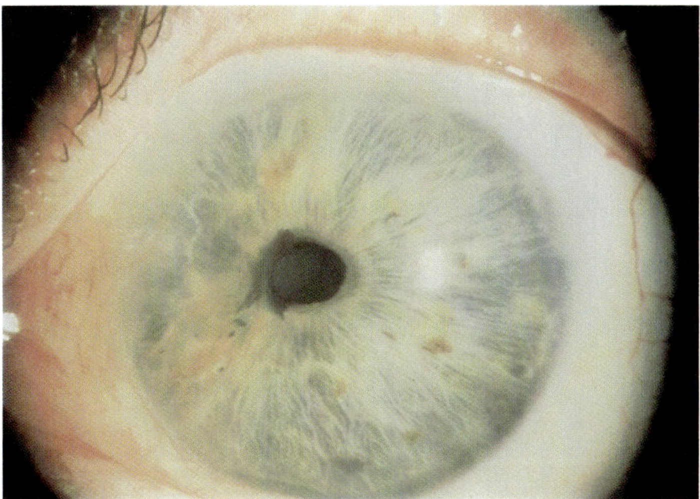

Figure 15-15 Posterior polymorphous dystrophy showing iridocorneal adhesion and corectopia.

must be managed, and corneal transplants may be required. Prognosis for PK is related to the presence of visible peripheral anterior synechiae and glaucoma. PPMD may recur in the graft. Simultaneous peripheral crescentic lamellar keratoplasty and central PK show encouraging preliminary results.

Rasheed K, Rabinowitz YS. Surgical treatment of advanced pellucid marginal degeneration. *Ophthalmology.* 2000;107:1836–1840.

Ectatic Disorders

Keratoconus

Keratoconus is a common disorder (prevalence of about 50 per 100,000) in which the central or paracentral cornea undergoes progressive thinning and bulging, so the cornea takes on the shape of a cone (Fig 15-16). The hereditary pattern is not prominent or predictable, but positive family histories have been reported in 6%–8% of cases. Clinically unaffected first-degree relatives have a higher chance of showing subclinical topographic abnormalities associated with keratoconus than does the general population. A putative locus for keratoconus has been identified on chromosome 21. This is interesting because Down syndrome (trisomy of chromosome 21) is strongly associated with keratoconus.

PATHOGENESIS Etiology is unknown and likely multifactorial because of the wide variety of associated syndromes and the low recurrence rate following transplantation. Histopathologically, keratoconus shows the following:

- Fragmentation of Bowman's layer
- Thinning of the stroma and overlying epithelium

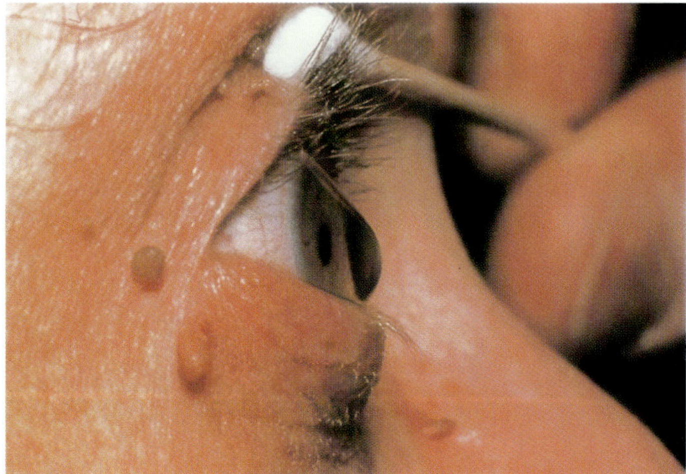

Figure 15-16 Keratoconus.

- Folds or breaks in Descemet's membrane
- Variable amounts of diffuse scarring

CLINICAL FINDINGS Nearly all cases are bilateral, but one eye may be much more severely involved. Sometimes the less affected eye shows only high astigmatism, which may be considered the minimal manifestation of keratoconus. The disease tends to progress during the adolescent years and then to stabilize when the patient has attained full growth, although progression can occur at any time. Early biomicroscopic and histopathologic findings include fibrillation of Bowman's layer, leading to breaks followed by fibrous growth and dysplasia through the break. As progression occurs, the apical thinning of the central cornea worsens, and extreme degrees of irregular astigmatism can develop. No associated inflammation occurs.

Scissoring of the red reflex on ophthalmoscopy or retinoscopy is a very early sign of keratoconus. *Rizzutti's sign,* a conical reflection on the nasal cornea when a penlight is shone from the temporal side, is another early finding (Fig 15-17). Iron deposits are often present within the epithelium around the base of the cone and constitute a *Fleischer ring* (Fig 15-18). This ring is brown in color and best appreciated with the cobalt blue filter. Fine, relucent, and roughly parallel striations *(Vogt lines),* or stress lines, of the stroma can be observed. Focal ruptures and flecklike scars occur in Bowman's layer.

Spontaneous perforation in keratoconus is extremely rare. However, a tear can occur in Descemet's membrane at any time, resulting in the sudden development of corneal edema, or *acute hydrops.* Allergy and eye rubbing are risk factors for the development of hydrops. The break in the posterior cornea usually heals spontaneously in 6–12 weeks; the corneal edema then disappears, but stromal scarring may be left in its wake. Some patients regain good vision following the resolution of hydrops, depending largely on the extent and location of the scar.

An increased prevalence of keratoconus has been reported in Down syndrome, atopy, Marfan syndrome, floppy eyelid syndrome, Leber congenital hereditary optic neuropathy,

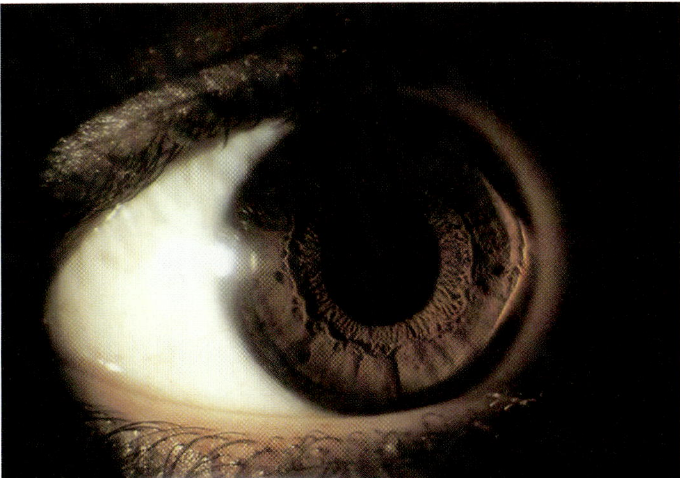

Figure 15-17 Rizzutti's sign.

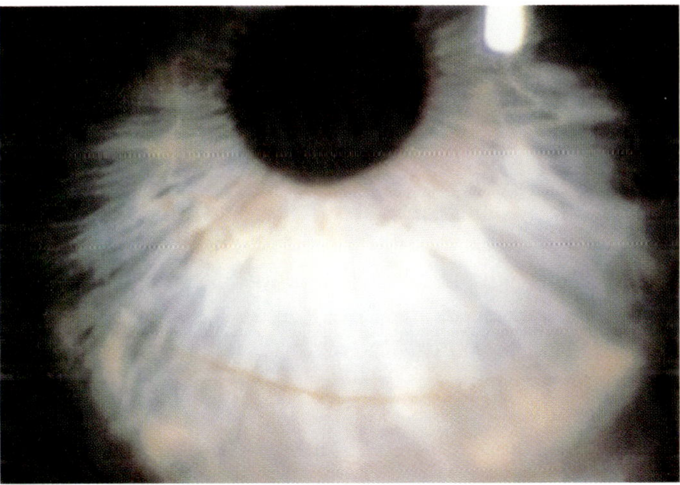

Figure 15-18 Keratoconus showing a Fleischer ring. *(Photograph courtesy of Vincent P. deLuise, MD.)*

and mitral valve prolapse. Keratoconus also occurs commonly in numerous congenital anomalies of the eye.

LABORATORY EVALUATION Computerized videokeratography is helpful in detecting early keratoconus, in following its progression, or in helping to fit contact lenses. Placido-based topography shows inferior steepening in the power map, but pachymetry mapping shows the thin zone to be paracentral (Fig 15-19). Algorithms to diagnose forme fruste, or subclinical, keratoconus are continually being perfected to detect keratoconus suspects and screen them from prospective refractive surgery. A measurement of steepness above the posterior best-fit sphere on Orbscan topography that is greater than 50 to 75 has

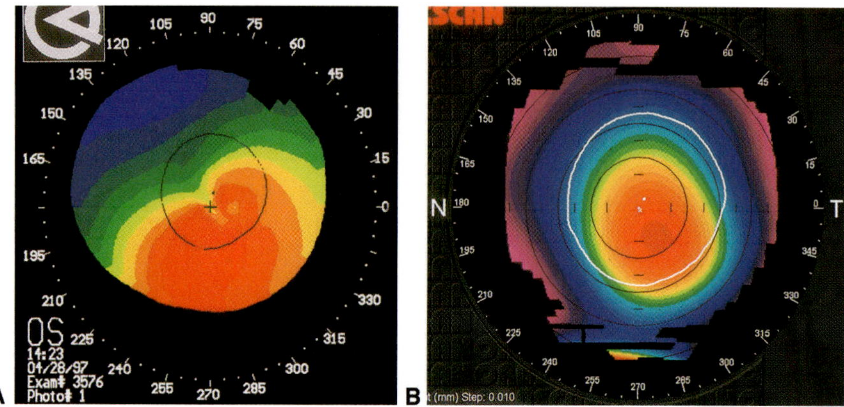

Figure 15-19 Keratoconus. **A,** Placido disk computerized videography showing inferior steepening. **B,** Orbscan computerized videography showing a pachymetry map of the same eye as in **A.** Note that the thinnest zone is near the visual axis and not at the steepest point.

been suggested to be predictive of keratoconus. (See Chapter 2 in this volume and BCSC Section 3, *Clinical Optics,* Chapter 9.)

MANAGEMENT Some cases of keratoconus are mild enough, at least for a time, that vision can be corrected adequately with glasses. However, hard or gas-permeable contact lenses are far more helpful in all but the mildest cases. Their ability to neutralize the irregular corneal astigmatism often produces dramatic improvement in vision. The majority of patients with keratoconus without central corneal scarring can be fitted successfully with contact lenses using advanced techniques, and a central subepithelial scar can, on occasion, be removed (nodulectomy), allowing continued wear of contact lenses. A multicenter study is presently examining the natural history of keratoconus and whether the type of contact lens fit (flat or vaulting the cone) determines if vision improves or leads to earlier or more frequent surgery.

When contact lenses are no longer satisfactory, PK is the treatment of choice. The prognosis for keratoplasty in keratoconus is excellent. Deep LK has recently been reported. Thermokeratoplasty, corneal flattening by heat application, may regularize the corneal surface, but the procedure is difficult and fraught with complications. It is most often used to flatten the cornea at the time of PK to make trephination easier.

Although some surgeons have reported performing PRK or LASIK or placing intracorneal rings in patients with subclinical, or forme fruste, keratoconus, the disease is presently considered a contraindication for refractive procedures because of unpredictability and the potential for poor results in either the short or long term in these patients. Penetrating keratoplasty has been reported after performance of LASIK in keratoconus patients because of long-term loss of best-corrected visual acuity. However, some surgeons use PTK for central scarring.

Hydrops is treated conservatively with topical hypertonic agents and patching or a soft contact lens for several months. A cycloplegic agent may be needed for ciliary pain. Hydrops is not an indication for immediate surgery.

Maguire LJ. Computerized corneal analysis. In: *Focal Points: Clinical Modules for Ophthalmologists*. San Francisco: American Academy of Ophthalmology; 1996: vol 14, no 5.

Rabinowitz YS. Keratoconus. *Surv Ophthalmol.* 1998;42:297–319.

Zadnik K, Barr JT, Edrington TB, et al. Baseline findings in the Collaborative Longitudinal Evaluation of Keratoconus (CLEK) Study. *Invest Ophthalmol Vis Sci.* 1998;39:2537–2546.

Keratoglobus

Keratoglobus is a very rare, bilateral, noninflammatory condition that differs from keratoconus and pellucid marginal degeneration (see the following section) in typically being present at birth (Table 15-2). It is usually not hereditary. Keratoglobus is similar in appearance to keratoconus but manifests a globular rather than a conical deformation of the cornea (Fig 15-20).

Table 15-2 Noninflammatory Ectatic Disorders Compared and Contrasted: Typical Clinical Presentation and Appearance

	Keratoconus	Keratoglobus	Pellucid Marginal Degeneration
Frequency	Most common	Rare	Less common
Laterality	Usually bilateral	Bilateral	Bilateral
Age at onset	Puberty	Usually at birth	Age 20–40 years
Thinning	Inferior paracentral	Greatest in periphery	Inferior band 1–2 mm wide
Protrusion	Thinning at apex	Generalized	Superior to band of thinning
Iron line	Fleischer ring	None	Sometimes
Scarring	Common	Mild	Only after hydrops
Striae	Common	Sometimes	Sometimes

(Modified from Krachmer JH, Mannis MJ, Holland EJ, eds. *Cornea.* St Louis: Mosby; 1997:1092.)

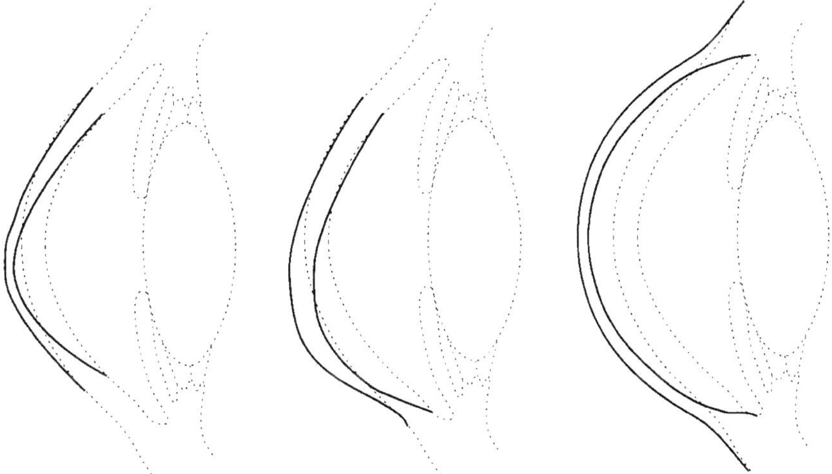

Figure 15-20 The presence of corneal thinning and the type of contour abnormality can be helpful in recognizing the type of ectatic disorder. From left: keratoconus, pellucid marginal degeneration, keratoglobus. *(Reproduced with permission from Krachmer JH, Mannis MJ, Holland EJ, eds. Cornea. St Louis: Mosby; 1997:1092.)*

PATHOGENESIS Keratoglobus is strongly associated with blue sclera and Ehlers-Danlos syndrome type VI (see Chapter 13), and it may represent a defect in collagen synthesis. Histopathologically, it is characterized by absent or fragmented Bowman's layer, thinned stroma with normal lamellar organization, and thin Descemet's membrane. Unlike keratoconus, keratoglobus is not associated with atopy, hard contact lens wear, or tapetoretinal degeneration.

CLINICAL FINDINGS Both corneas have a globular shape with very deep anterior chamber. The corneal curve may be as steep as 50–60 D, and generalized thinning appears, especially in the midperiphery; this is in contrast to keratoconus, which has maximal thinning at or near the apex of the protrusion. Spontaneous rupture of Descemet's membrane and corneal hydrops can occur, but iron lines, stress lines, and anterior scarring are not seen. The corneal diameter may be slightly increased. Fleischer rings are usually not present, but prominent folds and areas of thickening in Descemet's membrane are common. Keratoglobus may be associated with blue sclera, hyperextensibility of the joints, sensorineural deafness, fractures, and corneal perforation with minimal trauma (fragile cornea).

MANAGEMENT Prognosis for successful PK is much poorer in keratoglobus, and lamellar surgery should be considered in those cases requiring intervention to maintain functional vision. Spontaneous corneal rupture has been reported, so patients must be counseled regarding the importance of protection with eye wear. High myopia is treated with spectacles to prevent amblyopia.

Pellucid Marginal Degeneration

Pellucid marginal degeneration is somewhat common, nonhereditary, and bilateral. Clear, inferior, peripheral corneal thinning takes place in the absence of inflammation. Etiology is unknown.

CLINICAL FINDINGS Protrusion of the cornea occurs above the band of thinning. At times, a clear distinction between pellucid marginal degeneration and keratoconus is not possible. A cornea with keratoconus will show protrusion at the point of maximal thinning, but pellucid marginal degeneration can be superior or inferior and will show protrusion above the area of maximum thinning. No vascularization or lipid deposition occurs, but posterior stromal scarring has been noted within the thinned area. Most patients are diagnosed between 20 and 40 years of age, and men and women are affected equally. Decreased vision results from high irregular astigmatism (Figs 15-21, 15-22). Acute hydrops has been reported, and, although rare, spontaneous corneal perforation has also occurred.

MANAGEMENT Treatment consists of contact lenses early in the disease, although lens fitting is more difficult in pellucid marginal degeneration than in keratoconus. Eventually, PK may be required to restore vision. Because of the location of the thinning, the grafts tend to be large and close to the limbus, making surgery technically more difficult and the graft more prone to rejection. Recently, wedge resection or lamellar tectonic grafts have been advocated.

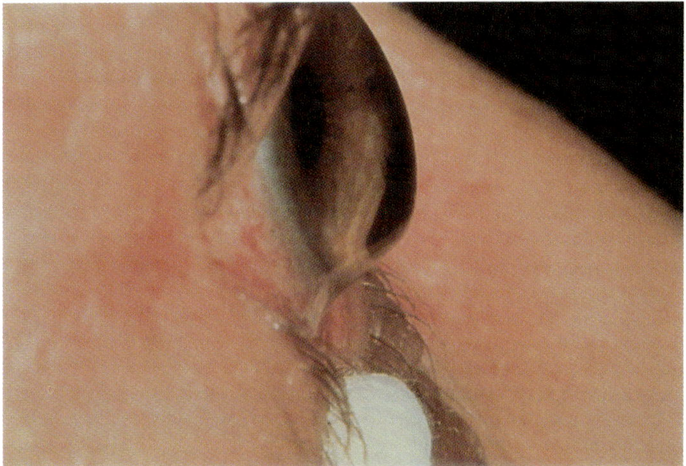

Figure 15-21 Pellucid marginal degeneration. *(Photograph courtesy of Vincent P. deLuise, MD.)*

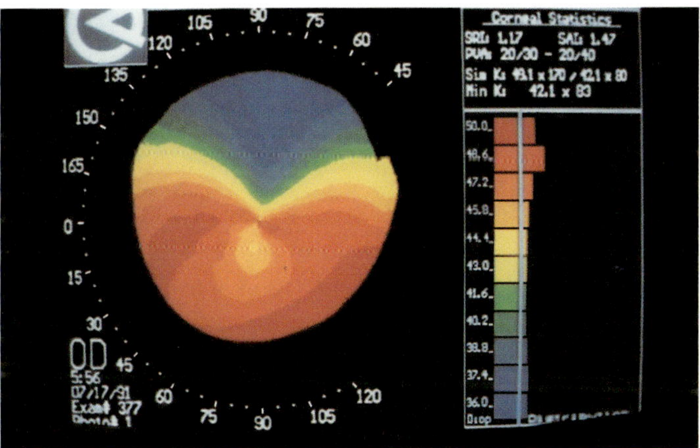

Figure 15-22 Topogram of pellucid marginal degeneration. Note inferior steepening.

Feder RS. Noninflammatory ectatic disorders. In: Krachmer JH, Mannis MJ, Holland EJ, eds. *Cornea.* Vol 2. St Louis: Mosby; 1997:1091–1106.

Metabolic Disorders With Corneal Changes

Many of the corneal manifestations of systemic disease are alterations in corneal clarity caused by abnormal storage of metabolic substances within the epithelium, stroma, or endothelium. Abnormal substances typically accumulate in lysosomes or lysosome-like intracytoplasmic structures as a result of a single enzyme defect. Most of these disorders are autosomal recessive, with the notable exceptions of Hunter syndrome (MPS type II) and Fabry disease, which are both X-linked recessive.

Sugar J. Metabolic disorders of the cornea. In: Kaufman HE, Barron BA, McDonald MB. *The Cornea.* 2nd ed. Boston: Butterworth-Heinmann; 1998:391–410.

Disorders of Carbohydrate Metabolism

Mucopolysaccharidoses

Systemic mucopolysaccharidoses (MPS) are rare inherited lysosomal storage diseases that result from the absence of lysosomal acid hydrolases, the enzymes that usually catabolize the glycosaminoglycans (GAGs) dermatan sulfate, heparan sulfate, and keratan sulfate.

PATHOGENESIS Although there are at least eight separate syndromes, several features are common to all. Heparan sulfate, dermatan sulfate, and keratan sulfate, the GAGs normally present in highest concentration, are the accumulated metabolites. All syndromes are autosomal recessive, with the exception of the X-linked recessive Hunter syndrome, which rarely involves the cornea until old age, if at all. Hurler (MPS IH) and Scheie (MPS IS) and the intermediate syndrome (Hurler-Scheie, MPS IH/S) are all allelic for the enzyme α-L-iduronidase, with different nucleotide substitutions leading to different amino acid substitutions and markedly reduced enzyme activity (<0.1% of normal). Recent work suggests that functional inactivation of an elastin-binding protein in Hurler syndrome may adversely affect elastic fiber assembly and contribute to the clinical phenotype. Normally, GAGs constitute the ground substance of the cornea, but in these diseases microscopic deposits of mucopolysaccharide are found in the keratocytes and stroma and, in some cases, in the corneal epithelium and endothelium.

CLINICAL FINDINGS Differential findings are listed in Table 15-3. These various conditions are characterized by corneal clouding, retinopathy, and optic atrophy, although Sanfilippo syndrome only occasionally has corneal opacities, and Hunter syndrome only rarely has corneal clouding. This clouding generally involves the entire cornea and may or may not be present at birth. It is often slowly progressive from the periphery toward the center and can cause serious reduction in visual acuity.

LABORATORY EVALUATION Microscopic differentiation of the syndromes is not possible. Scheie syndrome has been studied most intensely with regard to its corneal manifestations. Histiocytes laden with abnormally accumulated storage material (gargoyle cells) are noted. Electron microscopic and x-ray diffraction studies demonstrate an abnormally large range of stromal fibril size (20–52 nm, in contrast to a normal 26 nm) and disruption of the extracellular matrix by sulfated glycosaminoglycan deposits. Chorionic villus sampling has been used in some of these conditions for prenatal diagnosis.

Conjunctival biopsy can confirm classic histopathology, but specific diagnosis requires biochemical assay for enzymes in tears, leukocytes, cultured fibroblasts, or amniotic cells and for elevated urinary GAG levels.

MANAGEMENT These conditions, as well as those discussed in the following sections, are sometimes amenable to PK, unless impairment of the patient's mental status or retinal or optic nerve abnormalities preclude visual improvement. The prognosis for successful keratoplasty is considered guarded, as the abnormal storage material may accumulate again in the graft. Some regression of corneal clouding following successful donor stem-

Table 15-3 Differential Features of the Systemic Mucopolysaccharidoses

	Identified Genes	No. Per 1 Million Births	Genetics	Median Age at Diagnosis	Systemic Features		Ocular Features			Urinary Amp Excess			Defective Enzyme
					Skeletal Dysplasia	Mental Retardation	Corneal Clouding	Retinal Pigmentary Degeneration	Optic Atrophy	Heparan Sulfate	Dermatan Sulfate	Keratan Sulfate	
IH: Hurler	4p16.3	9.0	AR	1–2	+++	+++	+++	R	R	++	+++	−	α-L-Iduronidase
IS: Scheie (formerly MPS V)			AR	1–2	+	+	+++	R	R	++	+++ (partial)	−	α-L-Iduronidase
II: Hunter	Xq28	6.2		2–3									
A: Severe phenotype			XR		+++	+++	−	R	R	++	++	−	L-Iduronate 2-sulfatase
B: Mild phenotype			XR		++	+	+*	R	R	++	++	−	L-Iduronate 2-sulfatase
III: Sanfilippo													
A: Sulfatase-deficient	17q25.3	7.8	AR	3–5	+	+++	−	R	R	+++	−	−	Glucosamine-N-sulfatase
B: Glucosaminidase-deficient		4.3	AR	3–5	+	+++	−	R	R	+++	−	−	α-N-acetyl-glucosaminidase
C: Acetyl-CoA-α-glucosaminidase-N-acetyltransferase-deficient		0.7	AR	10–12	+	+++	−	R	R	+++	−	−	Acetyl-CoA-α-glucosaminide N-acetyltransferase
D: N-acetylglucosaminidase-6-sulfate-sulfatase-deficient		0.9	AR	3–5	+	+++	−	R	R	+++	−	−	N-acetylglucosamine-6-sulfatase
IV: Morquio	16q24.3	5.0	AR	3–5	+++	+	++	NR	R	−	−	+++	N-acetylgalactosamine-sulfatase
V: Vacant; now MPS IS													
VI: Maroteaux-Lamy	5q11–q13	4.0											
A: Severe phenotype			AR	1–2	+++	−	++	NR	R	−	+++	−	N-acetylgalactosamine-4-sulfatase
B: Mild phenotype			AR	1–2	+	−	++	NR	NR	−	+++	−	N-acetylgalactosamine-4-sulfatase
VII: Sly		0.5	AR	0–1	+	+	++	NR	NR	+++	+++	−	β-Glucuronidase

* Positive by slit-lamp biomicroscopy in some older patients.
AR = autosomal recessive; XR = X-linked recessive; R = reported; NR = not reported; − = absent/not elevated; + = mild; ++ = moderate; +++ = marked.

cell bone-marrow transplantation occurs in about one third of patients. Gene transfer therapy is under investigation in animal models.

Hinek A, Wilson SE. Impaired elastogenesis in Hurler disease: dermatan sulfate accumulation linked to deficiency in elastin-binding protein and elastic fiber assembly. *Am J Pathol.* 2000;156:925–938.

Diabetes mellitus

The most common disorder of carbohydrate metabolism, diabetes mellitus has nonspecific corneal manifestations of punctate epithelial erosions, basement membrane changes resembling EBMD, Descemet's folds, and decreased corneal sensation. Diabetes is discussed at length in BCSC Section 12, *Retina and Vitreous*, although the emphasis is on retinal rather than corneal aspects of the disease.

PATHOGENESIS Diabetic patients have ultrastructural abnormalities of the basement membrane complex that contribute to problems of epithelial–stromal adhesion. These abnormalities include thickening of the multilaminar basement membrane, reduced hemidesmosome number, and decreased penetration of anchoring fibrils. Accumulation of polyols such as sorbitol by the action of aldose reductase on excess glucose may contribute to the alterations in the epithelium and endothelium and the corneal hypoesthesia seen in diabetic patients.

CLINICAL FINDINGS Corneal epithelial surface changes and hypoesthesia occur with increasing severity (eg, type I, insulin-dependent diabetes mellitus, as opposed to type II, non–insulin-dependent diabetes mellitus) and increasing duration of disease. Removal of diabetic epithelium at surgery results in the loss of the basal cells and basement membrane, leading to prolonged healing difficulties. Faint vertical folds in Descemet's membrane and deep stroma (Waite-Beetham lines) are not specific to diabetes mellitus but may represent early endothelial dysfunction and increased stromal hydration.

LABORATORY EVALUATION Glycosolated hemoglobin is related to poor control of diabetes and may correlate with poor corneal healing in addition to progressive retinopathy.

MANAGEMENT Diabetes is not a contraindication to PK or other corneal surgery. Topical aldose reductase inhibitors may prove beneficial in treating diabetic epitheliopathy. Measures that can improve diabetic epitheliopathy include the following:

- Minimizing epithelial debridement at surgery
- Increasing lubrication
- Avoiding toxic medications
- Using therapeutic contact lenses

Disorders of Lipid Metabolism and Storage

Hyperlipoproteinemias

These common conditions are associated with premature coronary artery and peripheral vascular disease. Recognition of the ocular hallmarks of these diseases as well as xanthelasma and corneal arcus can result in early intervention and reduced morbidity.

PATHOGENESIS Extracellular deposits consist of cholesterol, cholesterol esters, phospholipids, and triglycerides.

CLINICAL FINDINGS Table 15-4 gives Fredrickson's classification of five types of hyperlipoproteinemia. Types II and III are associated with early-onset xanthelasma and corneal arcus, or arcus juvenilis. Types II, III, and IV can have xanthomas involving the conjunctiva. Type III has been linked to 19q13.2 (apolipoprotein E mutation). Corneal arcus is a very common degenerative change of older patients and does not require systemic evaluation. Schnyder crystalline corneal dystrophy is thought to be a localized defect of lipid metabolism, but laboratory evaluation is needed to rule out concurrent systemic abnormality (see discussion earlier in this chapter).

LABORATORY EVALUATION A fasting and alcohol-restricted lipid profile that includes cholesterol, triglycerides, and high- and low-density lipoproteins (HDL and LDL, respectively) is required. Patients can then be classified phenotypically to assess their risk for atherosclerotic disease when corneal arcus is present in individuals younger than 50 years of age or is significantly asymmetric.

MANAGEMENT Early detection gives the patient time to be referred for diet or drug treatment.

Hypolipoproteinemias

Abnormal reductions in serum lipoprotein levels occur in five disorders:

- Lecithin–cholesterol acyltransferase (LCAT) deficiency
- Tangier disease
- Fish eye disease
- Familial hypobetalipoproteinemia
- Bassen-Kornzweig syndrome

The last two disorders do not result in corneal disease; discussion here focuses on the other three disorders.

PATHOGENESIS LCAT facilitates the removal of excess cholesterol from peripheral tissues to the liver, and a deficiency would be expected to lead to accumulation of free cholesterol

---

Table 15-4 Genetically Determined Hyperlipoproteinemias

Primary Type	Prevalence	Lipoprotein Abnormality	Increased Lipid Fraction	Lipemia Retinalis	Corneal Arcus	Xanthelasma	Inheritance
I	Very rare	Chylomicrons	Triglyceride	+	−	−	8p22 AR
II	0.5%	β-lipoprotein	Cholesterol	−	+	+	2p24 AD
III	Rare	Broad-β band	Cholesterol	+	+	+	19q13.2 AR apolipo-protein E
IV	1.0%	Pre-β lipoprotein	Triglyceride	+	−	−	AD
V	Rare	Chylomicrons Pre-β	Triglyceride	+	−	−	AD

(Modified from Bron AJ. Dyslipoproteinemias and their ocular manifestations. *Birth Defects Orig Artic Ser.* 1976; 12:257.)

in the tissues. Atherosclerosis, renal insufficiency, and diffuse corneal clouding ensue. LCAT deficiency and fish eye disease are allelic variants of the same genetic locus on chromosome 16q22.1, but fish eye disease has normal levels of LCAT that do not function to aid HDL in esterifying cholesterol. Tangier disease has a complete absence of serum high-density α-lipoproteins and maps to 9q22–q31.

CLINICAL FINDINGS All three cornea-affecting hypolipoproteinemias are rare, autosomal recessive conditions. Familial LCAT deficiency is characterized by peripheral arcus and nebular stromal haze made up of myriad minute focal deposits of lipid that appear early in childhood but do not interfere with vision. Fish eye disease has obvious corneal clouding from minute gray-white-yellow dots that progress from the periphery to decrease vision. One source describes the eye as resembling that of a boiled fish. Tangier disease, named after the Chesapeake Bay island, features very large orange tonsils; enlarged liver, spleen, and lymph nodes; hypocholesterolemia; abnormal chylomicron remnants; and markedly reduced HDL in the plasma. Corneas show diffuse clouding and posterior focal stromal opacities but no arcus. Neuropathy leads to lagophthalmos and corneal sequelae. Heterozygotes show low α-lipoproteins in the serum.

LABORATORY EVALUATION AND MANAGEMENT The serum lipid profile shows characteristic low levels of HDL. Recognition can allow the clinician to make appropriate referrals and encourage the patient to seek genetic counseling.

Sphingolipidoses

These rare inherited disorders of complex lipids (gangliosides and sphingomyelin) involve the cornea in three conditions:

- Fabry disease (angiokeratoma corporis diffusum)
- Multiple sulfatase deficiency
- Generalized gangliosidosis (GM$_1$ gangliosidosis type I)

PATHOGENESIS These disorders of lipid storage are autosomal recessive, with the exception of Fabry, which is X-linked recessive. They principally affect the retina and may lead to central nervous system dysfunction. Fabry disease is again an important exception. It is caused by a deficiency of α-galactosidase A, leading to the accumulation of ceramide trihexoside in the renal and cardiovascular systems. Multiple sulfatase deficiency combines features of metachromatic leukodystrophy and mucopolysaccharidosis. Affected children have subtle diffuse corneal opacities, optic atrophy, and progressive psychomotor retardation. They die in the first decade. Generalized gangliosidosis is characterized by deficiencies of β-galactosidases and the accumulation of gangliosides in the central nervous system and keratan sulfate in somatic tissues. It has been linked to chromosome 3p12–3p13. Although Tay-Sachs disease (hexosaminidase A deficiency with accumulation of GM$_2$ ganglioside) primarily involves the retina, the corneal endothelial cells can appear distended and filled with single membrane–bound vacuoles. Recent work suggests that impaired elastic-fiber assembly may result in some of these disorders.

CLINICAL FINDINGS In these conditions, the cornea exhibits distinctive changes, consisting of whorl-like lines (cornea verticillata) in the basal layers of the epithelium that appear to flow together to the inferior central corneal epithelium (Fig 15-23).

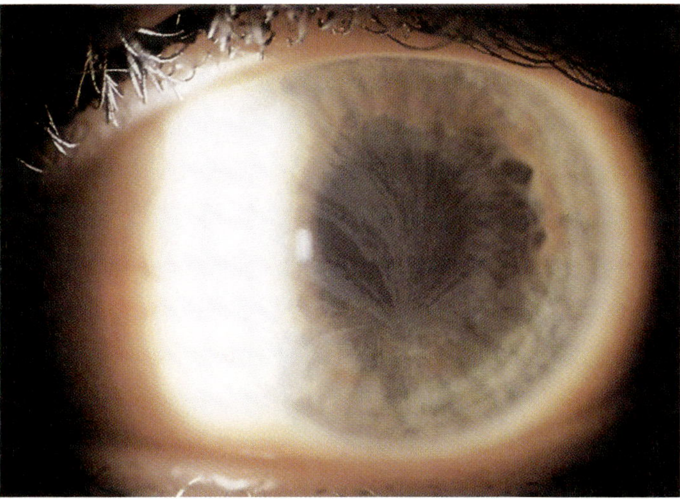

Figure 15-23 Whorl-like deposits of sphingolipid in basal layer of corneal epithelium in patient with Fabry disease; identical deposits occur in otherwise asymptomatic female carriers of this disease.

Periorbital edema occurs in 25% of cases, posterior spokelike cataracts in 50%, and conjunctival aneurysms in 60%. Other ocular signs include papilledema, retinal or macular edema, optic atrophy, and retinal vascular dilation. The corneal changes resemble those seen in patients on long-standing oral chloroquine or amiodarone treatment. A careful drug history will help make this differentiation.

Hemizygous males with Fabry disease are more seriously affected and show the typical corneal changes. The heterozygous female is usually asymptomatic but still shows the same corneal changes. Fabry disease is also characterized by renal failure, peripheral neuropathy with painful dysesthesias in the lower extremities, and skin lesions. The skin lesions are small, round vascular eruptions that later become hyperkeratotic. They consist of an accumulation of sphingolipid within the vascular endothelium.

Corneal opacities have been reported in Gaucher disease, but this is a rare finding.

LABORATORY EVALUATION In Fabry disease, α-galactosidase is markedly decreased in urine and plasma. Conjunctival biopsy may be positive before cornea verticillata are apparent. Prenatal diagnosis can be performed with chorionic villus sampling.

MANAGEMENT If a female patient is diagnosed as an asymptomatic heterozygous Fabry carrier, genetic counseling should be considered. The prognosis for successful PK in these conditions is generally poor. Clinical trials of enzyme replacement with infusion of α-galactosidase A are under way.

Guemes A, Kosmorsky GS, Moodie DS, et al. Corneal opacities in Gaucher disease. *Am J Ophthalmol.* 1998;126:833–835.

Hinek A, Zhang S, Smith AC, et al. Impaired elastic-fiber assembly by fibroblasts from patients with either Morquio B disease or infantile GM1-gangliosidosis is linked to deficiency in the 67-kD spliced variant of beta-galactosidase. *Am J Hum Genet.* 2000;67:23–36.

Mucolipidoses

These autosomal recessive conditions have features common to both mucopolysaccharidoses and lipidoses.

PATHOGENESIS These diseases are inherited defects of carbohydrate and lipid metabolism combined. Consequently, they have something in common with the mucopolysaccharidoses as well as the sphingolipidoses. Mucopolysaccharides accumulate in the cornea and viscera, and sphingolipids are deposited in the retina and central nervous system. Currently recognized diseases in this class are the following:

- Mucolipidosis (MLS) I (dysmorphic sialidosis)
- MLS II (inclusion-cell [I-cell] disease)
- MLS III (pseudo-Hurler polydystrophy)
- MLS IV
- Goldberg syndrome
- Mannosidosis
- Fucosidosis

These conditions are all autosomal recessive. MLS IV has been mapped to chromosome 19p. Histopathologic examination of corneal scrapings has revealed the accumulation of intracytoplasmic storage material. In fucosidosis, histopathologic study has revealed that, in spite of clinically normal corneas, corneal endothelial cells show the presence of cytoplasmic, membrane-bound, confluent areas of fibrillar, granular, and multilaminated deposits. A retinal cherry-red spot and retinal degeneration are also associated with many of these disorders. All are caused by a defect in lysosomal acid hydrolase enzymes.

CLINICAL FINDINGS With the exception of mannosidosis and fucosidosis, which are oligosaccharidoses, all of these conditions are characterized by varying degrees of corneal clouding, which can often be progressive. A recent report described a patient with fucosidosis who was afflicted with recurrent episodes of severe ocular pain, tearing, and ipsilateral facial flushing. These findings were thought to be suggestive of reflex sympathetic dystrophy (pain and sympathetic hyperactivity).

LABORATORY EVALUATION Plasma cells are vacuolated and plasma lysosomal hydrolases are elevated. In MLS IV, with corneal clouding from birth, conjunctival biopsy shows fibroblast inclusion bodies that are

- Single membrane–limited cytoplasmic vacuoles containing both fibrillogranular material and membranous lamellae
- Lamellar and concentric bodies resembling those of Tay-Sachs disease

There is no evidence of mucopolysacchariduria or cellular metachromasia. Chorionic villus sampling has been reported in MLS II for prenatal diagnosis.

MANAGEMENT Both PK and LK have been associated with generally poor results, probably because resurfacing is impaired by the abnormal epithelial cells. Although donor limbal stem-cell transplantation has been advocated, tissue matching may be required, as graft rejection in these vascularized recipient beds is possible. Bone-marrow transplantation has been reported.

Bietti crystalline corneoretinal dystrophy

This very rare autosomal recessive condition is characterized by peripheral corneal opacities and tapetoretinal dystrophy. It is presumed to be caused by a defect in lipid metabolism and has been mapped to chromosome 4q35–4qter.

PATHOGENESIS Lysosomes of fibroblasts in the choroid and skin and circulating lymphocytes contain crystalline deposits, but no abnormal accumulation of cholesterol or cholesterol esters has been documented.

CLINICAL FINDINGS Retinal crystals that are pathognomonic appear to decrease with time. Peripheral, sparkling, yellow-white spots are seen at the corneal limbus in the superficial stroma and subepithelial layers of the cornea in 75% of patients. These spots may fade with time.

LABORATORY EVALUATION AND MANAGEMENT Visual fields, dark adaptation testing, and ERG may be normal in early cases, but advanced cases may have decreased ERG and retinal findings of atypical retinitis pigmentosa. No specific treatment is reported.

> Kenyon KR, Navon SE. Corneal manifestations of metabolic diseases. In: Krachmer JH, Mannis MJ, Holland EJ, eds. *Cornea.* Vol 2. St Louis: Mosby; 1997:897–924.

Disorders of Amino Acid Metabolism

Cystinosis

This rare autosomal recessive disorder is characterized by the accumulation of the amino acid cystine within lysosomes. It affects 3.5 infants per 1 million births. Cystinosis has been mapped to chromosome 17p13; the defective gene is *CTNS.*

PATHOGENESIS A defect in transport across the lysosomal membrane leads to accumulation of cystine.

CLINICAL FINDINGS Cystinosis is a systemic metabolic defect that can present as an infantile, intermediate, or adult form. The age at diagnosis averages 1 year but can range into the teenage years. The *infantile,* or *nephropathic,* form features dwarfism and progressive renal dysfunction, with the deposition of fine polychromatic cystine crystals in the conjunctiva, corneal stroma, and other parts of the eye. This form is uniformly fatal in the first decade of life in the absence of renal transplantation. The *intermediate,* or *adolescent,* form has less severe renal involvement, with death occurring in the second or third decade. In the *adult* form, life expectancy is normal. Crystals can be seen in the corneal stroma on slit-lamp examination and in the trabecular meshwork on gonioscopy. Although the crystals usually do not affect visual acuity, these patients are often photophobic.

LABORATORY EVALUATION Cystine crystals may be seen in conjunctival biopsy or in the buffy coat of blood or bone marrow.

MANAGEMENT Topical cysteamine drops reduce the density of the crystalline deposits and diminish corneal pain, possibly as a result of a decrease in the development of corneal erosions. Presumably, the topically administered cysteamine reacts with the intracellular cystine, forming a cysteine-cysteamine disulfide that resembles lysine and is transported through the lysosome by the normal lysine transport system. The crystals have been observed to recur in patients who have undergone PK for clouding associated with the corneal deposits. These refractile polychromatic crystals are densest in the peripheral cornea but are seen throughout the anterior stroma, even within the central cornea (Fig 15-24).

The normal cornea and conjunctiva are transparent and any deposits—whether from the tear film, limbus, or aqueous humor—are easily discerned. Table 15-5 summarizes the differential diagnosis based on the depth of corneal involvement, color and refractile character, and conjunctival involvement.

Gahl WA, Kuehl EM, Iwata F, et al. Corneal crystals in nephropathic cystinosis: natural history and treatment with cysteamine eyedrops. *Mol Genet Metab*. 2000;71:100–120.

Tyrosinemia

Richner-Hanhart syndrome (tyrosinemia type II) is characterized by systemic findings, including hyperkeratotic lesions of palms, soles, and elbows, as well as eventual mental retardation.

PATHOGENESIS This autosomal recessive disorder occurs secondary to an enzymatic defect of tyrosine aminotransferase that leads to excess tyrosine in the blood and urine. The elevated tyrosine probably has a direct action on lysosomal membranes, leading to release of their enzymes with characteristic changes. The gene locus is at 16q22.1–q22.3.

CLINICAL FINDINGS Ocular changes include marked photophobia, tearing, conjunctival injection, and tarsal papillary hypertrophy. Patients develop recurrent episodes of pseudodendrites, which usually do not stain well with fluorescein or rose bengal. Continued episodes of epithelial breakdown can result in corneal vascularization and scarring. It is important to consider this disorder in the young child who may carry a diagnosis of recurrent herpes simplex virus keratitis.

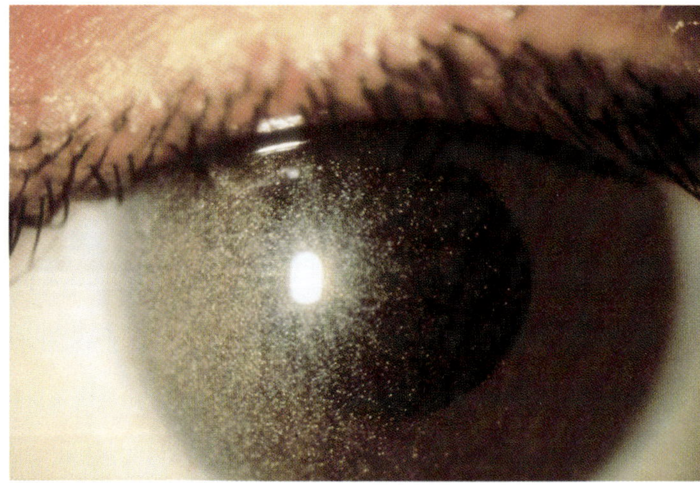

Figure 15-24 Cystinosis. Refractile polychromatic crystals are clustered in the peripheral cornea.

Table 15-5 Corneal Deposits in Differential Diagnosis

Type	Superficial	Stromal	Deep Stromal/Endothelial	Conjunctiva
Pigmented	Cornea verticillata (Fabry disease, amiodarone) Striate melanokeratosis Iron lines Pigmented (noncalcific) band keratopathy Spheroidal degeneration Adrenochrome Alkaptonuria	Phenothiazines Blood staining Bilirubin Siderosis (iron) Corneal tattoo	Mercury Wilson disease (copper) Chalcosis (copper) Chrysiasis (systemic gold) Argyriasis (topical silver) Krukenberg spindle	Tetracycline Adrenochrome Argyriasis
Nonpigmented	Subepithelial mucinous dystrophy Coats white ring Calcific band keratopathy Ciprofloxacin	Granular dystrophy Macular dystrophy Fleck dystrophy Lipid deposition Mucopolysaccharidoses	Cornea farinata Pre-Descemet's dystrophy X-linked ichthyosis Argyriasis (silver)	Gout (urate)
Refractile/ crystalline	Meesmann dystrophy Superficial amyloid Tyrosinemia type II Intraepithelial ointment Gout (urate)	Lattice dystrophy Schnyder dystrophy Bietti crystalline corneoretinal dystrophy Immunoglobulin deposition Cystinosis Infectious crystalline keratopathy	Polymorphic amyloid degeneration	Cystinosis

(Modified from Bridges WZ, Palay DA. Corneal deposits. In: Krachmer JH, Mannis MJ, Holland EJ, eds. *Cornea.* Vol 1. St Louis: Mosby; 1997:418.)

LABORATORY EVALUATION Hypertyrosinemia and tyrosinuria with normal phenylalanine level and biopsy showing soluble tyrosine aminotransferase (TAT) deficiency are diagnostic.

MANAGEMENT Restriction of dietary intake of tyrosine and phenylalanine can reduce both the corneal and systemic changes, including mental retardation. The institution of appropriate dietary restrictions even later in life can improve the mental status.

Alkaptonuria

Alkaptonuria is a rare autosomal recessive disorder with a defect of tyrosine metabolism that maps to gene locus 3q21–q23. An unusually high frequency occurs in the Dominican Republic and Slovakia.

PATHOGENESIS Homogentisate 1,2-dioxygenase, the enzyme necessary to degrade tyrosine and phenylalanine, is deficient. Phenylalanine and tyrosine cannot be metabolized beyond homogentisic acid, which is oxidized and polymerized into alkapton, a brown-black material similar to melanin. Alkapton then deposits in connective tissues as dark pigment known as *ochronosis*. Corneal lesions consisting of homogentisic acid are easily seen by light microscopy. Recent electron microscopic studies have shown extracellular deposits of finely granular ochronotic pigment in and around collagen fibrils. Intracellular membrane-bound ochronotic pigment granules were observed in macrophages in fibroblasts, along with two other forms of extracellular ochronotic pigment.

CLINICAL FINDINGS Patients develop arthropathy, renal calculi, and pigmentation of cartilaginous structures, including earlobes, trachea, nose, tendons, dura mater, heart valves, and prostate. Eventually, medial and lateral rectus muscle tendons and the sclera adjacent to the tendon insertions develop smudgelike pigmentation. Darkly pigmented, dotlike opacities may appear in the corneal epithelium or in Bowman's layer near the limbus.

LABORATORY EVALUATION Urine turns dark on standing and alkalinization. Homogentisic acid oxidase deficiency can be demonstrated.

MANAGEMENT No specific therapy is available, although high-dose ascorbic acid is reported to reduce arthropathy in young patients. It is hoped that specific gene therapy will be available to treat this disorder in the future.

Cheskes J, Buettner H. Ocular manifestations of alkaptonuric ochronosis. *Arch Ophthalmol.* 2000;118:724–725.

Disorders of Protein Metabolism

Amyloidosis

The amyloidoses are a heterogeneous group of diseases characterized by the accumulation of amyloid in various tissues and organs. Table 15-6 summarizes ocular findings in the amyloidoses.

PATHOGENESIS Amyloid is an eosinophilic hyaline material with five basic staining characteristics:

- Positive staining with Congo red dye

Table 15-6 Amyloid in the Eye

Type	Heredity	Ocular Distribution	Associated Conditions	Genetic Linkage
Primary localized amyloidosis	Nonfamilial	Conjunctival plaque Polymorphic amyloid degeneration	None	
	Familial	Lattice corneal dystrophy types I and III Avellino and granular dystrophy Gelatinous droplike dystrophy		5q31 (keratoepithelin gene) 1p32–q12 (M1S1 gene)
Primary systemic amyloidosis	Nonfamilial	Skin and conjunctiva (very rare)	Occult plasma cell dyscrasias	
	Familial	Ophthalmoplegia (orbital and muscle infiltrates), ptosis, vitreous veils, dry eye, pupil abnormalities	Cardiomyopathy Peripheral neuropathy Gastrointestinal disease Skin involvement	18q11.2–q12.1 (transthyretin gene) Many others
		Lattice corneal dystrophy type II, cranial neuropathies	Meretoja syndrome (facial palsies, skin nodules, rarely renal involvement)	9q34 (gelsolin gene)
Secondary localized amyloidosis	Nonfamilial	Conjunctiva Skin Cornea	Trachoma, psoriasis, trauma, phlyctenulosis, retinopathy of prematurity, keratoconus, bullous keratopathy, interstitial keratitis, leprosy, contact lens wear, trichiasis, tertiary syphilis, uveitis, climatic droplet keratopathy	
	Familial	None		
Secondary systemic amyloidosis	Nonfamilial	Rarely vitreous body (corneal deposits are not amyloid)	Multiple myeloma	
		Conjunctiva, skin (rare)	Infectious diseases (tuberculosis, leprosy, syphilis) Inflammatory diseases (rheumatoid arthritis, other connective tissue disorders) Hodgkin disease	
	Familial	(Corneal nerve enlargement is not amyloid)	MEN type IIa	10q11.2 (RET oncogene)

- Dichroism and birefringence
- Metachromasia with crystal violet dye
- Fluorescence in ultraviolet light with thioflavine T stain
- Typical filamentous appearance by electron microscopy

Protein AP derives from α-globulin and is found in all amyloid fibrils. In addition, amyloid fibrils are composed of immunoglobulin light chains or fragments of light chains (especially of the variable region) and nonimmunoglobulin protein. Amyloid composed of immunoglobulin is designated *AL* for amyloid fibril protein and the L chain amyloid protein. Nonimmunoglobulin amyloid is designated *AA* for amyloid fibril protein and SAA, its serum-related protein. Protein AF has several subtypes found in the various dystrophies. These noncollagenous proteins can be deposited in the cornea and conjunctiva and in intraocular or adnexal structures.

CLINICAL FINDINGS A useful classification of amyloidosis considers four types. Each type will be considered separately:

- Primary localized amyloidosis
- Primary systemic amyloidosis
- Secondary localized amyloidosis
- Secondary systemic amyloidosis

Ocular amyloidosis is classified as either primary (idiopathic) or secondary (to some chronic disease) and either localized or systemic.

Primary localized amyloidosis This form of ocular amyloidosis is the most common. Conjunctival amyloid plaques occur in the absence of systemic involvement (Fig 15-25). Primary familial amyloidosis of the cornea (gelatinous droplike dystrophy), in which puddinglike translucent nodules occur as cobblestone masses on the central corneal surface (see Figure 15-8), and lattice corneal dystrophy, a special form of primary localized

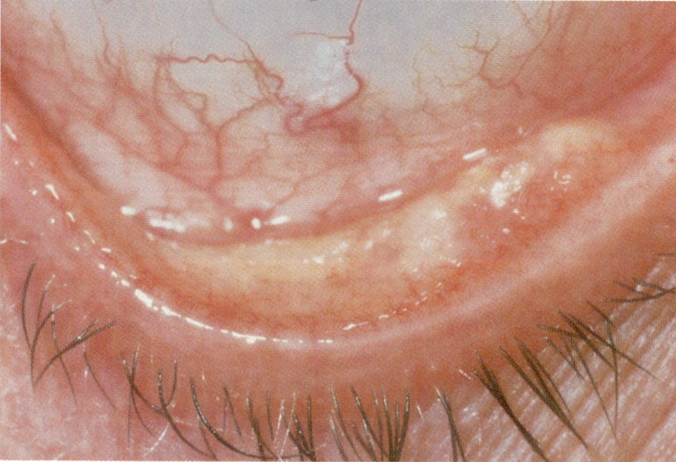

Figure 15-25 Conjunctival amyloidosis. *(Photograph courtesy of Vincent P. deLuise, MD.)*

amyloidosis, are discussed earlier in this chapter. Polymorphic amyloid degeneration is discussed in Chapter 17.

Primary systemic amyloidosis In this heterogeneous group of diseases, waxy ecchymotic eyelid papules occur in association with vitreous veils and opacities as well as pupillary anomalies such as light-near dissociation. Orbital involvement, extraocular muscle involvement with ophthalmoplegia, and scleral infiltration with uveal effusion have been reported. The most common form of primary systemic amyloidosis is an autosomal dominant group of diseases linked to 18q11.2–q12.1, with more than 40 different mutations of the transthyretin (TTR, prealbumin) gene described. Corneal involvement occurs in lattice dystrophy type II (Meretoja syndrome), as discussed earlier in this chapter.

Secondary localized amyloidosis This form develops in eyes with long-standing chronic inflammatory disease such as trachoma; interstitial keratitis; tumors; or connective tissue disorders, usually rheumatoid arthritis. Corneal involvement may be seen in keratoconus, trachoma, phlyctenulosis, bullous keratopathy, interstitial keratitis, leprosy, contact lens wear, trichiasis, tertiary syphilis, uveitis, and climatic droplet keratopathy. Secondary deposition takes the form of a degenerative pannus, lamellar deposits in the deep stroma, or perivascular deposits. Deposits are typically yellowish pink or yellow-gray, depending on the associated disease.

Secondary systemic amyloidosis This form features amyloid AA and is seen in association with rheumatoid arthritis, Mediterranean fever, bronchiectasis, and Hansen disease (leprosy). The eyelids can be affected but less commonly than with primary systemic amyloidosis. Amyloid does not deposit in the cornea in secondary systemic amyloidosis.

Goodfriend AN, Ching SST. Corneal and conjunctival degenerations. In: Krachmer JH, Mannis MJ, Holland EJ, eds. *Cornea*. Vol 2. St Louis: Mosby; 1997:1119–1137.

Online Mendelian Inheritance in Man (OMIM). McKusick-Nathans Institute for Genetic Medicine, Johns Hopkins University (Baltimore, MD) and National Center for Biotechnology Information, National Library of Medicine (Bethesda, MD), 2000. Website updated daily: www.ncbi.nlm.nih.gov/omim.

Disorders of Immunoglobulin Synthesis

The excess synthesis of immunoglobulins by plasma cells in multiple myeloma, Waldenström macroglobulinemia, and benign monoclonal gammopathy may be associated with crystalline corneal deposits.

PATHOGENESIS Monoclonal proliferation of plasma cells (B lymphocytes) leads to overproduction of both light (κ or λ) chains and heavy (α, γ, ε, δ, or μ) chains (together, M proteins), overproduction of light chains with or without production of heavy chains (Bence Jones protein), or overproduction of heavy chains without light chains (heavy chain disease). Pathogenesis is related either to direct tissue invasion, particularly of the bone marrow, or to hyperviscosity syndrome. Secondary hypercalcemia may occur. Deposition of paraproteins in the cornea is very rare and is related to diffusion of the proteins, probably from the limbal vessels or, alternately, from the tears or aqueous humor, followed by precipitation perhaps related to corneal temperature or local tissue factors.

CLINICAL FINDINGS Ophthalmic findings include the following:

- Crystalline deposition in all layers of the cornea or in the conjunctiva
- Copper deposition in the cornea
- Sludging of blood flow in the conjunctiva and retina
- Pars plana proteinaceous cysts
- Infiltration of the sclera
- Orbital bony invasion with proptosis

Corneal deposits are numerous, scintillating, and polychromatic. They are typical of IgG-κ chain deposition and possibly related to the size of the paraprotein and the chronicity of the disease.

Waldenström macroglobulinemia is characterized by malignant proliferation of plasma cells generating IgM, causing hyperviscosity syndrome, principally in older men. It has been associated with needlelike crystals and amorphous deposits subepithelially and in deep stroma.

Benign monoclonal gammopathy is a frequent finding in people over age 60 (up to 6%). The systemic evaluation in these cases is negative, but a mild increase in paraprotein is detected (<3 g/dL). Slit-lamp findings of iridescent crystals resemble myeloma and are also very infrequent (about 1%–2% of affected patients).

Cryoglobulins are proteins that precipitate on exposure to cold. They occur nonspecifically in autoimmune disorders, immunoproliferative disorders, or hepatitis B infection. Ophthalmic findings include retinal hyperviscosity signs, occasional crystalline corneal deposits, amorphous limbal masses, and signs of autoimmune disease.

LABORATORY EVALUATION Corneal crystalline deposits have many causes, and evaluation depends on appearance and location in the cornea (see Table 15-5). Serum protein electrophoresis, complete blood count (CBC), and general screening for albumin/globulin and calcium levels are performed when clinical suspicion of immunoglobulin excess arises. Further testing for systemic evaluation depends on clinical suspicion and the initial findings.

MANAGEMENT No ophthalmic treatment is needed unless the amorphous depositions interfere with vision and need to be removed with LK. Crystals will resolve slowly after successful treatment of an underlying malignancy.

Noninflammatory Disorders of Connective Tissue

Table 15-7 summarizes the connective tissue disorders associated with corneal changes.

Ehlers-Danlos syndrome

This heterogeneous group of diseases is characterized by hyperextensibility of joints and skin, easy bruisability, and formation of "cigarette paper" scars. It was discussed briefly in Chapter 13 in connection with blue sclera.

PATHOGENESIS The many (more than 20) known types of Ehlers-Danlos syndrome are classified as autosomal dominant and recessive and X-linked recessive. Eight genetic loci

Table 15-7 Connective Tissue Disorders Associated With Corneal Changes

Name and MIM No*	Corneal Findings	Other Ocular Findings	Genetics/Map/Other Information
Apert syndrome(101200)	Exposure keratitis with severe proptosis Keratoconus (very rare) Megalocornea (very rare)	Strabismus (exotropia with V pattern) Absence of extraocular muscles, proptosis, ocular hypopigmentation, optic atrophy Rare: nystagmus, ptosis, cataract, ectopia lentis, coloboma of iris	AD Gene maps to 10q26. Mutations in fibroblast growth factor receptor–2
Carpenter syndrome Acrocephalo-polysyndactyly type II (201000)	Exposure keratitis secondary to severe proptosis Microcornea (rare) Corneal leukoma (rare)	Epicanthal folds, antimongoloid slant, hypertelorism or hypotelorism, optic atrophy, strabismus	AR
Crouzon syndrome (123500)	Exposure keratitis with severe proptosis Keratoconus (very rare) Microcornea (very rare)	Strabismus (exotropia with V pattern) Exophthalmos, hypertelorism, optic atrophy in 30% Rare: nystagmus, glaucoma, cataract, ectopia lentis, aniridia, anisocoria, myelinated nerve fibers	AD Gene maps to 10q26. Mutations in fibroblast growth factor receptor–2
Ehlers-Danlos syndrome (more than 20 known types)	Brittle cornea, keratoglobus in type VI Keratoconus in types I and VI	Epicanthal folds, blue sclerae, retinal detachment, ectopia lentis, glaucoma, angioid streaks (rare)	Inheritance varies by type. Type VI is AR and maps to 1p36.3–1p36.2. Mutations in lysyl hydroxylase Multiple genes identified.
Hallerman-Streiff-François syndrome Oculomandibulo-dyscephaly (234100)	Sclerocornea	Congenital cataracts, spontaneous resorption of lens cortex with secondary membranous cataract formation, glaucoma, uveitis, retinal folds, optic nerve cysplasia, microphthalmos	Sporadic Rarely AD Increased anesthetic risk secondary to tracheomalacia
Marfan syndrome (154700)	Megalocornea Flat cornea Keratoconus (uncommon)	Ectopia lentis, strabismus, cataracts, myopia, retinal detachment, glaucoma	AD 15q21.1 Mutations in fibrillin-1
Oculodentoosseous dysplasia (164200, AD) (25750, AR)	Microcornea	Hypotelorism, convergent strabismus, anterior segment dysgenesis, glaucoma, cataracts, remnants of the hyaloid system	AD gene maps to 6q22.q24. Rarely AR

(Continued)

Table 15-7 Connective Tissue Disorders Associated With Corneal Changes (Continued)

Name and MIM No*	Corneal Findings	Other Ocular Findings	Genetics/Map/Other Information
Osteogenesis imperfecta Type I (259400) Type II (166210) Type III (259420) Type IV (166220)	Decreased central corneal thickness Keratoconus Megalocornea (rare) Posterior embryotoxon (rare)	Blue sclerae Rare: congenital glaucoma, cataract, choroidal sclerosis, subhyaloid hemorrhage, hyperopia, ectopia lentis	AD in types I–IV *Types I–III:* Gene maps to 17q21.31–q22 and 7q22.1. *Type IV:* Gene maps to 17q21.31–q22. Mutations in COL1A2 Collagen type I, α-2 polypeptide; COL1A1 Collagen I, α-1 polypeptide
Pierre Robin malformation (261800)	Megalocornea (rare)	Congenital glaucoma, high myopia, vitreoretinal degeneration, retinal detachment, esotropia, congenital cataracts, microphthalmos	Sporadic Stickler syndrome in one third of cases Other syndromes *NB: Increased anesthetic risk secondary to glossoptosis.*
Rothmund-Thomson syndrome (268400)	Degenerative lesions of cornea	Cataracts	AR 70% female 8q24.3
Treacher Collins syndrome (Mandibulofacial dysostosis) (154500)	Microcornea	Coloboma of lower eyelids, dysplasia of bony orbit, absent lower eyelid cilia, absent lower lacrimal puncta, iris coloboma, microphthalmos, strabismus, antimongoloid slant	AD Gene maps to 5q32–q33.1.
Onychoosteodysplasia (Nail-patella syndrome) (161200)	Microcornea	Cataracts, microphthalmos	AD Gene maps to 9q34.1.

* From *Online Mendelian Inheritance in Man,* OMIM. McKusick-Nathans Institute for Genetic Medicine, Johns Hopkins University (Baltimore, MD) and National Center for Biotechnology Information, National Library of Medicine (Bethesda, MD), 2000. www.ncbi.nlm.nih.gov/omim.

(Modified from Traboulsi EI, Kattan HM. Skeletal and connective tissue disorders with anterior segment manifestations. In: Krachmer JH, Mannis MJ, Holland EJ, eds. *Cornea.* Vol 2. St Louis: Mosby; 1997:927–928.)

have been identified to date. Specific defects occur in collagen type I and III synthesis, and there can be lysyl hydroxylase deficiency.

CLINICAL FINDINGS Ehlers-Danlos syndrome VI (EDS VI), or the ocular-scoliotic type, is autosomal recessive and associated with only moderate joint and skin extensibility, brittle cornea easily ruptured on minor trauma, blue sclera, keratoconus and keratoglobus, and severe scoliosis. Type VIA shows lysyl hydroxylase deficiency, but type VIB shows normal production of lysyl hydroxylase.

LABORATORY EVALUATION Traditionally, the clinical diagnosis is confirmed by an insufficiency of hydroxylysine on analysis of hydrolyzed dermis and/or reduced enzyme activity in cultured skin fibroblasts. However, it can also be confirmed by the altered urinary ratio of lysyl pyridinoline to hydroxylysyl pyridinoline that is characteristic for EDS VI.

MANAGEMENT Recognition of the syndrome and awareness of its association with mitral valve prolapse, spontaneous bowel rupture, complications of strabismus surgery, and potential confusion of the brittle cornea with child abuse are essential. Scleral patch grafts for ruptures have been successful. Genetic counseling should be considered.

Marfan syndrome

This common autosomal dominant disorder is associated with disorders of the eye (ectopia lentis), heart (dilation of the aortic root and aneurysms of the aorta), and skeletal system (arachnodactyly, pectus excavatum, and kyphoscoliosis). It maps to chromosome 15q21.1 (fibrillin gene).

PATHOGENESIS Fibrillin and glycoprotein make up the microfibrillar system of the extracellular matrix. Fibrillin is found in corneal basement membrane, zonular fibers of the lens and capsule, and sclera. Defects in fibrillin synthesis lead to thinning of the sclera (blue sclera), lens subluxation, and flattening of the cornea. BCSC Section 11, *Lens and Cataract*, discusses and illustrates the lens subluxation caused by Marfan syndrome.

CLINICAL FINDINGS Megalocornea and keratoconus are uncommon, but excessive flattening (35 D range) occurs in up to 20% of patients.

MANAGEMENT Cardiac evaluation should be completed, as premature mortality is associated with aortic complications. Open-angle glaucoma and cataract occur at a higher rate and earlier age than in the normal population and require attention as usually dictated by those conditions.

Disorders of Nucleotide Metabolism

Gout

Hyperuricemia is a heterogeneous group of disorders of purine metabolism that result in increased uric acid. Discrete deposits of urate crystals into the joints or kidney is called *gout*.

PATHOGENESIS Hyperuricemia may be familial, as a result of an enzyme deficiency (eg, hypoxanthine phosphoribosyltransferase in Lesch-Nyhan syndrome). More commonly, it is polygenic or secondary to obesity, cytotoxic chemotherapy, myeloproliferative disease, diuretic therapy, or excessive alcohol consumption.

CLINICAL FINDINGS Acute inflammation of the sclera, episclera, or conjunctiva can occur. Fine corneal epithelial and stromal deposits may appear in the absence of inflammation. See Table 15-5 for differential diagnosis of corneal deposits. An orange-brown band keratopathy or a typical whitish band keratopathy is seen rarely.

LABORATORY EVALUATION Serum uric acid level is typically elevated. However, in urate keratopathy, uric acid level may be normal in the presence of keratopathy if there is no concurrent inflammation.

MANAGEMENT Acute treatment is with indomethacin, colchicine, or phenylbutazone; long-term reduction in uric acid levels should be pursued with drugs such as allopurinol. Superficial deposits can be removed mechanically with scraping or keratectomy.

Porphyria

The porphyrias are a group of disorders characterized by excess production and excretion of porphyrins—pigments involved in the synthesis of heme.

PATHOGENESIS *Porphyria cutanea tarda,* the form most commonly associated with ocular surface problems, is either sporadically or autosomal dominantly inherited (chromosome 1p34). The enzyme uroporphyrinogen decarboxylase is deficient, resulting in an accumulation of porphyrins in the liver and in the circulation. Typically, a second insult to the liver such as alcoholism or drug metabolism brings on the condition in late middle age.

The pathogenesis is related to porphyrin accumulation in the skin and mucous membranes and to significant iron overload. A severe form of porphyria, called *hepatoerythropoietic porphyria (HEP),* is a homozygous presentation of the same enzymatic defect, but the onset of the disease occurs in infancy.

CLINICAL FINDINGS Sun-exposed surfaces develop hyperpigmentation, erythema, scleroderma-like changes, increased fragility, and vesicular and ulcerative lesions. Interpalpebral injection occurs, and the conjunctiva may develop vesicles, necrosis, scarring, and symblepharon mimicking bullous pemphigoid. Necrotizing scleritis has been reported. The cornea may be affected by exposure or by thinning and perforation at the limbus. Skin and ocular lesions may fluoresce.

LABORATORY EVALUATION Urine turns dark on standing. Reduced liver and red cell uroporphyrinogen decarboxylase is confirmatory, and hepatic biopsy shows liver parenchyma cells filled with porphyrins that fluoresce bright red in ultraviolet light.

MANAGEMENT Protection from ultraviolet light and reduction of iron by phlebotomy are the principal treatments. No specific ocular treatment is available, and corneal thinning and perforation are treated in standard ways.

Disorders of Mineral Metabolism

Wilson disease

Inherited as an autosomal recessive metabolic defect linked to chromosome 13q14.3–q21.1, Wilson disease, or *hepatolenticular degeneration,* is caused by multiple allelic substitutions or deletions in DNA coding for an ATPase, Cu^{2+}-transporting, β-polypeptide.

PATHOGENESIS Copper is deposited in the liver, then in the kidneys, and eventually in the brain and the cornea at Descemet's membrane.

CLINICAL FINDINGS Muscular rigidity increases, and tremor and involuntary movement gradually occur in a fluctuating course resembling parkinsonism. Unintelligible speech and mild dementia usually occur concomitantly. Equal numbers of patients (40%) present with hepatic or nervous system symptoms. In the cornea, a golden brown, ruby red, or green pigment ring (Kayser-Fleischer ring) appears in peripheral Descemet's membrane (Fig 15-26). Not all patients with bona fide Wilson disease will manifest a Kayser-Fleischer ring, which appears first superiorly, gradually spreading and widening to meet deposits inferiorly. It consists of deposits of copper in the posterior lamella of Descemet's membrane. Gonioscopy may assist in visualizing the ring.

Differential diagnosis includes primary biliary cirrhosis, chronic active hepatitis, exogenous chalcosis, and progressive intrahepatic cholestasis of childhood. These and other non-Wilsonian hepatic disorders can also be associated with Kayser-Fleischer rings, but only Wilson disease has decreased serum ceruloplasmin and neurologic symptoms.

LABORATORY EVALUATION Patients with Wilson disease can be differentiated from others with Kayser-Fleischer rings by their inability to incorporate radioactive copper into ceruloplasmin. Low serum ceruloplasmin, high nonceruloplasmin-bound serum copper, and high urinary copper suggest the diagnosis, which can be established with liver biopsy. Nonspecific findings of proteinuria, aminoaciduria, glycosuria, uricaciduria, hyperphosphaturia, and hypercalciuria are seen.

MANAGEMENT Wilson disease can be treated with penicillamine. The Kayser-Fleischer ring disappears gradually with therapy including liver transplantation, and the disappearance of the rings can be used to help monitor therapy. Recently, electrophysiologic abnormalities from retinal dysfunction have been shown to reverse after disease treatment.

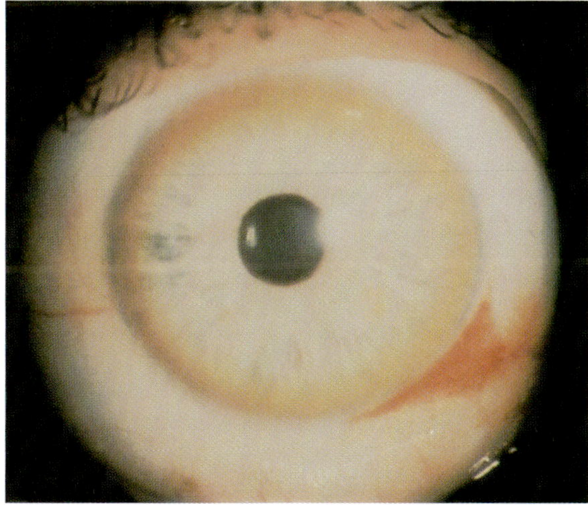

Figure 15-26 Kayser-Fleischer ring of Wilson hepatolenticular degeneration; deposits of copper in Descemet's membrane.

Hypercalcemia

Disorders of calcium and phosphate metabolism are associated with formation of *band keratopathy.* See Chapter 17.

Hemochromatosis

Systemic iron overload is not associated with corneal deposits or changes. In rare cases, congenital spherocytosis has been associated with deep intraepithelial reddish brown deposits in an oval shape of unknown pathogenesis. Iron depositions are discussed further in Chapter 17.

Corneal and External Disease Signs of Systemic Neoplasia

Chapter 11 discusses neoplastic disorders in greater depth. See also BCSC Section 7, *Orbit, Eyelids, and Lacrimal System.*

Enlarged corneal nerves

Several conditions feature enlarged corneal nerves. The most important is multiple endocrine neoplasia (MEN) type IIB (Sipple-Gorlin syndrome). This autosomal dominant (chromosome 10q11.2) disease is characterized by medullary carcinoma of the thyroid gland, pheochromocytoma, and mucosal neuromas in patients who frequently have a marfanoid habitus. Besides the thickened corneal nerves, conjunctival and eyelid neuromas and keratoconjunctivitis sicca may occur. Recently, patients with MEN type IIA and type III have also been noted to have enlarged corneal nerves. Other causes of prominent corneal nerves from either true enlargement or increased visibility are listed in Table 15-8.

Table 15-8 Prominent Corneal Nerves

Enlarged Corneal Nerves	More Visible Corneal Nerves
Multiple endocrine neoplasia type IIB (Sipple-Gorlin syndrome)	Keratoconus
Phytanic acid storage disease (Refsum syndrome)	Ichthyosis
Hansen disease (leprosy, beading of nerves)	Fuchs corneal dystrophy
Familial dysautonomia (Riley-Day syndrome)	Corneal edema
Neurofibromatosis	Congenital glaucoma
Acanthamoeba perineuritis	

PART VIII

Degenerative Disorders of the Conjunctiva, Cornea, and Sclera

CHAPTER 16

Degenerative and Aging Processes of the Conjunctiva, Cornea, and Sclera

Degenerations of the ocular surface may occur from the physiologic changes associated with aging, or they may follow an environmental insult to the eye such as exposure to ultraviolet light.

Degeneration of a tissue is a physiologic decomposition of tissue elements and deterioration of tissue functions. Table 16-1 summarizes the differences between degenerations and corneal dystrophies.

Aging of the Conjunctiva

The conjunctiva loses transparency as an individual ages. The epithelium thickens and may become keratinized in exposed zones. The substantia propria becomes thinner and less elastic. In older persons, the conjunctival vessels can become more prominent. Saccular telangiectases, fusiform dilatory changes, or tortuosities may appear. These changes are not necessarily uniform and tend to be more pronounced in the area of the interpalpebral fissure. Furthermore, increased laxity is often apparent in the inferior bulbar conjunctiva. This condition, termed *conjunctivochalasis*, appears as redundant, loose, nonedematous conjunctiva interposed between the lower eyelid and globe.

Aging of the Cornea

Over time, the cornea gradually becomes flatter, thinner, and slightly less transparent. Its refractive index increases, and Descemet's membrane becomes thicker, increasing from 3 μm at birth to 10 μm in adults as a result of the increased thickness of its posterior nonbanded zones. Occasional peripheral guttata, sometimes known as Hassall-Henle bodies, can form with age. Age-related attrition of corneal endothelial cells results in a loss of about 100,000 cells during the first 50 years of life, from a cell density of about 4000 cells/mm² at birth to a density of 2500–3000 cells/mm² in adults. The average rate of endothelial cell density decrease throughout adult life is approximately 0.6% per year.

Table 16-1 Differences Between Corneal Degenerations and Corneal Dystrophies

Degeneration	Dystrophy
Opacity often peripherally located	Centrally located
May be asymmetric	Bilateral and symmetric
Presents later in life, associated with aging	Presents early in life, hereditary
Progression can be very slow or rapid	Progression usually slow

Bourne WM, Nelson LR, Hodge DO. Central corneal endothelial cell changes over a ten-year period. *Invest Ophthalmol Vis Sci.* 1997;38:779–782.

Degenerative Changes in the Cornea

The cornea of the aging eye is more susceptible to degenerative changes, which occur most often near the limbus. Peripheral corneal degeneration can be divided into two general categories:

- Deposition of lipid or other substances
- Connective tissue changes with thinning

The peripheral cornea differs from the central cornea in several unique anatomic and physiologic features. Contiguity with the limbal vasculature is the most important difference. Unlike the central cornea, the peripheral cornea can be adversely affected by the pathologies associated with blood vessels, such as inflammatory infiltrations and depositions of serum proteins or other substances. Because of its proximity to limbal vessels, the peripheral cornea is inevitably involved in the early stage of any condition causing corneal vascularization.

The peripheral cornea is also close to the surrounding conjunctiva, episclera, and sclera, and it is secondarily affected by the primary diseases of these adjacent tissues. Conjunctival inflammatory conditions such as pterygium and trachoma often involve the peripheral cornea. Mechanical disruption of normal corneal wetting by the adjacent swollen conjunctiva can lead to drying of the peripheral cornea and dellen formation.

Corneal epithelial stem cells are located in the limbal basal epithelium. These cells are the proliferative source of corneal epithelium and are responsible for the renewal of the corneal surface. Disruption of this important corneal physiologic barrier may lead to conjunctival invasion, resulting in surface irregularity and vascularization, as in pterygium and keratinization of the eyelid margin.

Aging of the Sclera

Age-related changes in the sclera involve connective tissue changes and atrophy of scleral fibrocytes. The most common alteration is lipid deposition in the deeper layers, which can give the anterior sclera a yellowish color. A gradual loss of elasticity can result in increased rigidity that can affect estimation of the intraocular pressure.

CHAPTER 17

Clinical Approach to Depositions and Degenerations of the Conjunctiva, Cornea, and Sclera

Conjunctival Degenerations

Pinguecula

A pinguecula is a common conjunctival condition that occurs typically at the nasal and temporal anterior bulbar conjunctiva.

PATHOGENESIS This degenerative lesion of the bulbar conjunctiva occurs as a result of the effects of ultraviolet (UV) light (actinic exposure), but it may also be related to other insults such as welding. The epithelium overlying a pinguecula may be normal, thick, or thin. Calcification occurs occasionally.

CLINICAL FINDINGS Pingueculae appear adjacent to the limbus in the interpalpebral zone, more often nasally, and have the appearance of yellow-white, amorphous subepithelial deposits. They may enlarge gradually over long periods of time. Recurrent inflammation and ocular irritation may be encountered.

LABORATORY EVALUATION Histopathologically, the subepithelial collagen fibers become fragmented, curled, and more basophilic with hematoxylin-eosin stain. The fibers also stain with elastic tissue stains but are not elastic tissue. These fibers are insensitive to treatment with elastase, which does not prevent positive staining for elastin. This particular kind of degeneration of collagen, in which it takes on staining characteristics of elastic tissue, is referred to as *elastoid* or *elastotic degeneration* or, simply, *elastosis*.

MANAGEMENT Lubricant therapy to alleviate ocular irritations is often used clinically. Excision is indicated only when pingueculae constitute cosmetic problems or in the rare instances in which they become chronically inflamed or interfere with successful contact lens wear. The inflammation of a pinguecula should be distinguished from nodular scleritis or episcleritis. Judicious use of topical steroids can be considered in patients with chronic inflammation.

Pterygium

A pterygium is a wing-shaped growth on the bulbar conjunctiva.

PATHOGENESIS The occurrence of pterygia is strongly correlated with UV exposure, although dryness, inflammation, and exposure to wind and dust or other irritants may also be factors. UV-B is mutagenic for the p53 tumor suppressor gene in limbal basal stem cells. Without apoptosis, transforming growth factor–beta is overproduced and leads to collagenase up-regulation, cellular migration, and angiogenesis. The ensuing pathologic changes consist of elastoid degeneration of collagen and the appearance of subepithelial fibrovascular tissue. The cornea shows destruction of Bowman's layer by fibrovascular ingrowth, frequently with mild inflammatory changes. The epithelium may be normal, thick, or thin, and it occasionally shows dysplasia.

CLINICAL FINDINGS A pterygium is a wing-shaped fold of conjunctiva and fibrovascular tissue that has invaded the superficial cornea. Pterygia are nearly always preceded and accompanied by pingueculae. It is not known why some patients develop pterygia, whereas others have only pingueculae, but the prevalence of pterygia increases steadily with proximity to the equator. Regular and irregular astigmatism occurs in proportion to pterygium size. A pigmented iron line *(Stocker's line)* may be seen in advance of a pterygium on the cornea (Fig 17-1).

MANAGEMENT Excision is indicated if the visual axis is threatened or in cases of considerable irritation. See Chapter 21.

Conjunctival Concretions

Concretions appear histopathologically to be epithelial inclusion cysts filled with epithelial and keratin debris. Yellow-white deposits are sometimes found in the palpebral conjunctiva of patients who are elderly or who have had chronic conjunctivitis. Secondary calcification occurs occasionally, in which case the lesions are sometimes referred to as *conjunctival lithiasis.* The subconjunctival deposition of tetracycline mimics concretions.

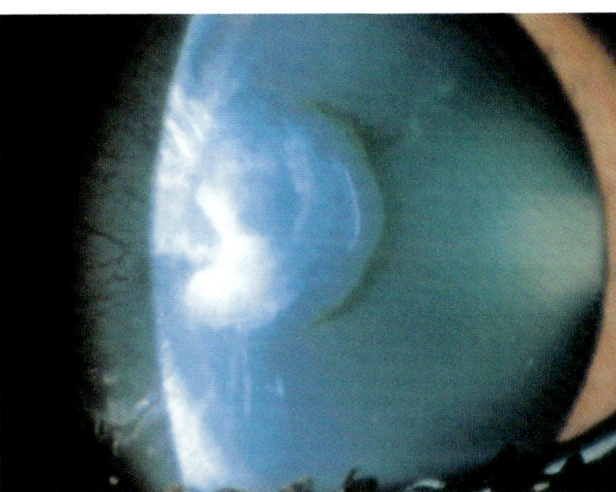

Figure 17-1 Stocker's line at the head of a pterygium. *(Photograph courtesy of Vincent P. deLuise, MD.)*

Concretions are almost always asymptomatic but may erode the overlying epithelium to cause foreign-body sensation. If symptomatic, concretions can be easily removed under topical anesthesia.

Conjunctivochalasis

Conjunctivochalasis is a loose adherence of the lower conjunctiva; it occurs commonly with chronic inflammation or aging and is often overlooked and asymptomatic. Occasionally, the redundant conjunctiva overlies the lower eyelid margin to such an extent that various clinical problems appear. These range from the aggravation of dry eye in the mild stages, to secondary tearing due to occlusion of the lower punctum when the chalasis is prominent medially, to exposure-related pain and irritation in its severe stages. One recently proposed grading system recommends specifying the following:

- Location (temporal, nasal, middle, or whole lid)
- Height (relative to the tear meniscus)
- Whether or not the chalasis occludes the punctum, changes in downgaze, or changes with digital pressure

Lubricants, anti-inflammatory agents, antihistamines, and nocturnal patching have been offered as treatments. If these modalities fail, then cautious surgical excision or conjunctival fixation to the sclera may be needed.

Meller D, Tseng SC. Conjunctivochalasis: literature review and possible pathophysiology. *Surv Ophthalmol.* 1998;43:225–232.

Corneal Degenerations

Epithelial and Subepithelial Degenerations

Coats white ring

A small (1 mm or less in diameter) circle of discrete gray-white dots is sometimes seen in the superficial stroma. Referred to as *Coats white ring*, it represents iron-containing fibrotic remnants of a metallic foreign body. These rings probably develop when a rust ring from an iron foreign body is not entirely removed. No treatment is required (Fig 17-2).

Spheroidal degeneration

This common degeneration is often bilateral, interpalpebral, and more common in males. It is characterized by the appearance in the cornea, and sometimes in the conjunctiva, of translucent, golden brown, spheroidlike deposits in the superficial stroma. The condition has been reported under different names, including corneal elastosis, keratinoid degeneration, climatic droplet keratopathy, Bietti nodular dystrophy, proteinaceous degeneration, and Labrador keratopathy.

In *primary spheroidal degeneration,* the deposits are bilateral and initially located in the nasal and temporal cornea. They are related to advancing age and can extend onto

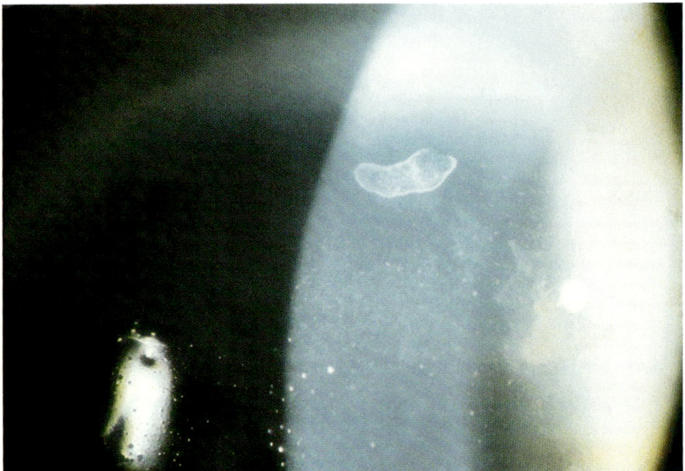

Figure 17-2 Coats white ring (not to be confused with map-dot-fingerprint dystrophy). *(Photograph courtesy of W. Craig Fowler, MD.)*

the conjunctiva. The degeneration is unrelated to the coexistence of other ocular disease. In rare cases, generally in childhood, the spheroidal deposits extend across the interpalpebral zone of the cornea, producing a noncalcific band-shaped keratopathy.

Secondary spheroidal degeneration is associated with ocular injury or inflammation. The deposits aggregate near the area of corneal scarring or vascularization. All cases show extracellular proteinaceous deposits with characteristics of elastotic degeneration, which are thought to be secondary to the combined effects of genetic predisposition, actinic exposure, age, and perhaps various kinds of environmental trauma other than sunlight. The composition is not lipid despite its "oil droplet" appearance. The pattern is similar to other UV light–associated degenerations such as pingueculae. No medical therapy is of value. In cases of central involvement, superficial keratectomy or excimer excision may be indicated. Recurrence after conjunctival resection is common.

Stromal Degenerations: Age-Related (Involutional) Changes

White limbal girdle

Two forms of the white limbal girdle of Vogt have been described. *Type I* is a narrow, concentric, whitish superficial band running along the limbus in the palpebral fissure. A lucid interval appears between the limbus and the girdle. This girdle is a degenerative change of the anterior limiting membrane, with chalklike opacities and small clear areas like Swiss cheese. *Type II* consists of small white flecklike and needlelike deposits that are often seen at the nasal and temporal limbus in older patients. No clear interval separates this girdle from the limbus. The histopathologic picture represents epithelial elastotic degeneration of collagen, sometimes with particles of calcium.

Corneal arcus (arcus senilis)

PATHOGENESIS Arcus senilis is most often an involutional change modified by genetic factors. However, arcus is sometimes indicative of a hyperlipoproteinemia (low-density lipoprotein) with elevated serum cholesterol, especially in patients under 40 years of age (see Chapter 15). It is also a prognostic factor for coronary artery disease in this age group. Arcus occurs occasionally as a congenital anomaly *(arcus juvenilis),* usually involving only a sector of the peripheral cornea and not associated with abnormalities of serum lipid.

CLINICAL FINDINGS Arcus is a deposition of lipid in the peripheral corneal stroma. It starts at the inferior and superior poles of the cornea and, in the late stages, encircles the entire circumference. Incidence is 60% in individuals between the ages of 50 and 60; it approaches 100% in persons over 80. Frequency is higher in the black population. The arcus has a hazy white appearance, a sharp outer border, and an indistinct central border; it is denser superiorly and inferiorly. A lucid interval is usually present between the peripheral edge of the arcus and the limbus. Unilateral arcus is a rare condition associated with contralateral carotid artery disease or ocular hypotony. Arcus is also seen in Schnyder central crystalline dystrophy.

LABORATORY EVALUATION The lipid can be demonstrated histopathologically only by the use of fat stains of frozen sections because standard fixation techniques dissolve it. The lipid is found to be concentrated mainly in two areas of the peripheral cornea stroma: one adjacent to Bowman's layer and another near Descemet's membrane.

Crocodile shagreen

Anterior crocodile shagreen, or *mosaic degeneration,* is a central corneal opacity at the level of Bowman's layer characterized by mosaic, polygonal, gray opacities separated by clear zones. Histologically, Bowman's layer is thrown into ridges and may be calcified. Posterior crocodile shagreen shows similar changes in the deep stroma near Descemet's membrane. The posterior variety of crocodile shagreen resembles central cloudy dystrophy of François (see Figure 13-4).

Cornea farinata

This involutional change is probably dependent on a dominantly transmitted genetic predisposition. The deep corneal stroma shows many opacities in the shapes of dots and commas. They are very nebulous and subtle and often can be seen with retroillumination. The condition does not affect vision and has no clinical significance, except that it is sometimes mistaken for a progressive dystrophy. The deposits may consist of lipofuscin, a degenerative pigment that appears in some aged cells. Pre–Descemet's dystrophy is probably a morphologic variant of cornea farinata. Although these conditions are most likely related, it is unclear whether they are degenerations or dystrophies.

Polymorphic amyloid degeneration

This bilaterally symmetric, slowly progressive corneal degeneration appears late in life. The corneal opacities emerge as either stellate flecks in mid to deep stroma or irregular filaments. Both forms may occur together, but usually one predominates. These deposits are usually axial, polymorphic, and filamentous. The opacities are gray to white and somewhat refractile but appear translucent in retroillumination. The intervening stroma appears clear. Visual acuity is usually normal. The corneal deposits consist of amyloid and can resemble some of the deposits seen in early lattice corneal dystrophy.

Stromal Degenerations: Peripheral Cornea

Senile furrow degeneration

This condition is an appearance of thinning that is seen in older people in the lucid interval of a corneal arcus. There is no inflammation, vascularization, or tendency to perforate. Vision is rarely affected unless astigmatism occurs because of the thinning. Although slight thinning is occasionally present, it is usually more apparent than real. The epithelium is intact. No treatment is required.

Terrien marginal degeneration

PATHOGENESIS The cause is unknown, although association with vernal keratoconjunctivitis has been reported.

CLINICAL FINDINGS This condition is a quiet, essentially noninflammatory, unilateral or asymmetrically bilateral, slowly progressive thinning of the peripheral cornea. Sex prevalence is roughly equal, and cases usually occur in the second or third decade of life. The corneal thinning can be localized or involve extensive portions of the peripheral cornea.

Terrien marginal degeneration begins superiorly, spreads circumferentially, and rarely involves the inferior limbus. The central wall is steep, and the peripheral wall slopes gradually. The epithelium remains intact, and a fine vascular pannus traverses the area of stromal thinning. A line of lipid deposits appears at the leading edge of the pannus (central edge of the furrow). Spontaneous perforation is rare, although perforation can easily occur with minor trauma. Corneal topography reveals flattening of the peripheral thinned cornea, with steepening of the corneal surface approximately 90° away from the midpoint of the thinned area (Fig 17-3). This pattern usually results in high against-the-rule or oblique astigmatism. Spontaneous ruptures in Descemet's membrane can result in interlamellar fluid or even a corneal cyst.

An inflammatory condition of the peripheral cornea that may resemble Terrien marginal degeneration occurs, in rare instances, in children and young adults. Also known as *Fuchs superficial marginal keratitis,* it features progressive thinning without epithelial ulceration and can lead to perforation.

LABORATORY EVALUATION AND MANAGEMENT Electron microscopic studies have revealed histiocytes that may be responsible for phagocytosis of corneal collagen. Surgical correction is indicated when perforation is imminent due to progressive thinning or when marked astigmatism significantly limits visual acuity. Crescent-shaped lamellar or full-thickness corneoscleral patch grafts may be utilized and have been reported to arrest the progression of severe against-the-rule astigmatism for up to 20 years. Annular lamellar keratoplasty grafts may be required in severe cases of 360° marginal degeneration.

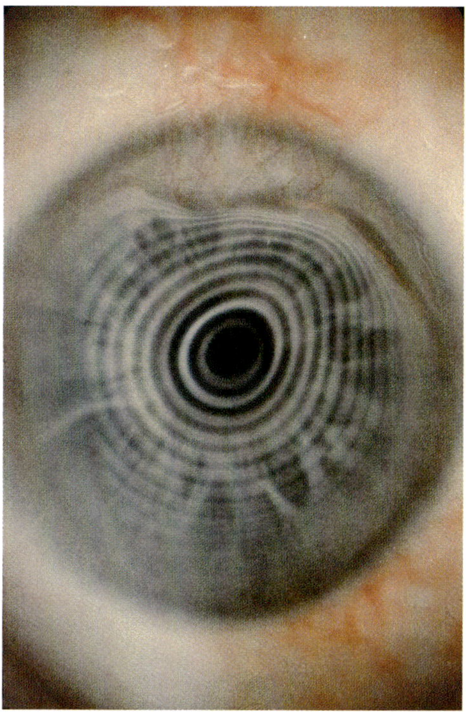

Figure 17-3 Terrien marginal degeneration with superior thinning. *(Photograph courtesy of W. Craig Fowler, MD.)*

Stromal Degenerations: Postinflammatory Changes

Salzmann nodular degeneration

This noninflammatory corneal degeneration sometimes occurs as a late sequel to old, long-standing keratitis, or it may be idiopathic. Causes include phlyctenulosis, trachoma, and interstitial keratitis. The degeneration may not appear until years after the active keratitis has subsided. It can be bilateral and is more common in middle-aged and older women. The nodules are gray-white or blue-white and elevated, and they may be associated with recurrent erosion. They often develop in a roughly circular configuration in the central or paracentral cornea and at the ends of vessels of a pannus. Histopathologic examination reveals localized replacement of Bowman's layer by hyaline and fibrillar material, probably representing basement membrane and material similar to that found in spheroidal degeneration. Treatment is with superficial keratectomy. This degeneration may recur after keratoplasty (Fig 17-4).

Amyloid degeneration

Acquired (secondary localized) corneal amyloidosis may be associated with corneal inflammation (such as trachoma, keratoconus, Hansen disease, or phlyctenulosis) or intraocular disease (such as uveitis, retinopathy of prematurity, or glaucoma) or may be secondary to trauma. Clinically, amyloid deposits usually occur as raised, yellow-pink nodular masses in the cornea. Less commonly, they may appear as perivascular deposits. In most cases, corneal vascularization is associated with the amyloid. The

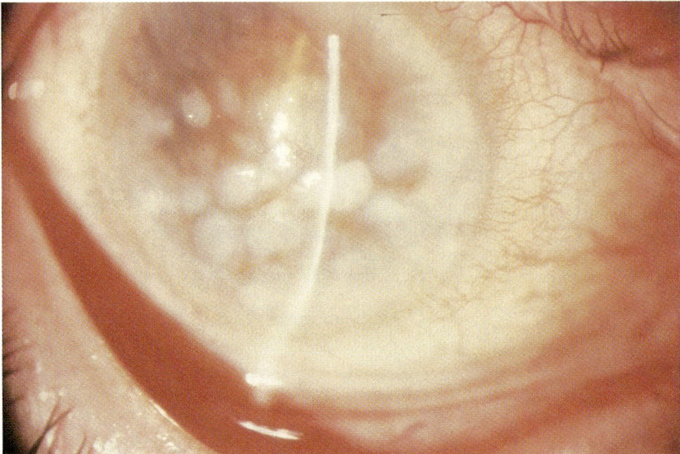

Figure 17-4 Salzmann corneal nodules. *(Photograph courtesy of W. Craig Fowler, MD.)*

deposits may be refractile with retroillumination. See the discussion on amyloidosis in Chapter 15.

Corneal keloid

These white, sometimes protuberant, glistening corneal masses often resemble dermoids and can involve the entire corneal surface. They are thought to be secondary to a vigorous fibrocytic response to corneal perforation or injury. The resemblance to corneal dermoids can make diagnosis difficult. Subtle differences between corneal keloids and dermoids include the glistening and jellylike quality of the keloids. Definitive diagnosis can be made by performing corneal biopsy. Study of enucleation specimens has revealed associated findings, including cataract, anterior staphyloma, ruptured lens capsule with lens fragments in the wound, buphthalmos, chronic glaucoma, and angle-closure glaucoma. Proper diagnosis may result in the use of appropriate procedures other than enucleation to treat this condition. Congenital corneal keloid is discussed in Chapter 13.

Lipid keratopathy

Yellow or cream-colored lipids containing cholesterol, neutral fats, and glycoproteins are deposited in the superficial or deeper cornea, usually in areas of vascularized corneal scars. The epithelium is involved secondarily, after prolonged corneal inflammation with corneal vascularization (eg, herpes simplex or herpes zoster keratitis or trachoma). This form would best be described as *secondary lipid keratopathy*. Lipid keratopathy has been reported, in rare instances, with no evidence of an antecedent infection, inflammatory process, or corneal damage. These cases would best be described as *primary lipid keratopathy*.

Calcific band keratopathy (calcium hydroxyapatite deposition)

PATHOGENESIS This calcific degeneration of the superficial cornea involves mainly Bowman's layer. There are six main causes:

- Chronic ocular disease (usually inflammatory) such as uveitis in children, interstitial keratitis, severe superficial keratitis, and phthisis bulbi
- Hypercalcemia caused by hyperparathyroidism, vitamin D toxicity, milk–alkali syndrome, sarcoidosis, and other systemic disorders
- Hereditary transmission (primary hereditary band keratopathy, with or without other anomalies)
- Elevated serum phosphorus with normal serum calcium, which sometimes occurs in patients with renal failure
- Chronic exposure to mercurial vapors or to mercurial preservatives (phenylmercuric nitrate or acetate) in ophthalmic medications (the mercury causes changes in corneal collagen that result in the deposition of calcium)
- Silicone oil instillation in an aphakic eye

Other rare associated disorders have been reported, including iris melanoma. Band keratopathy may also result from the deposition in the cornea of urates, which appear brown, unlike the gray-white calcific deposits, and may be associated with gout or hyperuricemia.

CLINICAL PRESENTATION Calcific band keratopathy begins as fine, dustlike, basophilic deposits in Bowman's layer. These changes are usually first seen peripherally. A peripheral clear zone representing a lucid interval is seen between the limbus and the peripheral edge of the keratopathy. Eventually, the deposits may coalesce to form a horizontal band of dense calcific plaques across the interpalpebral zone of the cornea (Fig 17-5).

MANAGEMENT Underlying conditions, such as keratoconjunctivitis sicca or renal failure, should be treated or controlled as much as possible, which may reduce or control the deposition of calcium or at least help reduce the recurrence of band keratopathy. The calcium can usually be removed from Bowman's layer by chelation with a neutral solution of disodium ethylenediaminetetraacetic acid (EDTA) 150 mg/mL (Endrate, 20 mL per vial). A proper concentration can be made by mixing one 20 mL vial with 100 mL of

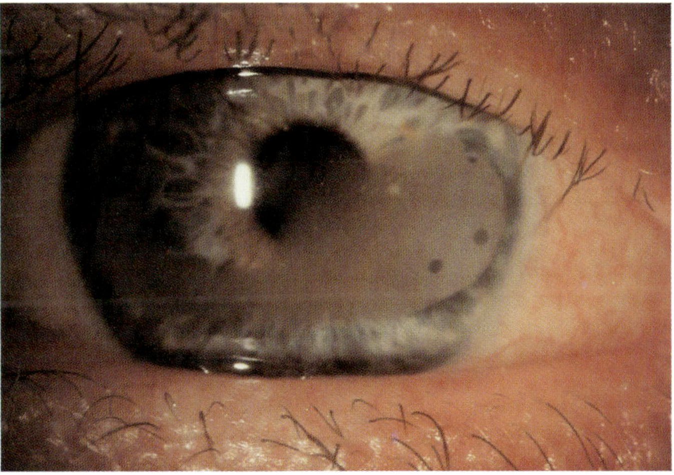

Figure 17-5 Band keratopathy. *(Photograph courtesy of Vincent P. deLuise, MD.)*

sterile ophthalmic irrigation solution, and this mixture can be warmed to speed up the chemical chelation of calcium. The epithelium overlying the calcium needs to be removed prior to applying the chelating solution. Any cylindrical tube that approximates the corneal diameter can facilitate the process by acting as a reservoir to confine the chelating solution to the desired treatment area. With the reservoir in place, very gentle surface agitation with truncated Weck-cel sponges may further enhance the release of the impregnated calcium. If used at all, scraping should be gentle so as to prevent damage to Bowman's layer. A fibrous pannus may be present along with extensive calcific band keratopathy, especially if silicone oil is responsible, and neither EDTA nor scraping will remove such fibrous tissue. A soft contact lens can be helpful postoperatively until the epithelium has healed. The problem can recur but may not do so for years, at which time the treatment may be repeated. Phototherapeutic keratectomy using excimer laser is not advised as a primary treatment because calcium ablates at a different rate from stroma, which could produce a severely irregular surface. If residual opacification remains after the initial EDTA chelation, then PTK may be employed.

Endothelial Degenerations

Peripheral corneal guttata (Hassall-Henle bodies)

These small, wartlike excrescences appear in the peripheral portion of Descemet's membrane as a normal aging change. They occur on the posterior aspect of the membrane and protrude toward the anterior chamber. With the slit lamp, Hassall-Henle bodies have the appearance of small, dark dimples within the endothelial mosaic, and they are best seen by specular reflection. Rarely seen before age 20, they then increase steadily in number with age. They are pathologic when they appear in the central cornea and are then referred as *cornea guttata*. Central cornea guttata associated with progressive stromal and eventually epithelial edema represent Fuchs endothelial-epithelial dystrophy (see Chapter 15). They are the result of localized overproduction of basement membrane by endothelial cells and so have the same collagenous structure as does normal Descemet's membrane.

Melanin pigmentation

Deposits of melanin on the corneal endothelium can be observed in patients with glaucoma associated with pigment dispersion syndrome. Typically, the cluster of vertically oriented pigments is known as *Krukenberg spindle* (see Table 17-2).

Drug-Induced Deposition and Pigmentation

In rare instances, ophthalmic ointments can become entrapped in the epithelium after corneal abrasions have healed. Clear globules appear within the epithelium. These deposits are usually well tolerated; however, some vascular ingrowths may occur if they are located near the limbus. Subepithelial deposits of tetracycline ointment in the fornix sometimes may simulate amyloid deposition.

Corneal Epithelial Deposits

Cornea verticillata

Amiodarone, a coronary artery dilator, produces lysosomal deposits in the basal epithelial layer, creating a whorl-like pattern resembling that seen in Fabry disease with accumulation of sphingolipid. Such a distinctive pattern of deposits can also be seen with long-term chloroquine, chlorpromazine, or indomethacin therapy. It is unusual for these deposits to result in reduction of visual acuity or ocular symptoms, although this has occurred in some patients.

The development of deposits is not necessarily an indication to stop these medications, although the deposits will resolve with discontinuation of the responsible agents. Chronic administration of chloroquine can lead to a retinopathy that has no specific relationship with the corneal deposits. Systemic drugs associated with corneal deposits are summarized in Table 17-1. Toxic ulcerative keratopathy related to topical ophthalmic medications or, frequently, the preservatives within them, is a significant cause of ocular morbidity as a result of exogenously administered ophthalmic medications. See also the discussion of persistent epithelial defect in Chapter 5 and material on toxic medication reaction in Chapter 19.

Ciprofloxacin deposits

Topical ciprofloxacin therapy can result in the deposition of a chalky white precipitate within an epithelial defect. The precipitate is composed of ciprofloxacin crystals. Although white plaques predominate, a crystalline pattern may be also observed.

Table 17-1 Drugs Associated With Corneal Deposits

Epithelial Deposits	Stromal Deposits
Aminoquinolones	Antacids
Amodiaquine	Gold
Chloroquine	Indomethacin
Hydroxychloroquine	Phenothiazines
Amiodarone	
Clofazimine	Phenylbutazone
Chlorpromazine	
Indomethacin	Practolol
Naproxen	Retinoids
Perhexiline	Silver
Suramin	
Tamoxifen	
Thioxanthines	
Chlorprothixine	
Thiothixine	
Tilorone	

(Adapted from Arffa RC, Eve FR. Systemic associations of corneal deposits. *Int Ophthalmol Clin.* 1991;31:89–110.)

Pigmentation

Corneal pigmentation may result from deposits of melanin, blood or blood products, or a variety of metallic compounds. Table 17-2 lists pigments that may be of diagnostic importance, with their locations and associated conditions. See also Table 15-5.

Argyriasis

Silver compounds (particularly Argyrol) were commonly used in the preantibiotic era for the treatment of external infections. Their chronic use can result in a condition known as *argyriasis*, consisting of a slate gray or silver discoloration involving the bulbar and palpebral conjunctiva. This condition can be permanent.

Adrenochrome

Long-standing administration of epinephrine compounds may lead to black or very dark brown deposits in the conjunctiva and cornea. Composed of adrenochrome, an oxidation product of the basic epinephrine compound, these melanin-like deposits can accumulate in conjunctival cysts and concretions in the conjunctiva (Fig 17-6). They may discolor the cornea or contact lenses as well. The deposits are harmless, although they are occasionally misdiagnosed as conjunctival melanoma or other conditions.

Table 17-2 Corneal Pigmentations

Pigment	Clinical Condition	Location in Cornea
Melanin	Krukenberg spindle	Endothelium, in a vertically oriented ellipse; sometimes associated with pigmentary glaucoma
Melanin-like pigment (oxidized epinephrine)	Adrenochrome deposition	Between basement membrane and Bowman's layer or in conjunctival cysts; occurs in patients using topical epinephrine compounds for glaucoma
Melanin-like pigment (alkapton)	Ochronosis	Epithelium and superficial stroma, peripherally; occurs in the metabolic disease alkaptonuria
Iron	Blood staining	Chiefly stroma; epithelium in some cases; occurs in some cases of hyphema
Iron (foreign body)	Siderosis	Chiefly stroma; epithelium in some cases
Iron	Ferry's line	Corneal epithelium anterior to filtering bleb
Iron	Fleischer ring (or line) (Fig 15-18)	Corneal epithelium surrounding base of cone in keratoconus
Iron	Hudson-Stähli line	Corneal epithelium at junction of upper two thirds with lower one third of the aging cornea
Iron	Stocker's line (Fig 17-1)	Corneal epithelium anterior to head of pterygium
Copper	Kayser-Fleischer ring (Fig 15-26)	Descemet's membrane peripherally, in patients with Wilson hepatolenticular degeneration
Copper	Chalcosis	Descemet's membrane
Silver	Argyriasis	Deep stroma and Descemet's membrane
Gold	Chrysiasis	Deep stroma (more in periphery)
Carbon	Corneal tattoo	Stroma

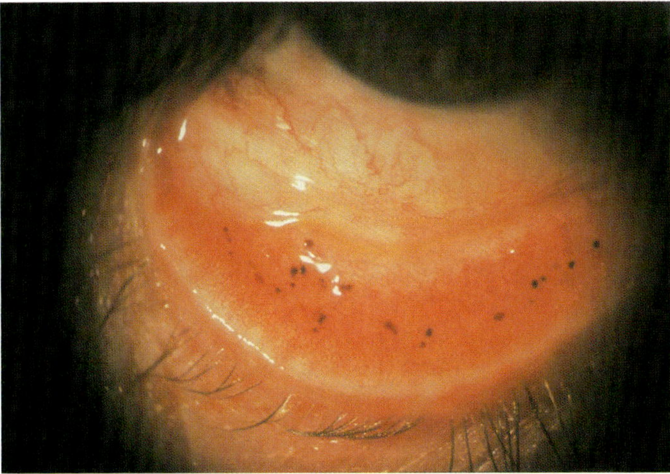

Figure 17-6 Adrenochrome deposits in inferior cul-de-sac. *(Photograph courtesy of Vincent P. deLuise, MD.)*

Arffa RC. *Grayson's Diseases of the Cornea.* 4th ed. St Louis: Mosby; 1997.

Kaiser PK, Pineda R, Albert DM, et al. "Black cornea" after long-term epinephrine use. *Arch Ophthalmol.* 1992;110:1273–1275.

Iron deposits

Iron deposition in the corneal stroma can occur as a result of a retained metallic foreign body or corneal blood staining from prolonged hyphema with secondary glaucoma. A Fleischer ring, representing iron deposition in keratoconus, is one of many corneal iron lines associated with epithelial irregularities (see Figure 15-18). This sign is exceedingly useful in the diagnosis of mild or early cases of keratoconus. Many times, it can be seen only by using red-free or cobalt blue illumination prior to the instillation of fluorescein. The Hudson-Stähli line, generally located at the junction of the upper two thirds and lower third of the cornea, is ubiquitous. Most iron lines are related to abnormalities of tear pooling related to surface irregularities. Iron lines are also associated with kerato-refractive procedures. Following radial keratotomy in approximately 80% of patients, visually insignificant iron lines are noted centrally and are commonly characterized as a "tear star." Common conditions associated with corneal iron lines are listed in Table 17-2.

Arffa RC, Eve FR. Systemic associations of corneal deposits. *Int Ophthalmol Clin.* 1991;31: 89–110.

Scleral Degenerations

Senile Plaques

Scleral rigidity increases in elderly persons, along with a relative decrease in scleral hydration and the amount of mucopolysaccharide. These changes are accompanied by subconjunctival deposition of fat, which gives the sclera a yellowish appearance. Calcium may also be deposited either diffusely among the scleral collagen fibers in granular or crystalline form or focally in a plaque anterior to the horizontal rectus muscle insertions. The plaques are visible as ovoid or rectangular zones of grayish translucency (Fig 17-7). Histologically, the midportion of the involved sclera contains a focal calcified plaque surrounded by relatively acellular collagen. The plaques do not elicit inflammation and rarely extrude. If sufficiently dense, they may be visualized on CT scan.

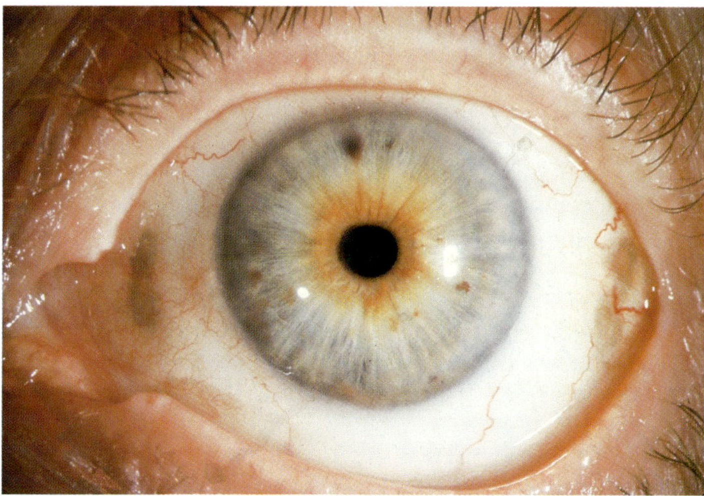

Figure 17-7 Senile scleral plaques anterior to horizontal rectus muscle insertions.

Toxic and Traumatic Injuries of the Anterior Segment

CHAPTER 18

Wound Healing of the Conjunctiva, Cornea, and Sclera

The reader is referred to BCSC Section 4, *Ophthalmic Pathology and Intraocular Tumors*, for an in-depth discussion (with illustrations) of ophthalmic wound healing in the anterior segment. The ensuing sections will cover the basic cellular and tissue responses to wounding and explain the clinical relevance of these basic mechanisms.

Wound Healing of the Conjunctiva

The conjunctival epithelium heals like other mucous membranes. Abrasions stimulate sliding and proliferation, and conjunctival epithelial defects (in a healthy ocular surface) often heal within 1 or 2 days. The substantia propria (conjunctival stroma) heals with revascularization of the wound, associated with budding of nonfenestrated capillaries. The processes of angiogenesis, inflammation, and matrix turnover are integral and co-dependent processes in wound healing. Corticosteroids can retard wound healing by down-modulating every one of these processes. The superficial layer of the conjunctiva, normally composed of loose tissue, may not regenerate after wounding exactly as it was prior to trauma. Rather, the deeper, fibrous layer can predominate in a healed conjunctival wound, making the conjunctiva more adherent to the sclera. This is one reason why eyes that have had prior conjunctival surgery (posterior incisions for cataract surgery or pars plana vitrectomy) have conjunctival scarring that can pose a problem for the glaucoma surgeon who needs to dissect large flaps for filtration surgery.

Wound Healing of the Cornea

Unlike the conjunctiva, corneal wound healing is generally avascular unless there is profound concurrent inflammation or ocular surface/epithelial disease. The basic mechanisms of corneal reepithelialization are similar to that seen in other mucous membranes and consist of epithelial migration and proliferation. Corneal epithelial cells do not have a high turnover unless wounded. Like other stratified epithelia, the corneal epithelium is self-renewing, with a normal turnover of approximately 5–7 days. After injury, it is believed that limbal stem cells migrate centrally and differentiate into cells that are capable of very rapid turnover; these cells can then repopulate and fill in the defect (first centripetally, and later by repopulating the area of defect by moving from the basal layer to the more superficial layer of the epithelium). Corneal wound healing is also discussed in Chapter 19 of this section.

Stromal Wound Healing

Unlike most other tissues, the cornea is avascular and thus heals through *fibrosis* rather than fibrovascular proliferation. After a penetrating injury of the stroma, keratocytes (the corneal stromal fibroblasts) immediately adjacent to the wound margin undergo apoptosis (die); next, the defect is soon filled with a fibrin clot. Neutrophils, carried by both the tears and the limbal vasculature, are the first cells recruited to the site (within 2–6 hours); they engage in proteolytic debridement of cellular and extracellular debris. They also release metalloproteinases (collagenases) that can degrade the stromal matrix—a process that if too exuberant leads to a corneal melt, but that when controlled is central to the wound-healing response.

Subsequently, the fibroblasts of the stroma become activated, eventually migrating across the wound and laying down collagen and fibronectin. The direction of the fibroblasts and collagen is not always parallel to the native stromal lamellae. Hence, cells are directed anteriorly and posteriorly across a wound that is always visible microscopically as an irregularity in the stroma, and clinically as an opacity. If the wound edges are separated, as may occur in a poorly apposed corneal transplant wound, the gap is not completely filled by proliferating fibroblasts, leaving a partially filled crater that is largely covered (plugged) by proliferating epithelial cells.

If the epithelium does not cover the wound within days, the subjacent stromal healing is limited and the wound remains weak. It is believed that growth factors from the epithelium stimulate and sustain the healing response by keratocytes. In the late months of healing, the initial fibrillar collagen in the stroma is replaced by stronger collagen. Bowman's layer (which is not a true membrane, but rather compacted collagen of the anterior stroma) does not regenerate when incised or destroyed. With an ulcer that has caused significant stromal loss, the epithelium eventually covers the surface, but little of the lost stromal volume is replaced by fibrous tissue; thus, the area remains thin. Many nerve fibers interdigitate between both keratocytes and corneal epithelial cells, suggesting that these cell types may exchange information through these nerve fibers.

Endothelial Wound Healing

Endothelial repair processes are of great clinical concern for two reasons: first, because maintenance of a continuous endothelial cell monolayer is critical to stromal deturgescence and hence to optical clarity and, second, because the human corneal endothelial cells do not replicate. A variety of inflammatory and mechanical insults can incite these repair responses.

Immediately after a *perforating* injury (in which the endothelial barrier is violated), the cut edges of Descemet's membrane retract and curl anteriorly toward the stroma. Adjacent endothelial cells are lost, and a fibrin clot forms in the wound. Within hours, adjoining endothelial cells attenuate with extensive cytoplasmic processes and migrate into the wound. In the adult human, almost the entire healing effort occurs by means of cellular reorganization, enlargement, and migration to reconstitute an intact monolayer. These remaining endothelial cells then lay down a thin Descemet's membrane that covers the posterior extent of the wound. If the margin of the wound is not covered by Descemet's membrane, the stromal fibroblasts may continue to proliferate into the anterior chamber as a fibrous ingrowth (membrane formation)—a process that may complicate surgical wounds.

Once Descemet's membrane has been resurfaced by a continuous endothelial monolayer, the cells become contact-inhibited and form contiguous cellular junctions. The cells that have been involved in the healing process are now much larger than those in the uninvolved areas. Once the integrity of the endothelial cell layer has been restored, its pump and barrier functions soon begin to stabilize, as shown by stromal deturgescence and increasing clarity. As a nonspecific response to any form of endothelial trauma, the regenerating endothelium deposits new layers of Descemet's membrane material. This process can be seen regularly in clear-cornea phacoemulsification surgery, where the corneal stroma overlying the area of anterior chamber entry (endothelial wound) is often edematous immediately after surgery but clarifies with decreased edema over the first few weeks following surgery as the endothelial cells in the area regain normal function.

The normal process of wound healing is not guaranteed; for example, when wound apposition is poor, local endothelial cells may become multilayered and undergo fibroblastic transformation, causing abnormal basement membrane material to be deposited. Although these endothelial cells also appear capable of eventually reverting to a more normal cellular morphology, months to years may be required for transformation into endothelium with new Descemet's membrane of normal morphology and thickness.

Pathophysiology of corneal edema: the sequelae of endothelial dysfunction

The endothelium functions as a permeability barrier between the aqueous humor and the corneal stroma and as a pump to maintain the cornea in a partially dehydrated state. Water is pumped across the endothelial apical plasma membrane into the aqueous humor in an energy-dependent process. The endothelium derives oxygen from the aqueous humor to maintain normal pump function. Two forces allow the corneal stroma to naturally take in and release water:

- The glycosaminoglycans exert an osmotic pressure that pulls water into the stroma
- The pump function osmotically draws water out of the stroma

The endothelial barrier is leaky, and the leak rate normally equals the metabolic pump rate, so that the endothelium maintains a stromal water content of 78% and an average corneal thickness of 0.52 mm.

If endothelial function fails, water diffuses into the stroma, disrupting the orderly structure of the collagen fibrils and causing light scattering and corneal opacification. The water may also pass through the stroma to accumulate as microcysts and bullae beneath and within the epithelium, which forms a virtually impermeable barrier with its zonula occludens junctions.

Wound Healing of the Sclera

When stimulated by wounding, the episclera migrates down the scleral wound, supplying vessels, fibroblasts, and activated macrophages. The sclera differs from the cornea in that the collagen fibers are randomly distributed, not laid down in orderly lamellae, and the principal glycosaminoglycan is dermatan sulfate rather than the keratan sulfate and chondroitin sulfate present in the cornea. The sclera is avascular and acellular. If the uvea is also damaged, uveal fibrovascular tissue may enter the scleral wound. The result is a scar with a dense adhesion between uvea and sclera.

Gipson IK, Joyce NC. Anatomy and cell biology of the cornea, superficial limbus, and conjunctiva. In: Albert DM, Jakobiec FA, eds. *Principles and Practice of Ophthalmology.* Vol 2. 2nd ed. Philadelphia: Saunders; 2000:612–629.

Zieske JD, Gipson IK. Agents that affect corneal wound healing: modulation of structure and function. In: Albert DM, Jakobiec FA, eds. *Principles and Practice of Ophthalmology.* Vol 1. 2nd ed. Philadelphia: Saunders; 2000:364–372.

Clinical Aspects of Toxic and Traumatic Injuries of the Anterior Segment

Injuries Caused by Temperature and Radiation

Thermal Burns

Heat

Rapid-reflex eyelid closure, Bell's phenomenon, and reflex movement away from the source of intense heat usually limit damage to the globe from flames. Burns from molten metal that stays in contact with the eye are more likely to cause corneal injuries that result in permanent scarring. Heat is a major inducer of inflammation and stromal protease expression and can lead to collagen melt if severe. The major objectives of therapy for burns caused by heat are the following:

- Relieve discomfort
- Prevent secondary corneal inflammation, ulceration, and perforation from infection or from exposure caused by eyelid damage
- Minimize eyelid scarring and resultant malfunction

A cycloplegic agent can help relieve discomfort from secondary ciliary spasm or iridocyclitis. Prophylactic antibiotics (topical and/or systemic) can help prevent infection of burned eyelids and/or reduce the chances of infectious corneal ulceration. Limited debridement of devitalized tissues and granulation tissue, used with full-thickness skin grafts and tarsorrhaphy, helps minimize eyelid scarring and ectropion. Burned ocular tissue can be protected temporarily by covering the eye with a lubricant and a piece of sterile plastic wrap. Topical corticosteroids help suppress any associated iridocyclitis, but they can also inhibit corneal wound healing and must be used with great caution.

Hair curling irons are a common household cause of corneal burns. Fortunately, burns caused by curling irons are usually limited to the epithelium and generally require only a brief period of antibiotic and cycloplegic therapy.

Freezing

Transient corneal stromal edema induced by cold has been reported in a variety of settings, including individuals with Raynaud disease. Associated conjunctival vascular changes consistent with the Raynaud phenomenon have been documented under cold stress. Transient cold-induced corneal edema has also been reported in several patients with cranial nerve V (trigeminal) dysfunction. Research suggests that sensory denervation of the eye influences ocular temperature regulation as well as altering the morphological characteristics, and likely the function, of corneal cells including the endothelium.

Ultraviolet (UV) Radiation

The corneal epithelium is highly susceptible to injury from UV radiation. Symptoms usually occur a few hours after exposure, when the injured epithelial cells are shed. The condition, although painful, is generally self-limited, and the epithelium heals within 24 hours.

The most common causes of ocular UV injuries are unprotected exposure to sunlamps, arc welding, and prolonged outdoor exposure to reflected sunlight. *Snow blindness*, which occurs in skiers and mountain climbers, is caused by UV light reflected from snow. Appropriate protection with UV-filtering eyewear can prevent such injuries. Treatment consists of patching to minimize discomfort from eyelid movement and cycloplegia. If discomfort is severe, patients may require systemic analgesics.

Ionizing Radiation

Exposure to ionizing radiation may be associated with nuclear explosions, x-rays, and radioisotopes. The amount of exposure is related to the amount of energy, the type of rays emitted, and proximity to the ionizing source. Tissue destruction may be the result of direct killing of cells, cellular DNA changes that produce lethal or other mutations, or radiation damage to blood vessels, with secondary ischemic necrosis. Longer wavelengths penetrate less deeply, causing a more intense reaction in superficial layers. Shorter wavelengths penetrate to deeper tissues and may not cause extensive damage to superficial tissues.

Most cases of ocular exposure to ionizing radiation involve both the conjunctiva and cornea and possibly the lacrimal gland(s). Conjunctival edema and chemosis occur acutely, often followed by scarring, shrinkage, loss of tear production, and alterations in conjunctival blood vessels with telangiectasia. Necrosis of the conjunctiva and underlying sclera can occur if radioactive material is embedded in the conjunctiva. Acute corneal changes are typified by punctate epithelial erosions. Explosions involving ionizing radiation may lead to perforation of ocular tissues with immediate radiation necrosis.

Management of acute problems includes removal of all foreign bodies. Depending on the severity of the injury, a bandage soft contact lens, tissue adhesive, or tectonic graft may be necessary. Poor wound healing is a hallmark of ionizing radiation injuries. Late complications are related to lack of tears, loss of corneal sensation, loss of corneal epithelium and its failure to heal, secondary microbial keratitis, vascularization, and keratitis. Management of these sequelae includes the use of artificial tears and tarsorrhaphy. Late changes in the conjunctiva preclude its use for a conjunctival flap. If the fellow eye has

not been injured, a contralateral autologous conjunctival flap may be helpful. The prognosis for penetrating keratoplasty in these situations is poor.

Miller D, ed. *Clinical Light Damage to the Eye.* New York: Springer-Verlag; 1987.

Chemical Injuries

Chemical trauma to the external eye is a common problem that can range in severity from mild irritation to complete destruction of the ocular surface epithelium, corneal opacification, loss of vision, and even loss of the eye. The offending chemical may be in the form of a solid, liquid, powder, mist, or vapor. Chemical injuries can occur in the home, most commonly from detergents, disinfectants, solvents, cosmetics, drain cleaners, oven cleaners, ammonia, bleach, and other common household alkaline agents. Fertilizers and pesticides are common offending agents in agricultural chemical injuries. Chemical injuries occurring in industry are usually caused by caustic chemicals and solvents. Some of the worst ocular chemical injuries result when strong alkalis (lye) or acids are used for assault.

Whenever possible, the offending chemical agent should be identified, because the severity of a chemical injury depends on the pH, the volume and duration of contact, and the inherent toxicity of the chemical. The most severe chemical injuries are caused by strong alkalis and, to a lesser extent, acids. These solutions cause damage by drastically altering the concentration of highly reactive hydrogen and hydroxyl ions in affected tissues.

Alkali Burns (Figs 19-1, 19-2)

Strong alkalis raise the pH of tissues and cause saponification of fatty acids in cell membranes and ultimately cellular disruption. Once the surface epithelium is damaged, alkaline solutions readily penetrate the corneal stroma, where they rapidly destroy the proteoglycan ground substance and collagen fibers of the stromal matrix. Strong alkaline substances may also penetrate into the anterior chamber and produce tissue damage and intense inflammation (Fig 19-3).

The visual prognosis is often determined by the extent of ocular surface injury and the presence and degree of skin burns and their effect on eyelid function. The most unfavorable visual prognosis is associated with extensive limbal epithelial damage and intraocular chemical penetration. The limbus contains corneal epithelial stem cells; hence, damage to this area can lead to a disruption in the normal repopulation of the corneal epithelium seen after less severe injuries. Repopulation of the corneal surface epithelium with cells that do not have the proper degree of differentiation leads to "conjunctivalization" of the cornea, which is associated with vascularization, persistence of goblet cells in the cornea, poor epithelial adhesion, and possibly chronic inflammation if the original trauma is severe. Intraocular chemical penetration is often accompanied by cataract formation and secondary glaucoma; the latter is thought to result from damage to the outflow tract and conjunctival cicatrization, which can affect outflow facility. In the most severe cases, phthisis of the globe may occur.

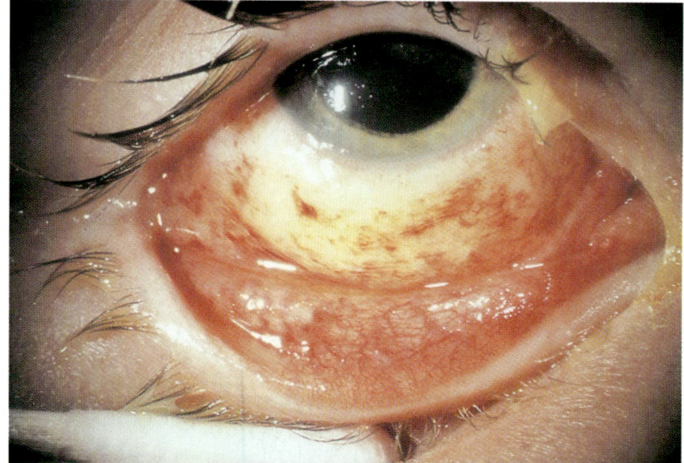

Figure 19-1 Mild alkali burn. Note inferior scleral ischemia.

Figure 19-2 Moderate alkali burn with corneal edema and haze.

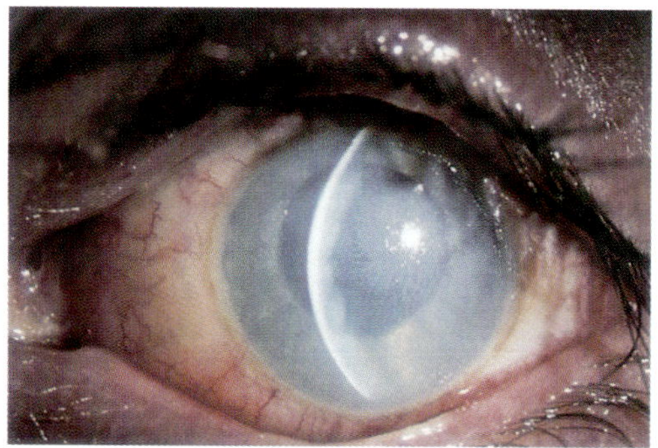

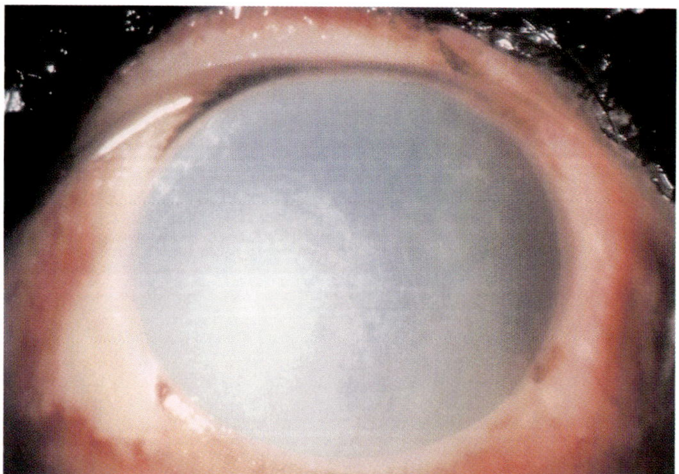

Figure 19-3 Severe alkali burn with epithelial loss and stromal necrosis.

Wagoner MD, Kenyon KR. Chemical injuries of the eye. In: Albert DM, Jakobiec FA, eds. *Principles and Practice of Ophthalmology.* Vol 2. 2nd ed. Philadelphia: Saunders; 2000:943–959.

Acid Burns

Acids denature and precipitate proteins in tissues they contact. Acidic solutions tend to cause less severe tissue damage than alkaline solutions because of the buffering capacity of tissues as well as the barrier to penetration formed by precipitated protein. Acids do not directly cause loss of the proteoglycan ground substance in the cornea, though they too can incite severe inflammation with secondary up-regulation in protease expression that can damage the corneal matrix.

Management of Chemical Injuries

Beyond the immediate steps that need to be taken to minimize ongoing exposure to the offending agent (see below), there is no general consensus regarding the optimal management of chemical injuries. Few clinical trials have been performed in humans, and many of the current recommendations for management are based on animal models of acute alkaline injury.

The most important step in the management of chemical injuries is *immediate and copious irrigation* of the ocular surface with water or normal saline solution. If these liquids are not available, any other generally nontoxic and unpolluted solutions (eg, soda pop) can also be used to avoid delaying treatment. If possible, this irrigation should be initiated at the site of the chemical injury and continued until the patient is evaluated by an ophthalmologist. The eyelid should be immobilized with a retractor or eyelid speculum, and topical anesthetic should be instilled. Irrigation may be accomplished using handheld intravenous tubing, an irrigating eyelid speculum, or a Medi-flow lens (a special scleral contact lens that connects to IV tubing). Irrigation should continue until the pH of the conjunctival sac normalizes. The conjunctival pH can be checked easily with a urinary pH strip. If this is not available, it is better to "overtreat" for prolonged periods of irrigation than to "guess" that the pH has normalized.

Because they can continue to release the toxic chemical, particulate chemicals should be removed from the ocular surface with cotton-tipped applicators and forceps. Double eversion of the upper eyelid should be performed to search for material in the upper fornix (see Figure 19-9). Some have proposed that severe chemical injuries may be approached by performing a paracentesis of the anterior chamber, removing 0.1–0.2 mL of aqueous humor, and reforming the chamber with balanced salt solution to try to normalize the anterior chamber pH. However, this procedure can sometimes lead to more inflammation and should be reserved for the most severe cases.

The next phases of management should be directed at *decreasing inflammation, monitoring IOP, limiting matrix degradation,* and *promoting reepithelialization of the cornea.* An intense polymorphonuclear (PMN) leukocyte infiltration of the corneal stroma has been noted in histologic sections of corneas subjected to acute alkali burns. PMNs may be a major source of proteolytic enzymes capable of dissolving corneal stromal collagen and ground substance. Corticosteroids are excellent inhibitors of PMN function, and intensive topical steroid administration is recommended for the acute phase (first 2 weeks) following chemical injuries. The dosage should be markedly reduced after 2 weeks, because steroids can inhibit wound healing and increase the risk of infection.

A deficiency of calcium in the plasma membrane of PMNs inhibits their ability to degranulate, and both tetracycline and citric acid are potent chelators of extracellular calcium. Therefore, oral tetracyclines (eg, doxycycline) have theoretical benefits for inhibiting PMN-induced collagenolysis.

Topical cycloplegics are recommended for patients with significant anterior chamber reaction. IOP is best controlled by use of oral carbonic anhydrase inhibitors in order to avoid toxicity from topical glaucoma medications. However, if the corneal epithelium is healing normally, topical therapies may be used as well. BCSC Section 10, *Glaucoma*, discusses medications for IOP control in depth.

Measures to promote wound healing and inhibit collagenolytic activity may help prevent stromal ulceration. Severe alkali burns in rabbit eyes have been found to reduce aqueous humor ascorbate levels to one third of normal levels. Reduced aqueous humor ascorbate has been correlated with corneal stromal ulceration and perforation. Systemic administration of ascorbic acid to rabbits with acute corneal alkaline injuries has restored the aqueous humor ascorbate level to normal and significantly reduced the incidence of ulceration. High-dose ascorbic acid is believed to promote collagen synthesis in the alkali-burned eye because ascorbic acid is required as a cofactor for this synthesis. There is currently no widely accepted standard for administration of ascorbate to corneas after chemical injury, but one recommendation is for patients to receive 2 grams of oral ascorbic acid (vitamin C) per day. This therapy is potentially toxic to the kidneys; thus, patients with compromised renal function are not good candidates for this approach.

There are several strategies for promoting epithelial healing in acute chemical injury. Patients should be treated initially with intensive nonpreserved lubricants. Necrotic epithelium should be debrided to allow for its replacement by healthier epithelium. A bandage contact lens or tarsorrhaphy may be beneficial for protecting ocular surface epithelium once it has begun to move onto the peripheral cornea. A tarsorrhaphy has the advantage of not increasing the risk of corneal infection, which is a concern with contact lens use in eyes with poor epithelia.

Autologous conjunctival or limbal transplants from a patient's uninvolved fellow eye may restore the integrity of the damaged corneal epithelium. Amniotic membrane transplantation, though currently not a standard of care, may be helpful in suppressing inflammation and thereby promoting reepithelialization and prevention of symblepharon formation. Limbal stem-cell transplantation may be performed as soon as 2 weeks after chemical injury if no signs of corneal epithelialization have appeared. However, in general, the prognosis of limbal grafts is better when the eye is not very inflamed. Corneal transplantation has a poor prognosis and is often delayed for years after a severe alkali injury. Even then, stromal vascularization in the host bed is associated with a much higher risk of rejection in these cases. Keratoprosthesis surgery has also been used in eyes with a history of chemical injury; as with other types of surgery in these eyes, the prognosis is best when the inflammation has been brought under control.

Kenyon KR, Tseng SC. Limbal autograft transplantation for ocular surface disorders. *Ophthalmology.* 1989;96:709–723.

Letko E, Stechschulte SU, Kenyon KR, et al. Amniotic membrane inlay and overlay grafting for corneal epithelial defects and stromal ulcers. *Arch Ophthalmol.* 2001;119:659–663.

Wagoner MD. Chemical injuries of the eye: current concepts in pathophysiology and therapy. *Surv Ophthalmol.* 1997;41:275–313.

Animal and Plant Substances

A variety of other external agents have been reported to result in trauma to the cornea.

Insect Injuries

Bee and wasp stings to the cornea and/or conjunctiva are rare. Acutely, conjunctival hyperemia and chemosis usually occur, sometimes associated with severe pain, corneal edema, and infiltration with subsequent decreased vision. The variability of the acute response is thought to reflect differences in the quantity of the venom injected and whether the reaction to the venom is primarily toxic or immunologic. Rarely, other sequelae have been documented, including hyphema, lenticular opacities, iritis, secondary glaucoma, and heterochromia.

Initial therapy with cycloplegics and topical, and occasionally systemic, steroids has been beneficial. Removal of externalized stingers may be attempted. After the acute episode, retained stingers may remain inert in the cornea for years. Tarantula hairs have also become embedded in the cornea, and these may elicit a focal inflammatory response, remain inert, or migrate.

Vegetation Injuries

Ocular contact with the sap (latex) from a variety of trees can cause toxic reactions manifested by acute keratoconjunctivitis, epithelial defects, and stromal infiltration. The pencil tree and the manchineel tree, widely distributed in tropical regions, are known offenders. The dieffenbachia plant is known to cause keratoconjunctivitis associated with calcium oxalate corneal crystals. Corneal foreign bodies from coconut shell, sunflower stalk, and ornamental cactus have all been documented.

Initial management for all such plant materials should include irrigation removal of foreign bodies when possible and administration of topical cycloplegics with prophylactic antibiotic coverage as indicated by the clinical situation. Corticosteroids are best avoided, as they suppress immunity to microbes in general and may promote fungal infection specifically.

Surgical removal of foreign bodies may be required in the setting of uncontrolled inflammatory response or associated secondary microbial infections. Clinicians should be aware that plant sources are common causes of fungal keratitis. Hence, in a patient with a severe injury from plant sources or in cases that fail to improve after supportive therapy, the possibility of infection should be entertained and appropriate workup (including culturing and/or biopsy) is indicated. See Chapter 7 for an in-depth discussion of microbial keratitis.

Toxic Keratoconjunctivitis From Medications

A commonly encountered and frequently unrecognized clinical problem is that of epithelial keratopathy secondary to ocular medications and their preservatives. Topical anesthetics have repeatedly been shown to be toxic if used for prolonged administration. However, sometimes even a single application of a topical anesthetic may cause transient epithelial irregularity, while prolonged use can lead to frank epithelial loss, stromal edema, infiltration, and corneal opacities. Medical personnel with easy access to anesthetics are especially susceptible to this sometimes factitious disorder.

One of the most toxic ingredients in these preparations is the preservative. The corneal epithelium and conjunctiva act as depots for preservatives, with residual amounts detectable in the epithelium days after a single topical application. Benzalkonium chloride is a common preservative that has been studied extensively. Corneal application can cause severe epithelial changes with loss of microvillae, plasma membrane disruption, and subsequent cell death.

PATHOGENESIS Toxic conjunctivitis or keratoconjunctivitis may occur as a complication of exposure to various substances. Topically applied ophthalmic medications can result in a dose-dependent cytotoxic effect on the ocular surface. The epithelium of the conjunctiva and cornea may show punctate staining or erosive changes indicative of direct toxicity. A conjunctival reaction may be observed in the form of either a papillary reaction (vascular dilation) or follicular response (lymphocytic and plasma cell hyperplasia). An immune response can also produce subepithelial corneal infiltrates.

CLINICAL PRESENTATION Although these reactions generally occur after long-term use (weeks to months) of a drug, they may take place sooner in individuals with delayed tear clearance from aqueous tear deficiency or tear drainage obstruction. Toxic reactions of the ocular surface can take different forms. A generalized injection of the tarsal and bulbar conjunctiva may be associated with a mild to severe papillary reaction of the tarsal conjunctiva, mucopurulent discharge, and punctate keratopathy. Occasionally, the discharge may be severe and mimic bacterial conjunctivitis. Infrequently, the reaction occurs in only one eye even though the medication has been applied to both.

In its mildest form, *toxic keratitis* consists of punctate epithelial erosions of the inferior cornea. A diffuse punctate epitheliopathy, occasionally in a whorl pattern, may be observed in more severe cases. This pattern is sometimes called *vortex* or *hurricane* keratopathy. The most severe cases may involve a corneal epithelial defect of the inferior or central cornea, stromal opacification, and neovascularization. This severe type of corneal disease is seen with extensive damage to the limbal stem cells. A sign of limbal stem-cell deficiency is effacement of the palisades of Vogt. Prolonged use of medication or administration of antifibrotic agents (eg, topical mitomycin drops, which have a radiomimetic effect on surrounding cells) may be the cause. Even when used in correct dosages for brief periods, mitomycin has been associated with prolonged, irreversible stem-cell damage with resultant chronic keratopathy. Localized application of mitomycin using a cellulose microsponge to the surgical field (as in trabeculectomy or pterygium excision) is believed to incur a lower risk than more widespread topical administration and is the preferred method of antifibrotic therapy.

A different type of toxic keratitis manifests as peripheral corneal infiltrates located in the epithelium and anterior stroma, leaving a clear zone between them and the limbus. Conjunctival and/or corneal toxic reactions are typically seen following use of aminoglycoside antibiotics, antiviral agents, or medications preserved with benzalkonium chloride or thimerosal.

Chronic follicular conjunctivitis is another manifestation of external ocular toxicity. Generally, the follicular reaction involves both the upper and lower palpebral conjunctiva, but the follicles are usually most prominent on the inferior tarsus and fornix. Bulbar follicles are uncommon but highly suggestive of a toxic etiology when present. The medications most commonly associated with toxic follicular conjunctivitis include atropine, antiviral agents, miotics (particularly phospholine iodide), sulfonamides, epinephrine (including dipivefrin), apraclonidine (Iopidine), and vasoconstrictors. Inferior punctate epithelial erosions may occasionally accompany toxic follicular conjunctivitis.

With ongoing use of topical medications, the conjunctiva shows an increased number of chronic inflammatory cells and fibroblasts. Although any medication may potentially cause this low-grade inflammatory response, it is most common with the chronic use of miotics for treatment of glaucoma. Asymptomatic subconjunctival fibrosis is not uncommon with chronic topical drug use, but a small minority of affected patients will develop an insidiously progressive and more severe type of subconjunctival scarring that can lead to forniceal contraction, symblepharon formation, and, eventually, corneal pannus. This entity is called *pseudopemphigoid*, or *drug-induced cicatricial pemphigoid*.

MANAGEMENT Treatment of toxicity requires discontinuation of the offending topical medications. Severe cases may take months to resolve completely; thus, the failure of symptoms and signs to resolve within a period of days to a few weeks is not inconsistent with a toxic etiology. Patients who are experiencing significant ocular irritation may find relief with nonpreserved topical lubricant drops or ointment. It is important to stress that toxic reactions to ocular medications can lead to irreversible changes, as may occur rarely with use of cholinergic (pilocarpine-like) and other medications.

Pseudopemphigoid should be confirmed with a conjunctival biopsy, which will often (but not always) demonstrate the characteristic diffuse immunofluorescent staining indicative of antibody deposition at the conjunctival basement membrane. Withdrawal of the medication is generally followed by a lag of weeks to months before stabilization of progressive scarring can be achieved. If clinical observation and photographic documentation demonstrate clinical progression despite discontinuation of the medication, chemotherapy may be necessary (see Chapter 9).

Grant WM, Schuman JS. *Toxicology of the Eye*. 4th ed. Springfield, IL: Thomas; 1993.

Liesegang TJ. Conjunctival changes associated with glaucoma therapy: implications for the external disease consultant and the treatment of glaucoma. *Cornea* 1998;17:574–583.

Concussive Trauma

Conjunctival Hemorrhage

Blood under the conjunctiva creates a dramatic appearance that can alarm the patient. Most frequently, patients present with intraconjunctival or subconjunctival hemorrhage without a history of antecedent trauma. When trauma has occurred, damage to deeper structures of the eye must be ruled out. Subconjunctival hemorrhage is usually not associated with an underlying systemic disease and rarely has an identifiable cause. Occasionally, a history of vomiting, coughing, or other forms of the Valsalva maneuver can be elicited.

Most patients simply require reassurance that things are not as bad as they appear to be. However, if a patient suffers from repeated episodes of spontaneous subconjunctival hemorrhage or indicates the presence of a possible bleeding diathesis (easy bruising, frequent bloody noses), a careful medical evaluation may be warranted. Recurrent subconjunctival hemorrhages can be seen in association with systemic illness such as uncontrolled hypertension, diabetes mellitus, or a bleeding diathesis. No therapy is necessary for the hemorrhage, as it usually resolves in 7–12 days. Patients should be warned that the hemorrhage may spread around the circumference of the globe before it resolves and that it may change in color from red to yellow to green during its dissolution.

Corneal Changes

Blunt trauma to the cornea can result in abrasions, edema, tears in Descemet's membrane, and corneoscleral lacerations, usually located at the limbus. Traumatic posterior annular keratopathy or traumatic corneal endothelial rings have also been described. The rings, composed of disrupted and swollen endothelial cells, are whitish gray in appearance and occur directly posterior to the traumatic impact. The endothelial rings appear within several hours of a contusive injury and usually disappear within a few days.

Traumatic Mydriasis and Miosis

Blunt injury to the globe may result in traumatic mydriasis or, less commonly, miosis. Traumatic mydriasis is often associated with iris sphincter tears that can permanently alter the shape of the pupil. Miosis tends to be associated with anterior chamber inflammation. Pupillary reactivity may be sluggish in both situations. Cycloplegia is essential to prevent formation of posterior synechiae.

Traumatic Iritis

Photophobia, tearing, and ocular pain may occur within the first 24 hours after injury. The inflammation of traumatic iritis is often associated with diminished vision and perilimbal conjunctival injection. The anterior chamber reaction can be surprisingly minimal but is usually present if carefully sought. IOP is characteristically reduced, but it may be elevated if associated trabecular meshwork dysfunction occurs.

Treatment should consist of, at the very least, a topical cycloplegic agent to relieve patient discomfort. Prepresbyopic patients should be counseled to expect a loss of near vision resulting from the paralysis of accommodation. Topical corticosteroids may be used if significant inflammation is present and if compliance can be expected. Once the iritis has diminished, cycloplegia may be discontinued, and topical corticosteroids should be tapered slowly over a number of weeks to prevent rebound iritis. Long-acting agents such as atropine 1%, homatropine 5%, or scopolamine 0.25% can be administered in the office if the potential for noncompliance is significant. Rarely, traumatic iritis may trigger chronic or bilateral uveitis. See BCSC Section 9, *Intraocular Inflammation and Uveitis*, for a more detailed discussion of uveitis.

Rosenbaum JT, Tammaro J, Robertson JE Jr. Uveitis precipitated by nonpenetrating ocular trauma. *Am J Ophthalmol.* 1991;112:392–395.

Iridodialysis and Cyclodialysis

Iridodialysis

Blunt trauma may cause traumatic separation of the iris root from the ciliary body. Frequently, anterior segment hemorrhage ensues, and the iridodialysis may not be recognized until the hyphema has cleared. A small iridodialysis requires no treatment. A large dialysis may cause polycoria and monocular diplopia, necessitating early surgical repair before the tissue becomes fibrotic.

Cyclodialysis

Traumatic cyclodialysis is characterized by a separation of the ciliary body from its attachment to the scleral spur, resulting in a cleft. Gonioscopically, this cleft appears at the junction of the scleral spur and the ciliary body band. Sclera may be visible through the disrupted tissue. A cyclodialysis cleft can cause increased uveoscleral outflow and aqueous hyposecretion, leading to chronic hypotony and macular edema. If treatment with topical cycloplegics does not suffice, closure may be attempted by using argon laser, diathermy, cryotherapy, or direct suturing. If repair is necessary, it should be done at the time of resolution of the hyphema.

Traumatic Hyphema

Traumatic hyphema occurs most commonly in young males. It results from injury to the vessels of the peripheral iris or anterior ciliary body. Trauma causes posterior displacement of the lens–iris diaphragm and scleral expansion in the equatorial zone, which leads to disruption of the major iris arterial circle, arterial branches of the ciliary body, and/or recurrent choroidal arteries and veins (Fig 19-4). Histopathologic studies of gross hyphemas reveal a red blood cell aggregate surrounded by a pseudocapsule of fibrin/platelet coagulum.

Anterior segment bleeding can often be seen on penlight examination as a layering of blood inferiorly in the anterior chamber (Fig 19-5). At other times the bleeding is so subtle that it can be detected only as a few circulating red blood cells on slit-lamp examination (microscopic hyphema). At presentation, more than 50% of hyphemas occupy less than one third of the height of the anterior chamber; fewer than 10% fill the whole chamber. The prognosis is good in patients who do not develop complications, but it is

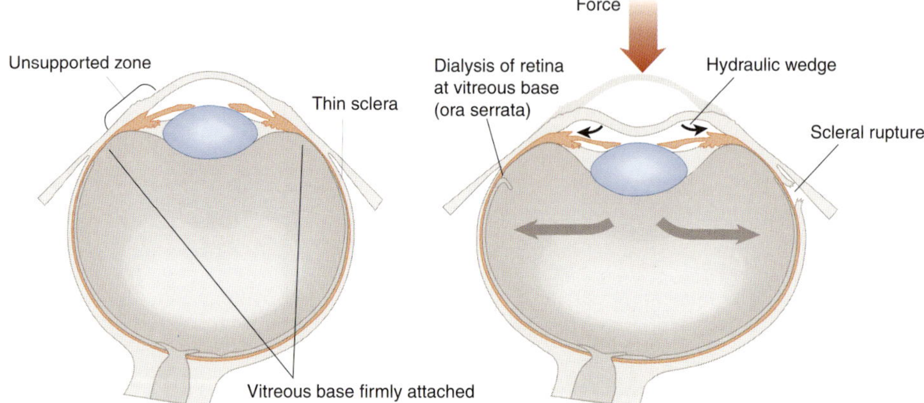

Figure 19-4 Mechanism of hyphema and blunt force injury to the eye. Blunt force applied to the eye displaces the aqueous volume peripherally, causing an increase in hydraulic pressure at the lens, iris root, and trabecular meshwork. If this "wedge of pressure" exceeds the tensile strength of ocular structures, the vessels in the peripheral iris and face of the ciliary body may rupture, leading to hyphema. The force may cause scleral ruptures, typically at the limbus and posterior to the muscle insertions where the sclera is thinner and unsupported by the orbital bones. Severe trauma leads to subluxation of the lens, retinal dialysis, optic nerve avulsion, and/or vitreous hemorrhage. *(Illustration by C.H. Wooley.)*

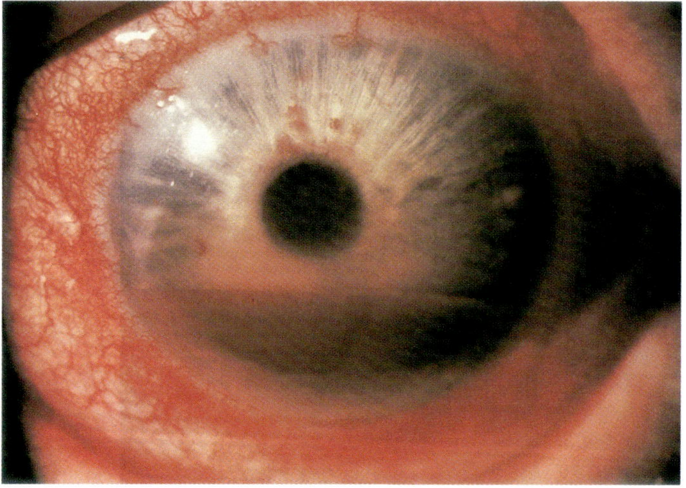

Figure 19-5 Layered hyphema from blunt trauma.

not dependent on the size of the hyphema itself. Even "eight-ball," or total, hyphemas can resolve without sequelae, unless secondary complications result (Fig 19-6). Hyphema is frequently associated with corneal abrasion, iritis, and mydriasis, as well as significant injuries to the angle structures, lens, posterior segment, and orbit.

Spontaneous hyphema is much less common and should alert the examiner to the possibility of clotting abnormalities, herpetic disease, intraocular lens problems, or ru-

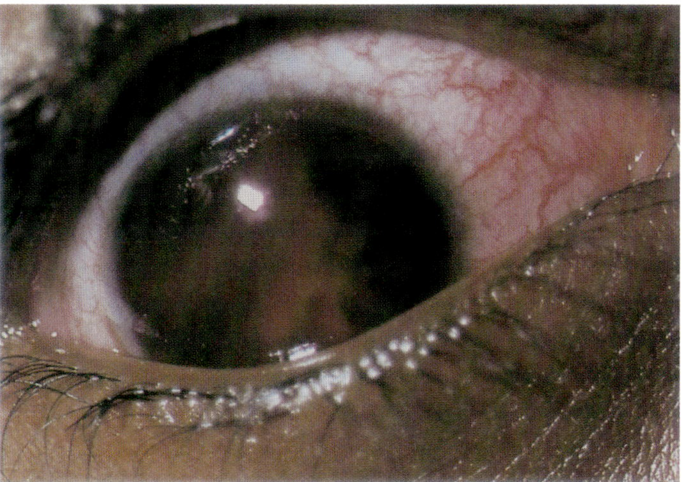

Figure 19-6 Total, or "eight-ball," hyphema.

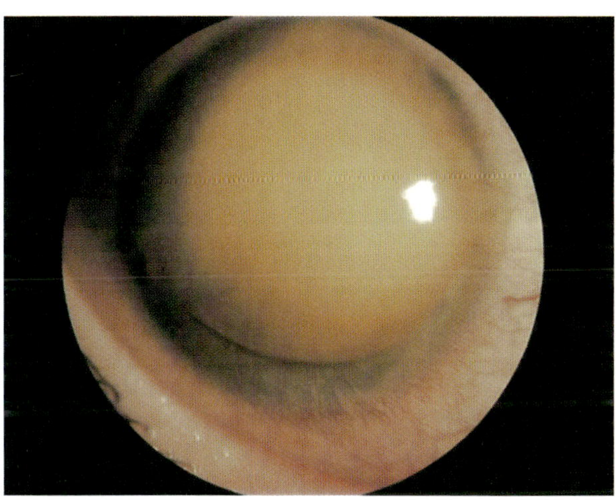

Figure 19-7 Dense corneal blood staining after a traumatic hyphema. *(Photograph courtesy of Vincent P. deLuise, MD.)*

beosis iridis in adults. Juvenile xanthogranuloma, retinoblastoma, and leukemia are associated with spontaneous hyphema in children.

Rebleeding

The major concern after a traumatic hyphema is rebleeding. Complications associated with secondary hemorrhage include glaucoma, optic atrophy, and corneal blood staining (Fig 19-7). The rate of rebleeding varies from 3% to 30%.

Rebleeding may complicate any hyphema, regardless of size, and occurs most frequently between 2 and 5 days after injury. The timing of the rebleeding may be related to the lysis and clot retraction that occur during this period. Numerous studies have documented the importance of rebleeding as a prognostic factor for poor visual outcome.

Approximately 50% of patients with rebleeding develop elevated IOP. The combination of elevated IOP, endothelial dysfunction, and anterior chamber blood predisposes the eye to corneal blood staining, which is difficult to detect when blood is in apposition to the endothelium. On slit-lamp examination, early blood staining is detected by yellow granular changes and reduced fibrillar definition in the posterior corneal stroma. Blood staining leads to a reduction in corneal transparency that may persist for years and can lead to the development of amblyopia in children. Histologically, red blood cells and their breakdown products can be seen within the corneal stroma. Corneal blood staining slowly clears in a centripetal pattern starting in the periphery (Fig 19-8).

Medical management

The overall treatment plan for traumatic hyphema should be directed at minimizing the possibility of secondary hemorrhage. Elevated IOP may require treatment in order to reduce the chances of corneal blood staining and optic atrophy. Specifics of medical management remain controversial; however, most patients are treated with the following:

- A protective shield over the injured eye
- Moderate restriction of physical activity
- Elevation of the head of the bed
- Frequent observation

Analgesics that do not contain aspirin should be used for pain relief, because aspirin has been demonstrated to increase the risk of rebleeding. Hospitalization often facilitates daily examination and is necessary if satisfactory home care and outpatient observation cannot be ensured.

Most ophthalmologists administer long-acting topical cycloplegic agents initially for comfort, to facilitate posterior segment evaluation, and to eliminate iris movement. Others, however, think these agents should be instituted only after the hyphema has cleared. Miotics are rarely used, because they may increase inflammation. Topical cor-

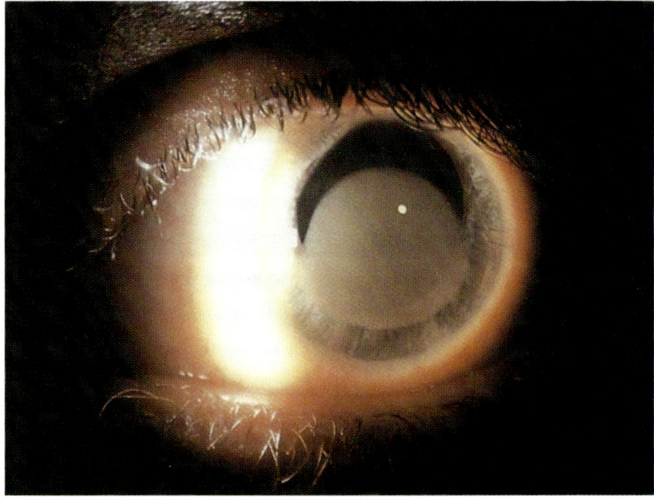

Figure 19-8 Blood staining of the cornea. Opacity consists of free hemoglobin and small amounts of hemosiderin and develops in association with large or protracted hyphemas, especially in the presence of endothelial dysfunction or increased intraocular pressure. Blood staining clears beginning in the peripheral cornea.

ticosteroids are of benefit in cases with significant anterior chamber inflammation. Topical β-adrenergic antagonists, α-agonists, and carbonic anhydrase inhibitors are the mainstays of IOP control but should be used only after the patient has been checked for sickle cell trait or disease. Intravenous and oral hyperosmotic agents may be required.

Prospective studies have supported the efficacy of antifibrinolytic agents in reducing the incidence of rebleeding. It is postulated that these agents act to inhibit fibrinolysis at the site of the injured blood vessel. However, the side effects of antifibrinolytic agents include nausea, vomiting, postural hypotension, muscle cramps, conjunctival suffusion, nasal stuffiness, headache, rash, pruritus, dyspnea, toxic confusional states, and arrhythmias as well as the risk of increased IOP on discontinuation. Patients on aminocaproic acid should be hospitalized; but patients using oral corticosteroids, which may also reduce the rate of rebleeding, may be treated as outpatients.

Aminocaproic acid (Amicar) is used in an oral dosage of 50 mg/kg every 4 hours for 5 days (up to 30 g/day). A recent randomized clinical trial has demonstrated a rebleeding rate of 7.1% with the use of aminocaproic acid or systemic prednisone in a series of 112 patients. Rebleeding rates in untreated patients have ranged from 20% to 33% in various studies. In predominantly white populations, a significantly lower incidence of secondary hemorrhage (4.1%–5.4%) has been noted. Tranexamic acid is an antifibrinolytic agent similar to aminocaproic acid that has been used successfully to reduce the rate of rebleeding in studies performed outside the United States.

Surgery

Surgery may be required to prevent corneal blood staining and optic atrophy from persistently elevated IOP. The timing of surgery is controversial, but immediate surgery is indicated at the earliest detection of blood staining. Some authors suggest that surgery may be indicated if the IOP averages greater than 25 mm Hg for 6 days when the blood is in direct apposition to the endothelium. In healthy individuals, surgical intervention should be considered when the IOP is greater than 50 mm Hg despite maximal medical management. Patients with preexisting optic nerve damage or hemoglobinopathies may require earlier intervention. See Table 19-1 for guidelines on surgical intervention.

Surgical techniques are multiple and varied. The simplest technique is paracentesis and anterior chamber irrigation with balanced salt solution. The goal is to remove circulating red blood cells that may obstruct the trabecular meshwork; removal of the entire clot is neither necessary nor wise. This procedure can be repeated. Intraocular diathermy may also be employed to control active intraoperative bleeding. Large limbal incision techniques with clot expression, if necessary, are best performed 4–7 days after the initial injury, when clot consolidation is at its peak. Automated cutting/aspiration instruments can be used to remove blood and clots through quite small incisions. Iris damage, lens injury, and additional bleeding are the major complications of surgical intervention.

Sickle cell complications

When an African-American patient develops a traumatic hyphema, a sickle cell workup or, if indicated, a hemoglobin electrophoresis should be performed to evaluate the patient for the possibility of sickle cell hemoglobinopathy. Sickle cell patients and carriers of the sickle cell trait are predisposed to sickling of red blood cells in the anterior chamber. Rigid sickled cells are restricted in their outflow through the trabecular meshwork and

Table 19-1 Guidelines for Surgical Intervention in Traumatic Hyphema

To prevent optic atrophy
Operate before IOP averages >50 mm Hg for 5 days
Operate before IOP averages >35 mm Hg for 7 days

To prevent corneal bloodstaining
Operate before IOP averages >25 mm Hg for 6 days
Operate if there is any indication of early bloodstaining

To prevent peripheral anterior synechiae
Operate before a total hyphema persists for 5 days
Operate before a diffuse hyphema involving most of the anterior chamber angle persists for
9 days

In hyphema patients with sickle hemoglobinopathies
Operate if IOP averages ≥25 mm Hg for 24 hours
Operate if IOP has repeated transient elevations >30 mm Hg

(Adapted with permission from Deutsch TA, Goldberg MF. Traumatic hyphema: medical and surgical management. *In: Focal Points: Clinical Modules for Ophthalmologists.* San Francisco: American Academy of Ophthalmology; 1984: no 5.)

may raise the IOP dramatically. In addition, the optic nerve appears to be at greater risk for damage in sickle cell patients, even with modest IOP elevation.

All efforts must be made to normalize IOP in these patients. Carbonic anhydrase inhibitors and osmotic agents must be used with caution because of their tendency to reduce pH and lead to hemoconcentration, both of which may exacerbate sickling of red blood cells. Surgical intervention has been recommended if the average IOP remains 25 mm Hg or more after the first 24 hours or increases transiently and repeatedly over 30 mm Hg, despite medical intervention.

Crouch ER Jr, Williams PB, Gray MK, et al. Topical aminocaproic acid in the treatment of traumatic hyphema. *Arch Ophthalmol.* 1997;115:1106–1112.

Deutsch TA, Weinreb RN, Goldberg MF. Indications for surgical management of hyphema in patients with sickle cell trait. *Arch Ophthalmol.* 1984;102:566–569.

Fong LP. Secondary hemorrhage in traumatic hyphema. Predictive factors for selective prophylaxis. *Ophthalmology.* 1994;101:1583–1588.

Kearns P. Traumatic hyphema. A retrospective study of 314 cases. *Br J Ophthalmol.* 1991; 75:137–141.

Teboul BK, Jacob JL, Barsoum-Homsy M, et al. Clinical evaluation of aminocaproic acid for managing traumatic hyphema in children. *Ophthalmology.* 1995;102:1646–1653.

Volpe NJ, Larrison WI, Hersh PS, et al. Secondary hemorrhage in traumatic hyphema. *Am J Ophthalmol.* 1991;112:507–513.

Nonperforating Mechanical Trauma

Conjunctival Laceration

In managing conjunctival lacerations associated with trauma, the physician must be certain that the deeper structures of the eye have not been damaged and that no foreign body is present. It is often useful to explore the limits of a conjunctival laceration using sterile forceps or cotton-tipped applicators. The slit lamp is used following the instillation of a topical anesthetic. If any question remains as to whether the globe has been penetrated, consideration must be given to performing a peritomy in the operating room to better explore and examine the injured area. In general, conjunctival lacerations do not need to be sutured.

Conjunctival Foreign Body

Foreign bodies on the conjunctival surface are best recognized with slit-lamp examination. Foreign bodies can lodge in the inferior cul-de-sac or can be located on the conjunctival surface under the upper eyelid (Fig 19-9). It is imperative to evert the upper eyelid to examine the superior tarsal plate and eyelid margin in all patients with a history that suggests a foreign body. If several foreign bodies are suspected or particulate matter is present, double eversion of the eyelid with a Desmarres retractor or a bent paper clip is advised to allow the examiner to effectively search the entire arc of the superior cul-de-sac (Fig 19-10).

Following eversion of the upper eyelid, copious irrigation should be used to cleanse the fornix. This procedure should then be repeated using a Desmarres retractor for the upper and lower eyelids. Glass particles, cactus spines, or insect hairs are often difficult to see, but a careful search of the cul-de-sac with high magnification aids in identification and removal. Using slit-lamp magnification, the clinician can use a moistened cotton-tipped applicator to gently remove superficial foreign material. Occasionally, saline lavage of the cornea or cul-de-sac washes out debris that is not embedded in tissue.

When a patient complains of foreign body sensation, topical fluorescein should be instilled to check for the fine, linear, vertical corneal abrasions that are characteristic of retained foreign bodies on the eyelid margin or superior tarsal plate. If such vertical lines are noted, their source must be identified, as they are a fairly specific localizing sign. Foreign matter embedded in tissue is removed with a sterile, disposable hypodermic needle. Glass or particulate matter may be removed with a fine-tipped jeweler's forceps or blunt spatula. If a foreign body is suspected but not seen, the cul-de-sac should be irrigated and wiped with a moistened cotton-tipped applicator.

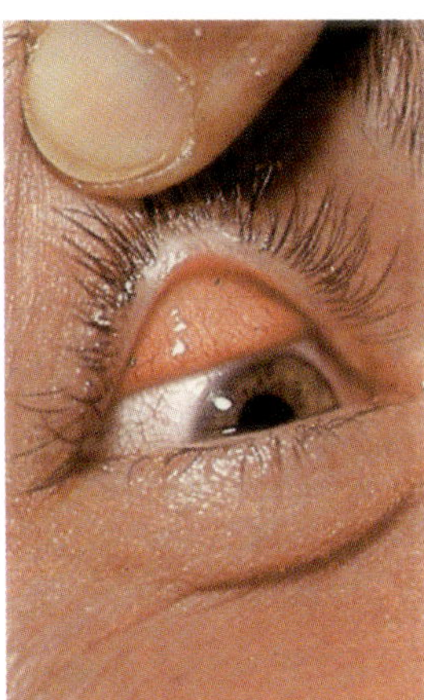

Figure 19-9 Foreign bodies seen on the everted surface of the upper eyelid.

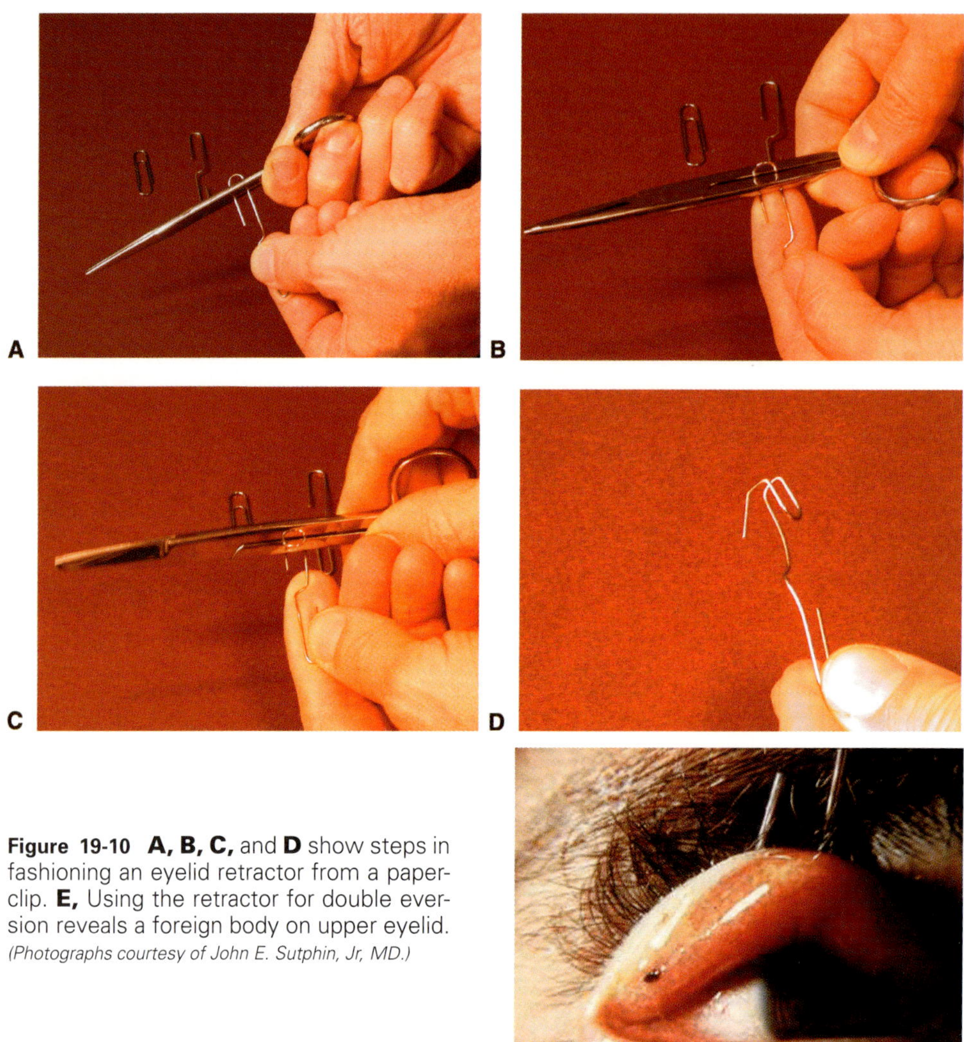

Figure 19-10 **A, B, C,** and **D** show steps in fashioning an eyelid retractor from a paper-clip. **E,** Using the retractor for double eversion reveals a foreign body on upper eyelid. *(Photographs courtesy of John E. Sutphin, Jr, MD.)*

Corneal Foreign Body

Corneal foreign bodies are identified most effectively during slit-lamp examination. Before removing the corneal foreign body, the clinician should assess the depth of corneal penetration. If anterior chamber extension is present or suspected, the foreign body should be removed in a sterile operating-room environment with sufficient microscopic magnification and coaxial illumination, adequate anesthesia, and appropriate instruments. Overly aggressive attempts to remove deeply embedded foreign bodies at the slit lamp may result in leakage of aqueous humor. If such a leak occurs and cannot be adequately tamponaded with a therapeutic bandage contact lens, tissue adhesive and/or urgent surgical repair is required.

If several glass foreign bodies are present, all of the exposed fragments should be removed. Fragments that are deeply embedded in the cornea are often inert and can be left in place. Careful gonioscopic evaluation of the anterior chamber is essential to ensure that the iris and the angle are free of any retained glass particles.

When an iron foreign body has been embedded in the cornea for more than a few hours, an orange-brown "rust ring" results (Fig 19-11). Corneal iron foreign bodies can usually be removed at the slit lamp under topical anesthesia with a disposable hypodermic needle. The rust ring can be removed using a battery-powered dental burr with a sterile tip. It is advisable to remove as much metallic material as possible, because material left in the cornea may lead to persistent epithelial defects and poor healing secondary to chronic, smoldering inflammation. Corneal perforation is a rare complication of foreign body removal.

Therapy following the removal of a corneal foreign body includes topical antibiotics, cycloplegia, and the application of a firm pressure patch. Reexamination the following day is usually indicated. If the residual corneal abrasion does not heal or if additional curettage is needed to remove a rust ring, cycloplegic and antibiotic drops are again instilled prior to reapplication of a new pressure patch.

Corneal Abrasion

Corneal abrasions are usually associated with immediate pain, foreign body sensation, tearing, and discomfort with blinking. Abrasions may be caused by contact with a finger, fingernail, fist, or even the edge of a piece of paper. The abrasion can also be caused by a propelled foreign body or by contact lens wear, either because of improper fit or excessive wear. Occasionally, a patient may not recall a definite history of trauma but still presents with signs and symptoms suggestive of a corneal abrasion. Herpes simplex virus keratitis must be excluded as a possible diagnosis in such cases.

A slit-lamp examination is essential to determine the presence, extent, and depth of the corneal defect. It is very important to make a distinction between a "clean" corneal

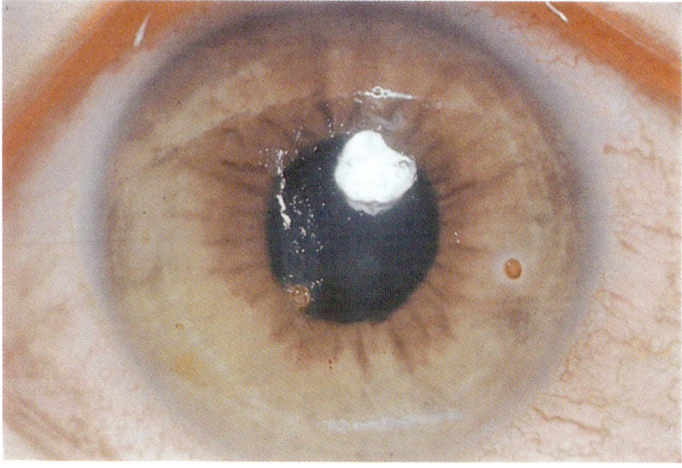

Figure 19-11 Corneal rust ring and multiple retained iron foreign bodies.

abrasion, which generally has sharply defined edges and little to no associated inflammation (when seen acutely), versus a true corneal ulcer. Foreign body sensation is an exceedingly specific localizing symptom for a corneal epithelial defect. It is important to evert the upper eyelid and examine the superior cul-de-sac to rule out a retained foreign body.

Patching may not be necessary for small, superficial abrasions, as the primary indication for pressure patching is to relieve discomfort, but patches prevent eyelid movement from continually abrading the denuded surface. Many patients find patches uncomfortable: the clinician should decide whether a given patient will be more uncomfortable from the abrasion or from the patch. Alternatively, abrasions may be managed with a therapeutic contact lens, usually with antibiotic prophylaxis until the surface heals. However, the decision to use these lenses must take into account the possibility of related complications such as tight lens syndrome. Many small abrasions can be managed with antibiotic drops or ointment alone. Extensive corneal abrasions usually require topical antibiotics, cycloplegics, and pressure patching. Abrasions caused by organic material require closer follow-up to monitor for infection.

Patients with contact lens–associated epithelial defects should never be patched because of the possibility of promoting a secondary infection. These patients should be treated with topical antibiotic drops or ointment.

Posttraumatic Recurrent Corneal Erosion

A corneal abrasion can precipitate future recurrent corneal erosions. See Chapter 5 for a discussion of the pathogenesis, diagnosis, and treatment of recurrent corneal erosions.

Perforating Trauma

It is important to differentiate a *penetrating* wound from a *perforating* wound. A penetrating wound passes *into* a structure; a perforating wound passes *through* a structure. For example, an object that passes through the cornea and lodges in the anterior chamber perforates the cornea but penetrates the eye.

Evaluation

History

If a patient presents with both eye and systemic trauma, diagnosis and treatment of any life-threatening injury take precedence over evaluation and management of the ophthalmic injury. Once the patient is medically stable, the ophthalmologist should then elicit a complete presurgical history (Table 19-2). Even though the diagnosis of perforating injury in many cases may be obvious from casual eye examination, a detailed history of the nature of the injury should include questions about factors known to predispose to ocular penetration so that this diagnosis will not be overlooked in more subtle cases. Such factors include

---

Table 19-2 Penetrating/Perforating Ocular Injury History

Nature of injury
Concomitant life-threatening injury
Time and circumstances of injury
Suspected composition of intraocular foreign body (brass, copper, iron, vegetable, soil-
  contaminated)
Use of eye protection
Prior treatment of injury

Past ocular history
Refractive history
Eye diseases
Current eye medications
Previous surgery

Medical history
Diagnoses
Current medications
Drug allergies
Risk factors for HIV/hepatitis
Currency of tetanus prophylaxis
Previous surgey
Recent food ingestion

- Metal on metal strike
- High-velocity projectile
- High-energy impact on globe
- Sharp injuring object
- Lack of eye protection

Examination

Evaluation of the patient with suspected perforating injury to the eye should include a complete general and ophthalmologic examination. As soon as possible, the examiner should determine visual acuity, which is the most reliable predictor of final visual outcome in traumatized eyes. In unilateral injury, presence of an afferent pupillary defect should be sought. Unfortunately, both parts of the examination may be omitted by busy emergency room staff, so the ophthalmologist must both check the visual acuity and pupils and help educate nonophthalmic practitioners about the importance of these assessments. The ophthalmologist should then look for key signs that are suggestive or diagnostic of perforating ocular injury (Table 19-3).

If a significant perforating injury is suspected, forced duction testing, gonioscopy, tonometry, and scleral depression should be avoided. Ancillary tests that may be useful in this setting are summarized in Table 19-4. Regardless of the results of laboratory tests, all cases should be managed with safeguards appropriate for patients known to have bloodborne infections (see universal precautions, Chapter 2).

Table 19-3 Ocular Signs of Perforating Trauma

Suggestive	Diagnostic
Deep eyelid laceration	Exposed uvea, vitreous, retina
Orbital chemosis	Positive Seidel test
Conjunctival laceration/hemorrhage	Visualization of intraocular foreign body
Focal iris–corneal adhesion	Intraocular foreign body seen on x-ray or
Shallow anterior chamber	ultrasonography
Iris defect	
Hypotony	
Lens capsule defect	
Acute lens opacity	
Retinal tear/hemorrhage	

Management

Preoperative management

If surgical repair is required, the timing of the operation is crucial. Although studies have not documented any disadvantage in delaying the repair of an open globe for up to 36 hours, intervention ideally should occur as soon as possible. Prompt repair can help minimize numerous complications:

- Pain
- Prolapse of intraocular structures
- Suprachoroidal hemorrhage
- Microbial contamination of the wound
- Proliferation of the microbes projected into the eye
- Migration of epithelium into the wound
- Intraocular inflammation
- Lens opacity

In a late-night or weekend injury, these concerns must be balanced against the benefits of keeping the patient NPO, having a well-rested surgeon, and using experienced ophthalmic operating-room staff during regular hours.

The deleterious effects of a small delay in repair can be offset by the following temporizing measures that can be taken during the preoperative period:

- Apply a protective shield
- Avoid administering topical medications
- Keep the patient on NPO status
- Provide appropriate medications for sedation, pain control, and antiemesis
- Administer facial nerve block to reduce eyelid squeezing
- Take external eye cultures
- Initiate intravenous antibiotics (such as tobramycin with either clindamycin or vancomycin)
- Provide tetanus prophylaxis
- Seek anesthesia consultation

Injuries with soil-contaminated retained intraocular foreign bodies require attention to the risk of *Bacillus* endophthalmitis. Because this organism can destroy the eye within 24 hours, intravenous and/or intravitreal therapy should be considered with an antibiotic effective against *Bacillus* species, usually clindamycin or vancomycin or oral fluoroquinolones such as levoflaxacin. Surgical repair should be undertaken with minimal delay in cases at risk for contamination with this organism.

Nonsurgical options

Some penetrating injuries are so minimal that they spontaneously seal prior to ophthalmic examination, with no intraocular damage, prolapse, or adherence. These cases may require only systemic and/or topical antibiotic therapy along with close observation. If a corneal wound is leaking (Fig 19-12), but the chamber remains formed, the clinician can attempt to stop the leak with pharmacologic suppression of aqueous production (topical

---

Table 19-4 Ancillary Tests in Perforating Eye Trauma

Useful in many cases
  CT scan
  Plain-film x-rays
  CBC, differential, platelets
  Electrolytes, blood urea nitrogen, creatinine
  Test for HIV status, hepatitis

Useful in selected cases
  MRI (especially in cases of suspected organic foreign objects in the eye or orbit, but this should
    never be used if a metallic foreign object is suspected)
  Prothrombin time, partial thromboplastin time, bleeding time
  Sickle cell
  Drug and/or ethanol levels

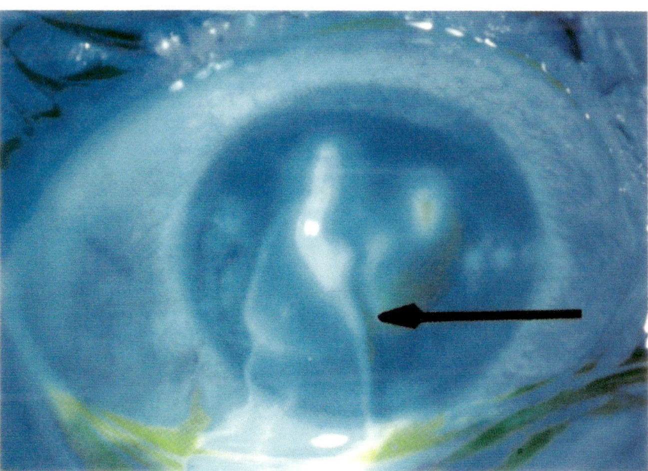

Figure 19-12 Leakage of aqueous from the anterior chamber following a corneal laceration. Concentrated fluorescein on the edge of the aqueous rivulet (Seidel test) indicates an active flow of fluid from a leaking anterior chamber.

or systemic), patching, and/or a therapeutic contact lens. Generally, if these measures fail to seal the wound in 3 days, closure with cyanoacrylate glue or sutures is recommended. Although cyanoacrylate tissue adhesives are not approved by the FDA for use in the eye, they have been used extensively over the past two decades to seal perforations. Several glues are available, such as Histocryl and Bucrylate. A therapeutic contact lens must be used after application of glue, since polymerization of the glue produces a rough surface that abrades the palpebral conjunctiva.

Surgical repair

The eye can sustain severe internal damage with even a small, seemingly insignificant wound. The management of a typical corneoscleral laceration with uveal prolapse generally requires surgery (Fig 19-13). The primary goal of initial surgical repair of a corneoscleral laceration is to restore the integrity of the globe. The secondary goal, which may be accomplished at the time of the primary repair or during subsequent procedures, is to restore vision through repair of both external and internal damage to the eye.

If the prognosis for vision in the injured eye is hopeless and the patient is at risk for sympathetic ophthalmia, enucleation must be considered. Primary enucleation should be performed only for an injury so devastating that restoration of the anatomy is impossible, when it may spare the patient another procedure. In the overwhelming majority of cases, however, the advantages of delaying enucleation for a few days far outweigh any advantage of primary enucleation. This delay (which should not exceed the 14 days thought necessary for an injured eye to incite sympathetic ophthalmia) allows for assessment of postoperative visual function, vitreoretinal or ophthalmic plastic consultation, and stabilization of the patient's medical condition. Most important, delay in enucleation following unsuccessful repair and loss of light perception allows the patient time to acknowledge that loss and accompanying disfigurement and to consider enucleation in a nonemergency setting.

Anesthesia General anesthesia is almost always required for repair of an open globe, because retrobulbar or peribulbar anesthetic injection increases orbital pressure, which may cause or exacerbate the extrusion of intraocular contents. A nondepolarizing muscle relaxant is preferred because of the theoretical possibility that cocontraction of the extraocular contents may occur. After the surgical repair is complete, a periocular anesthetic injection may be used to control postoperative pain.

Steps in the repair of a corneoscleral laceration All attempts at repair of a corneoscleral laceration should be performed in the operating room with use of the operating microscope and trained ophthalmic personnel. Table 19-5 summarizes the basic steps in restoring the integrity of the globe with a corneoscleral laceration. No attempt should be made to fixate an open globe with rectus muscle sutures. Because eyelid surgery can put pressure on an open globe and because certain eyelid lacerations may actually improve globe exposure, repair of adnexal injury should follow repair of the globe itself.

The corneal component of the injury is approached first. If vitreous or lens fragments have prolapsed through the wound, these should be cut flush with the cornea, taking

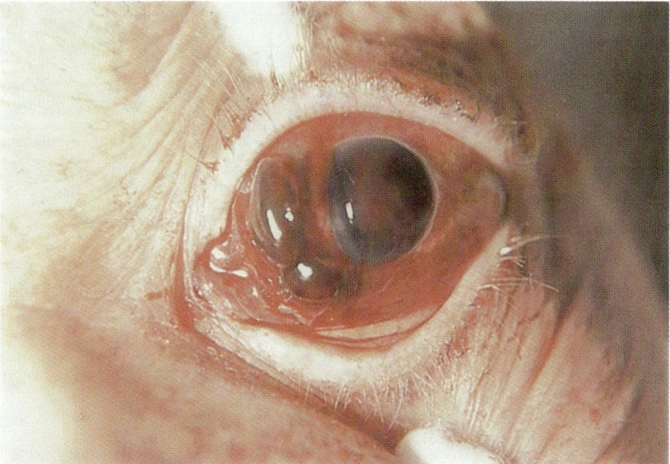

Figure 19-13 Ruptured globe secondary to blunt trauma.

Table 19-5 Essential Steps in Surgical Repair of a Corneoscleral Laceration

1. General anesthesia
2. Excision of anteriorly prolapsed vitreous, lens fragments, transcorneal foreign bodies
3. Repositioning of anteriorly prolapsed uvea, retina
4. Closure of corneal component of laceration at limbus, landmarks
5. Completion of watertight corneal closure (10-0 nylon)
6. Peritomy as necessary for exposure of scleral component
7. Stepwise excision of posteriorly prolapsed vitreous
8. Stepwise repositioning of posteriorly prolapsed uvea, retina
9. Stepwise closure of scleral component (9-0 nylon or 8-0 silk)
10. Conjunctival closure
11. Subconjunctival antibiotics, steroids

---

care not to exert traction on the vitreous or zonular fibers. If uvea or retina (seen as translucent, tan tissue with extremely fine vessels) protrudes, it should be reposited using a gentle sweeping technique through a separate limbal incision, with the assistance of viscoelastic injection to temporarily reform the anterior chamber (Fig 19-14). If epithelium has obviously migrated onto a uveal surface or into the wound, an effort should be made to peel this tissue off. Only in cases of frankly necrotic uveal prolapse should uveal tissue be excised.

Points at which the laceration crosses landmarks such as the limbus are then closed with 10-0 nylon suture, followed by closure of the remaining corneal components of the laceration. It may be necessary to reposit iris tissue repeatedly after each suture is placed to avoid entrapment of iris in the wound. Despite these efforts, uvea may still remain apposed to the posterior corneal surface. Many surgeons place very shallow sutures at this stage of the closure, in order to avoid impaling uvea with the suture needle. Then, after the closure is watertight, the uvea can be definitively separated from the cornea with viscoelastic injection, followed by replacement of shallow sutures with new ones of ideal,

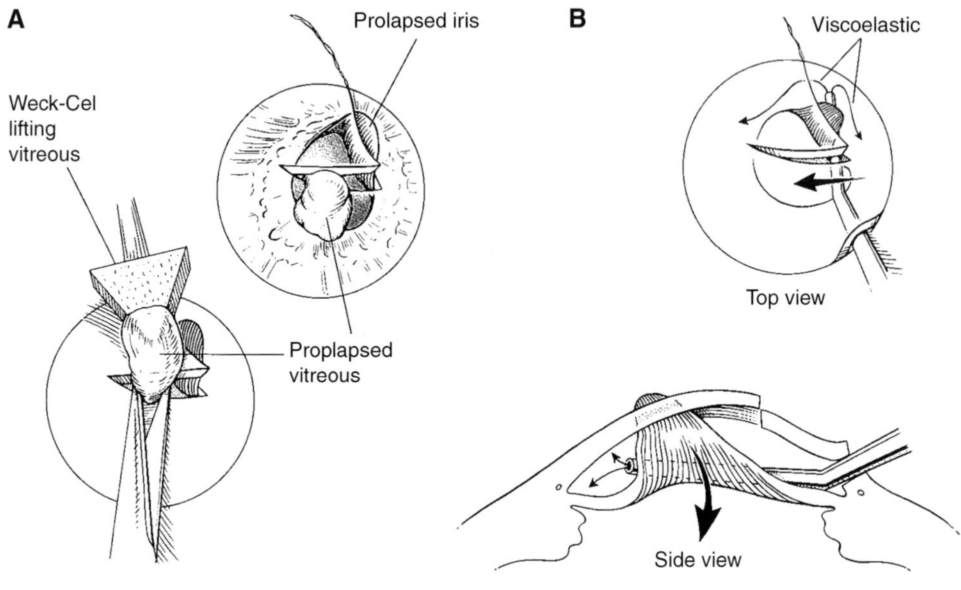

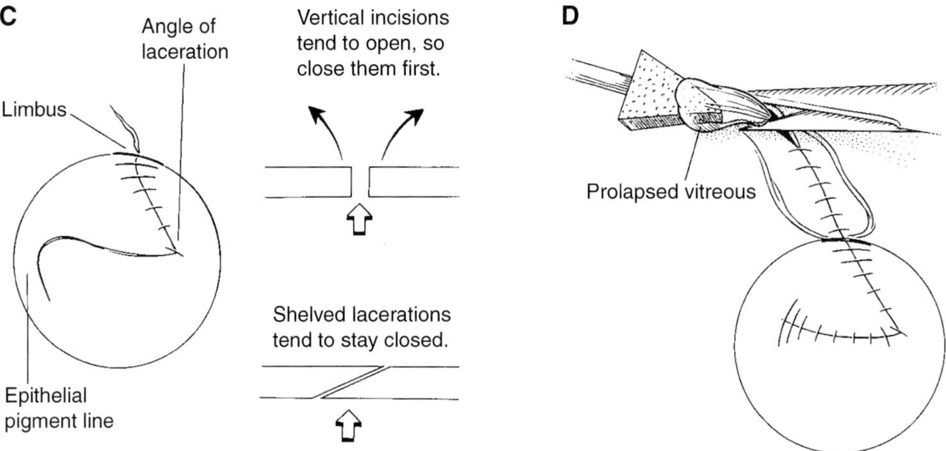

Figure 19-14 Restoring anatomic relationships in corneoscleral laceration repair. **A,** Prolapsed vitreous or lens fragments are excised. **B,** Iris is reposited by means of viscoelastic and a cannula inserted through a separate paracentesis. **C,** Landmarks such as limbus, laceration angles, or epithelial pigment lines are closed. Vertical lacerations are closed first to create a watertight globe more quickly, followed by shelved lacerations. **D,** The scleral part of the wound is exposed, prolapsed vitreous is severed, and the wound is closed from the limbus, working posteriorly. *(Reproduced with permission from Hamill MB. Repair of the traumatized anterior segment. In:* Focal Points: Clinical Modules for Ophthalmologists. *San Francisco: American Academy of Ophthalmology; 1992: vol 10, no 1. Illustrations by Christine Gralapp.)*

near-full-thickness depth (Fig 19-15). Suture knots should be buried in the corneal stroma, not in the wound.

When watertight closure of the wound proves difficult to achieve because of unusual laceration configuration or loss of tissue, X-shaped sutures or other customized (ad hoc) techniques may suffice. Cyanoacrylate glue or even primary penetrating keratoplasty may be required in extremely difficult cases. A conjunctival flap should not be used to treat a wound leak.

When the anatomy of the wound allows, a topographic closure is best for reducing long-term complications. Wider spaced, longer sutures are used in the peripheral cornea to flatten locally and steepen centrally. Closer, shorter sutures are used centrally, avoiding the visual axis to close the wound without excessive flattening (Fig 19-16).

The scleral component of the laceration is then approached with gentle peritomy and conjunctival separation only as necessary to expose the wound. Prolapsed vitreous

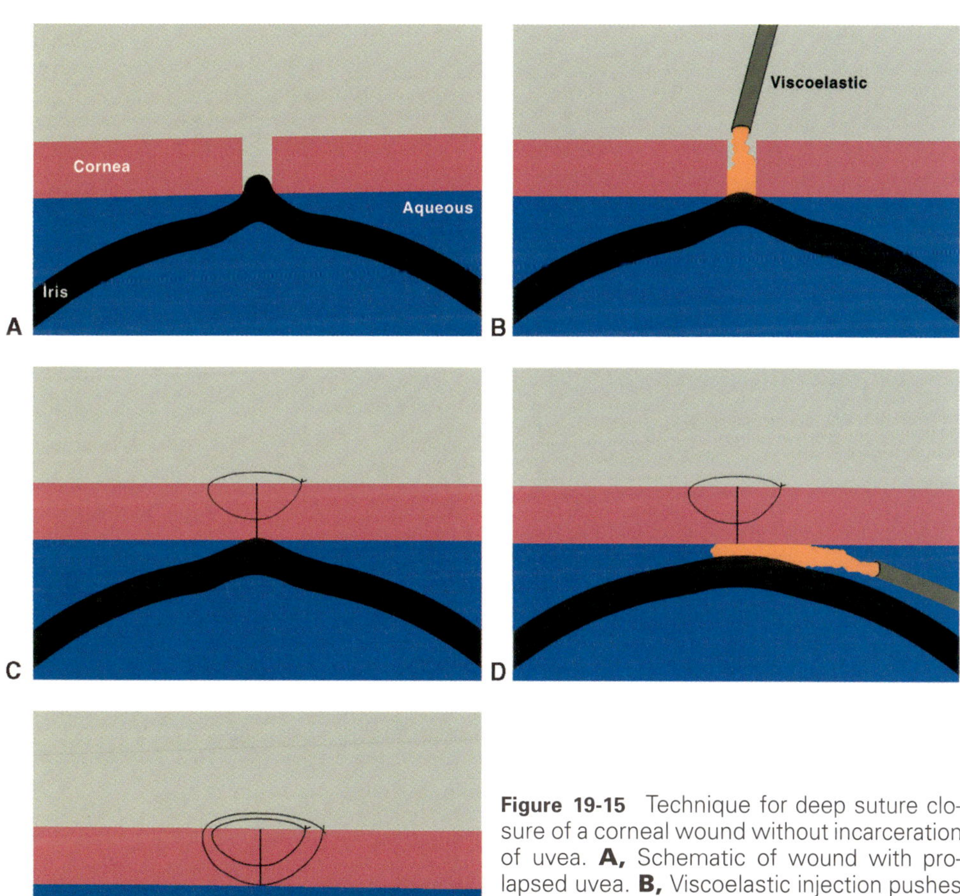

Figure 19-15 Technique for deep suture closure of a corneal wound without incarceration of uvea. **A,** Schematic of wound with prolapsed uvea. **B,** Viscoelastic injection pushes uvea posteriorly. **C,** Shallow suture closure produces watertight wound despite uveal apposition. **D,** Viscoelastic definitively separates uvea from cornea. **E,** Shallow sutures are replaced with deep ones.

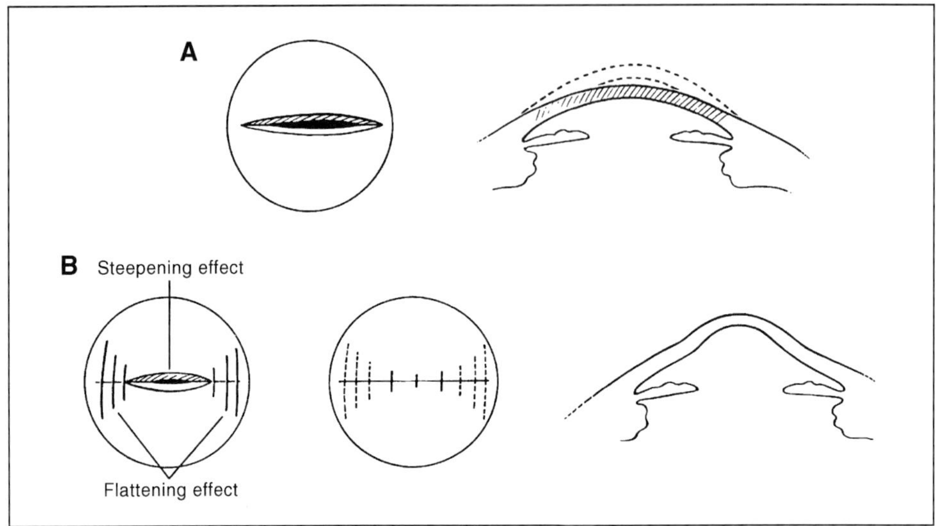

Figure 19-16 Restoring functional architecture in corneal wound closure. **A,** Laceration has a flattening effect on the cornea. **B,** Long compressive sutures are taken in the periphery to flatten the peripheral cornea and steepen the central cornea. Subsequently, short, minimally compressive sutures are taken in the steepened central cornea to preserve sphericity despite the flattening effect of sutures. *(Reproduced with permission from Hamill MB. Repair of the traumatized anterior segment. In: Focal Points: Clinical Modules for Ophthalmologists. San Francisco: American Academy of Ophthalmology; 1992: vol 10, no 1.)*

is excised, and prolapsed nonnecrotic uvea and retina are reposited with a spatula or similar instrument. The scleral wound is closed with 9-0 nylon or 8-0 silk suture. Often, dissection of Tenon's capsule and management of prolapsed tissue must be repeated incrementally after each suture is placed.

Some posterior wounds are more easily approached with loupes and a headlight, since the open globe should not be rotated too far. If the laceration extends under an extraocular muscle, the muscle may be removed at its insertion and reinserted following repair. Closure of the laceration should continue posteriorly only to the point at which it becomes technically difficult or requires undue pressure on the globe. Very posterior lacerations benefit from effective physiologic tamponade by orbital tissue and are best left alone.

Once the globe is watertight, a decision must be made whether intraocular surgery (if necessary) should be attempted immediately or postponed. Subconjunctival injections of antibiotics to cover both gram-positive and gram-negative organisms are given prophylactically at the conclusion of primary repair. Intravitreal antibiotics such as vancomycin 1 mg and amikacin 200 µg may be used after contaminated wounds involving the vitreous.

Secondary repair of intraocular trauma Following primary repair of a corneoscleral laceration the following secondary measures may be indicated:

- Removal of intraocular foreign bodies
- Iris repair
- Cataract extraction
- Mechanical vitrectomy
- Intraocular lens (IOL) insertion
- Cryotherapy of retinal tears

Deciding whether to pursue such intervention at the time of initial repair is a complex process. The expertise of the surgeon; the quality of the facility, technical equipment, and instruments; the adequacy of the view of the anterior segment structures; and issues of informed consent should be considered.

For example, the average anterior segment surgeon should not attempt automated vitrectomy with retina present in the anterior chamber, and even the most expert cataract surgeon might not attempt a lens extraction with no view of the lens. On the other hand, opacity of a damaged lens may increase, intraocular inflammation may worsen, opportunity for placement of an IOL in the capsular bag may be lost, and the patient may experience increased pain and expense if these procedures are delayed.

As always, the welfare of the patient should determine the proper course. In general, if a foreign body is visible in the anterior segment and can be grasped, it is reasonable to remove it, either through the wound or through a separate limbal incision. If removal of opacified lens material is attempted, it is helpful to know whether the posterior capsule has been violated and lens-vitreous admixture has occurred. BCSC Section 11, *Lens and Cataract,* also discusses the issues of cataract surgery and IOL placement following trauma to the eye.

Sometimes the leaflets of a damaged anterior capsule can be manipulated to form a partial or complete circular capsulorrhexis, which will facilitate placement of an IOL in the bag. If the posterior capsule is ruptured, a capsulorrhexis allows more stable ciliary sulcus fixation of an IOL. In the older patient, a firm nucleus may be extracted with a lens loop or emulsified, but it probably should not be extracted with pressure on the globe. However, the soft lens material of the average young trauma patient is most easily removed using a mechanical vitrector in the aspiration mode, cutting only when vitreous is encountered.

The primary surgical goal is to remove all lens cortical and nuclear material as well as vitreous in the anterior segment, preserving as much lens capsule and zonular support as possible, all without causing additional vitreous traction. If a reasonable refractive history has indicated similarity between the two eyes, and the axial length and keratometry of the fellow eye are known, primary placement of an IOL should be considered. If adequate capsular support is present, placement within the capsular bag is preferred to sulcus fixation. Most surgeons prefer not to place an anterior chamber IOL in these typically young patients.

Iris repair can be undertaken either primarily or secondarily. Closure of iris lacerations may not only restore iris function and improve vision but may also keep the iris in its proper plane, decreasing the formation of anterior or posterior synechiae. The McCannel technique using 10-0 polypropylene suture requires only a small additional limbal incision to be made (Fig 19-17). Iridodialysis, usually resulting from blunt trauma, may cause monocular diplopia and an eccentric pupil if left untreated. The McCannel technique can also be used to repair iridodialysis (Fig 19-18). In the event that corneal opacity prevents safe repair of internal ocular injury, repairs can be combined later with penetrating keratoplasty or with placement of a temporary keratoprosthesis, if posterior segment repair is planned.

Postoperative management

After repair of penetrating anterior segment trauma, therapy is directed at prevention of infection, suppression of inflammation, control of IOP, and relief of pain. Intravenous antibiotics are usually continued for 3–5 days, and topical antibiotics are generally used for about 7 days. Topical corticosteroids and cycloplegics are tapered off, depending on the degree of inflammation. A massive fibrinous response may respond well to a short course of systemic prednisone.

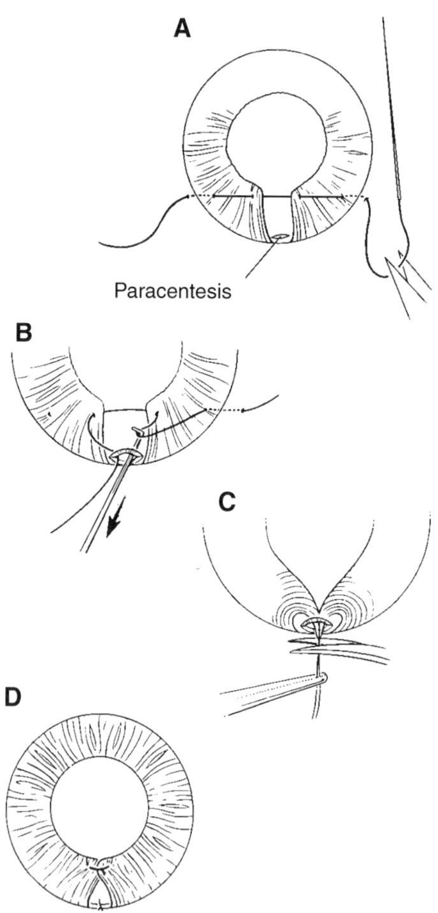

Figure 19-17 The McCannel technique for repairing iris lacerations. With large lacerations, multiple sutures may be used. **A,** A limbal paracentesis is made over the iris discontinuity. Then a long Drews needle with 10-0 polypropylene is passed through the peripheral cornea, the edges of the iris, and the peripheral cornea opposite, and the suture is cut. **B,** A Sinskey hook, introduced through the paracentesis and around the suture peripherally, is drawn back out through the paracentesis. **C,** The suture is securely tied. **D,** After the suture is secure, it is cut, and the iris is allowed to retract. *(Reproduced with permission from Hamill MB. Repair of the traumatized anterior segment. In: Focal Points: Clinical Modules for Ophthalmologists. San Francisco: American Academy of Ophthalmology; 1992: vol 10, no 1. Illustrations by Christine Gralapp.)*

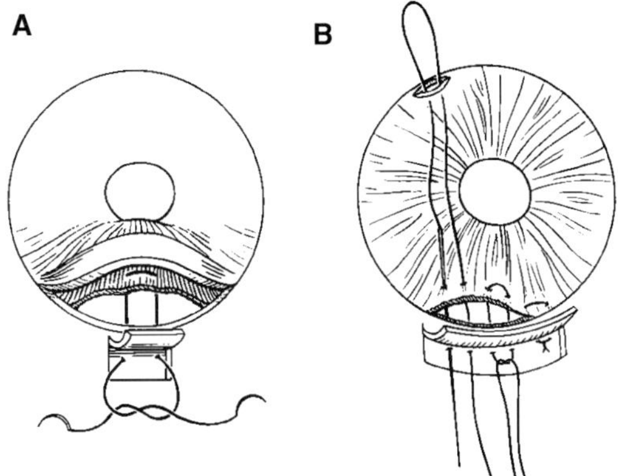

Figure 19-18 Repair of iridodialysis. **A,** A cataract surgery–type incision is made at the site of iridodialysis or iris disinsertion. A double-armed, 10-0 polypropylene suture is passed through the iris root, out through the angle, and tied on the surface of the globe under a partial-thickness scleral flap. The corneoscleral wound is then closed with 10-0 nylon sutures. **B,** In an alternative technique, multiple 10-0 Prolene sutures on double-armed Drews needles are passed through a paracentesis opposite the site of iris disinsertion to avoid the need to create a large corneoscleral entry wound. *(Reproduced with permission from Hamill MB. Repair of the traumatized anterior segment. In:* Focal Points: Clinical Modules for Ophthalmologists. *San Francisco: American Academy of Ophthalmology; 1992: vol 10, no 1. Illustrations by Christine Gralapp.)*

Corneal sutures that do not loosen spontaneously are generally left in place for at least 3 months and then removed incrementally over the next few months. Fibrosis and vascularization are indicators that enough healing has occurred to render suture removal safe.

These traumatized eyes are at increased risk of retinal detachment, so frequent examination of the posterior segment is mandatory. If media opacity precludes an adequate fundus examination, evaluation for an afferent pupillary defect and B-scan ultrasonography are helpful in monitoring retinal status.

Refraction and correction with contact lenses or spectacles can proceed when the ocular surface and media permit. Because of the risk of amblyopia in a child or loss of fusion in an adult, visual rehabilitation should not be unnecessarily delayed.

Barr CC. Prognostic factors in corneoscleral lacerations. *Arch Ophthalmol.* 1983;101:919–924.

Catalana RA, ed. *Ocular Emergencies.* Philadelphia: Saunders; 1992.

Hamill MB. Repair of the traumatized anterior segment. In: *Focal Points: Clinical Modules for Ophthalmologists.* San Francisco: American Academy of Ophthalmology; 1992: vol 10, no 1.

Kenyon KR, Starck T, Hersh PS. Anterior segment reconstruction after trauma. In: Brightbill FS, ed. *Corneal Surgery: Theory, Technique, and Tissue.* 2nd ed. St Louis: Mosby; 1993: 352–359.

Lin DT, Webster RG Jr, Abbott RL. Repair of corneal lacerations and perforations. *Int Ophthalmol Clin.* 1988;28:69–75.

Shingleton BJ, Hersh PS, Kenyon KR, eds. *Eye Trauma.* St Louis: Mosby; 1991.

Spoor TC. *An Atlas of Ophthalmic Trauma.* London: Martin Dunitz; 1997.

Surgical Trauma

Corneal Epithelial Changes From Intraocular Surgery

The corneal epithelium functions as a barrier to corneal absorption of fluid from tears, including medication instilled topically, and pathogens residing on the ocular surface. Breakdown of the epithelial barrier function, resulting in epithelial edema and stromal swelling, can follow any of these surgical missteps:

- Inadvertent intraoperative trauma to the epithelium by the surgical instruments
- Desiccation of the epithelium through inadequate intraoperative hydration
- Toxic keratopathy resulting from excessive preoperative instillation of topical ophthalmic preparations (and their preservatives)
- Accidental instillation of preoperative periocular facial scrub detergents

Although epithelial damage allows fluid to reach the stroma, it is resisted by the intraocular pressure and pumped out by the endothelium. Thus, endothelial damage has a far greater effect on corneal edema than does epithelial damage. Intraoperative damage to the corneal endothelium and/or Descemet's membrane can result in a positive stromal fluid pressure and subsequent epithelial edema. Epithelial edema begins in the basal cell layers of the epithelium, then spreads through the epithelium, occasionally resulting in subepithelial bullae.

The transparency of the corneal epithelium is a result of the homogeneity of the refractive index throughout the epithelium. With epithelial edema, this layer loses its homogeneity, and the corneal surface becomes irregular, leading to symptoms of glare, photophobia, and haloes around lights from light scattering. In bright light, edematous epithelium causes more light scattering and can have a marked effect on vision. Surface irregularities caused by epithelial edema are more damaging to vision than stromal edema or scarring. The influence of epithelial surface irregularities on visual acuity is often underestimated, whereas the role of stromal scarring and edema is overestimated.

Descemet's Membrane Changes During Intraocular Surgery

The distensibility of Descemet's membrane permits stretching or distortion, followed by return to its original shape. When the stroma imbibes fluid and thickens, the increased volume is distributed posteriorly, producing bowing and folding of Descemet's membrane (striate keratopathy). Detachment of Descemet's membrane can occur when an instrument or intraocular lens is introduced through the surgical incision or when fluid is inadvertently injected between the membrane and the corneal stroma, resulting in stromal swelling and epithelial bullae localized in the area of detachment. Descemet's membrane can be reattached with air tamponade or nonexpansile concentrations of sulfur hexafluoride (SF6) in the anterior chamber. Recurrence may require suturing after replacement of Descemet's membrane.

Corneal Endothelial Changes From Intraocular Surgery

Corneal hydration involves the following factors:

- Stromal swelling pressure
- Barrier function of the epithelium and endothelium
- The endothelial pump
- Evaporation from the corneal surface
- Intraocular pressure

Causes of corneal edema following surgical procedures are often multifactorial: related to the health of the patient's endothelium as well as to iatrogenic factors such as surgical technique, duration of surgery, and intraocular irrigating solutions.

Any decompression operation may result in corneal edema. Patients with underlying corneal endothelial dysfunction such as Fuchs corneal dystrophy are at risk to develop postoperative corneal edema, even after smooth, atraumatic surgery.

Cataract surgery/IOL implantation

Manipulation of instruments in the eye through a limbal or clear corneal incision during cataract surgery can impair the functional reserve of an already partially compromised endothelium, leading to localized edema at the site. During phacoemulsification, heat transferred from the probe to the cornea can result in stromal shrinkage. A wound that is too tight to allow adequate irrigation fluid flow through the probe or the occlusion of irrigation or aspiration tubing can cause such heat transfer. A phaco tip held too close to corneal endothelium during surgery allows the ultrasonic energy to injure and cause loss of endothelial cells. Corneal edema in these cases may appear on the first postoperative day or months to years after surgery.

Uncomplicated intracapsular cataract extraction or complicated extracapsular cataract extraction may result in vitreous touch to the corneal endothelium. Persistent corneal edema can occur in the region of vitreocorneal adherence either early or late. Early recognition and treatment with anterior vitrectomy as soon as corneal edema develops can help prevent irreversible corneal edema. More advanced cases with prolonged corneal edema may require a penetrating keratoplasty combined with vitrectomy.

Current irrigating solutions are superior to those used in the past. They are pH balanced with bicarbonate buffers, have no epinephrine, and contain glutathione. Endothelial cell loss rates of 8% or less have been reported in multiple series. Preserved solutions either irrigated or inadvertently injected into the anterior chamber can be toxic to the corneal endothelium and cause temporary or permanent corneal edema. Subconjunctival antibiotic injections have been reported to enter the anterior chamber through scleral tunnel incisions acting as one-way valves.

The presence of iris-fixated or closed-loop flexible anterior chamber intraocular lenses has historically been associated with significant chronic corneal edema and development of pseudophakic bullous keratopathy. Reduced visual acuity, foreign body sensation, photophobia, epiphora, and occasional infectious keratitis are usually associated.

Laser burns

Endothelial damage occurs following argon laser procedures as a result of the thermal effects of iris photocoagulation. Endothelial burns are usually dense white with sharp margins; they may result in focal endothelial cell loss. An increase in mean endothelial cell size and endothelial cell loss associated with the use of greater laser power has also been reported. In follow-up periods of up to 1 year, endothelial cell loss following laser iridectomy has not been found to be statistically significant, however.

Conjunctival and Corneal Changes From Extraocular Surgery

Conjunctival chemosis with prolapse may result from orbital surgery or trauma. Exposed conjunctiva should generally not be excised but rather reposited and kept in place with patching or, if recurrent, mattress sutures.

Orbital surgery and trauma can cause proptosis of the globe leading to exposure keratopathy. Therapy includes lubricants, eyelid patching or taping, moist-chamber dressings, and temporary tarsorrhaphy.

PART X

Surgery of the Ocular Surface

CHAPTER 20

Introduction to Surgery of the Ocular Surface

The term *ocular surface* describes the entire epithelial surface of the external eye, encompassing the corneal epithelium as well as the bulbar and palpebral conjunctival epithelium. Moreover, this term stresses the interdependence of the corneal and conjunctival epithelia in maintaining the health of the external eye. Initially, the ocular surface was considered as an anatomic classification based solely on the physical continuity of the stratified nonkeratinizing epithelium of the conjunctiva, limbus, and cornea. More recently, clinical and research insights have offered compelling evidence of important functional relationships within this anatomic entity. This rethinking of the ocular surface as a functional unit has stimulated a complete reorganization of the current approach to the management of ocular surface disease (Table 20-1).

Corneal and Conjunctival Epithelial Wound Healing

The mechanisms of wound healing of the corneal stroma and sclera have been covered in Chapter 18 and are also discussed in BCSC Section 4, *Ophthalmic Pathology and Intraocular Tumors*. Observations of the normal replacement process of corneal epithelium provide valuable insights into the rationale for various ocular surface replacement techniques. Numerous studies have demonstrated that central corneal epithelial mass is maintained by continued centripetal movement of peripheral corneal epithelium toward the visual axis, as well as by anterior movement from the basal epithelial cells.

Role of Stem Cells

Because the corneal epithelium is a highly differentiated cell type that is self-renewing, its stem cells are essential for epithelial replacement and migration. It is believed that the limbal basal layer contains the stem cells of the corneal epithelium that normally repopulate the corneal surface. After severe injuries, this normal process is augmented appreciably in eyes that have a normal reservoir of functioning stem cells. When there is concurrent damage to the limbal stem cells, the conjunctival cells also become involved in repopulating the corneal surface. However, this is a pathological process often associated with vascularization and poor epithelial adhesion.

Table 20-1 Indications for Ocular Surface Reconstruction

Conjunctival Autograft	Limbal Autograft or Allograft*	Mucous Membrane or Amniotic Membrane[†] Transplantation
Recurrent pterygium	Chemical injury	Fornix reconstruction (bilateral)
Cicatricial strabismus (bilateral)	Thermal burn	Chemical injury[‡]
Fornix reconstruction (unilateral)	Contact lens keratopathy	Immune melts
Postexcision of conjunctival tumor	Persistent epithelial defect (various etiologies)	
Symblepharon repair	Post–multiple surgery limbal depletion	
	Chronic medication toxicity	
	Stevens-Johnson syndrome	
	Ocular cicatricial pemphigoid	
	Aniridia	
	Atopy	

* Limbal autograft preferable in unilateral or asymmetric cases; limbal allograft reserved for bilateral cases.
[†] May be used in conjunction with limbal autograft or allograft.
[‡] Indicated for fornix reconstruction after cicatrization.

Conjunctival Epithelium

Healthy conjunctival epithelium also has the ability to directly replace damaged corneal epithelium; but, as mentioned above, conjunctival epithelial cells cannot completely restore its function because they do not have the pluripotency of limbal stem cells and cannot differentiate into the corneal phenotype. Following complete traumatic loss of corneal and limbal epithelium, the remaining conjunctival epithelium resurfaces the corneal epithelium by an advancing wave of adjacent conjunctiva. Some of these cells demonstrate morphological changes, but they do not acquire all the biochemical markers of mature corneal epithelia. It was long believed that conjunctival cells retained the capacity for phenotypic change into corneal epithelium, but we now know that this is not the case. The absolute necessity of repopulating the corneal surface epithelium with stem cells forms the rationale for syngeneic or allogeneic limbal stem-cell transplantation.

Maintenance of the Ocular Surface and Its Response to Wound Healing

In the mechanically abraded cornea (eg, total epithelial debridement during vitrectomy surgery), reepithelialization and restoration of a relatively normal corneal surface usually occur quickly. In eyes that have suffered severe chemical injury, however, where the insult is to a wide array of cells (corneal, limbal, and conjunctival), the process of cell migration and differentiation may become defective. Consequently, the wave of cells that repopulate the corneal surface often maintain conjunctival characteristics, with variable goblet cells and neovascularization. Based on these observations, autologous conjunctival transplantation has limited value in repopulating the corneal surface unless associated limbal cells are also harvested for grafting. However, conjunctival grafting can be successful in suppressing inflammation and scarring in the traumatized conjunctiva, and thereby providing (indirectly) more support for the proliferating corneal cells. The success of this procedure is contingent on procurement of normal or near-normal donor tissue.

If the goal of surgery is the restoration of a more functional conjunctival mucosal surface, as in bilateral conjunctival cicatricial disorders or in severe epitheliopathy in keratoconjunctivitis sicca (eg, Sjögren syndrome), then a buccal mucosal graft or amniotic membrane transplant may be employed. Such grafts can restore more normal forniceal architecture and reduce ocular surface inflammation and corneal damage resulting from abnormal eyelid–globe relationships (eg, entropion, trichiasis), chronic exposure (lagophthalmos), and direct corneal trauma (palpebral conjunctival keratinization). In advanced cases of mucosal (conjunctival) disease, complications caused by recurrent corneal epithelial breakdown, secondary infectious keratitis, vascularization, and scarring may lead to corneal blindness.

Mucosal membrane grafting is not, however, by itself effective in repopulating the cornea with normal cells. Rather, its contribution to the health of the corneal surface is indirect: it improves ocular surface wetting by narrowing the palpebral fissure, thereby reducing exposure and evaporation; and it enhances eyelid movement and distribution of the tear film over the cornea. Preserved amniotic membrane is another tissue that can be used for ocular surface reconstruction, either by itself to prevent further stromal degradation or in conjunction with limbal autograft or allograft to repopulate the corneal stem cells.

CHAPTER 21

Surgical Procedures of the Ocular Surface

This chapter covers some of the common surgeries performed on the ocular surface as well as a few nonsurgical techniques such as the use of bandage contact lenses and cyanoacrylate adhesives. Part XI of this volume discusses corneal transplantation, and Part XII covers keratorefractive surgery.

Conjunctival Biopsy

Indications

A conjunctival biopsy can be helpful in the evaluation of chronic conjunctivitis and unusual ocular surface diseases, including the following:

- Superior limbic keratoconjunctivitis
- Conjunctival lymphoid tumors
- Cicatricial pemphigoid
- Graft-versus-host disease
- Squamous lesions of the conjunctiva (eg, conjunctival intraepithelial neoplasia)

Surgical Technique

After a topical anesthetic agent is administered, a pledget wet with proparacaine or similar agent is applied to the lesion or site for approximately 30 seconds. Subconjunctival anesthesia can also be given but is usually unnecessary. A drop of topical phenylephrine can blanch the conjunctival vessels and reduce bleeding. The surgeon uses forceps and scissors to snip a conjunctival specimen. Lesions are completely excised (excisional biopsy) if possible. A wedge or block is excised for a subepithelial lesion. Tissue crushing must be minimized by grasping only the edge of the biopsy specimen. Gentle cauterization can be used to facilitate hemostasis. It is best to cauterize after excision to minimize burning of the specimen, which severely hinders histological evaluation.

Tissue Processing

The sample is placed on a carrier template and inserted into the appropriate fixative, such as formalin (for histology), glutaraldehyde (for electron microscopy), or saline (for frozen-section or immunopathologic processing).

Preferred Practice Patterns Committee, Cornea Panel. *Conjunctivitis.* San Francisco: American Academy of Ophthalmology; 1998.

Tarsorrhaphy

Tarsorrhaphy is the surgical fusion of the upper and lower eyelid margins. The exact mechanisms that make this procedure so effective in the treatment of many corneal disorders remains to be fully determined; nevertheless, tarsorrhaphy is one of the safest and most effective procedures for healing difficult-to-treat corneal lesions. It is most commonly performed to protect the cornea from exposure caused by inadequate eyelid coverage, as may occur in Graves disease or facial nerve (CN VII) dysfunctions such as Bell's palsy. It can also be used to aid in the healing of indolent corneal ulceration sometimes seen with tear film deficiency, stem-cell dysfunction, or CN V dysfunction (neurotrophic lesions). Tarsorrhaphies may be temporary or permanent, in which case raw tarsal edges are created to form a lasting adhesion. They may be total or partial, depending on whether all or only a portion of the palpebral fissure is occluded. Finally, they are classified as lateral, medial, or central, according to the position in the palpebral fissure. BCSC Section 7, *Orbit, Eyelids, and Lacrimal System,* discusses eyelid anatomy and surgical procedures in detail.

Postoperative Care

Antibiotic ointment is usually applied to the wound twice a day for the first 5 days. If anterior lamellar sutures over a pledget are used, ointment is applied until they are removed 2 weeks later. Ointment containing corticosteroids should be avoided, because it may interfere with rapid healing. The clinician should use slit-lamp examination of the cornea to guide administration of lubricants.

A tarsorrhaphy can be released under local anesthesia. A muscle hook is placed under the tissue, and a blade is used to incise the tarsorrhaphy adhesion parallel to the upper and lower eyelid margins. Iris scissors can also be used to cut along the margin. If the status of the corneal exposure is uncertain, the tarsorrhaphy can be opened in stages, a few millimeters at a time. If the tarsorrhaphy has been performed properly, eyelid margin deformity will be minimal.

Alternatives to Tarsorrhaphy

Other therapeutic modalities can help protect the integrity of the ocular surface. Periorbital injection of botulinum toxin type A (Botox) to paralyze the orbicularis and levator muscles can cause pharmacological ptosis and provide temporary protective effects. Application of cyanoacrylate tissue adhesive (discussed later in this chapter) to the eyelid margins may also provide temporary closure of the eyelids for therapeutic purposes.

Pterygium Excision

A pterygium is an abnormal overgrowth of conjunctiva onto the cornea, almost always in the palpebral fissure (see Chapter 17). Indications for pterygium excision include persistent discomfort, vision distortion, significant (>3–4 mm) and progressive growth toward the corneal center/visual axis, and restricted ocular motility.

Microsurgical excision of a pterygium aims to achieve a normal, topographically smooth ocular surface. A common surgical technique is to remove the pterygium using a flat blade to dissect a smooth plane toward the limbus. Although it is preferable to dissect down to bare sclera at the limbus, it is not necessary to dissect excessive Tenon's tissue medially, as this can sometimes lead to bleeding from inadvertent trauma to subjacent muscle tissue. After excision, light thermal cautery is usually applied to the sclera for hemostasis. Options for wound closure include (Fig 21-1)

- Bare sclera: No sutures or fine, absorbable sutures are used to appose the conjunctiva to the superficial sclera in front of the rectus tendon insertion, leaving an area of exposed sclera. (This technique, however, has an unacceptably high recurrence rate of 40%–50%.)
- Simple closure: The free edges of the conjunctiva are secured together (effective only when the conjunctival defect is very small).
- Sliding flap: An L-shaped incision is made adjacent to the wound to allow a conjunctival flap to slide into place.
- Rotational flap: A U-shaped incision is made adjacent to the wound to form a tongue of conjunctiva that is rotated into place.
- Conjunctival graft: A free graft, usually from the superior bulbar conjunctiva, is excised to correspond to the size of the wound and is then moved and sutured into place. This technique is described in more detail below.

Conjunctival Transplantation

Only those cases in which conjunctival inflammation, scarring, or loss is *not* complicated by extensive damage or destruction of the limbal epithelial stem cells are appropriate for conjunctival autograft transplantation (see Table 20-1). This technique is essentially an ocular surface patch graft designed to

- Replace a focal or localized defect in the conjunctiva (such as after pterygium excision)
- Relieve the restriction of extraocular muscle movement caused by scarring of conjunctival and Tenon's tissue (after pterygium removal, strabismus surgery, or bulbar tumor excision)
- Eliminate problems of conjunctival fornix scarring

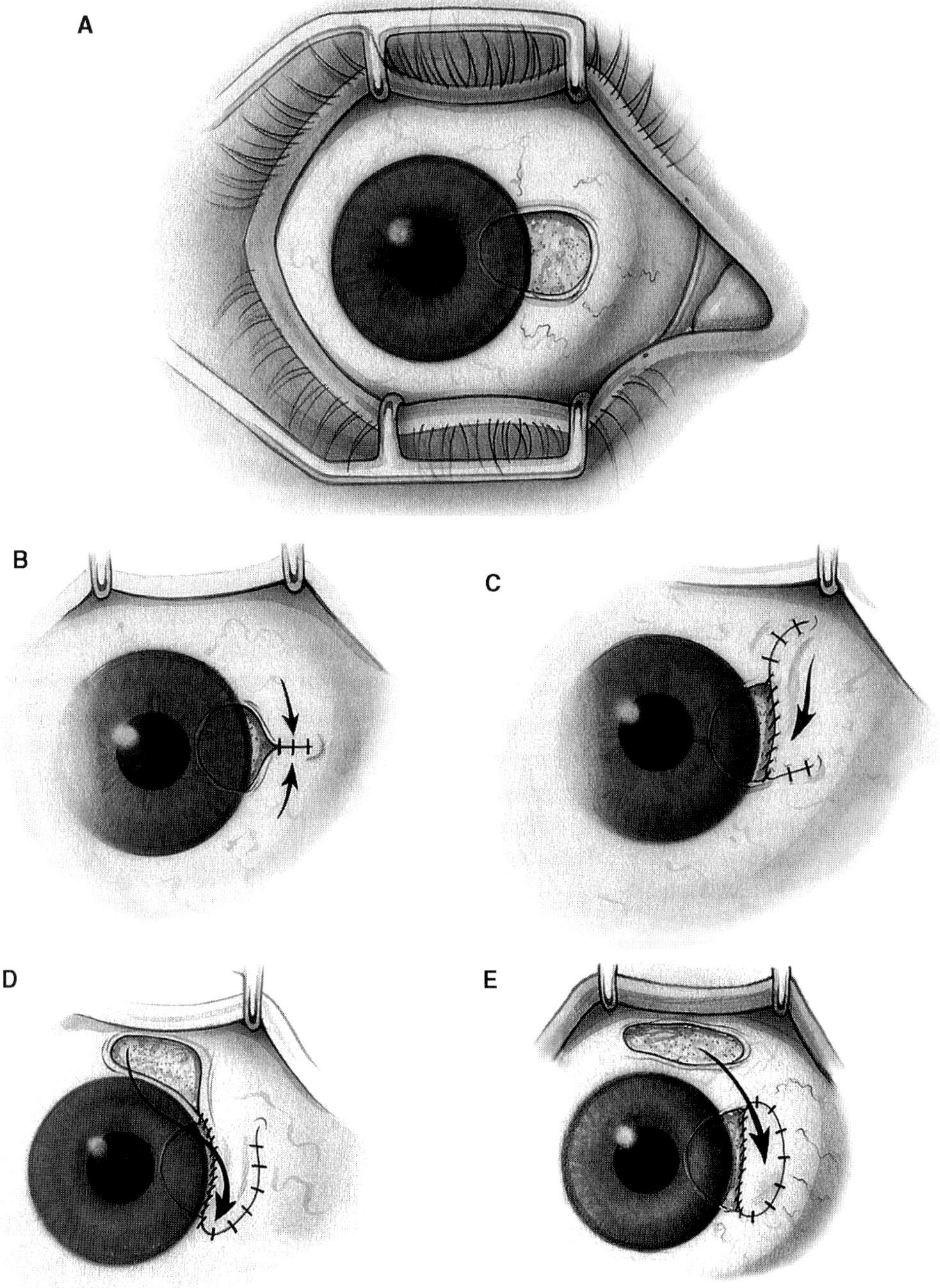

Figure 21-1 Surgical wound closures following pterygium excision. **A,** Bare sclera, although sutures can be placed to tack down conjunctival wound edges. **B,** Simple closure with fine, absorbable sutures. **C,** Sliding flap that is closed with interrupted and/or running suture. **D,** Rotational flap from the superior bulbar conjunctiva. **E,** Conjunctival autograft that is secured with interrupted and/or running suture. *(Reproduced with permission from Gans LA. Surgical treatment of pterygium. In:* Focal Points: Clinical Modules for Ophthalmologists. *San Francisco: American Academy of Ophthalmology; 1996: vol 14, no 12. Illustration by Christine Gralapp.)*

Conjunctival Transplantation for Pterygium

The most common indication for conjunctival transplantation is the management of advanced primary and recurrent pterygium. This technique reduces the risk of pterygium recurrence to approximately 2%–5% and ameliorates the restriction of extraocular muscle function frequently encountered after pterygium excision. Because the superior bulbar conjunctiva is usually normal and undamaged, conjunctival autograft tissue can be obtained from this area in the same eye.

Various techniques of conjunctival transplantation have been used to manage pterygium. The procedure is performed on an outpatient basis, using topical plus peribulbar or retrobulbar anesthesia, especially in recurrent cases complicated by scarring. A traction suture (eg, 6-0 on a spatulated needle) placed at the 12 o'clock position, which can then be clamped down in various positions to the surgical drape, facilitates maximal exposure of the pterygium and the graft site. The pterygium is usually excised with a #57 blade or a crescent (flat) blade. The size of the defect is then measured with calipers. It is best to allow a little extra tissue for grafting, so the harvested tissue should be approximately 0.5–1.0 mm larger than the size of the defect.

The eye is then turned down to expose the superior bulbar conjunctiva. The area to be harvested is then marked with multiple focal cautery spots or with a surgical pen. The most important aspect of the harvesting is to procure conjunctival tissue with only minimal or no Tenon's included. After the graft is freed, it is transferred to the recipient bed and secured to adjacent conjunctiva (with or without incorporating episclera) with absorbable (eg, 8-0 Vicryl) sutures. Some surgeons make a special point of harvesting limbal stem cells along with the conjunctiva and orienting the donor material in the host bed so that the stem cells are adjacent to the site of corneal lesion excision. The donor site is usually left bare. Postoperatively, topical antibiotic-corticosteroid ointment is administered frequently for approximately 4–6 weeks until inflammation subsides. The surgeon should emphasize to the patient that compliance with this regimen minimizes the chance of recurrence.

Complications

A large body of literature supports the use of mitomycin-C (MMC) in pterygium surgery to minimize recurrence rates. Although low concentrations of MMC used at the time of surgery (applied to the area of resection with a surgical sponge) have been shown to be effective in reducing recurrence, it is important to note that any use of topical mitomycin-C can be toxic and may cause visually significant complications such as aseptic scleral necrosis and infectious sclerokeratitis. The critical point regarding these complications is that they may occur many months, or even years, after the use of MMC. If surgery is being performed in a case of recurrent pterygium, and MMC use is contemplated, it is safer to apply it intraoperatively rather than to give the patient topical MMC to use postoperatively; the latter is prone to abuse.

The risk of recurrent pterygium following conjunctival autografting is very low, between 2% and 5%. Self-limited problems include conjunctival graft edema, corneoscleral dellen, and epithelial cysts. Cases of recurrent pterygium after conjunctival autograft transplantation may be substantially improved by either repeated conjunctival autograft or modified limbal autografts. Most studies suggest that the rate of recurrence with MMC is similar to that with conjunctival grafting.

Other Indications for Conjunctival Grafting

Conjunctival autografts can also be used for fornix reconstruction when conjunctival fibrosis and cicatrization lead to fornix foreshortening, symblepharon formation, cicatricial entropion, trichiasis, and ocular surface keratinization and vascularization. Occasionally, unilateral fornix foreshortening occurs after localized disease, retinal detachment surgery, or excision of ocular surface tumors. It can be remedied by placement of a conjunctival autograft from the opposite eye. Usually, however, conditions associated with fornix obliteration (cicatricial pemphigoid, Stevens-Johnson syndrome) are bilateral so that uninvolved conjunctiva is not available for grafting. Mucous membrane transplantation using buccal mucosa or amniotic membrane has become the preferred ocular surface replacement technique in such instances.

Limbal Transplantation

When stem cells are destroyed by disease or injury, the corneal surface becomes covered with conjunctival epithelium, which is less transparent, more irregular, and more prone to erosion and vascularization than normal corneal epithelium (see Chapters 18 and 20 for discussion of this phenomenon). This condition can be diagnosed clinically by the absence of the limbal palisades of Vogt, or cytologically with impression cytology or biopsy of the limbal region to show goblet cells. Loss of limbal stem cells is seen most often in chemical injury, but it can also occur as a result of contact lens overwear, multiple surgical procedures, large ocular surface abrasions, repeated infections, or use of topical medications.

If total loss of limbal stem cells occurs unilaterally, an autograft of limbal epithelium from the fellow eye can repopulate the diseased cornea with normal corneal epithelium (Fig 21-2). In this procedure, corneal epithelium, conjunctiva, and superficial pannus are removed from within 2 mm outside the limbus of the recipient eye, and two thin limbal autografts from the fellow eye are then attached to the limbus and allowed to regenerate and proliferate.

If total loss of limbal stem cells occurs bilaterally, the options for ocular surface transplantation are more limited. The appropriate selection of procedures depends on the relative health of the stem-cell population in the prospective donor eye. A limbal stem-cell allograft from a living related donor may be considered. A similar procedure, *keratoepithelioplasty*, uses peripheral cornea or corneolimbal rims from an eye bank donor eye. Even though host cells may eventually reject or replace such a tissue, good long-term results have been reported. Although technical difficulties, poor epithelial viability, and rejection problems necessitating systemic immunosuppression have limited the usefulness of this modality, dramatic success has been observed in selected desperate cases. In contrast, the use of *cultured* limbal epithelium is still not routinely available, even though it is technically feasible and has been used with success. For cases of bilateral stem-cell loss, the most promising technique for transferring donor stem cells is limbal allograft transplantation. Use of allogeneic (cultured cell or tissue) grafts requires systemic immune modulation to minimize the chance of rejection of the highly immunogenic limbal tissue.

Tsubota K, Satake Y, Kaido M, et al. Treatment of severe ocular-surface disorders with corneal epithelial stem-cell transplantation. *N Engl J Med*. 1999;340:1697–1703.

Conjunctival Flap

Indications

The conjunctival flap procedure covers an unstable or painful corneal surface with a hinged flap of more durable conjunctiva. Conjunctival flap surgery is performed less frequently now than in the past because of broadened indications for penetrating keratoplasty (see Chapters 22 and 23), more effective antimicrobial agents, availability of bandage contact lenses, and improved management of corneal inflammatory diseases. Nevertheless, this procedure remains an effective method for managing inflammatory and structural corneal disorders when restoration of vision is not an immediate concern. It should not be used for active microbial keratitis or corneal perforation, because residual infectious organisms may proliferate under a flap if an ulcer is not sterilized first. Any corneal perforation must first be sealed, or it will continue to leak under the flap. The principal indications for this procedure are

- Chronic sterile epithelial and stromal ulcerations (stromal herpes simplex virus keratitis, chemical and thermal burns, keratoconjunctivitis sicca, postinfectious ulcers, neurotrophic keratopathy)
- Closed but unstable corneal wounds
- Painful bullous keratopathy in a patient who is not a good candidate for penetrating keratoplasty
- A phthisical eye being prepared for a prosthetic shell

Reduced visualization of the anterior chamber and creation of a potential barrier against drug penetration are among the disadvantages of conjunctival flap surgery. However, a successful conjunctival graft, free of buttonholes, will thin out and enable useful vision.

Surgical Technique

A thin hood, or *Gundersen flap* (Fig 21-3), is highly successful if attention is paid to several fundamental principles:

- Complete removal of the corneal epithelium and debridement of necrotic tissue
- Creation of a mobile, thin conjunctival flap that contains minimal Tenon's capsule
- Absence of any conjunctival buttonhole that may lead to flap retraction
- Absence of any traction on the flap at its margins

Retrobulbar, peribulbar, or general anesthesia may be used. The corneal epithelium and all necrotic tissue are removed, and the eye is retracted inferiorly with an intracorneal traction suture at the superior limbus. Elevation of the flap with subconjunctival injection

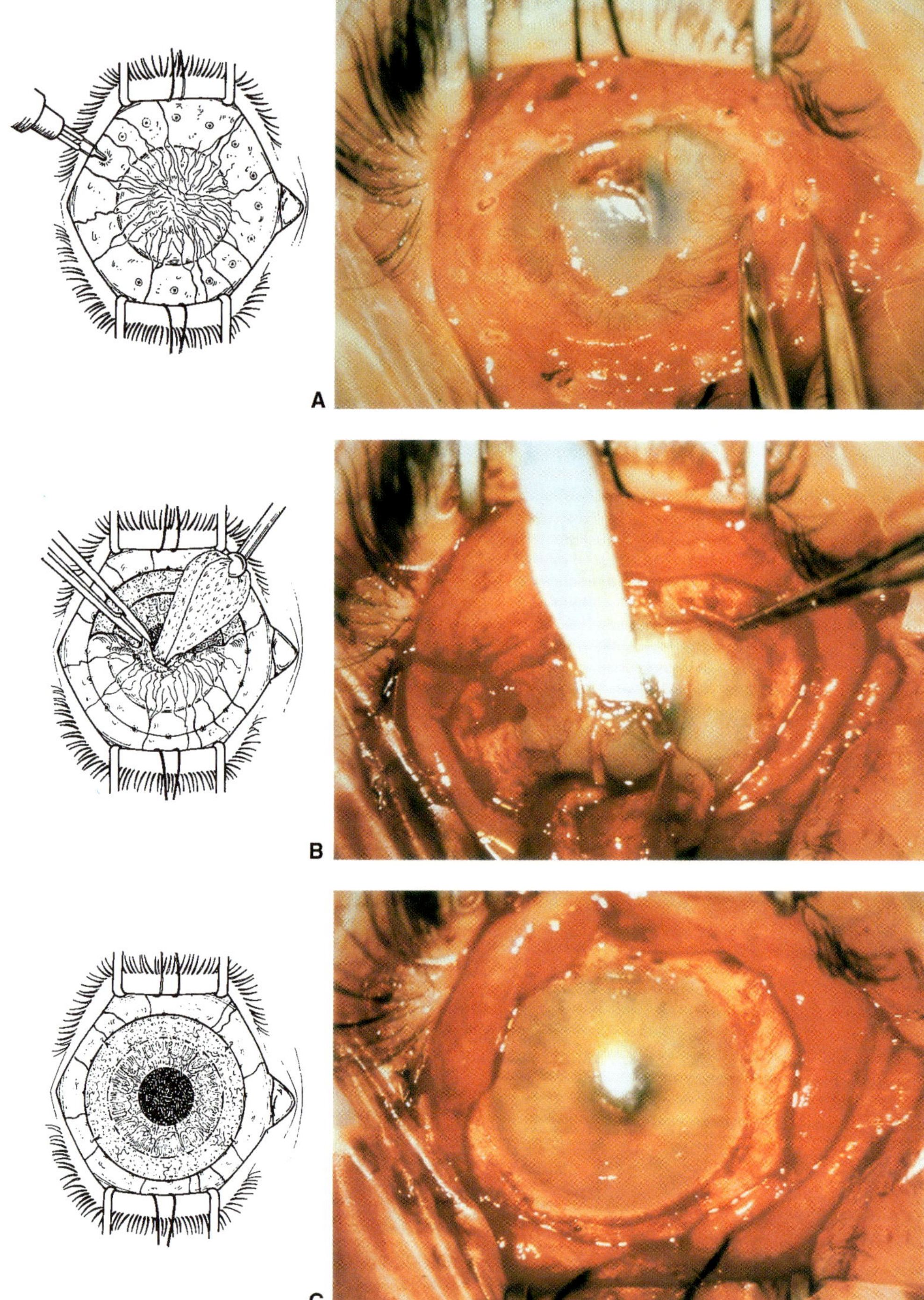

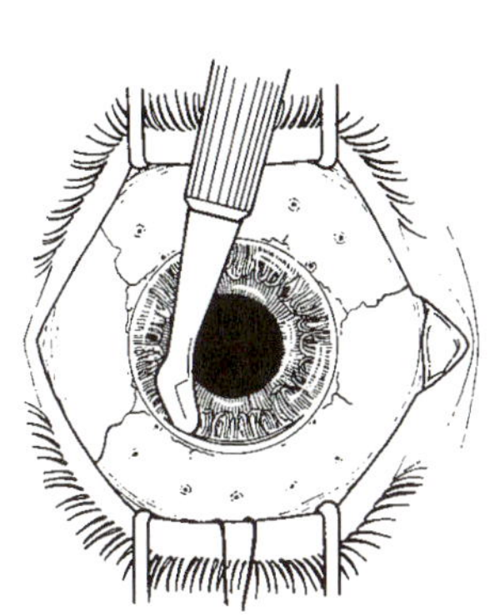 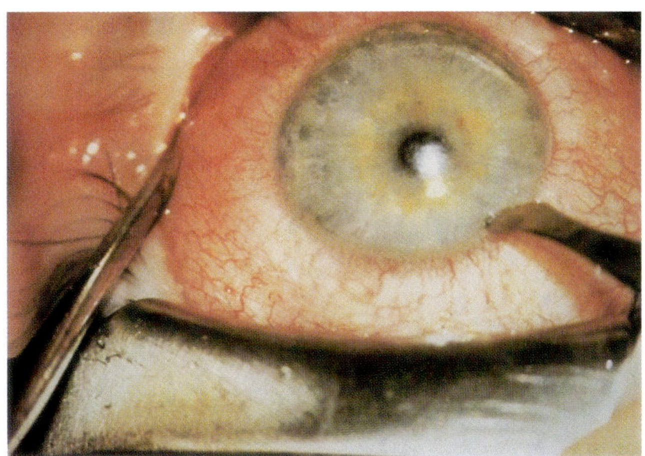

D

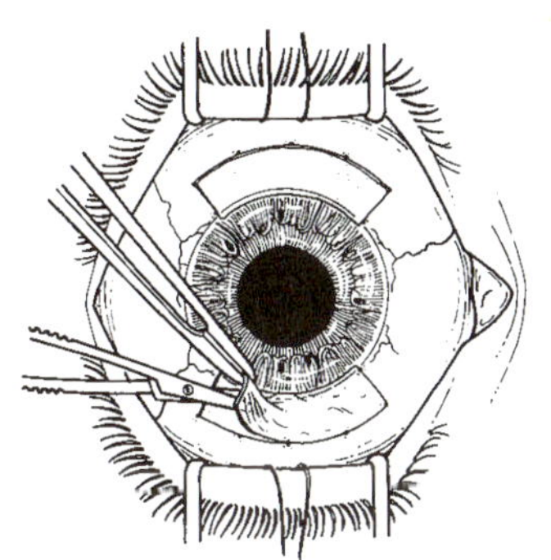 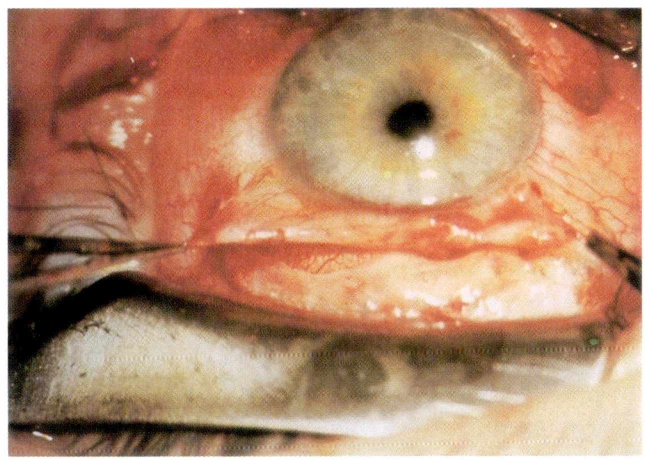

E

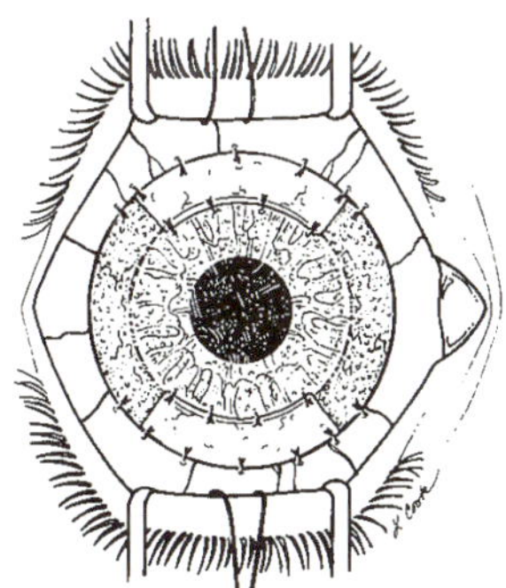

F

Figure 21-2 Limbal autograft procedure. **A,** With disposable cautery, the area of bulbar conjunctiva to be resected is marked approximately 2 mm posterior to the limbus. **B,** After conjunctival resection, abnormal corneal epithelium and fibrovascular pannus are stripped by blunt dissection using cellulose sponges and tissue forceps. **C,** Additional surface polishing smooths the stromal surface and improves clarity. **D,** Superior and inferior limbal grafts are delineated in the donor eye with focal applications of cautery approximately 2 mm posterior to the limbus. The initial incision is made superficially within clear cornea using a disposable knife. **E,** The bulbar conjunctival portion of the graft is undermined and thinly dissected from its limbal attachment. **F,** The limbal grafts are transferred to their corresponding sites in the recipient eye and are secured with interrupted sutures, 10-0 nylon at the corneal edge and 8-0 Vicryl at the conjunctival margin. *(Reproduced by permission from Kenyon KR, Tseng SC. Limbal autograft transplantation for ocular surface disorders. Ophthalmology. 1989;96:709–723.)*

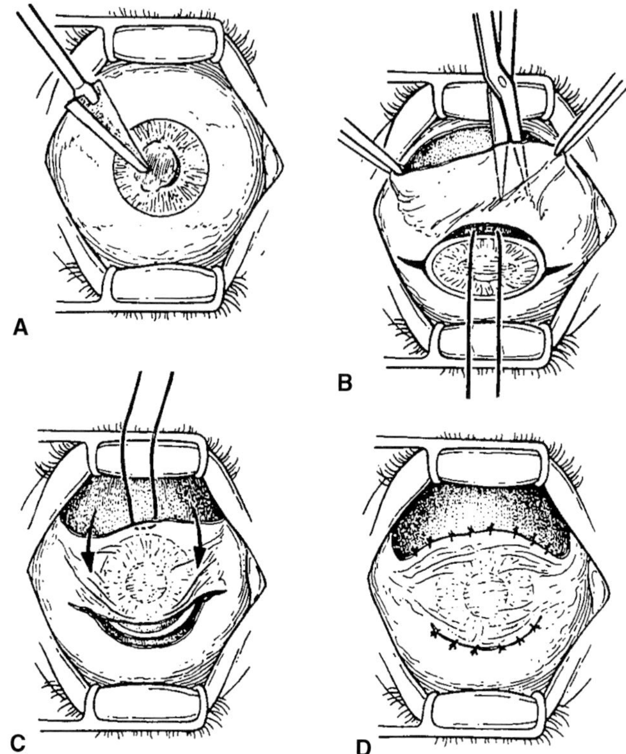

Figure 21-3 Surgical steps for the Gundersen conjunctival flap. **A,** Removal of the corneal epithelium. **B,** A 360° peritomy with relaxing incisions, placement of superior limbal traction suture, superior forniceal incision, and dissection of a thin flap. **C,** Positioning of flap. **D,** Suturing of flap into position with multiple interrupted sutures. *(Reproduced by permission from Mannis MJ. Conjunctival flaps. Int Ophthalmol Clin. 1988;28:165–168.)*

of lidocaine with epinephrine enhances anesthesia, facilitates dissection, and reduces bleeding. The needle for this injection should not pierce the conjunctiva in the area to be used for the flap.

The dissection may start from either the limbus or superior fornix. Dissection of conjunctiva from underlying Tenon's fascia must be performed carefully under direct visualization to prevent conjunctival perforation, especially in eyes with previous conjunctival surgery. Once the flap has been dissected, a 360° peritomy is performed, followed by scraping of all remaining limbal epithelium. Additional undermining of the flap allows it to cover the entire cornea and to rest there without traction. Any residual tension may foster later retraction of the flap. After the flap is positioned over the prepared cornea, it is sutured to the sclera just posterior to the limbus superiorly and inferiorly.

Partial conjunctival flap

A partial, or *bridge,* flap may be used for temporary coverage of a peripheral wound or area of ulceration. Retraction is common despite adequate relaxation of the base. The flap should be well undermined to relieve tension and decrease the chance of retraction.

Bipedicle flap

This partial, or *bucket handle,* flap can be used for small central or paracentral corneal lesions that do not require complete corneal coverage. The advantage is that the view of the anterior chamber and the remaining uninvolved cornea is not obstructed. The flap is fashioned similar to the Gundersen flap but with only enough dissection required to cover the lesion, plus a small margin (the width of the flap should be 1.3–1.5 times the width of the lesion). Anesthesia is administered, and the epithelium beneath the site of the flap is removed. After marking the bulbar conjunctiva with methylene blue, the surgeon can create the flap and mobilize it into position for suturing with interrupted nylon suture.

Advancement flap

Peripheral limbal or paralimbal corneal lesions can be covered with a simple advancement conjunctival flap. A limbal incision is created with relaxing components, and the conjunctiva is simply advanced onto the cornea to cover the defect. Scleral patch grafts and onlay grafts may also be used in conjunction with this technique. The disadvantage of this type of flap is a tendency to retract with time.

Single-pedicle flaps

Also known as *racquet flaps,* these flaps can be used for peripheral corneal lesions that are not large enough to require a total flap. Although a single-pedicle flap is more difficult to dissect than an advancement flap, it is less likely to retract.

Complications

Retraction of the flap is the most common complication, occurring in about 10% of cases. Other complications include hemorrhage beneath the flap and epithelial cysts. In some cases, inclusion cysts enlarge to the point of requiring excision or marsupialization. Ptosis, usually of the levator dehiscence type, may also occur postoperatively. Unsatisfactory cosmetic appearance can be improved with a painted contact lens. Progressive corneal disease under the flap is a concern with infective and autoimmune conditions.

Considerations in Removal of the Flap

If penetrating keratoplasty (PK) is to be performed in an eye with a conjunctival flap, the flap may be removed as a separate procedure or at the time of PK. Simple removal of the flap (without keratoplasty) is usually unsatisfactory in restoring vision, as the underlying cornea is almost always scarred and/or thinned. Because the conjunctival flap procedure tends to destroy or displace most limbal stem cells, a limbal autograft after removal of the flap may be necessary to provide a permanent source of normal epithelium before an optical corneal transplant.

Abbott RL, Beebe WE. Corneal edema. In: Abbott RL, ed. *Surgical Intervention in Corneal and External Diseases.* Orlando: Grune & Stratton; 1987:81–84.

Mannis MJ. Conjunctival flaps. *Int Ophthalmol Clin.* 1988;28:165–168.

Mucous Membrane Grafting

Indications

The goal of surgery is to reconstruct a more functional conjunctival mucosal surface so as to ameliorate the fornix obliteration or eyelid margin keratinization that usually occurs with bilateral cicatricial conjunctival disorders such as Stevens-Johnson syndrome or ocular cicatricial pemphigoid (see Table 20-1). Buccal mucosa or preserved amniotic membrane can be employed. Mucous membrane grafting has rarely been used as a treatment for unilateral chemical injury and is performed only in desperate cases of bilateral injury where advancement of Tenon's capsule is not possible and allograft limbal tissue is not available. Nonetheless, this technique has long been a popular method of correcting eyelid position abnormalities caused by cicatrizing conjunctival disorders. Although good results have been reported in inactive cicatricial disorders such as late-stage, nonprogressive Stevens-Johnson syndrome, there is some reluctance to apply this technique to advanced (stage III or IV) ocular cicatricial pemphigoid for fear of exacerbating this relentlessly progressive inflammatory disorder. This fear may no longer be warranted, however: advances in immunosuppressive treatment have brought promise that mucous membrane grafting for the eyelid abnormalities associated with late-stage ocular cicatricial pemphigoid can achieve substantial success.

The purpose of grafting mucosal membranes is to achieve better ocular surface wetting by improving eyelid movement and distribution of the tear film over the cornea, thereby reducing exposure and evaporation. This procedure also provides favorable extracellular matrix substrate for better epithelial migration and adhesion. However, mucous membrane grafting is not effective in replacing normal stem cells. In a small series of patients with advanced ocular cicatricial pemphigoid and Stevens-Johnson syndrome, combinations of allograft limbal transplantation, amniotic membrane transplantation, and tarsorrhaphy, followed by the use of serum-derived tears and systemic immunosuppression, were shown to reconstruct the ocular surface. These therapeutic modalities appear to provide an alternative to other difficult procedures such as keratoprosthesis for treating patients with desperate cicatricial keratoconjunctivitis (see Chapter 23).

There are many surgical techniques for mucosal grafting, and the reader should consult a surgical textbook or video for specifics. Regardless of the particular technique, potential complications include buttonholing, retraction, trichiasis, surface keratinization of the graft, ptosis, phimosis, depressed eyelid blink, incomplete eyelid closure, submucosal abscess formation, and persistent nonhealing epithelial defects of the cornea.

Dua HS, Azuaro-Blanco A. Amniotic membrane transplantation. *Br J Ophthalmol.* 1999; 83:748–752.

Superficial Keratectomy and Corneal Biopsy

Indications

This procedure consists of excision of the superficial layers of cornea (epithelium, Bowman's layer, or superficial stroma) without replacement of tissue. The primary indications are

- Removal of hyperplastic or necrotic tissue (eg, corneal dermoid, pterygium, Salzmann degeneration, epithelial basement membrane reduplication)
- Excision of retained foreign material in the cornea
- Need for tissue for diagnosis (histopathology or microbiology)
- Excision of scarring or superficial corneal dystrophic tissue

If corneal biopsy is performed for histopathology, preservation of tissue integrity and anatomical orientation is crucial. A small specimen can be placed on a filter or thin card to maintain the tissue orientation before fixation or cryosection. For microbiology workup, the biopsied specimens can be minced or homogenized prior to inoculation of the culture media or tissue smearing for histochemical stainings.

Surgical Techniques

Mechanical keratectomy

If the corneal lesion is superficial, it may be possible to scrape or peel it away without sharp dissection. When deeper dissection is required, the surgeon can mark the area freehand with an adjustable-depth blade or use a trephine. Care must be taken to maintain the surgical plane and to avoid inadvertent perforation; keeping the dissection plane dry can be very helpful. A lamellar keratectomy can also be performed using a microkeratome, a diamond burr on a surgical drill, or an excimer laser.

Phototherapeutic keratectomy (PTK)

The excimer laser can remove tissue with much greater precision than is possible with mechanical techniques. One problem with PTK, however, is that scar tissue may ablate at a different rate from normal tissue, which results in an uneven surface even if the original surface was smooth. Conversely, if the corneal surface is irregular to begin with and ablates homogeneously, the irregularity will persist. Frequent application of viscous liquid to the corneal surface during ablation fills in the gaps and helps to achieve a smooth surface. Most patients experience a hyperopic shift after PTK from the corneal-flattening effect of the procedure. Nevertheless, PTK may produce marked improvement in vision in selected patients with superficial stromal scarring or dystrophies and obviate the need for corneal transplant surgery.

Campos M, Nielsen S, Szerenyi K, et al. Clinical follow-up of phototherapeutic keratectomy for treatment of corneal opacities. *Am J Ophthalmol.* 1993;115:433–440.

Management of Descemetocele, Corneal Perforation, and Corneal Edema

Bandage Contact Lens

The application of an ultrathin, continuous-wear soft contact lens as a therapeutic bandage can protect the loosely adherent remaining or regenerating epithelium from the "windshield wiper" action of the blinking eyelids. Use of bandage contact lenses has significantly improved and simplified the management of recurrent erosions and persistent epithelial defect. Continuous bandaging can reduce stromal leukocyte infiltration and ensure the regeneration of basement membrane and restoration of tight epithelial–stromal adhesion without compromising the patient's vision and comfort.

Frequent irrigation and lubrication with unpreserved saline, prophylaxis with antibiotics, and close follow-up are crucial, especially in patients with decreased corneal sensitivity or dry eye. The choice of a soft contact lens for patients with severe dry eye can be difficult. In general, patients with dry eye run a high risk of infection with soft contact lenses. Punctal occlusion can facilitate lens retention and comfort. High-water-content lenses usually are not appropriate because rapid water evaporation further compounds the hypertonicity-induced surface damage in dry eyes. The use of a nonhydrophilic, acrylic scleral lens may circumvent the problems encountered with a hydrogel lens.

Even though a hydrogel lens can actually cause corneal hypoxia and increase corneal edema, continuous wear of this type of lens can provide symptomatic relief of painful bullous or filamentary keratopathy. Mild corneal edema can often be managed with hypertonic saline solution or ointment and judicious use of topical steroids if indicated. Chronic use of a bandage contact lens can lead to corneal pannus and compromise the success of future penetrating keratoplasty for visual rehabilitation. Tarsorrhaphy should be considered for patients who have contact lens complications or a high risk of infection.

Cyanoacrylate Adhesive

Tissue adhesives, particularly butylcyanoacrylate, have been used widely as an adjunct in the management of corneal ulceration and perforation. Early application of tissue adhesives in the management of stromal melting has greatly reduced the need for major surgical interventions such as therapeutic keratoplasty or conjunctival flap. Although cyanoacrylate tissue adhesives are not approved by the FDA for use on the eye, they have been employed extensively over the past two decades to seal perforations or near perforations.

Some perforations are so minimal that they seal spontaneously prior to any ophthalmologic examination, with no intraocular damage, prolapse, or adherence. These cases may require only treatment with systemic and/or topical antibiotic therapy, along with close observation. If a corneal wound is leaking but the chamber remains formed, leakage can be reduced or stopped with pharmacologic suppression of aqueous production (topical or systemic), patching, and/or a bandage contact lens. Generally, if these measures fail to seal the wound in 3 days, closure with cyanoacrylate glue or sutures is recommended. Perforations greater than 2–3 mm are usually not amenable to tissue adhesive.

Cyanoacrylate tissue adhesive applied to thinned or ulcerated corneal tissue may prevent further thinning and support the stroma through the period of vascularization and repair. The adhesive plug is also thought to retard the entry of inflammatory cells and epithelium into the area, thus decreasing the rate of corneal melting. After the lesion has been sealed, new stromal tissue may be laid down, and accompanying corneal vascularization may help to ensure the integrity of the area by providing nutrients and antiproteases. Tissue adhesives may be useful whether or not infection is present, since they are also bacteriostatic. However, adherence of bacteria to the pores in the glue has been reported. In any case, continued use of antimicrobial therapy is strongly recommended.

Surgical technique

Tissue adhesive can usually be applied on an outpatient basis for sterile ulcerations. However, if adherent or prolapsed uvea in the leakage site or a flat chamber is encountered, the procedure should be performed in the operating room using air or hyaluronate to reform the anterior chamber. The adhesive is applied under slit-lamp or microscopic observation using a topical anesthetic (0.5% proparacaine hydrochloride). An eyelid speculum is useful. Before the adhesive is applied, any necrotic tissue and corneal epithelium should be removed from the involved area and a 2 mm surrounding zone. The area is then dried using a cellulose sponge, and a small drop of the fluid adhesive is applied. The glue polymerizes completely within minutes and usually adheres well to the de-epithelialized surface.

The glue does not polymerize on plastic, so a simple way to handle it is to spread a small amount on a surface such as the inside of the sterile plastic wrapping of any medical product cut to a size slightly larger than the perforation. It should then be applied to the surface of the cornea in as thin a layer as possible using the plastic handle of a cellulose sponge or the wooden stick of a cotton-tipped applicator. The adhesive plug has a rough surface and can be irritating, so a bandage contact lens is used to protect the upper tarsal conjunctiva and to prevent the plug from being dislodged by eyelid blinking.

Reconstructive Lamellar and Patch Grafts

See Chapter 23 for discussion and illustration of lamellar keratoplasty and penetrating keratoplasty.

Corneal Tattoo

Indications and Options

Corneal tattooing has been used for centuries to improve the cosmetic appearance of a blind eye with an unsightly leukoma. It has also been used occasionally in seeing eyes to reduce the glare from scars and to eliminate monocular diplopia in patients with large iridectomies or traumatic loss of iris. Congenital iris coloboma is another indication.

Modern technology allows the ophthalmologist to manage these conditions adequately with anterior segment reconstruction, tinted contact lenses, or thin scleral shells. However, corneal tattooing may still be a reasonable alternative in high-risk cases of leukoma or leukocoria where corneal transplantation would lead to rejection and graft failure or in eyes without visual potential. The most common complications of corneal tattooing are ocular discomfort, conjunctival injection, and mild keratitis. However, corneal ulceration, iridocyclitis, and even endophthalmitis have also been reported.

Surgical Technique

Both eyes are prepared in sterile fashion and draped so that the color of the normal iris can be used for comparison. Topical and retrobulbar or peribulbar anesthesia is administered, and the corneal epithelium is removed in the area to be tattooed. A paste is made by mixing sterile saline or water with dry powder pigments that have been sterilized with ethylene oxide. India ink is the most commonly used material. Other pigments available for mixing to match the iris of the normal eye include black (iron oxide), brown (iron oxide), white (titanium dioxide), and blue (titanium dioxide and phthalocyanine). Staining solutions must be sterilized before use.

The conventional method of corneal tattooing is similar to dermatographic methods. A trephine of 3–4 mm is centered on the central optical zone to mark the pupil, and multiple beveled stabs are made with a surgical blade to embed the pigments into the anterior stroma. Pigment can also be placed under a lamellar flap or into a lamellar dissection. In lamellar intrastromal keratography, the staining pigment is spread in a dissected pocket.

The color match is tested by first working in an area of the superior cornea that will be covered by the eyelid. The color is compared with that of the iris of the fellow eye and modified until satisfactory. Because the pigment can become embedded in conjunctival openings, care is taken not to break the conjunctival surface in exposed areas. Postoperatively, the eye is patched with antibiotic ointment and checked daily until the epithelial surface is intact, usually within 3–5 days.

Anastas CN, McGhee CN, Webber SK, et al. Corneal tattooing revisited: excimer laser in the treatment of unsightly leucomata. *Aust NZ J Ophthalmol.* 1995;23:227–230.

Reed JW. Corneal tattooing to reduce glare in cases of traumatic iris loss. *Cornea.* 1994;13:401–405.

PART XI

Corneal Transplantation

CHAPTER 22

Basic Concepts of Corneal Transplantation

Transplantation Immunobiology

Histocompatibility and Other Antigens

Antigens found within the host are known as *endogenous antigens.* The most important group of endogenous antigens is the *homologous antigens,* which are genetically controlled determinants specific to a given species. *Histocompatibility antigens,* homologous antigens found on the surfaces of most cells, are an expression of genetic material on human chromosome 6 in a region referred to as the *major histocompatibility complex (MHC).* In humans, the MHC is known as the *human leukocyte antigen (HLA) system.*

HLA antigens are found on the surface of all nucleated cells. They are determined by a series of four gene loci located on chromosome 6 known as *HLA-A, HLA B, HLA-C,* and *HLA-D.* Each zone controls several different antigenic specificities, over 95% of which can be recognized by serologic methods. The histocompatibility antigens are important clinically because they form the basis for graft rejection in organ transplantation and for sensitization to most antigens. It is possible that HLA antigens are genetic markers rather than actual transplantation antigens and that strong transplantation antigens are closely linked with the HLA markers on the genetic material.

Some grafts are rejected even when donor–recipient pairs are HLA compatible. Although minor histocompatibility antigens such as ABO and Lewis antigens are less potent than major histocompatibility antigens, they nonetheless add to the overall antigenicity of a graft. Little is known about the number of minor histocompatibility antigens or their importance in transplantation immunology.

Immune Privilege

The cornea was the first successfully transplanted solid tissue. After other tissues had also been transplanted, it was soon observed that corneas were rejected less frequently than other transplanted tissues. The concept emerged that the cornea was the site of "immunologic privilege" and that corneal grafts were somehow protected from immunologic destruction. It is now evident that corneal grafts are not different from other tissue grafts and that the so-called immunologic privilege accorded corneal grafts is simply the result of their relative isolation from recipient lymphatic channels. The fact that vascularized recipients reject corneal grafts more frequently than nonvascularized recipients supports this finding.

Tolerance to a corneal graft may also be a result of anterior chamber–associated immune deviation (ACAID) that involves the development of suppressor T cells. ACAID is a down-regulation of delayed-type cellular immunity. Antigens released into the aqueous humor are, presumably, recognized by dendritic cells of the iris and ciliary body. These antigen-presenting cells can then enter the venous circulation and induce regulatory T cells in the spleen, bypassing the lymphatic system.

For an immune response to occur, an antigenic substance is introduced and "recognized" *(afferent limb),* producing the synthesis of specific antibody molecules and the appearance of effector lymphocytes that react specifically with the immunizing antigen *(efferent limb).* Although antibodies to foreign tissues are formed during graft rejection, they are not believed to be important in the usual type of rejection of allografts. Rather, extensive evidence indicates that cellular immune mechanisms are associated with allograft rejection. The term *delayed hypersensitivity,* or *Type IV,* reaction is used to describe such T lymphocyte–mediated responses. Other mechanisms are also probably involved.

See also discussion of immune-mediated disorders in Part IV of this volume. BCSC Section 9, *Intraocular Inflammation and Uveitis,* discusses and illustrates the principles of immunology in greater detail.

Pepose, JS, Holland GN, Wilhelmus KR, eds. *Ocular Infection and Immunity.* St Louis: Mosby; 1996:435–445.

Eye Banking and Donor Selection

Before reliable storage or preservation methods were available, it was imperative that corneas be transplanted immediately from donor to recipient. The McCarey-Kaufman tissue transport medium developed in the early 1970s significantly reduced endothelial cell attrition, allowing corneal buttons to be safely transplanted after being stored for up to 4 days at 4° C. Improvements in storage media over the past 2 decades have extended the viable storage period to as long as 2 weeks, not only increasing the availability of donor corneas but also allowing penetrating keratoplasty to be performed on a less exigent basis. The most commonly used preservation medium in the United States is Optisol GS, which includes such components as 2.5% chondroitin sulfate, 1% dextran, ascorbic acid, vitamin B_{12}, adenosine triphosphate precursors, and the antibiotics gentamicin and streptomycin. Currently under investigation is the addition of insulin, epidermal growth factor, broader spectrum antibiotics, and other components to storage media. These changes may further improve endothelial cell viability and function and enhance sterility in the future.

Organ culture storage techniques are commonly practiced in Europe and have the potential to provide improved donor quality in the future. Organ culture offers a relatively long storage time, which permits optimal use of available donor corneas in areas where there is a relative shortage. An added benefit of organ culture is the delivery of a donor cornea with a sterility control of the medium prior to transplantation. Its disadvantages include increased complexity and cost as well as a thick, opaque cornea at the time of surgical transplantation.

Although previous smaller studies have shown benefit from HLA matching, a recent multicenter study of high-risk grafts found no reduction in the incidence of rejection with the use of HLA-matched or cross-matched tissue. The effect of ABO blood type matching remains uncertain.

Criteria Contraindicating Donor Cornea Use

The Eye Bank Association of America (EBAA) has developed extensive criteria for screening donor corneas prior to distribution to avoid transmissible infections and other conditions. Contraindications include

- Death of unknown cause
- Unknown central nervous system disease or certain infectious diseases of the central nervous system (eg, Creutzfeldt-Jakob disease, subacute sclerosing panencephalitis, progressive multifocal leukoencephalopathy, congenital rubella, Reye syndrome, rabies, active viral encephalitis, encephalitis of unknown origin, or progressive encephalopathy)
- Active septicemia (bacteremia, fungemia, viremia)
- Social, clinical, or laboratory evidence suggestive of HIV infection, syphilis, or active viral hepatitis
- Leukemias or active disseminated lymphomas
- Active bacterial or fungal endocarditis
- Active ocular or intraocular inflammation such as iritis, scleritis, conjunctivitis, vitritis, retinitis, choroiditis
- Intrinsic malignancies: malignant anterior segment tumors, adenocarcinoma in the eye of primary or metastatic origin, and retinoblastoma (eyes with posterior choroidal melanoma may be considered acceptable, but most medical eye bank directors decline their usage)
- Congenital or acquired eye disorders that would preclude successful surgical outcome: any central donor corneal scar or pterygia involving the central 8 mm clear zone (optical area of the donor button), keratoconus, keratoglobus, or Fuchs dystrophy
- Prior refractive corneal surgery: RK, PRK, LASIK, lamellar inserts, etc
- Corneas from patients with prior intraocular surgery (cataract, IOL implants, glaucoma filtration) may be accepted if endothelial adequacy is documented by specular microscopy and meets the local eye bank's prescribed standards; laser surgical procedures such as ALT or retinal photocoagulation may be used if cleared by the eye bank's medical director
- Hepatitis B surface antigen–positive donors, hepatitis C seropositive donors, HIV seropositive donors, HIV or high risk for HIV meeting any of the EBAA's behavioral or history exclusionary criteria (eg, inmates, drug users, homosexuality, or guidelines as prescribed by the CDC)

Diseases known or suspected to be transmitted by corneal transplantation are listed in Table 22-1.

Table 22-1 Disease Transmission From Donor Corneas

Proven transmission by corneal transplantation
Rabies
Hepatitis B
Creutzfeldt-Jakob disease (previously disgnosed)
Retinoblastoma
Bacterial or fungal keratitis
Bacterial or fungal endophthalmitis
Corneal dystrophy (eg, Fuchs endothelial dystrophy)

Possible transmission by corneal transplantation
Human immunodeficiency virus (HIV)
Herpes simplex virus (HSV)
Prion diseases

Other diseases that exclude corneal donors
Hepatitis C, HTLV-I or -II infection, ocular adenocarcinoma, malignant tumors of the anterior
segment, Reye syndrome, subacute sclerosing panencephalitis, progressive multifocal
leukoencephalopathy, leukemias, active disseminated lymphomas, active infectious
endocarditis, active septicemias

Even with these standards, the ultimate responsibility for accepting donor tissue rests with the surgeon. Other factors to be considered include the following:

- Slit-lamp appearance of donor tissue
- Specular microscopic data (generally, endothelial cell counts <2000 cells/mm^2 are not used)
- Death-to-preservation time (optimal range <12–18 hours)
- Tissue storage time prior to keratoplasty
- Donor age

Most surgeons do not use corneas from donors younger than 6–24 months, as these corneas are extremely flaccid and can result in high corneal astigmatism and myopia postoperatively. Most eye banks establish a lower age limit of 24 months and an upper age limit of 70 years, as older corneas tend to have lower endothelial cell counts. The acceptable age of donors who provide tissue for transplantation is up to the individual surgeon, and older age limits for tissue usage are under investigation.

CHAPTER 23

Clinical Approach to Corneal Transplantation

Penetrating Keratoplasty

The term *penetrating keratoplasty (PK)* commonly refers to surgical replacement of a portion of the host cornea with that of a donor eye. If the donor is another person, the procedure is called an *allograft*; use of donor tissue from the same or fellow eye is called an *autograft* (see Corneal Autograft Procedures later in this chapter). Advances in microsurgery, suture materials, storage media, and postoperative medical management have allowed corneal transplant surgery to progress from the novelty it was in the mid-twentieth century to an accepted procedure performed approximately 45,000 times annually in the United States alone.

Indications

Indications for penetrating keratoplasty have expanded considerably in recent years (Table 23-1). Today the most common indication for PK is decreased visual acuity secondary to corneal opacity. Other objectives include correction of abnormal corneal contour, treatment of corneal thinning or perforation, relief of pain, removal of infectious or neoplastic foci, or cosmesis. Even though some ophthalmologists do not perform PK, all should be familiar with its postoperative complications because patients do not always return to their surgeons when problems arise, and many of these problems require immediate intervention to save the graft.

Table 23-1 Indications for Penetrating Keratoplasty (in Approximate Order of Prevalence)

Pseudophakic or aphakic corneal edema
Fuchs endothelial dystrophy
Keratoconus
Failed previous corneal transplant
Stromal corneal dystrophies
Corneal opacification following infection (viral keratitis, microbial keratitis, syphilitic keratopathy)
Immune-mediated corneal diseases and perforation
Corneal degenerations
Mechanical and chemical trauma
Congenital opacity

Preferred Practice Patterns, Cornea Panel. *Corneal Opacification and Ectasia.* San Francisco: American Academy of Ophthalmology; 2000.

Soong HK. Penetrating keratoplasty. In: *Focal Points: Clinical Modules for Ophthalmologists.* San Francisco: American Academy of Ophthalmology; 1992: vol 10, no 6.

Preoperative Evaluation and Preparation

A complete eye examination is necessary prior to keratoplasty, and a detailed social history helps predict whether the patient will be compliant with the postoperative regimen and report quickly if problems arise. Simple clinical tests, such as those for color recognition or an afferent pupillary defect, can be enormously important in the evaluation of patients with media opacity. Ocular surface problems such as dry eye, trichiasis, exposure, blepharitis, and rosacea must be recognized and treated prior to PK.

The preoperative evaluation addresses any neurologic or intraocular factors that could compromise the final visual result, such as other media opacity, uncontrolled glaucoma, amblyopia, macular abnormalities, retinal disease, or optic nerve damage. Preexisting glaucoma or ocular inflammation must be controlled before PK is considered. Active keratitis or uveitis is treated medically if possible, and the eye should ideally remain quiet for several months before PK. An inflamed eye at the time of surgery is associated with a higher incidence of postoperative complications, such as graft rejection and failure, glaucoma, and cystoid macular edema. For example, corneal perforations in an acutely inflamed eye should, if possible, be closed either with cyanoacrylate tissue adhesive or by means of a lamellar corneal graft in order to restore the integrity of the globe and allow the eye to become quiet. A vision-restoring penetrating keratoplasty may then be undertaken at a later date. A lamellar graft should at least be considered in any case with normal endothelium.

Fluorescein angiography can be helpful in detecting retinal problems such as cystoid macular edema and age-related macular degeneration through less-than-ideal media. If the media are completely opaque, ultrasonography will reveal some problems that affect the visual prognosis after PK. The potential visual acuity meter, laser interferometer, blue-field entoptic phenomenon testing, visual fields, and visually evoked cortical potentials may also help in preoperative assessment of the afferent system.

In general, deep corneal vascularization, ocular surface disease, active anterior segment inflammation, peripheral corneal thinning, previous graft failures, and increased IOP worsen the prognosis for PK and thus influence the appropriateness of this procedure for the affected patient.

Surgical Technique

Preparation of the donor cornea

Donor tissue is commonly prepared for trephination by centering the previously excised corneoscleral donor tissue, endothelial side up, in the concave well of a cutting block apparatus that approximates the cornea's shape. Various methods attempt to avoid slippage of the moist donor cornea at the time of cutting, as this can create edge angulation or button ovaling and lead to significant astigmatism. Sharp disposable blades are vertically advanced along a guiding shaft to punch the button in a precise, crisp, guillotine fashion. Less commonly, the donor button is excised from the epithelial side utilizing an artificial anterior chamber system (Hanna, Krumeich, or Lieberman). Although many systems are available, each has subtle advantages and disadvantages relative to experience, cost, convenience, availability, and clinical scenario. The main goal is to obtain a central donor button with uniform, vertical edges avoiding tissue distortion or endothelial damage. The remaining donor corneoscleral rim and some of the preservative medium fluid may then be submitted for culture.

Most surgeons size the donor button 0.25–0.50 mm larger than the diameter of the host corneal opening (eg, an 8.0 mm diameter corneal button into a 7.5 mm wound). This size disparity may reduce postoperative glaucoma, enhance watertight wound closure, prevent peripheral anterior synechiae formation and excessive postoperative corneal flattening, and provide the recipient eye with more endothelial cells. In keratoconus, especially in eyes with high axial length, sizing the donor tissue to match the exact size of the wound may flatten the corneal contour and thereby reduce postoperative myopia. When the graft-to-host size disparity is lessened, postoperative wound dehiscence may be more common. The use of same-size grafts can make watertight wound closure more difficult.

Preparation of the recipient eye

For safety purposes, it is recommended that all donor preparations be completed before trephination of the recipient eye. In some instances, additional scleral support may be needed, especially in aphakic or pseudophakic eyes that have undergone vitrectomy and in pediatric corneal transplants. This support is commonly obtained by suturing a Flieringa ring to the episclera. By structurally bracing the anterior globe after excision of the recipient button, the ring reduces scleral infolding, distortion of the wound opening, and forward bulging of the iris, lens, and/or vitreous. A combination scleral support ring with eyelid speculum (McNeil-Goldmann blepharostat) is available. The ring itself, however, can distort the corneal or scleral shape, leading to irregular trephination; and limbal-suction trephine systems preclude their use. As a result, many keratoplasties are now successfully performed without scleral support. Therefore, if a ring is utilized, a meticulous and evenly spaced suturing technique using equal and light tensioning should be employed with the same care given to suturing the graft. In cases of trauma, positive vitreous pressure, inflammation, or scleral flaccidity in which a ring was not used, a speculum that gently and controllably elevates the eyelids away from the globe surface (eg, Schott or Geuder), independent of the lid-spreading function, can be particularly advantageous. Ultimately, the surgeon's goal is to achieve a round bed with uniform, vertical edges and accurate and reproducible centration.

Available trephines can be classified into descriptive categories: Traditional circular cutting trephines (hand-held, motorized, suction-fixation, and special purpose type); single-point cutting trephines (Lieberman cam-guided corneal cutter); combination trephines (Hanna System and the Guided Trephine System by Krumeich); and noncontact trephines (lasers).

The more widely used methods include the traditional hand-held trephine, which offers convenience, low cost, sharp disposable blades, and simplicity of design. Hand fixation and rotation, however, may lead to tilting and irregularity of cut as well as unanticipated anterior chamber entry. The Barron corneal vacuum trephine system offers improved accuracy and consistency of cut, depth control, disposability, suture placement marking points, and relatively low cost. Its disadvantages include outward beveling of the posterior corneal edges in deep trephination, slightly reduced observation, and more complexity than a traditional trephine. The Hanna limbal fixation trephine system offers the advantage of less recipient edge undercutting, and precision of depth of cut. Its disadvantages include cost, complexity, and reduced visualization.

After trephination, the donor corneal button is placed onto the recipient's eye, endothelial side down. Use of viscoelastic material helps protect the donor endothelium during surgical manipulation, keeps the anterior chamber formed, and shields the iris while the donor button is being sutured into the wound.

Initial graft placement and suturing techniques

The donor button is secured with at least four interrupted cardinal sutures. The second cardinal suture is the most important because a mistake at this stage in anchoring the button 180° away from the first suture has the greatest mathematical potential, in principle, for misalignment error and subsequent astigmatism. Complete wound closure is achieved with either interrupted sutures, one or two continuous sutures, or a combination (see below). Although intraoperative keratoscopy may help control corneal astigmatism, astigmatism management falls primarily within the scope of postoperative care, which is discussed below.

The suture knots may be positioned in either donor or host tissue and are buried in the corneal stroma, not left in the wound interface. Knots buried on the recipient side tend to not destabilize the graft upon removal, but they may be relatively more exposed to limbal immune surveillance. Most corneal surgeons prefer deep partial-thickness corneal suture bites over full-thickness bites. By attempting to incorporate 95% of the donor's and host's relative corneal thickness, the adjoining position of Descemet's membranes may be aligned. Full-thickness bites may be associated with a higher chance of leakage along suture tracks and serve as a portal of entry for microorganisms or epithelial ingrowth. The advantages of deep suture placement with either technique are decreased posterior wound gape and enhanced wound stabilization and healing. Following suture placement, the wound is tested for aqueous leakage using either a methylcellulose spear to blot the wound or a Seidel test with fluorescein paper strips.

Interrupted sutures (Fig 23-1). Vascularized, inflamed, or thinned corneas tend to heal unevenly and unpredictably. Interrupted sutures, usually 16–24 in number, are the technique of choice in such corneas as well as in pediatric keratoplasties, where wound healing is rapid. The tension of each interrupted suture acts as an independent vector generating central steepening and local flattening. Sutures may be removed selectively in the presence of sufficient donor–recipient interface healing if they attract blood vessels or if they loosen because of wound contraction. Astigmatism may be reduced postoperatively by selective removal of sutures in the steep corneal meridian, although too-early removal risks wound dehiscence or slippage.

Continuous sutures In the absence of vascularization, focal inflammation, or thinning, single or double continuous sutures can be used to secure the PK (Figs 23-2, 23-3). If properly placed, continuous sutures may allow more even distribution of tension and healing around the wound. Suture passes may be placed radially to the donor–recipient wound or be introduced torque-free.

Of these two approaches, the single continuous technique with radial placement is technically easier to perform because the surgeon can align the passes with marks on the host. The potential disadvantage is that when tensioning is performed, a torque is imparted to the graft–host interface. In contrast, anti-torque sutures are typically placed at

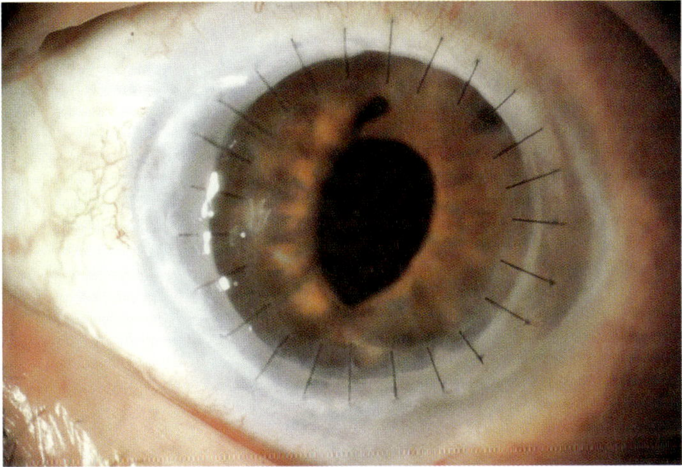

Figure 23-1 PK for syphilitic interstial keratopathy, with 24 interrupted 10-0 nylon sutures in place.

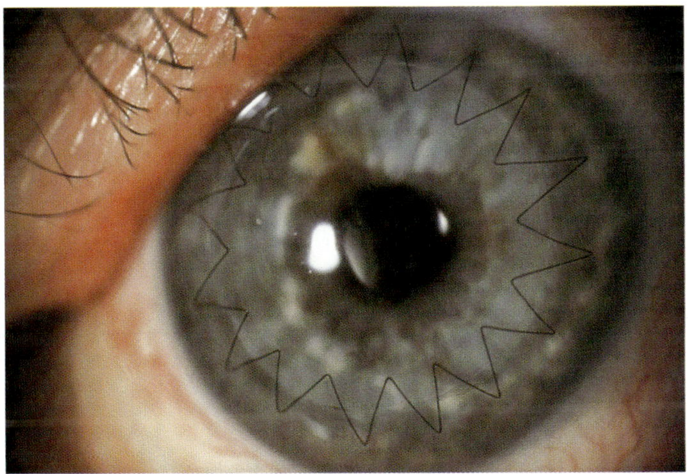

Figure 23-2 PK for pseudophakic corneal edema, with a single continuous 10-0 nylon suture in place.

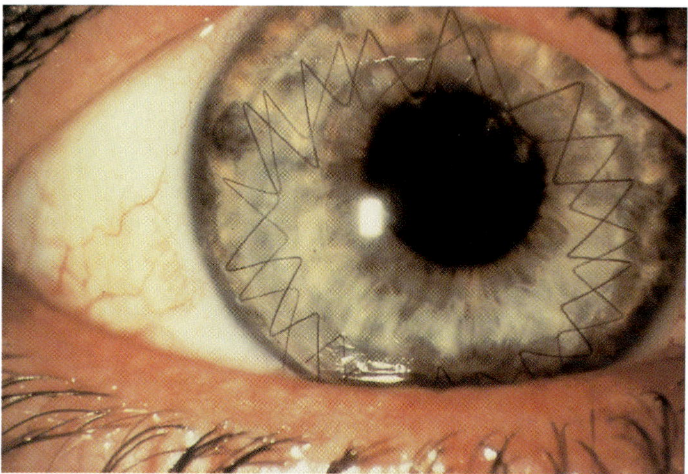

Figure 23-3 Double continuous suturing technique employs 10-0 nylon and 11-0 nylon running sutures in a patient with keratoconus.

an angle of 30°–45° to the donor–recipient interface in the direction of suture advancement. They create a series of isosceles triangles that theoretically negate torsional rotation of the graft.

Additional advantages of running sutures include their ease of removal postoperatively. Disadvantages include sectorial loosening or cheese wiring, which may compromise the entire closure. Further, interrupted suture closure may be more rapid than running suture closure when cardinal sutures are maintained or the patient is restless. Most surgeons feel, however, that less time is needed for continuous suturing than for interrupted sutures. Some surgeons employ double continuous sutures to give an added measure of wound protection should one running suture break or loosen. Moreover, the second running suture can be placed in a manner that counteracts the torque induced by the first.

The tension on a single, continuous suture is generally adjusted intraoperatively using a simple ring device or intraoperative keratoscope. Postoperatively, the suture may be adjusted at the slit lamp to reduce astigmatism by using a Tennant tying forceps after the installation of a topical antibiotic and anesthetic. Typically, the epithelium has healed over the suture loops and must be broken under each loop to allow adjustment. A small diameter spatula is gently swept under each loop; adjustment is limited by the position of the knot, which needs to remain internalized.

Combined sutures The combined interrupted and continuous suture technique offers several of the advantages of both methods (Fig 23-4). The interrupted sutures may be removed as early as 1 week after PK in order to reduce corneal astigmatism, while the continuous suture remains to protect against wound dehiscence. There is no consensus as to whether the combined technique or the running techniques are less astigmatic. Many variables contribute to astigmatism, but the key suturing principle is uniform

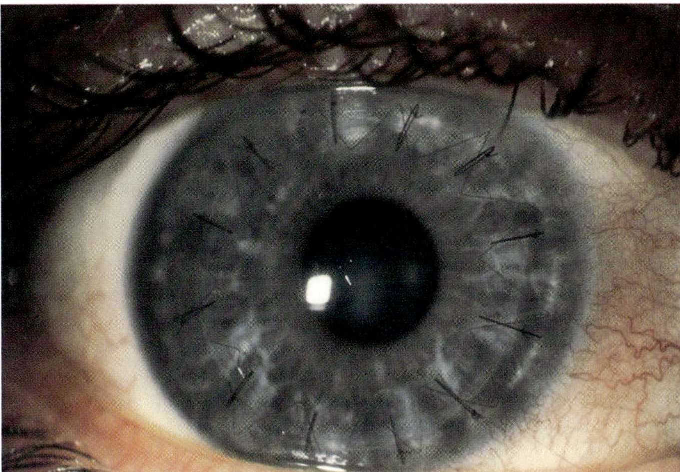

Figure 23-4 Combined suturing technique employs both interrupted 10-0 nylon and continuous 11-0 nylon sutures in a patient with Fuchs endothelial dystrophy.

placement to minimize uneven suture tension, tissue torque, and distortion, thereby achieving secure closure without override or posterior wound gape.

Combined Procedures

PK may be combined with other procedures such as cataract extraction, primary or secondary IOL implantation, IOL removal or exchange, glaucoma surgery, vitrectomy, and retinal procedures. A temporary intraoperative keratoprosthesis may or may not be used with these procedures. Synechialysis can be performed with caution, avoiding excessive bleeding, tearing, or tissue and inflammatory exudation. Iris defects may be repaired with 10-0 Prolene sutures to achieve pupil constriction, eliminate monocular diplopia, improve spectacle acuity, reduce glare, and minimize chances of iridocorneal adhesion. In eyes at risk for postoperative uveitis (eg, those with herpes simplex or interstitial keratitis), a peripheral iridectomy may reduce the chance of postoperative pupillary-block glaucoma.

Intraoperative Complications

Complications that can occur during PK include the following:

- Damage to the lens and/or iris from the trephine, scissors, or other instruments
- Irregular trephination
- Inadequate vitrectomy resulting in vitreous contact with graft endothelium
- Poor graft centration on the host bed
- Excessive bleeding from the iris and wound edge (in vascularized host corneas)
- Choroidal hemorrhage and effusion
- Iris incarceration in the wound
- Damage to the donor epithelium during trephination and handling

In aphakic eyes with large pupils or sector iris defects, the graft may drop back into the vitreous prior to suture fixation, especially if vitrectomy has previously been performed on the eye.

In severely edematous corneas, recipient Descemet's membrane may be inadvertently left behind after corneal excision, as it is easily stripped completely from the stroma. The recipient eye must be carefully examined for retained Descemet's membrane; otherwise, donor endothelium resting against host Descemet's membrane may severely compromise the graft.

Postoperative Care and Complications

The postoperative care of a corneal transplant is far more complex than that following cataract surgery. The long-term success of a PK is probably more dependent on the quality of the postoperative care than on the expertise of the operative technique. Routine postsurgical care—use of topical antibiotics and tapering topical steroids and frequent office visits—is directed at prevention and early recognition of the myriad complications that can occur after PK. This section covers some of the more common postsurgical complications. Astigmatism and graft rejection are discussed separately.

Wound leak

The wound is always checked carefully for leakage at the end of surgery. Small wound leaks that do not cause anterior chamber shallowing frequently close spontaneously. Patching, therapeutic contact lenses, and use of inhibitors of aqueous production may hasten wound closure. Resuturing is advised for leaks lasting longer than 3 days.

Flat chamber/iris incarceration in the wound

Both of these problems imply either poor wound integrity or excessive posterior pressure, and early surgical intervention is advised.

Glaucoma

High IOP may occur at any time after PK. Often, the first clinical sign is the loss of folds in Descemet's membrane, usually seen in the early postoperative period. Glaucoma should be treated aggressively with medical, laser, or surgical intervention as indicated. Unusual causes include epithelial downgrowth or fibrous ingrowth. (See BCSC Section 10, *Glaucoma.*)

Endophthalmitis

After PK, endophthalmitis may arise from intraoperative contamination, donor button contamination, or postoperative invasion by organisms. Extremely aggressive intervention can save the eye in some cases. (See BCSC Section 9, *Intraocular Inflammation and Uveitis.*)

Primary endothelial failure

When the graft is edematous from the first postoperative day and remains so without inflammatory signs, a deficiency of donor endothelium is presumed (Fig 23-5). Most surgeons allow several weeks for spontaneous resolution of edema and then consider a regraft.

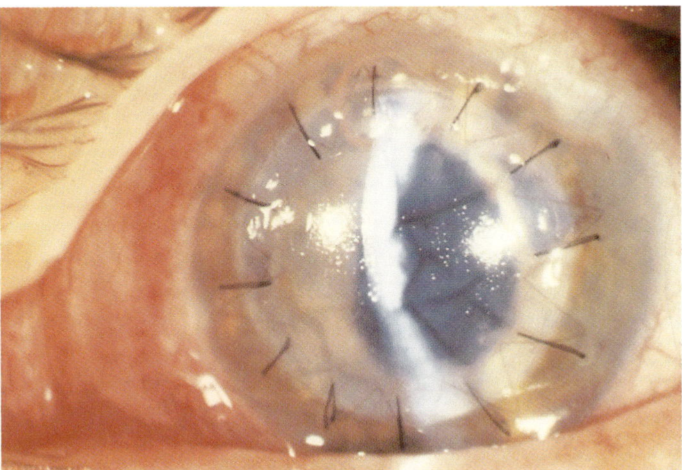

Figure 23-5 Primary endothelial failure after PK.

Persistent epithelial defect

Large epithelial defects are common after PK, but they should heal within 14–21 days. After this time, irreversible scarring and ulceration may occur. Ocular surface disease (such as dry eye, exposure, rosacea, blepharitis, or trichiasis) should be ruled out or treated. Lubrication, patching, therapeutic contact lenses, and tarsorrhaphy may be helpful in difficult cases.

Recurrence of primary disease

Bacterial, fungal, viral, and amebic keratitis, as well as stromal dystrophies, can recur in a graft (Fig 23-6). Treatment is directed at the causative agent in recurrent infections; regraft may be required for recurrent dystrophy.

Suture-related problems

Postoperative problems related to sutures include the following:

- Excessive tightness
- Loosening (usually as a result of wound contraction, suture breakage, or suture cheese wiring)
- Infectious abscesses (usually localized around loose, broken, or exposed sutures; see Figs 23-7 and 23-8)
- Noninfectious (toxic) suture infiltrates (Fig 23-9)
- Giant papillary conjunctivitis from exposed knots
- Vascularization along suture tracks

Loose and broken sutures do not contribute to wound stability and, therefore, are removed as soon as possible. Totally buried interrupted suture fragments may be left. Vascularization along the suture indicates that the wound is adequately healed in the vicinity and that sutures may be removed safely. Vascularized sutures are prone to loosen and may increase the chance of graft rejection.

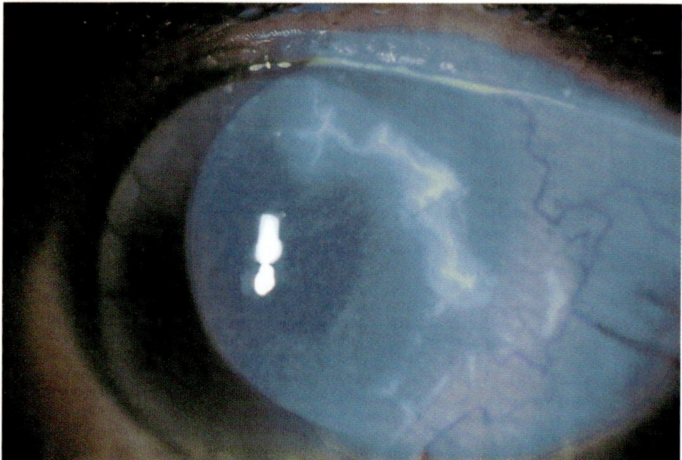

Figure 23-6 Herpes simplex virus keratitis recurring in a graft.

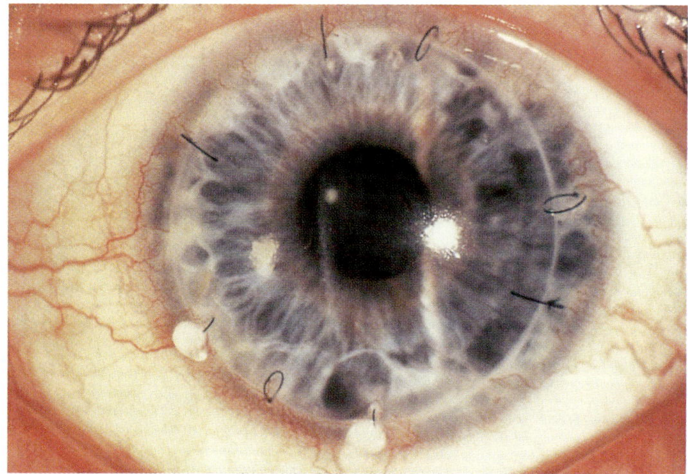

Figure 23-7 Broken and exposed sutures after PK. They should be removed immediately because of the risk of infection and rejection.

Microbial keratitis

The use of topical steroids, the presence of epithelial defects or edema, and exposed sutures predispose the PK patient to infectious keratitis, sometimes with unusual organisms. Decreased corneal sensation and topical steroid use may also delay presentation. Lesions must be scraped immediately for diagnosis, and broad-spectrum antibiotic therapy initiated, in order to preserve the graft. A peculiar form of keratitis, *infectious crystalline keratopathy*, is seen in grafts and other immunocompromised corneas (Fig 23-10). Branching colonies of organisms proliferate in the deep corneal stroma with no visible inflammatory response. Many organisms have been implicated, but streptococci are seen most frequently.

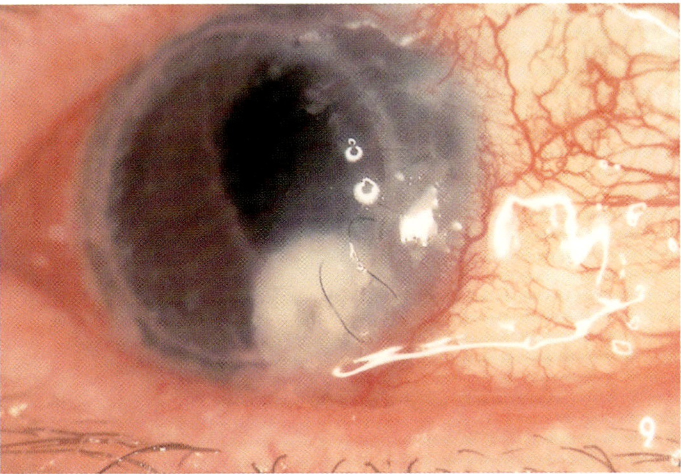

Figure 23-8 Suture abscess caused by *S pneumoniae,* 2 years after PK.

Late nonimmune endothelial failure

When a graft becomes edematous after months to years without inflammatory signs, two causes are possible. First, the tissue might have originally possessed a marginal number of endothelial cells, and the normal spreading of these cells has resulted in inability to maintain graft clarity. Alternatively, significant loss of endothelial cells might have occurred later in the postoperative period; possible causes include successfully treated rejection episodes, retention of an intraocular lens that causes endothelial damage, or persistent "ramping" loss along adhesional areas of peripheral anterior synechiae.

Control of Postoperative Corneal Astigmatism

A corneal transplant was once considered successful merely if the graft remained clear. Only later in the refinement of surgical procedures was the vexing and relatively common problem of high corneal astigmatism after surgery seriously addressed. Severe astigmatism may be associated with decreased visual acuity, anisometropia, aniseikonia, image distortion, and monocular diplopia, thus rendering an otherwise successful operation ineffective.

Astigmatism is the most frequent complication of PK. It may result in anisometropic asthenopic symptoms or in the inability to wear contact lenses. Many methods have been used to reduce the occurrence:

- Varying suture techniques
- Making intraoperative and postoperative adjustments
- Improving trephines to better match donor and host
- Matching donor 12 o'clock position to host 12 o'clock position
- Using computerized videokeratography for postoperative management

Use of *relaxing incisions* is the principal measure taken to reduce astigmatism. Incisions are placed inside the graft–host junction at the steep (plus cylinder) meridian in

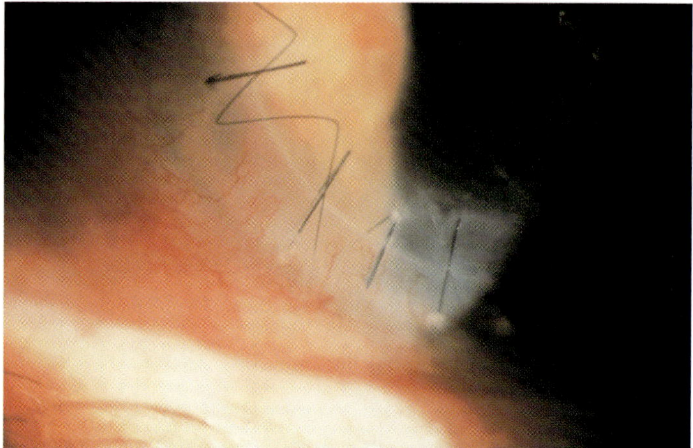

Figure 23-9 Deep, noninfectious toxic suture infiltrates after PK.

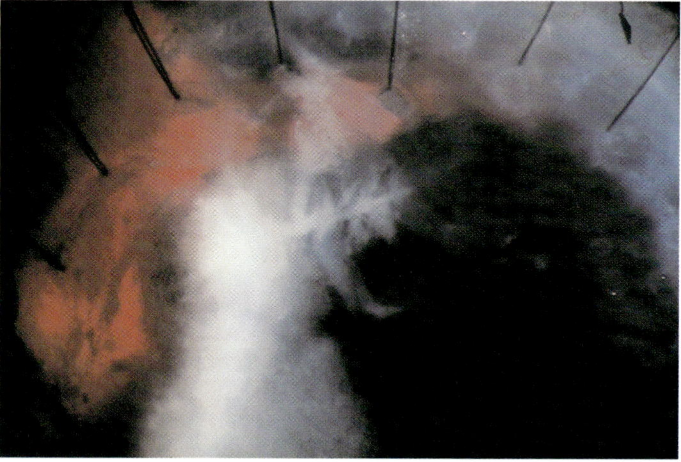

Figure 23-10 Infectious crystalline keratopathy after PK.

an arcuate manner for maximum effect. Incision placement in the wound is complicated by varying thickness and the possibility of perforation, and placement in the host is less predictable because the ring scar at the wound interferes with normal deflection of the cornea. The proper axis and length of incision are chosen based on evaluation of the peripheral cornea with Placido disk image or videokeratography. Similarly, LASIK and photorefractive astigmatic keratectomy techniques are being investigated. Flap timing and treatment algorithms are controversial.

Overcorrections can be treated by opening the wound, removing the epithelial plug, and resuturing. *Compression sutures* placed across the graft–host junction can be added in the opposite meridian from the relaxing incisions to increase the incisional wound gape and enhance the effect. The surgical goal is a moderate early overcorrection. Permanent sutures of 10-0 nylon or Mersilene are placed with a slipknot and adjusted to give the desired effect prior to burying the knots. Compression sutures can be removed to titrate the effect.

Wedge resection in the flat meridian is reserved for high degrees of astigmatism (>8 D) associated with marked flattening (<35 D) and hyperopic spherical equivalent. Wedge resection effectively shortens the radius of curvature in its axis, adding power to the cornea (Fig 23-11). The length (70°–90° of arc) and width (maximum of 1.5 mm) of resection determine the final results, but the operation is more complex and less predictable than use of relaxing incisions.

All of these procedures are associated with potential for micro- or macroperforation, infection, rejection, under- and overcorrections, chronic epithelial defects, and worsening of irregular astigmatism.

Krachmer JH, Mannis MJ, Holland EJ, eds. *Cornea.* St Louis: Mosby; 1997: vol 3, chap 137.

Tasman W, Jaeger EA, eds. *Duane's Clinical Ophthalmology.* Philadelphia: Lippincott; 1994: vol 6, chap 26.

Diagnosis and Management of Graft Rejection

Corneal allograft rejection rarely occurs within 2 weeks, and it may occur as late as 20 years after PK. Fortunately, most episodes of graft rejection do not cause irreversible graft failure if recognized early and treated aggressively with corticosteroids. Early recognition

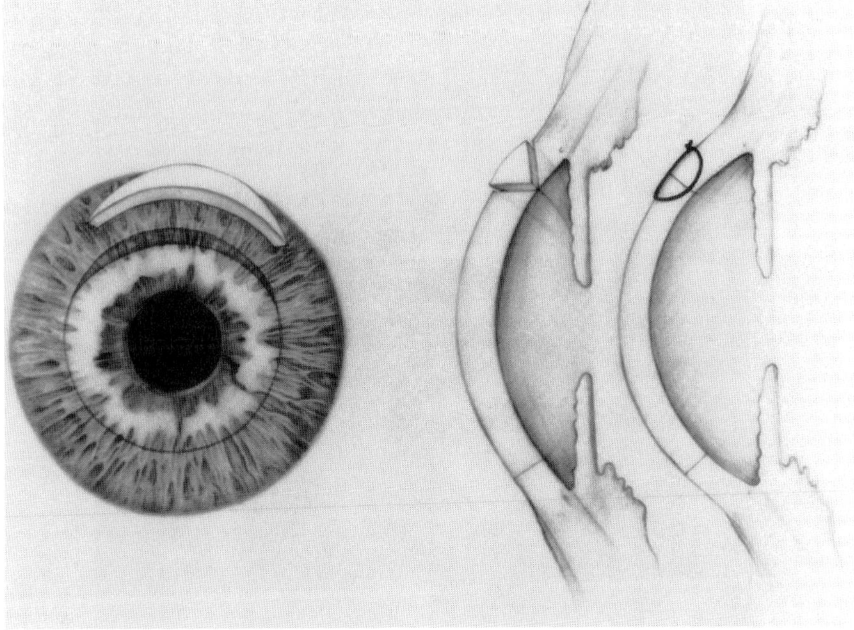

Figure 23-11 Wedge resection. A crescentic wedge of corneal tissue is removed from the flat corneal meridian to reduce postoperative astigmatism. *(Reproduced by permission from Schwab IR, ed. Refractive Keratoplasty. New York: Churchill Livingstone; 1987.)*

is the key to survival of an affected corneal graft. Corneal transplant rejection takes three clinical forms, which may occur either singly or in combination.

Epithelial rejection

The immune response may be directed entirely at the donor epithelium (Fig 23-12). Lymphocytes cause an elevated, linear epithelial ridge that advances centripetally. Because host cells replace lost donor epithelium, this form of rejection is problematic only in that it may herald the onset of endothelial rejection. Epithelial rejection has been reported at a rate of 10% of those patients experiencing rejection, and it is usually seen early in the postoperative period (1–13 months).

Subepithelial rejection

Corneal transplant rejection may also take the form of subepithelial infiltrates (Fig 23-13). When seen alone, they may cause no symptoms. It is not known whether these lymphocytic cells are directed at donor keratocytes or at donor epithelial cells. A cellular anterior chamber reaction may also accompany this form of rejection. Easily missed on cursory examination, subepithelial infiltrates can best be seen with broad, tangential light. They resemble infiltrates of adenoviral keratitis. Subepithelial graft rejection leaves no sequelae if treated, but it may presage the more severe endothelial graft rejection.

Isolated stromal rejection is not common but can be seen as stromal infiltrates and neovascularization. In very aggressive severe or prolonged bouts of graft rejection, the stroma can become necrotic.

Endothelial rejection

The most common form of graft rejection is endothelial rejection, with reported rates of 8%–37%. It is also the most serious form of corneal transplant rejection because endothelial cells destroyed by the host response can be replaced only by a regraft. Inflammatory precipitates are seen on the endothelial surface in fine precipitates, in random clumps, or in linear form (Khodadoust line, Fig 23-14). Inflammatory cells are usually

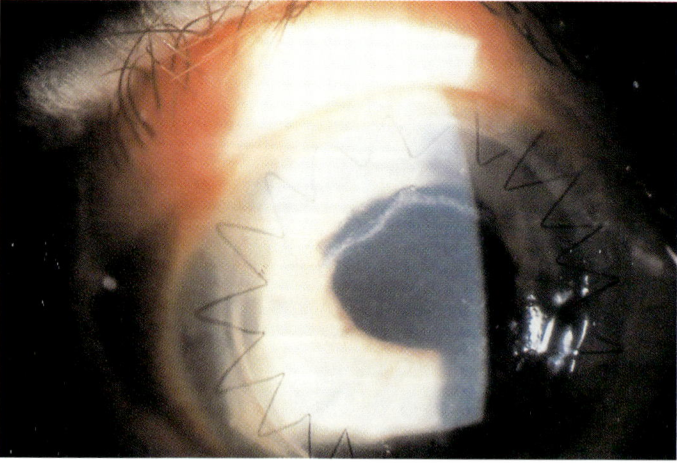

Figure 23-12 An epithelial rejection line after PK.

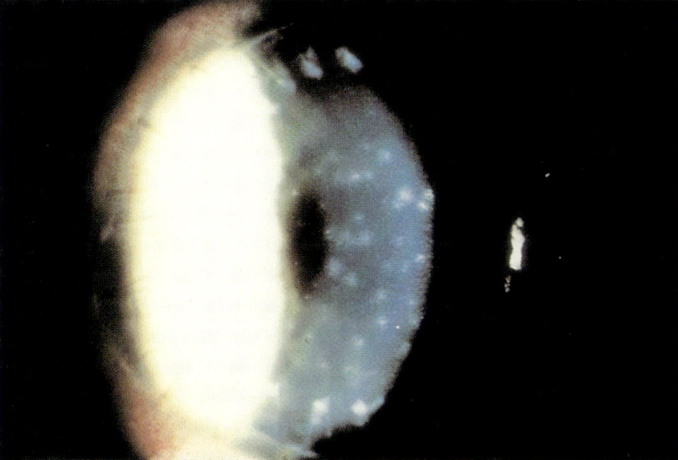

Figure 23-13 Corneal graft rejection manifested by subepithelial infiltrates.

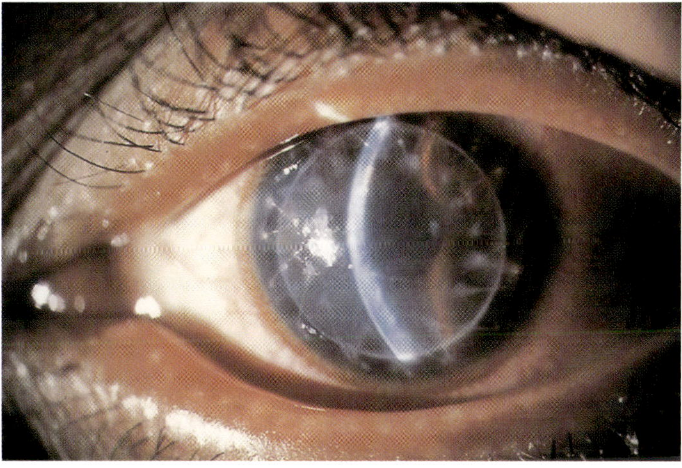

Figure 23-14 Endothelial graft rejection with stromal and epithelial edema on the trailing aspect of the migrating Khodadoust line.

seen in the anterior chamber as well. As endothelial function is lost, the corneal stroma thickens and the epithelium becomes edematous. Patients have symptoms related to inflammation and corneal edema such as photophobia, redness, irritation, haloes around lights, and fogginess of vision.

Treatment

Frequent administration of corticosteroid eyedrops is the mainstay of therapy for corneal allograft rejection. Either dexamethasone 0.1% or prednisolone 1.0% eyedrops are used as often as every 15 minutes to 2 hours, depending on the severity of the episode. Although topical corticosteroid ointments may be used on occasion, their bioavailability is not as beneficial as frequently applied eyedrops.

Corticosteroids may be given by periocular injection for severe rejection episodes or noncompliant patients. In particularly fulminant cases, systemic corticosteroids may be administered either orally or intravenously (80–120 mg methylprednisolone as a one-time dose). Oral or topical cyclosporine (2%) has been used prophylactically in high-risk grafts and may help reverse an ongoing graft-rejection episode.

Brightbill FS, ed. *Corneal Surgery: Theory, Technique, and Tissue.* 3rd ed. St Louis: Mosby; 1999.

The Collaborative Corneal Transplantation Studies Research Group. Effectiveness of histocompatibility matching in high-risk corneal transplantation. *Arch Ophthalmol.* 1992; 110:1392–1403.

Pediatric Corneal Transplants

Corneal transplantation in infants and children presents special problems. Development of amblyopia and the presence of concomitant ocular abnormalities often result in poor vision despite a technically successful graft. Nonetheless, improvements in pediatric anesthesia and the recognition that development of amblyopia following congenital and childhood diseases of the anterior segment is a major impediment to useful vision have led to PK being performed in neonates as early as 2 weeks after birth. Although there is no established scientific data, anesthesiologists believe that general anesthesia poses fewer risks after the first month of life. Increased understanding of the special problems associated with pediatric grafts and advances in surgical methods have improved the outlook for corneal transplants and have permitted earlier and more frequent surgical intervention. The best chance for a successful outcome in these cases comes with comanagement by the corneal specialist and the pediatric ophthalmologist.

Corneal grafting in children under the age of 2 is associated with rapid neovascularization, especially along the sutures. As the wound heals, erosions may occur along the sutures, leading to eye rubbing, epithelial defects, vascularization, and mucus accumulation. Suture erosion has been reported to occur as early as 2 weeks postoperatively in infants, which necessitates suture removal.

In general, suture removal is best performed in the operating room for pediatric cases. See Table 23-2 for guidelines for the timing of suture removal. In addition, it must

Table 23-2 Guidelines for Suture Removal in Pediatric Corneal Transplants

Age of Child	Timing of Suture Removal
6–9 months	Approximately 5 weeks postoperatively
12–24 months	6–8 weeks postoperatively
2–3 years	8–12 weeks postoperatively
4–6 years	4 months postoperatively
10 years until teens	6 months postoperatively
Teenage	Approximately 9 months postoperatively

be stressed that until all sutures are removed in infants or young children, frequent examinations are required.

Additional considerations in pediatric keratoplasty include measures to prevent globe collapse intraoperatively, as the eye wall is extremely flaccid at this age and collapses when the cornea is excised. Other common problems include anterior bulging of the lens–iris diaphragm (sometimes resulting in spontaneous delivery of the lens) and the propensity to develop large zones of iridocorneal adhesions. One measure to counteract this problem intraoperatively is the Cobo irrigating keratoprosthesis, which seals the recipient opening while simultaneously permitting infusion of BSS. This is particularly important in infants and young children because systemic hyperosmotic agents such as mannitol may cause hemodynamic instability related to fluid shifts and should therefore be used with caution.

Additional measures include a scleral ring, which many surgeons feel is crucial in pediatric grafts, particularly in neonates. Preoperative measures to reduce intravitreal pressure, including massage or ocular compression devices, should also be encouraged. Retrobulbar anesthesia, whether given supplementally or preoperatively, should generally be avoided because of the smaller orbital volume. Using a small-sized corneal opening may reduce the degree of anterior lens–iris bulge and the chance of peripheral synechiae formation. Preplaced mattress sutures in the recipient tissue can be brought up rapidly over the donor tissue and secured, allowing for quicker re-formation of the anterior chamber and placement of definitive 10-0 nylon sutures.

Early fitting with a contact lens (as early as the time of PK) and ocular occlusive therapy are necessary to stem the development of amblyopia in children with monocular aphakia.

Postoperative glaucoma, strabismus, self-induced trauma, and immune rejection are extremely common. The decision to perform penetrating keratoplasty in children must always involve the family. The surgeon must reserve additional time to discuss with the family many difficult issues including risks, prognosis, high costs, loss of time from work with associated loss of income, the extensive ongoing care required by the child, disruption of home life, and less time to attend to other dependents.

> Caldwell CB. Induction, maintenance and emergence. In: Gregory GA, ed. *Pediatric Anesthesia*. 3rd ed. New York: Churchill Livingston; 1994.

Corneal Autograft Procedures

The greatest advantage of a corneal autograft is the elimination of allograft rejection. Although cases with clinical circumstances appropriate for autograft are uncommon, an astute ophthalmologist who recognizes the possibility of a successful autograft can spare a patient the risk of long-term topical steroid use and the necessity of lifelong vigilance against rejection.

Rotational Autograft

A rotational autograft can be used to reposition a localized corneal scar that involves the pupillary axis. By making an eccentric trephination and rotating the host button prior to resuturing, the surgeon can place a paracentral zone of clear cornea in the pupillary axis. The procedure is particularly useful in children, who have a poorer prognosis for PK. Graft edema can still be a problem, since both the preexisting disease or scar and the rotational procedure usually cause endothelial cell loss. Residual postoperative astigmatism is also a problem because of the eccentric location of the graft.

> Bourne WM, Brubaker RF. A method for ipsilateral rotational autokeratoplasty. *Ophthalmology.* 1978;85:1312–1316.

Contralateral Autograft

A contralateral autograft is reserved for patients who have in one eye a corneal opacity with a favorable prognosis for visual recovery and in the other eye both a clear cornea and severe dysfunction of the afferent system (eg, retinal detachment, severe amblyopia). The clear cornea is transplanted to the first eye, and the cornea from the second eye is replaced either with the diseased cornea from the first eye or with an allograft, or the eye is eviscerated or enucleated. Such bilateral grafting carries the risk of bilateral endophthalmitis.

Lamellar Keratoplasty

Lamellar keratoplasty (LK) is a varying-thickness corneal allograft procedure. The high success rate of PK has reduced the need for LK in treating corneal disease. Antimicrobial agents, corticosteroids, bandage contact lenses, and tissue adhesives now control many disorders that were previously managed by this technique. Nevertheless, the corneal surgeon should be familiar with the special indications for and limitations of LK.

Indications

Lamellar corneal grafting may be indicated in patients who present with opacities or loss of tissue that, for the most part, does not involve the full thickness of the cornea (Fig 23-15). These conditions include

- Superficial stromal dystrophies and degenerations (eg, Reis-Bücklers dystrophy, Salzmann nodular degeneration, band keratopathy)
- Superficial corneal scars
- Recurrent pterygium in the presence of secondary stromal thinning
- Corneal thinning (eg, Terrien marginal degeneration, descemetocele formation, pellucid marginal degeneration)
- Superficial corneal tumors
- Congenital lesions (eg, dermoid)
- Corneal perforations that are not amenable to resuturing or that occur in patients with ocular surface disease (eg, keratoconjunctivitis sicca)
- Keratoconus

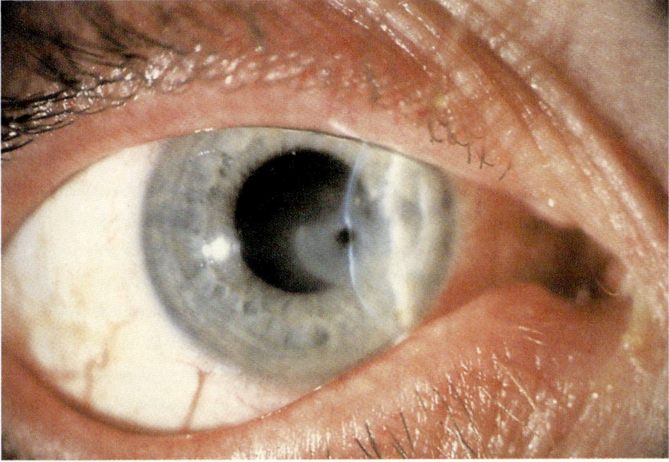

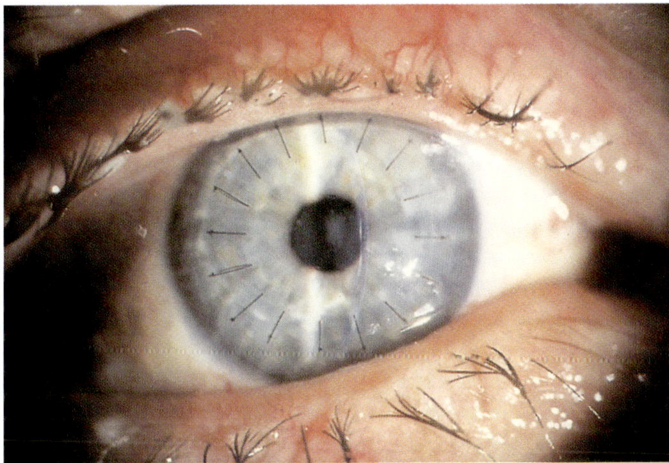

Figure 23-15 Descemetocele in a patient with rheumatoid arthritis *(top)*. Same patient after lamellar keratoplasty *(bottom)*.

Advantages

LK has the following advantages over PK:

- Minimal requirements for donor material (as preservation of endothelium is not mandatory)
- Reduced risk of entry into the anterior chamber
- Shorter wound healing and convalescence
- Reduced incidence of allograft rejection and, consequently, decreased need for topical steroids

LK is less risky than PK in patients who have ocular surface disease, show poor compliance with medical instructions, or experience difficulty in obtaining frequent follow-up.

Disadvantages

LK does not replace damaged endothelium, which severely restricts its indications. The procedure is technically more difficult than PK, and it may cause opacification and vascularization of the interface, which may limit visual function. Some authors consider herpes simplex virus keratitis to be a contraindication for LK.

Surgical Technique

Penetration into the anterior chamber remains the major operative complication, and it may at times require conversion to a PK. A few basic principles apply to the lamellar graft technique. The recipient cornea is dissected first, because a full-thickness graft may be necessary if the cornea sustains a large perforation during the lamellar dissection and to allow for accurate sizing of donor tissue. The donor lamellar graft may be taken from the whole globe. If possible, more than one donor eye should be available because of the difficulty of the lamellar dissection. In addition, preground stromal buttons for lamellar grafting are now available.

A microkeratome is capable of making both the recipient lamellar dissection and the donor dissection. The precision of this instrument has greatly reduced the opacification at the host–donor interface. The donor button can also be prepared by resecting Descemet's membrane from a corneal button using fine (Vannas) scissors.

Postoperative Care and Complications

Opacification and vascularization of the interface

Meticulous irrigation and cleaning of the lamellar bed at the time of surgery may reduce opacification and vascularization, which can occur despite corticosteroid therapy. Postoperatively, best-corrected visual acuity is usually limited to 20/40 or worse.

Allograft rejection

Because the endothelium is not transplanted, endothelial rejection cannot take place. Epithelial rejection, subepithelial infiltrates, and stromal rejection occasionally occur, but they respond to corticosteroid therapy. If graft edema occurs, another cause must be sought for endothelial dysfunction.

Inflammatory necrosis of the graft

Although inflammatory necrosis of the graft has previously been described as an allograft reaction, no immunohistopathologic evidence has confirmed this, and recent series have not demonstrated this phenomenon. The mechanism probably relates to the preexisting corneal disease. Prognosis for retention of a clear graft is poor despite corticosteroid therapy.

Current Developments

In *deep anterior lamellar keratoplasty (DALK)*, the objective is to create the smoothest recipient bed possible by removing all stromal tissue overlying the recipient pupillary zone while leaving the recipient Descemet's membrane and endothelium intact. Although this procedure is clinically preferable because endothelial allograft rejections are avoided, the disadvantages have been the development of interface haze caused by blunt dissection and perforation of the recipient bed. Recently, three techniques have become available that may provide a "sharp" dissection and avoid significant interface haze and reduce the risk of performation:

- The depth of the corneal dissection is visualized during surgery by filling the anterior chamber with air. The air-to-endothelial interface acts as an optical reference plane to monitor dissection depth through the operating microscope, minimizing the risk of performation.
- The depth of the corneal dissection is visualized during surgery by injection of air or viscoelastic just anterior to Descemet's membrane.
- A recipient lamellar bed is created with the femtosecond laser.

In *deep lamellar endothelial keratoplasty (DLEK)*, the posterior part of the cornea is replaced by donor tissue. Two approaches are currently employed: transplantation of a posterior lamellar disc underneath a sutured microkeratome flap; and transplantation of a posterior disc through a scleral pocket incision.

The advantages of the flap technique are, first, that most corneal surgeons have experience in performing microkeratome dissections and, second, that the posterior disc can be excised (and if necessary sutured) with routine trephination and suturing techniques. A disadvantage is that the procedure requires corneal surface incision(s) and sutures. Also, the posterior disc must have some thickness (~250 μm) for fixation into the recipient opening. As a result, postoperative irregular astigmatism, suture-related problems, and flap complications have occurred.

Posterior lamellar keratoplasty through a sclerocorneal pocket incision does not require corneal surface incisions or sutures. Three methods are currently available for excision of the recipient posterior corneal tissue, and three methods are available for implantation of the donor posterior disc. The recipient tissue may be excised by (1) using an intracorneal trephine and microscissors (when a relatively superficial dissection is employed); (2) using microscissors only (when the depth of the dissection is monitored by an optical reference plane, as just described for deep anterior lamellar keratoplasty); or (3) stripping Descemet's membrane from the recipient cornea—that is, "Descemetorhexis."

The donor tissue may be implanted by (1) using a spoon-shaped glide that carries the posterior donor disc on a layer of viscoelastic; (2) folding the donor disc prior to insertion and unfolding it inside the anterior chamber; or (3) injecting a donor Descemet's membrane roll into the anterior chamber and unrolling it inside the anterior chamber. With all methods, the donor tissue is positioned against the posterior recipient stroma and is fixed in place by the pump function of the donor endothelium without the use of sutures.

The advantage of the sclerocorneal pocket approach is that the anterior corneal surface is not compromised, resulting in low with-the-rule postoperative astigmatism. Suture-related complications are eliminated, and the risk of problems related to wound healing is minimized. A disadvantage is that the procedure requires training and has a learning curve. Currently, intrastromal lasers are being investigated to further facilitate the introstromal dissection.

Alio JL, Shah S, Barraquer C, et al. New techniques in lamellar keratoplasty. *Curr Opin Ophthalmol.* 2002;13:224–229.

Melles GR, Lander F, Rietveld FJ, et al. A new surgical technique for deep stromal anterior lamellar keratoplasty. *Br J Ophthalmol.* 1999;83:327–333.

Melles GR, Lander F, Rietveld FJ. Transplantation of Descemet's membrane carrying viable endothelium through a small scleral incision. *Cornea.* 2002;21:415–418.

Terry MA. The evolution of lamellar grafting techniques over twenty-five years. *Cornea.* 2000;19:611–616.

PART XII

Keratorefractive Surgery

CHAPTER 24

Basic Science of Keratorefractive Surgery

Refractive surgery encompasses a broad range of procedures to change the refraction of the eye. Such procedures include techniques to alter the basic shape of the cornea or its ability to refract light. A classification of terms used in "keratospeak" is summarized in Table 24-1.

Currently, the most prevalent refractive surgery is cataract removal with intraocular lens implantation. Other related techniques include removal of the natural lens to treat myopia *(clear lens extraction)*, removal and replacement of the natural lens with IOLs to treat either hyperopia or myopia, or insertion of an artificial lens without natural lens removal *(phakic IOL)*. All of these procedures are discussed in BCSC Section 11, *Lens and Cataract*. They are effective methods for correcting refractive errors, but their safety has not been established; the rate of complications, including retinal detachment and loss of corneal endothelial cells, remains to be determined.

Refractive surgery involving the cornea is changing rapidly as technology advances. Chapter 25 discusses the clinical aspects of keratorefractive incisional surgery, and Chapter 26 covers laser techniques. Schematic illustrations of the more frequent procedures are shown later in this chapter.

Corneal Optics

Corneal topography and wavefront analysis are covered in Chapter 2 of this book. Optical considerations in refractive surgery are discussed in BCSC Section 3, *Clinical Optics*.

Biomechanics of the Cornea

The cornea is a composite material consisting of collagen fibrils that stretch from limbus to limbus packaged in lamellae that are arranged in parallel fashion and embedded in an extracellular matrix of glycosaminoglycans. The layers slide easily over each other, indicating a very low shear resistance, but the stroma itself is an inelastic, anisotropic structure that distributes tensile stress unequally throughout its thickness, depending on the corneal hydration (Fig 24-1).

Table 24-1 Classification of Corneal Refractive Surgery

Type of Refractive Keratoplasty	Basic Surgical Technique	Variations of Surgical Technique or Material	Refractive Error Treated	Comment
Lamellar	Keratomileusis (KM, cutting corneal disc with microkeratome)	Microkeratome techniques • Manual or mechanical advance • Oscillating or rotating blade		Suture techniques: Appositional, overlay, no suture Computerized calculations and control
		Femtosecond laser		Approved in U.S.
		Methods of making refractive stomal cut • Barraquer's cryolathe	Myopia (MKM), hyperopia, aphakia	
		• Nonfreeze–microkeratome with suction mold (BKS)	Myopia, hyperopia, aphakia	
		• Excimer laser (ArF, 193 nm)	Myopia	Early clinical trials
		Source of tissue for disc • Patient (autoplastic) • Donor (homoplastic)		
	KM in situ (carving corneal bed)	Microkeratome (plano excision)	Myopia	
		Keratokyphosis (refractive mold in microkeratome)	Myopia	In laboratory development
		Excimer laser (ArF, 193 nm) • Flap disc (LASIK)	Myopia, hyperopia, astigmatism	Approved in U.S.
		Femtosecond laser	Myopia	In laboratory development
		Autokeratophakia (same as KM in situ, except stromal button is cut smaller with trephine and left in place)	Hyperopia	In development in Moscow
	Epikeratoplasty (Epi)	Human donor lenticule • Cryolathe	Aphakia, hyperopia	If contact lens and IOL contra-indicated, eg, infant aphakia FDA core study; in laboratory development
		• Suction mold (BKS) • Excimer laser • Lyophilized	Myopia	
		Synthetic (eg, collagen and coated hydrogel)		
		Plano lenticule	Astigmatism and myopia in keratoconus	If penetrating keratoplasty contraindicated

	Intracorneal lens or ring (ICL, ICR, keratophakia)	Microkeratome (lamellar bed)		
		• Hydrogel lenticule	Aphakia, myopia	Early clinical trials
		• Human donor lenticule	Aphakia, myopia	Seldom used
		Lamellar pocket		
		• High index of refraction (eg, fenestrated polysulfone)	Aphakia	In laboratory development
		• Fresnel hydrogel	Aphakia	In laboratory development
		Annular lamellar dissection		
		• Intracorneal ring —Fixed volume: PMMA, silicone	Myopia	Approved in U.S. for −1.00 to −3.00
		• Gel injection adjustable (volume) keratoplasty	Myopia	In laboratory development
		Peripheral rectangular segments	Hyperopia, presbyopia	In development, early clinical trials
		Autokeratophakia; folded corneal flap	Aphakia	Under development in Russia
	Lamellar keratotomy	Single deep microkeratome pass	Hyperopia	Discontinued
	Lamellar keratoplasty	Central	Irregular astigmatism (eg, keratoconus)	
		Crescentic	Astigmatism from marginal thinning (eg, Terrien degeneration)	
Keratotomy (refractive keratotomy)	Radial	Single nomogram	Myopia	
		Staged with repeated adjustments		
		Open and suture wounds		Reduce overcorrection
	Transverse (TK, AK)	Isolated straight or arcuate (T cuts)	Astigmatism: primary (naturally occuring); secondary (eg, postoperative, posttraumatic)	Incision made transverse to steep corneal meridian (axis of plus refractive cylinder)
		Combined with radial	Compound myopic astigmatism	
		• Between radial		
		• Interrupted transverse		
		• Interrupted radial		
		• Trapezoidal (Ruiz, semiradial)		
		Modification of penetrating keratoplasty (relaxing incision)		Often staged under keratoscopic or keratometric control
		• Wound seperation or incision in wound	Postoperative astigmatism	
		• Transverse incision in donor	Postoperative astigmatism	*(Continued)*

KEY: KM, keratomileusis; MKM, myopic keratomileusis; BKS, Barraquer-Krumeich-Swinger; ArF, argon-fluoride; PMMA, ploymethylmethacrylate; Epi, epikeratoplasty; IOL, intraocular lens; ICL, intracorneal lens; ICR, intracorneal ring; TK, transverse keratotomy; AK, astigmatic keratotomy; PK, penetrating keratoplasty.

Table 24-1   Classification of Corneal Refractive Surgery (Continued)

Type of Refractive Keratoplasty	Basic Surgical Technique	Variations of Surgical Technique or Material	Refractive Error Treated	Comment
Keratotomy (refractive keratotomy) *(cont)*	Transverse (TK, AK) *(cont)*	Modification of cataract surgery • Intraoperative —Astigmatism neutral cataract incision —Manipulation of incision to reduce preexisting astigmatism, adjust wound size, center incision on steep meridian —Scleral flap recession or resection —Transverse keratotomy • Postoperative —Transverse keratotomy —Wound revision		Limbal or corneal cataract incision acts like TK Length <5 mm Scleral tunnel Few or no sutures
			Naturally occurring astigmatism	
			Postoperative astigmatism	
			High against-the-rule astigmatism	
		Suture adjustment • Removal or cutting of interrupted • Distribution of tension on running • Placement of compression sutures	Postoperative astigmatism	Acts like keratotomy Acts like wedge resection
	Circumferential	Hexagonal —Nonconnected —With transverse (hex-T)	Hyperopia	Seldom used
		Circular, partial-thickness trephination with double running suture	Astigmatism	Seldom used
Keratectomy	Laser	Photorefractive keratectomy (PRK) (central sculpting, large area ablation, and multiple zone ablation) • Excimer laser (ArF, 193 nm) • 5th harmonic Nd:YAG laser (213 nm)	Myopia, astigmatism, hyperopia Primary (naturally occurring) Secondary (eg, after radial, Epi, PK)	FDA approved for −1.00 to −14.00 and +1.00 to +6.00 −0.50 to −5.00 D of astigmatism and +0.50 to +5.00
		Linear laser keratectomy (radial, transverse)	Myopia, astigmatism	Excimer laser (193 nm), femtosecond laser
		Intrastromal photodisruption with Nd:YAG laser • Picosecond ND-YLF (1053 nm) • Nanosecond frequency-doubled Nd:YAG laser (532 nm) • Femtosecond laser	Myopia	In laboratory development

			Purpose/indication	Status
		• Nanosecond Nd:YAG laser (1064 nm)		
		Laser adjustable synthetic Epi	To be evaluated	In laboratory development
	Mechanical	Crescentic wedge • Wedge resection after PK • Wound repair during or after cataract extraction	Astigmatism	
		Crescentic lamellar corneal tuck or flap for Terrien or pellucid marginal degenerations	Astigmatism	
		Mechanical central refractive superficial keratectomy • Rotating blades • Fine water stream		In design phase
Thermokeratoplasty	Noncontact: holmium YAG laser (2.06 μm)	Radial or circular pattern, peripheral or paracentral	Hyperopia/myopia	FDA approved for +0.75 to +2.50
		Treatment in flat meridian with or without concurrent treatment for myopia and hyperopia	Astigmatism	In clinical trials
	Contact: deep stromal hot needle thermocoagulation	Peripheral, intrastromal, radial pattern	Hyperopia	Seldom used
		Arcuate in flat meridian	Astigmatism	
	Diode laser (1.885 μm)	Circular pattern	Hyperopia	In clinical trials
Penetrating keratoplasty (refractive aspects)	Donor–host size disparity	Donor oversized	Hyperopia, aphakia	
		Donor undersized	Myopia, keratoconus	
	Suture adjustment during or after surgery	Selective removal of interrupted sutures in steep meridian		
		Adjustment of running suture		
		Early opening of wound in steep meridian		
		Early placement of interrupted sutures in flat meridian		
		Endothelial replacement only (with flap or from posterior)	Reduce anterior curvature	In clinical trials

KEY: KM, keratomileusis; MKM, myopic keratomileusis; BKS, Barraquer-Krumeich-Swinger; ArF, argon-fluoride; PMMA, ploymethylmethacrylate; Epi, epikeratoplasty; IOL, intraocular lens; ICL, intracorneal lens; ICR, intracorneal ring; TK, transverse keratotomy; AK, astigmatic keratotomy; PK, penetrating keratoplasty.

(Modified from Waring GO III. Making sense of keratospeak IV: classification of refractive surgery, 1992. *Arch Ophthalmol.* 1992;110:1385–1391. For IOL implants, see BCSC Section 11, *Lens and Cataract.*)

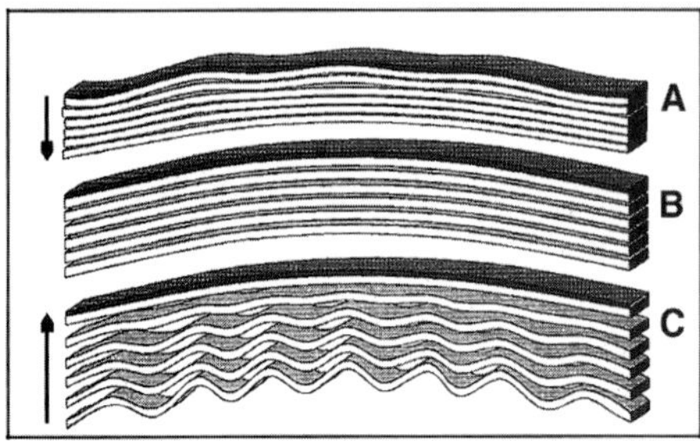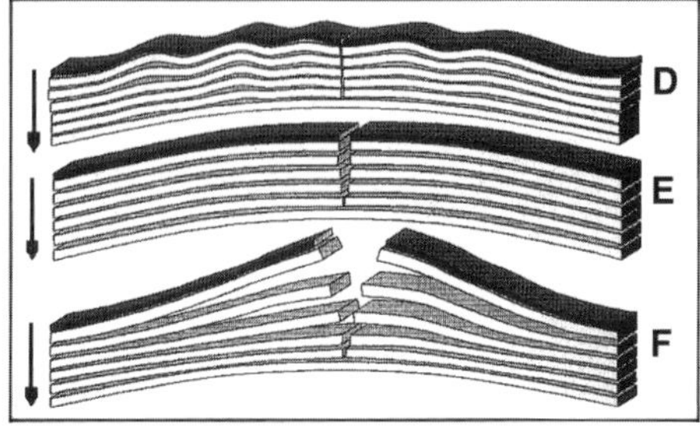

Figure 24-1 Diagram of the corneal stress model. For nonoperated eyes, the anterior curvature is not affected by IOP or corneal hydration as a result of the inelasticity of the cornea. However, the stress in the cornea is displaced posteriorly **(A)** or uniformly **(B)** when dehydrated and is anteriorly displaced in a normal or hydrated cornea **(C)**. After radial keratotomy, the anterior curvature remains either unchanged or mildly affected when in dehydrated **(D)** or normally hydrated **(E)** states. The anterior lamellae remain closely packed, and the inelastic nature of the intact posterior lamellae prevents changes in the shape of the cornea. When hydration increases, the loose anterior stroma absorbs water (swells) and the stress attempts to move anteriorly. However, since these layers have been cut, the cornea flattens its curvature and the posterior lamellae retain their shape by holding the stresses **(F)**. *(Reproduced with permission from Simon G, Ren Q. Biomechanical behavior of the cornea and its response to radial keratotomy. J Refract Corneal Surg. 1994;10:349.)*

When the cornea is in a dehydrated state, stress is distributed either principally to the posterior layers or uniformly over the entire structure. When the cornea is healthy or edematous, the anterior lamellae take up the strain. Stress within the tissue is partly related to IOP but not in a linear manner under physiologic conditions (normal IOP range).

Effects of Keratorefractive Surgery

Keratorefractive surgery can alter the corneal biomechanics in several ways:

- Incisional effect
- Tissue addition or subtraction
- Alloplastic material addition
- Laser effect
- Collagen shrinkage

The *optical zone* in refractive surgery generally refers to the boundary between operated and nonoperated cornea.

Incisional effect

Incisions perpendicular to the corneal surface will predictably alter its shape, depending on direction, depth, location, and number. All incisions cause a local flattening of the cornea. *Radial incisions* lead to flattening in both the meridian of the incision and 90° away. *Tangential incisions* (arcuate or linear, Fig 24-2) lead to flattening in the meridian of the incision and steepening in the meridian 90° away that may be equal to or less than the magnitude of the decrease in the primary meridian; this phenomenon is known as *coupling.*

The closer radial incisions approach the visual axis (ie, the smaller the optical zone), the greater their effect; similarly, the closer tangential incisions are placed to the visual axis, the greater the effect. The longer a radial incision, the greater its effect until approximately an 11 mm diameter is achieved, and then the effect reverses. The larger the angle severed by a tangential incision, the greater the effect.

For optimum effect, an incision should be 85%–90% deep to allow an intact posterior lamellae and maximum anterior bowing of the other lamellae. Nomograms for numbers of incisions and optical zone size can be calculated based on finite element analysis, but they are typically generated empirically. The important variables for radial and astigmatic surgery include patient age, optical zone size, number of incisions, and length of incisions for astigmatic surgery. Intraocular pressure and preoperative corneal curvature are not significant predictors of effect.

The effect of incisional surgery is dependent to a great deal on the hydration of the stroma and less on the IOP (see Figure 24-1). A hyperopic refractive shift can occur in patients exposed to high altitude or low Po_2 following radial keratotomy as a result of swelling in the vicinity of the wound. Daily fluctuation in refraction (typically hyperopic in the morning) in patients with radial keratotomy may also be related to stromal hydration effects rather than to diurnal variation in IOP.

One method that was tried for hyperopic correction, *hyperopic automated lamellar keratoplasty,* used a very deep lamellar pass (more than 70%) to allow the cornea to bow forward under physiologic conditions (Fig 24-3). However, this procedure is unpredictable, may lead to progressive ectasia, and is no longer used.

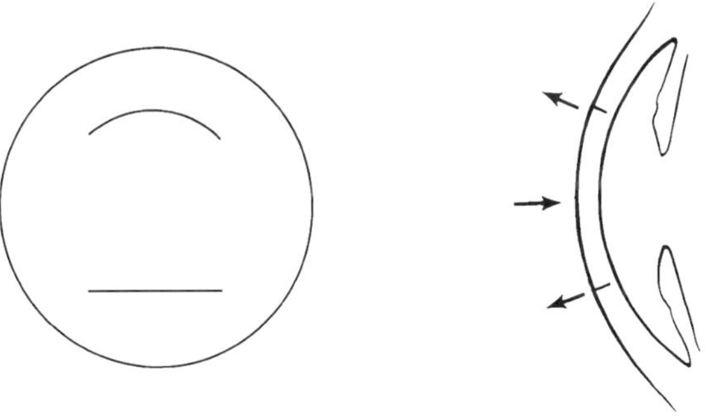

Figure 24-2 Astigmatic keratotomy: schematic arcuate *(above)* and transverse *(below)* incision. The peripheral cornea bulges in axis perpendicular to keratotomy.

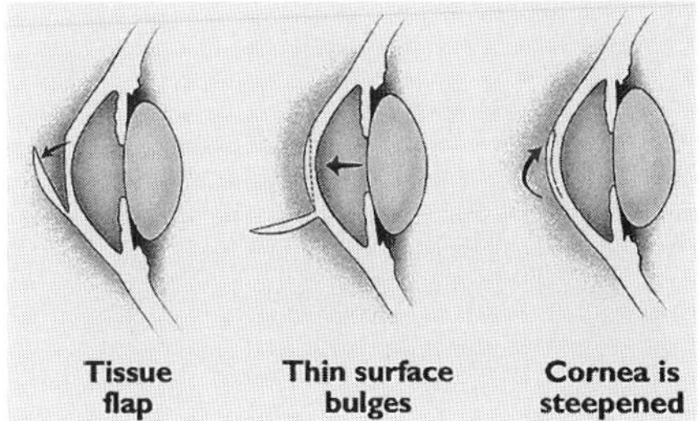

Figure 24-3 Automated lamellar keratoplasty (ALK) for hyperopia.

Tissue addition or subtraction

Lamellar surgery also alters the biomechanics of the cornea. *Keratomileusis* was originated by José Barraquer as "carving of the anterior surface" of the cornea. It is defined as a method of modifying the spherical or meridional surfaces of a healthy cornea by tissue subtraction (Fig 24-4). Tissue subtraction may be performed on the surface (photorefractive keratectomy, or PRK, Fig 24-5) or intrastromally (ALK and LASIK, Figs 24-6 and 24-7). The critical uncut depth of the cornea necessary to maintain normal integrity has not been determined but is presumed to be at least 250–300 μm or 50% of the stromal depth, whichever is greater.

Epikeratoplasty (sometimes called *epikeratophakia*) adds carved donor tissue to the surface to effect hyperopic (Fig 24-8) or myopic changes. *Hyperopic keratomileusis* requires the addition of tissue *(keratophakia)* centrally.

Alloplastic material addition

The biomechanics of the cornea can be altered by adding tissue or alloplastic material on the surface or into the corneal stroma to effect a change in the anterior shape or the refractive index of the cornea. Hydrogel and other material is placed onto or into the cornea (Fig 24-9). For example, the two arc segments of an *intrastromal corneal ring* are placed in two pockets of the stroma to directly alter the surface contour based on the profile of the individual rings (see Figure 25-2). These rings do not work by changing

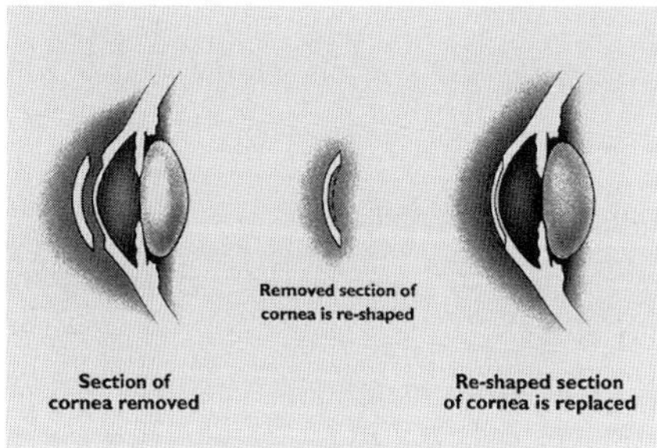

Figure 24-4 Keratomileusis.

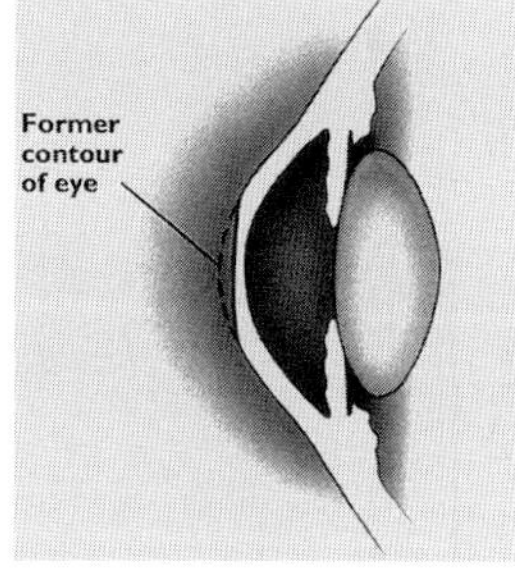

Figure 24-5 Photorefractive keratectomy (PRK) for myopia.

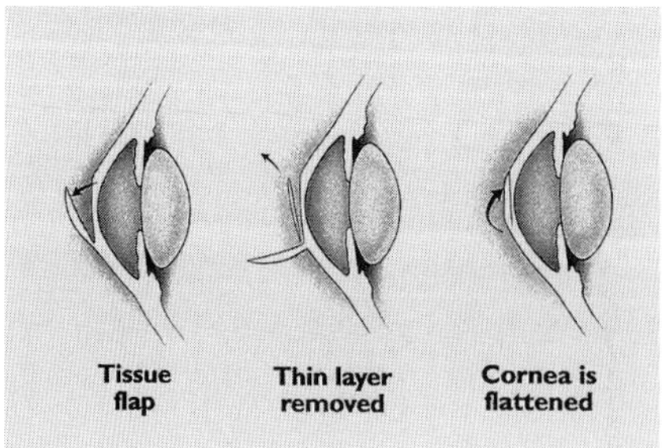

Figure 24-6 Automated lamellar keratoplasty (ALK) for myopia.

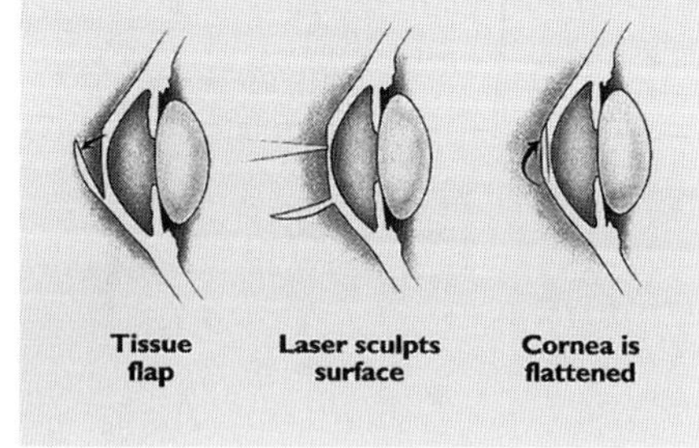

Figure 24-7 Laser in situ keratomileusis (LASIK).

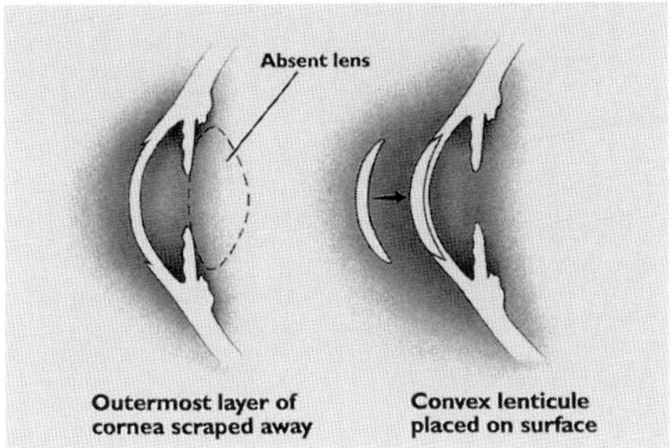

Figure 24-8 Epikeratoplasty for aphakia or hyperopia.

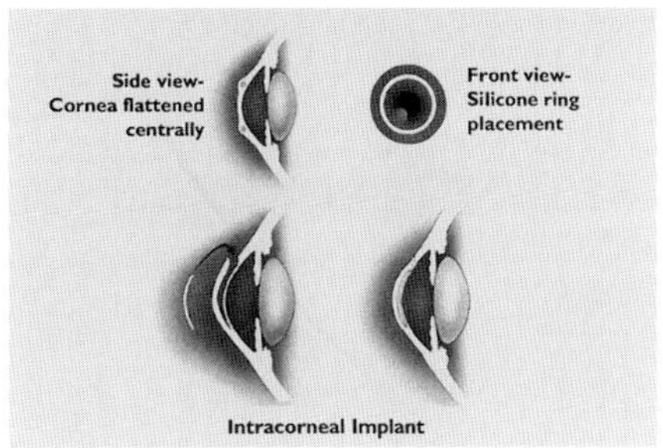

Figure 24-9 Intracorneal implants.

the circumferential measurement of the cornea (ie, by spreading the peripheral cornea to flatten the center). Rather, the manufacturer suggests that the rings work by stiffening or stretching the cornea much as a hammock spreader tightens and gives shape to the sagging mesh.

Laser effect

Photorefractive keratectomy (PRK) of the anterior surface is limited in the depth that can be removed while avoiding complications of forward bowing and scarring. For low amounts of correction (<7 D), the amount of tissue to remove centrally is estimated by *Munnerlyn's formula*:

> Ablation depth in micrometers (µm) equals diopters (D) of myopia divided by 3 times the square of the optical zone (mm)

Clinical experience has confirmed that the effective change is independent of the initial curvature of the cornea, although other formulas have been proposed that take into account preoperative curvature. Munnerlyn's formula also highlights some of the problems and limitations of PRK. The amount of ablation increases by the square of the optical zone, but the complications of glare, haloes, and regression increase when the optical zone decreases. To reduce these side effects, the optical zone should be 6 mm or larger.

Multizone keratectomies use several concentric optical zones to generate the total refraction required. This method can provide the full correction centrally, while the tapering peripheral zones reduce symptoms and allow higher degrees of myopia to be treated. For example, 12 D of myopia can be treated as follows: 6 D are corrected with a 4.5 mm optical zone, 3 D with a 5.5 mm optical zone, and 3 D with a 6.5 mm optical zone. Thus, the total 12 D correction is achieved in the center using a shallower ablation depth than would be necessary for a single pass (103 µm instead of 169 µm—see Figure 24-10). Similarly, *bitoric ablations* (combining a myopic with a hyperopic ablation profile) can reduce the amount of cornea removed centrally and provide a more physiologic postoperative topography (Fig 24-11).

Laser in situ keratomileusis (LASIK) combines a lamellar incision with ablation of the cornea, typically in the bed (see Figure 24-7). The same theoretical limits for residual

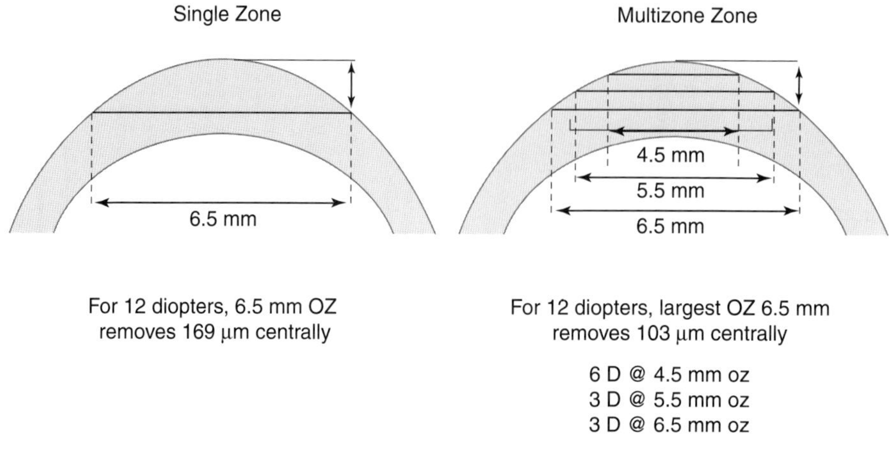

Figure 24-10 Multizone keratectomies. **A,** Depth of ablation required to correct 12 D of myopia in a single pass. **B,** Figure demonstrates how use of multiple zones reduces the ablation depth required. *(Illustration by C.H. Wooley.)*

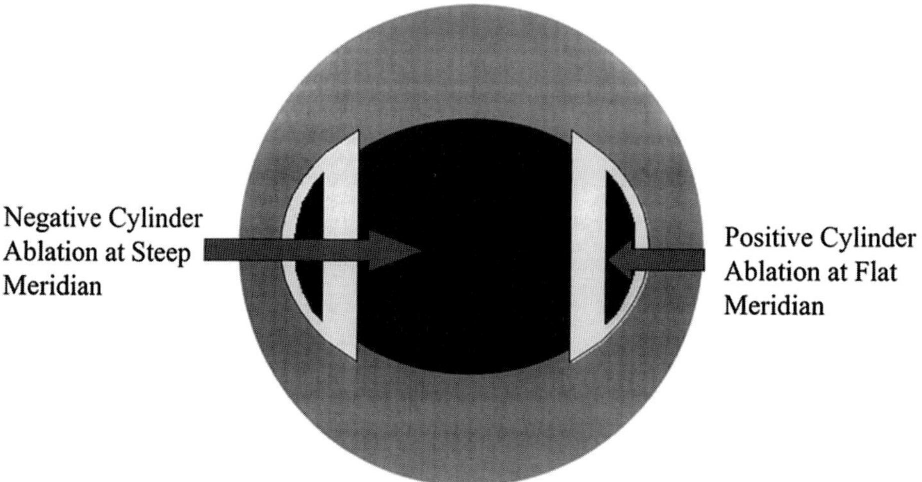

Figure 24-11 Bitoric ablation. *(From Chayet AS, Montes M, Gomez L. Bitoric laser in situ keratomileusis for the correction of simple myopic and mixed astigmatism. Ophthalmology. 2001;108:304.)*

posterior cornea apply as with PRK, and the calculated effect is based on a modification of Munnerlyn's formula empirically. To reduce the complications of surface irregular astigmatism, the flap is typically cut 130–160 μm thick, but not thicker, to allow for the bending at Bowman's layer necessary for correcting the refractive error. The thickness and diameter of the LASIK flap depend on instrumentation, corneal diameter, corneal curvature, and corneal thickness. Flatter corneas lead to smaller diameter and thinner flaps.

Hyperopic PRK uses a similar formula for determining the maximum ablation depth, but the optical zone is much larger. Consequently, the depth is much greater although located in the midperiphery (Fig 24-12).

Collagen shrinkage

Alteration in corneal biomechanics can also be achieved by shrinkage of collagen. Heating collagen to a critical temperature of 55°–60°C will cause it to shrink, inducing changes in the corneal curvature. *Thermokeratoplasty* is avoided in the central cornea because of scarring but can be used in the midperipheral cornea to induce peripheral flattening and central steepening to correct hyperopia (Fig 24-13). Collagen can be heated ab externo with holmium laser (Sunrise Hyperion system) or directly with a radio frequency diathermy probe.

Shrinkage can also be done in a linear manner to induce central flattening and correct myopia, but no clinical trials have been conducted. If the temperature is too high, local necrosis will occur, and if the source of heat is nonuniform or nonuniformly applied, irregular astigmatism will be induced.

Corneal Wound Healing

Chapter 18 has discussed the principles and mechanisms of corneal wound healing. All forms of keratorefractive surgery are exquisitely dependent on this process. Satisfactory results require either modifying or reducing wound healing or exploiting normal wound healing for the benefit of the patient. For example, astigmatic keratotomy requires initial

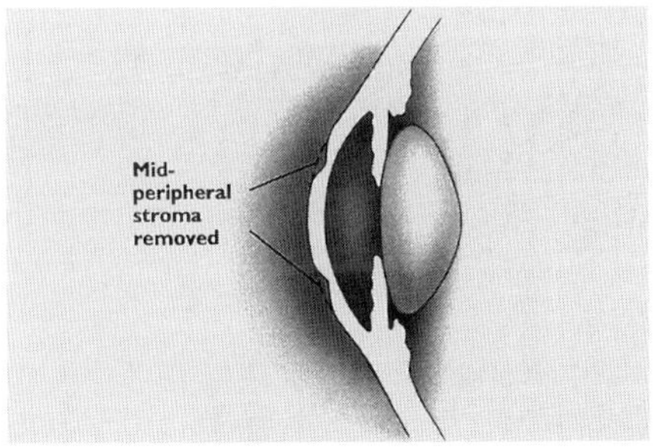

Figure 24-12 Hyperopic photorefractive keratectomy.

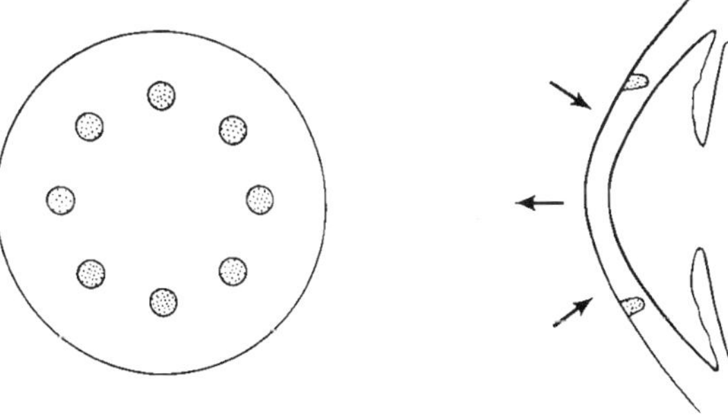

Figure 24-13 Thermokeratoplasty: heat shrinks the peripheral cornea, causing central steepening.

weakening followed by permanent healing with replacement of the epithelial plugs with collagen and remodeling of the collagen to ensure stability and avoid long-term hyperopic drift. PRK requires the epithelium to heal quickly with minimal stimulation of the underlying keratocytes to avoid corneal scar and haze. Lamellar keratoplasty requires intact epithelium and healthy endothelium early in the postoperative period to seat the flap; later, the cornea must heal in the periphery to secure the cap in place and avoid late-term displacement yet minimize irregular astigmatism.

Understanding of corneal wound healing has advanced tremendously with recognition of the multiple factors involved in a cascade of events initiated by corneal wounding. The cascade is somewhat dependent on the nature of the injury. Injury to the epithelium can lead to loss of underlying keratocytes from apoptosis. Remaining keratocytes respond by generating new glycosaminoglycans and collagen, to a degree dependent on the duration of the epithelial defect and the depth of the stromal injury. The tendency toward haze formation is greater with deeper ablations and prolonged absence of the epithelium. Despite loss of Bowman's layer, normal or even enhanced numbers of hemidesmosomes and anchoring fibrils form to secure the epithelium to stroma.

Controversy persists over the value of different agents to modulate wound healing in PRK. Typically, clinicians in the United States use steroids in a tapering manner following surgery to reduce haze formation and stabilize surgical effect. Topical nonsteroidal anti-inflammatory agents have also been tried with no established effect. Other agents such as transforming growth factor–β (TGF-β) have been proposed, but no information on their value is available at this time.

Haze formation does not seem to occur following lamellar keratoplasties, which may be related either to lack of significant epithelial injury and subcellular signaling or to the maintenance of some intact surface neurons. Lamellar surgery shows very little long-term evidence of healing between the disrupted lamellae and only typical stromal healing at the peripheral wound. The lamellae are initially held in position by negative stromal pressure generated by the endothelial cells aided by an intact epithelial surface. Even at 1 year, the lamellar interface can be broken and the flap lifted, indicating the minimal amount of healing that occurs. Aberrant healing can occur if the flap is placed with wrinkles or if epithelium grows into the interface.

Epithelium in the interface acts as a barrier to nutrient flow and must be removed at any sign of thinning, inflammation, or obstruction of visual axis. Interface debris can lead to inflammation or light scattering and should be minimized at the time of surgery. Hyperopic ALK also heals at the peripheral interface only, which may lead to late progressive effect. Epikeratoplasties from donor stroma will slowly repopulate with host keratocytes.

Laser Biophysics

Laser–Tissue Interactions

Three laser–tissue interactions are exploited for keratorefractive surgery. *Photothermal* uses a holmium:YAG laser focused into the anterior stroma with a wavelength of 2.13 μm that is absorbed by water, causing collagen shrinkage from heat. This technique is approved by the FDA for treating low hyperopia.

Photodisruption uses picosecond Nd:YAG laser or Nd:YSGG lasers to perform intrastromal ablations from optical breakdown within the corneal stroma and vaporization of tissue (Fig 24-14). The laser–tissue interaction is entirely intrastromal, and its refractive effect depends on collapse of the tissue above it. This technology is approved to create corneal flaps for LASIK.

Photoablation, the most important laser–tissue interaction in refractive surgery, breaks chemical bonds using excimer (for *excited* di*mer*) lasers or other lasers of the appropriate wavelength. Laser energy of more than 4 eV per photon is sufficient to break carbon–nitrogen or carbon–carbon bonds of tissue. Argon-fluoride (ArF) lasers are excimer lasers that use electrical energy to stimulate argon to form dimers with the caustic fluorine gas. They generate a wavelength of 193 nm with 6.4 eV per photon. The 193 nm light is in the ultraviolet C (high ultraviolet) range, approaching the wavelength of x-rays. In addition to having high energy per photon, light at this end of the electromagnetic spectrum also has very low tissue penetrance and is suitable for operating on the surface of tissue. Not only is the laser energy capable of precision with little thermal spread in tissue, but its lack of penetrance or lethality to cells makes the 193 nm laser nonmutagenic, enhancing its safety. (DNA mutagenicity is in the range of 250 nm.) *Solid-state lasers* can be designed to generate wavelengths of light near 193 nm without the need for toxic gas, possibly improving their reliability and decreasing their cost.

Types of Photoablating Lasers

Photoablating lasers can be divided into broad-beam lasers, scanning-slit lasers, and flying-spot lasers. *Broad-beam lasers* rely on internal optics to create a smooth and homogeneous multimode laser beam up to approximately 7 mm in diameter. They have very high energy per pulse and require a low number of pulses to ablate the cornea. *Scanning-slit lasers* use excimer technology to generate a smaller slit beam that is scanned over the surface to alter the lasing profile, improving the smoothness of the ablated cornea and allowing for larger-diameter ablation zones. *Flying-spot lasers* use smaller diameter beams (0.9–2.0 mm) that are scanned at a higher rate but require a tracking mechanism for precise placement to create the desired pattern of ablation. Wide-area beams and some scanning lasers require an iris or other masking to create the desired shape in the cornea. The flying-spot lasers and some of the scanning lasers use the pattern projected onto the surface to create the desired laser ablation profile without masking.

Surgical Guidelines

The following guidelines apply to all forms of refractive surgery and vary only by the specific refractive error to be corrected and the individual patient's special requirements (tolerance for risk, need for rapid rehabilitation, cost sensitivity, and perhaps wound-healing history). Until an ideal (that is, safe, predictable, and reversible) refractive procedure is developed, disagreement will persist among ophthalmologists as to which eyes and which patients are appropriate for refractive surgery.

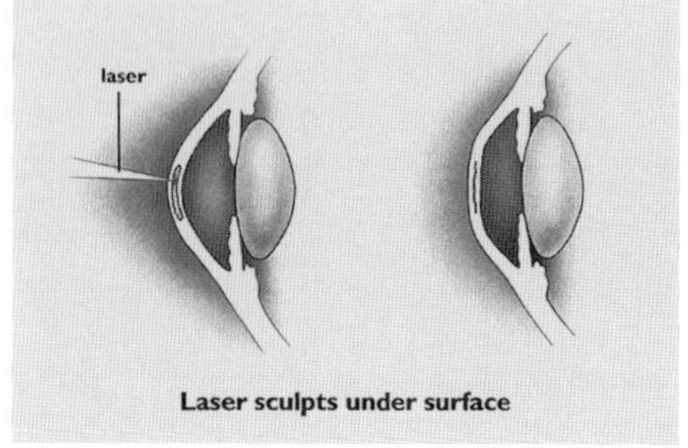

Figure 24-14 Intrastromal ablation.

Patient Selection

Most myopic patients who seek refractive surgery state that they wish to see well without dependence on spectacles or contact lenses. Most hyperopic patients wish to have more convenience. Some patients want the surgery for occupational or cosmetic reasons. Because the procedure is elective, the ophthalmologist must ensure that a prospective patient has a realistic understanding of the benefits and limitations of surgery.

Patients must understand that the outcome of surgery cannot be precisely predicted for an individual eye, that spectacles or contact lenses may still be required for best vision after surgery, and that contact lens wear may be more difficult because of changes in the shape of the cornea. Furthermore, patients must be informed that this surgery may necessitate the use of reading glasses at the age of 40–45 years.

Patients with specific occupational goals are encouraged to get prior assurance that surgical correction of refractive error will satisfy the employment requirements. Finally, the remote possibility of loss of vision or loss of the eye should be openly stated. The surgeon assumes responsibility for obtaining proper informed consent and is advised to do so well in advance of surgery.

Preoperative evaluation

The candidate for refractive surgery should have a stable refractive error and normal corneal structure, free of disorders such as keratoconus or unstable contact lens warpage. The patient should be old enough (18 years) for ocular stability and to understand and give consent for an elective procedure. The candidate should be psychologically stable, have reasonable goals, indicate understanding of the risks involved, and be available for follow-up care.

Contraindications

Any ocular disorders likely to elevate IOP or to require chronic topical corticosteroids should be absent. Systemic conditions that may alter wound healing (collagen vascular diseases, chronic exogenous steroids, immunocompromised status, pregnancy or nursing) are relative contraindications to surgery. Unreasonable expectations or unstable refraction (changing more than 1 D in the last 2 years) or keratometry are contraindications, along with active, recurrent, or residual external problems of the conjunctiva, cornea, and eyelids. Most surgeons obtain computerized corneal topography on all eyes prior to refractive surgery to rule out subclinical keratoconus and irregular astigmatism or contact lens warpage.

Patients should discontinue soft contact lenses 1–3 weeks before measurement for surgery. Hard or gas-permeable contact lenses should be discontinued for 6–12 weeks, with repeated measures of refraction and keratometry to ensure stability.

Centering Procedures

Placement of the refractive surgery is most critical. Misalignment leads to multiple problems of undertreatment, glare, haloes, induced astigmatism, and patient dissatisfaction. The pupil is the critical structure in the pathway of light to the retina and is consequently the basis for centering refractive procedures. It is important to make sure that the patient is fixing coaxially with the surgeon or fixation light of the specific device and that the eye is not tilted with respect to this axis. The head and eye should be level.

CHAPTER 25

Incisional, Inlay, and Onlay Procedures

Surgical Correction of Myopia

Radial Keratotomy

Corneal incisions were first used to correct refractive errors in the late 1890s. Refractive keratotomy for myopia then underwent a long period of international development. Although radial keratotomy (RK) had been the most common surgical procedure used to correct myopia since its modernization by Fyodorov in the 1970s (Fig 25-1), the popularity of this procedure has markedly decreased since the advent of other technologies to correct myopia.

PREOPERATIVE EVALUATION In addition to the patient selection criteria discussed in Chapter 24, RK is best limited to patients with 1.00–4.00 D of myopia or less. Otherwise, complications may result from more aggressive treatment with optical zones smaller than 3.0 mm or more than eight incisions. RK surgery has potential advantages over PRK and LASIK in that it does not involve treatment in the central visual axis or removal of tissue (see Chapter 26). Disadvantages of RK are the limited range of refractive error that can be treated, potential for long-term hyperopic drift, decreased ocular integrity, risk of intraoperative perforation, and risk of infectious keratitis or endophthalmitis. Further, RK may not be appropriate for individuals who spend time at high altitude because of possible hyperopic refractive shift.

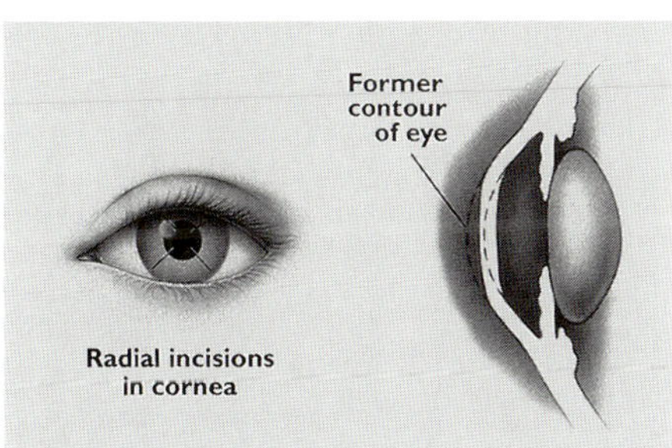

Figure 25-1 Radial keratotomy for myopia.

SURGICAL TECHNIQUES Radial corneal incisions sever collagen fibrils in the corneal stroma. This produces a wound gape (see Figure 24-1) that increases the radius of curvature in the central cornea, flattening it and decreasing its refractive power, thereby decreasing myopia.

The design of the diamond-blade micrometer knife (angle and sharpness of cutting edge, width of blade, and footplate design) influences both the depth and contour of incisions. The length of the knife blade is set based on the corneal thickness, which is usually measured with an ultrasonic pachymeter.

A vertical blade that is pushed centripetally (Russian technique) will cut deeper than an angled blade pulled centrifugally through the tissue (American technique).

VARIABLES AFFECTING OUTCOME

Surgical variables Four variables controlled by the surgeon affect the outcome of surgery:

- *Centering.* Corneal surgical procedures are preferably centered around the visual axis.
- *Optical zone diameter.* Smaller optical zones produce more flattening and reduction of myopic power.
- *Number of incisions.* Four, six, or eight incisions are typically used.
- *Depth of incisions.* The ideal depth of radial incisions is 80%–90% of the corneal thickness. Deeper incisions produce more flattening but less stability.

Patient variables The older the patient, the greater the effect achieved with the same surgical technique. The increase is approximately 0.50–1.00 D per decade.

Adjustments of variables Nomograms are available that suggest size of optical zone and number of incisions based on the patient's age and degree of myopia. It is much easier to enhance an undercorrection by lengthening, deepening, or adding incisions than to repair an overcorrection. Consequently, nomograms tend to result in a slight undercorrection. Enhancement or reoperation rate after RK is surgeon dependent.

EFFICACY AND PREDICTABILITY The ideal result after surgery is mild residual myopia, on the order of -0.50, because residual myopia delays the onset of symptomatic presbyopia and offsets the continued tendency toward hyperopia that occurs in some RK patients.

Based on the simple indicator of percentage of eyes with final spherical equivalent refractive error within ± 1.00 D, reported results range from 54% to 96%. Series that include reoperations for undercorrection generally show a higher percentage of eyes with the target refraction.

The percentage of patients who do not wear optical correction represents a reasonable measure of the overall success of surgery. Among 310 patients with bilateral radial keratotomy in the Prospective Evaluation of Radial Keratotomy (PERK) study, 70% reported not wearing spectacles or contact lenses for distance vision at 10 years, and 42% reported no correction at all.

POSTOPERATIVE REFRACTION, VISUAL ACUITY, AND CORNEAL TOPOGRAPHY RK changes not only the curvature of the central cornea but also its overall topography, creating a multifocal cornea. The result is a decrease in the direct correlation among refraction, central keratometry, and uncorrected visual acuity, presumably because the new corneal topography creates a more complex optical system, consisting of central flattening, paracentral steepening or flattening, and relative peripheral steepening. Thus, keratometric readings that sample only two points approximately 3.0 mm apart may indicate amounts of astigmatism different from those detected by refraction. Similarly, uncorrected visual acuity for a residual refractive error may vary, particularly depending on pupil diameter: the smaller the pupil, the smaller the multifocal effect of postoperative changes in the cornea.

STABILITY OF REFRACTION Almost all eyes show a decrease in myopia immediately followingradial keratotomy. Some regression occurs with healing, but most eyes are generally stable by 3 months after surgery. However, two phenomena of postoperative refractive instability—fluctuation of vision and a continued effect of surgery—may persist for several years.

Diurnal fluctuation of vision Diurnal fluctuation can occur because the cornea is flatter upon awakening and gradually steepens during the patient's waking hours. In a subset of the PERK study at 10 years, the mean change in the spherical equivalent of refraction between the morning (waking) and evening examinations was 0.31 ± 0.58–D increase in minus power in first eyes.

Continued effect of surgery The refractive error in 43% of eyes in the PERK study changed in the hyperopic direction by 1.00 D or more between 6 months and 10 years postoperatively. The hyperopic shift was statistically associated with the diameter of the clear zone. Duration of this ongoing effect is one of the major unknowns about RK.

COMPLICATIONS Probably the best measure of the safety of RK is the rate of loss of best spectacle-corrected visual acuity. From 1% to 3% of eyes lose two or more Snellen lines. The other 97%–99% of patients can put on spectacles postoperatively and obtain their baseline visual acuity.

Mild to moderate irregular astigmatism can cause visual distortion and glare, especially in eyes that have had one of the following:

- More than eight incisions
- Incisions extending inside a 3.0 mm central clear zone
- Intersecting radial and transverse incisions
- Hypertrophic scarring

Many patients report seeing a starburst pattern around lights at night that presumably results from light scattering off the radial scars. While most individuals find the effect comparable to looking through dirty spectacles or contact lenses, some have had to stop driving at night because of this complication. No clinical trials have objectively demonstrated an increase in disabling glare after RK. Common side effects that do not reduce corrected visual acuity include

- Postoperative pain for about 24 hours
- Undercorrection and overcorrection

- An increase in astigmatism of 1.00–3.00 D in approximately 15% of eyes
- Inclusion cysts and vascularization of stromal scars
- Slight, nonprogressive endothelial disruption beneath the incisions at the time of surgery

Potentially blinding complications occur rarely after RK. These include

- Perforation of the cornea, which can lead to endophthalmitis, epithelial ingrowth, and traumatic cataract.
- Traumatic rupture of the globe occurring through a keratotomy incision has been reported as long as 13 years after RK.
- Bacterial keratitis, which can occur immediately after surgery or up to 1–3 years later, presumably because the epithelium of the incision scars heals slowly and is constantly turning over, creating a site for bacterial adherence. Early-onset corneal ulcers are usually paracentral and deep, whereas late-onset ulcers are usually peripheral and superficial.

OCULAR SURGERY AFTER RADIAL KERATOTOMY Eyes that have unacceptable residual myopia after RK can undergo repeated surgery ("enhancement") by opening the incisions with a blunt instrument and deepening or extending them to a smaller clear zone, or by making additional incisions between the initial ones. Eyes that are unacceptably undercorrected or overcorrected can be managed by excimer laser treatment. Because unpublished reports suggest that corneal scarring may increase if PRK is performed after RK, LASIK may be preferable for treatment in such patients.

Linebarger EJ, Hardten DR, Lindstrom RL. Laser-assisted in situ keratomileusis for correction of secondary hyperopia after radial keratotomy. *Int Ophthalmol Clin.* 2000;40:125–132.

Salamon SA, Hjortdal JO, Ehlers N. Refractive results of radial keratotomy: a ten-year retrospective study. *Acta Ophthalmol Scand.* 2000;78:566–568.

Stevens SX, Young DA, Polack PJ, et al. Complications of radial keratotomy. In: Krachmer JH, Mannis MJ, Holland EJ, eds. *Cornea.* Vol 3. St Louis: Mosby; 1997:2101–2116.

Some eyes with marked irregular astigmatism and subjective glare following RK must undergo penetrating keratoplasty. Because the keratotomy wounds may open during PK, transverse sutures may need to be preplaced peripherally to reinforce the wounds prior to host trephination.

Cataract surgery may lead to temporary hyperopia following RK. In addition, IOL power calculation may be problematic and result in undercorrection and hyperopia. Calculation of implant power for cataract surgery after RK is done using a third-generation formula (eg, Haigis, Hoffer Q, Holladay 2, or SRK/T) rather than a regression formula (eg, SRK I or SRK II) and choosing the highest resulting IOL power. Keratometric power is determined in one of three ways: direct measurement using computerized videography; knowledge of pre-RK keratometry minus the refractive change; or adjustment of the base curve of a plano contact lens by the overrefraction (see BCSC Section 11, *Lens and Cataract*).

Seitz B, Langenbucher A. Intraocular lens calculations status after corneal refractive surgery. *Curr Opin Ophthalmol.* 2000;11:35–46.

Waring GO III. Radial keratotomy for myopia. In: *Focal Points: Clinical Modules for Ophthalmologists.* San Francisco: American Academy of Ophthalmology; 1992: vol 10, no 5.

Lamellar Procedures

José Barraquer pioneered the procedure called *keratomileusis,* in which a microkeratome removes a thin segment of tissue (called a lenticule) by cutting through the cornea in the plane perpendicular to the visual axis (see Figure 24-4). The posterior aspect of the lenticule can then be carved mechanically, either with or without freezing, or it can be modified with laser photoablation. Alternatively, the host bed can be modified by mechanical (automated lamellar keratectomy) or laser techniques, as in LASIK.

Myopic keratomileusis

Originally, the lenticule was quick-frozen and carved on a cryolathe, thawed, and replaced on the patient's cornea. Because of the resulting loss of keratocytes and epithelial cells, 6–8 months were required for the lenticule to clear. The improved technique of Barraquer-Krumeich-Swinger (BKS), which reshaped the lenticule over a vacuum mold without freezing, addressed this problem.

COMPLICATIONS Irregular astigmatism has been reported in 14% of eyes. Other problems include loss of lenticule, interface opacities, delayed epithelialization, corneal perforation, central ectasia, and loss of endothelial cells.

OCULAR SURGERY AFTER MYOPIC KERATOMILEUSIS Many times, secondary procedures such as homoplastic keratomileusis (with a donor lenticule), astigmatic relaxing incisions, or radial keratotomy are needed. Homoplastic keratomileusis has been used after LASIK procedures that are complicated by flap removal for infection or scarring. No information is available on the success of subsequent PK or cataract surgery after myopic keratomileusis.

FUTURE DEVELOPMENTS Myopic keratomileusis has been effectively replaced by LASIK (for myopia less than 15 D) or intraocular surgery for higher amounts of myopia (greater than 15 D). New manual and automated keratotomes are being developed.

American Academy of Ophthalmology. Keratophakia and keratomileusis: safety and effectiveness. Ophthalmic Procedures Assessment. *Ophthalmology.* 1992;99:1332–1341.

Automated lamellar keratoplasty (ALK)

In situ keratomileusis (now called ALK) uses a first pass with the keratome followed by a second, deeper pass to remove a lamellar (not lenticular) button of defined central thickness and diameter to correct higher degrees of myopia (see Figure 24-6). Initially, a manual keratome was used, but the advent of the automated keratome along with the use of a hinged flap and the avoidance of suturing improved the predictability and reduced the complications. The procedure has been mostly replaced by LASIK.

COMPLICATIONS In addition to the high reoperation rates, loss of best-corrected vision of two or more lines was reported in 6% of patients, usually secondary to irregular astigmatism. Other complications included loss of the cap, epithelial ingrowth into the interface (2%), overcorrection >1.00 D, infection, and decentration.

OCULAR SURGERY AFTER ALK Experience is limited, but one report mentions a dislocated cap during retinal detachment surgery 5 months after hyperopic ALK. Incisional astigmatic keratotomy and RK are less predictable following ALK.

FUTURE DEVELOPMENTS LASIK and intraocular surgery (for higher amounts of myopia and hyperopia) have effectively replaced ALK because of greater accuracy and safety.

American Academy of Ophthalmology. Automated lamellar keratoplasty. Preliminary procedure assessment. *Ophthalmology.* 1996;103:852–861.

Lyle WA, Jin GJ. Initial results of automated lamellar keratoplasty for correction of myopia: one year follow-up. *J Cataract Refract Surg.* 1996;22:31–43.

Epikeratoplasty

Also called *epikeratophakia*, this procedure to correct adult and pediatric aphakia, myopia, hyperopia, or keratoconus involves rehydration and suturing of a preprocessed, freeze-dried lenticule of human corneal tissue onto the bare Bowman's layer of the host cornea (see Figure 24-8). Because no viable donor cells are involved, classic graft rejection is not possible. Host epithelium migrates over the surface of the graft.

This procedure found its greatest use in the correction of adult and pediatric aphakia in patients who were poor candidates for an IOL. Complications such as persistent epithelial defects, ulceration, interface scarring, sloughing of tissue, epithelial ingrowth, loss of best-corrected visual acuity, and refractive under- or overcorrection, together with development of transscleral IOL placement techniques, have markedly reduced its use in recent years.

Epikeratoplasty never achieved predictable correction of myopia (reduction from -12.50 to -1.40 ± 3.64 D in a nationwide study), although dramatic results are seen in some patients. Its use in keratoconus was limited by its rather stringent indication: keratoconus without stromal scarring but so severe that correction with a contact lens was not possible. The lenticule used for keratoconus actually compressed and deformed the ectatic host cornea, which is not true in other indications for epikeratoplasty.

American Academy of Ophthalmology. Epikeratoplasty. Ophthalmic Procedure Assessment. *Ophthalmology.* 1996;103:983–991.

Alloplastic Intracorneal Implants

Materials used for keratorefractive surgery should correct a large range of spherical and cylindrical errors and be reversible. Alloplastic materials are desirable. Barraquer abandoned intracorneal methyl methacrylate discs in the 1960s because of necrosis anterior to the corneal implant. Other materials have been used, including perfilcon A, hydroxy ethyl methacrylate (HEMA), and other copolymers (soft contact lens material), which require a lamellar keratotomy to allow Bowman's layer to deform.

Polysulfone is a plastic with a high index of refraction (1.633) that can be placed in a stromal pocket without the lamellar keratotomy. However, it is impermeable and requires microperforations (which degrade the optics) to allow nutrients to move anteriorly. Copolymers are also in preliminary trials in primates for use as an epikeratoplasty lenticule. Processed collagen molded onto the cornea and allowed to heal, followed by final adjustment with laser, has been proposed as well.

Intracorneal ring (ICR)

Placement of a PMMA ring into the cornea has evolved into the placement of two segments of 150° arc for the correction of low myopia (Fig 25-2). The advantage of this technique is the maintenance of the cornea's inherent positive asphericity and the potential reversibility of the procedure.

PATIENT SELECTION Three different KeraVision Intacs ring segments of varying thickness have been approved by the FDA for correction of −1.00 to −3.00 D of myopia (Table 25-1). The astigmatic component should be less than 1 D.

SURGICAL TECHNIQUES A vacuum centering guide is used to pass a special stromal separator at approximately two thirds of the stromal depth with an inner diameter of 7.0 mm in two 180° arcs (clockwise and counterclockwise from a small superior radial incision). The ring segments are placed in each arc.

INSTRUMENTATION The procedure requires the vacuum-guided stromal separator to ensure that the two parts are in the same plane of appropriate depth.

VARIABLES AFFECTING OUTCOME The thickness of the ring is the only nomogram variable.

POSTOPERATIVE REFRACTION, VISUAL ACUITY, AND CORNEAL TOPOGRAPHY The advantage of the procedure is the maintenance of the cornea's inherent positive asphericity.

EFFICACY AND PREDICTABILITY In FDA clinical trials at 1 year, 92% of eyes were ±1.00 D, and 69% were ±0.50 D. Uncorrected vision of 20/20 occurred in 74%, and 20/40 in 97%, of 410 eyes. Better results were obtained with lower degrees of myopia requiring thinner segments. At 1 year, 20/20 uncorrected vision was achieved by 83.7% with 0.25 mm segments, 77.5% with 0.30 mm segments, and 60.6% with 0.35 mm segments. Normal prolate asphericity of the peripheral cornea is maintained.

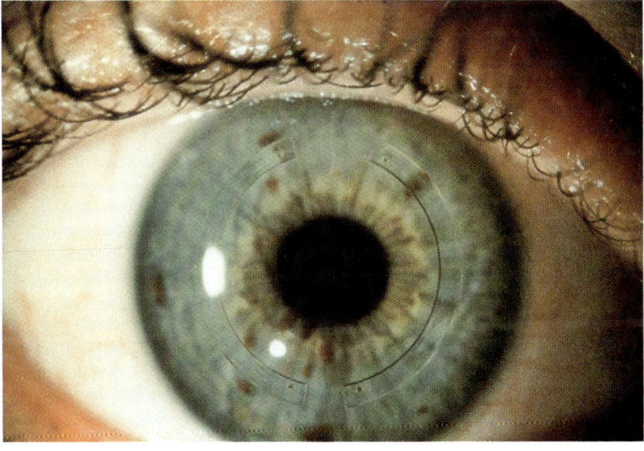

Figure 25-2 Intrastromal ring segments. *(Reproduced from* External Disease and Cornea: A Multimedia Collection. *San Francisco: American Academy of Ophthalmology; 2000.)*

Table 25-1 KeraVision® Intacs™: Recommended Prescribing Range in U.S.

Intacs Thickness	Recommended Prescribing Range
0.25 mm	− 1.00 to − 1.63 D
0.30 mm	− 1.75 to − 2.25 D
0.35 mm	− 2.38 to − 3.00 D

STABILITY OF REFRACTION By 1 year, almost 97% of patients demonstrated 1 D or less change in manifest refraction spherical equivalent from the prior refraction 3 months earlier. At 1 year, 100% stability was achieved only in the 0.25 mm thickness group. By 3 months after segment removal, 95% of 21 eyes returned to within 1 D of their preoperative manifest refraction spherical equivalent.

COMPLICATIONS Severe complications were reported in 1.1% of the 454 eyes that had Intacs surgery in Phase II and Phase III clinical trials and included infectious keratitis (0.2%), shallow placement of segment requiring removal (0.2%), corneal perforation (0.4%), and loss of two lines of best-corrected visual acuity, which subsequently returned (0.2%). Other ocular complications at 1 year included decrease of corneal sensation (5.5%), induced cylinder of 1–2 D (3.7%), neovascularization (2.7%), and persistent epithelial defect (0.2%). Thirty-nine of 449 eyes in the patients in the first U.S. trial underwent explantation (34 initial implant eyes and 5 contralateral eyes); 15 for undercorrection, overcorrection, or induced astigmatism and 19 for adverse visual symptoms like glare, haloes, and poor night vision. By 3 months after implant removal, all patients were within 1 D of the prior refractive error, and 96% of patients were within 0.50 D of prior refractive error. Best-corrected spectacle acuity returned to 20/20 in all cases. Another recent study reported an evening myopic shift similar to that found after RK.

OCULAR SURGERY AFTER ICR Patients' vision returned to preoperative status by 3 months following removal in most cases; all patients were correctable with glasses to 20/20.

FUTURE DEVELOPMENTS Applications for astigmatic correction and use in post-LASIK corneal ectasia and keratoconus are being evaluated. Additional ring thicknesses to correct higher amounts of myopia are being investigated.

Asbell PA, Ucakhan OO, Abbott RL, et al. Intrastromal corneal ring segments: reversibility of refractive effect. *J Refract Surg.* 2001;17:25–31.

Nose W, Neves RA, Burris TE, et al. Intrastromal corneal ring: 12-month sighted myopic eyes. *J Refract Surg.* 1996;12:20–28.

Surgical Correction of Hyperopia and Presbyopia

Epikeratoplasty for aphakia and hyperopia has been previously discussed under "Lamellar Procedures."

Hexagonal Keratotomy

Devised as an incisional correlate to radial keratotomy for the low hyperope, this procedure soon fell out of favor because it produces an unstable cornea with significant irregular astigmatism and wound-healing complications.

Hyperopic Keratomileusis

This procedure is similar to myopic keratomileusis except that the lenticule is reshaped to correct for hyperopia. Complications are also similar and results show unpredictability (51% within 3 D of emmetropia) and high complication rates (14%). With the advent of LASIK, this procedure has also fallen out of favor.

Keratophakia

This special form of keratomileusis uses a plus power donor corneal lenticule (up to 20 D) placed within a lamellar bed to increase the anterior curvature of the cornea. Initially, the lenticules were created on cryolathe and the lamellar dissection done with a manual keratome. Advances in the creation of the lenticule by the BKS device and automation of the keratectomy enhanced the predictability of the procedure. At best, 75% of patients are within 3 D of desired correction, and the complications are similar to other lamellar procedures. The procedure has been replaced by hyperopic LASIK, clear lens extraction, and holmium thermokeratoplasty.

Automated Lamellar Keratoplasty for Hyperopia

See the discussion of ALK under "Surgical Correction of Myopia." ALK for hyperopia creates a "controlled ectasia," similar to induced keratoconus, to steepen the anterior curve of the cornea (see Figure 24-3). Nomograms are used to predict the depth of lamellar cut that will produce the desired anterior bowing of the cornea. A maximum depth of 70% is recommended, limiting correction of hyperopia to approximately +6.00 D. Stability cannot be assessed, but the procedure appears to produce less irregular astigmatism than ALK for myopia, with none of the eyes losing two or more lines of best-corrected vision at 6 months. The procedure has been replaced by LASIK, holmium thermokeratoplasty, or conductive keratoplasty for correction of hyperopia (see Chapter 26). Conductive keratoplasty, which uses radiofrequency energy, has recently been approved by the FDA for hyperopia treatment.

> Manche EE, Judge A, Maloney RK. Lamellar keratoplasty for hyperopia. *J Refract Surg.* 1996;12:42–49.

Phakic IOLs

Phakic IOLs are undergoing Phase II and Phase III clinical trials for correction of myopia and hyperopia. Depending on the brand, the IOLs are placed either in the ciliary sulcus (Star ICL) or the anterior chamber (Artisan IOL) and correct up to 15 D of myopia and 12 D of hyperopia. Longer-term follow-up on endothelial cell loss and cataract formation is needed to assess safety (see BCSC Section 11, *Lens and Cataract*).

Refractive Lensectomy

A recent case series of patients undergoing refractive lensectomy with IOL implantation for hyperopia with an average spherical equivalent of 2.26 D of hyperopia showed 88% of patients within 1 D of intended postoperative spherical equivalent, and 88% with uncorrected vision of 20/40 or better. Loss of one line of best-corrected visual acuity occurred in 11%.

Fink AM, Gore C, Rosen ES. Refractive lensectomy for hyperopia. *Ophthalmology.* 2000; 107:1540–1548.

Presbyopia Correction

Intraocular lens

The FDA-approved Allergan Array multifocal lens is a posterior chamber IOL placed at the time of lens extraction. It affords the patient refractive correction for near, intermediate, and distance vision. Because side effects and complications include haloes and decreased quality of vision (especially in scotopic conditions), patients should be carefully selected in a manner similar to that used for refractive surgery patients. A 1% explantation rate is reported.

The AT-45 accommodating IOL is in Phase I FDA trials. This silicone plate haptic lens has a hingelike modification at the junction of the plate haptic and optic that allows the lens to flex forward with accommodation.

Intrastromal lens

High-index, 2.0 mm intrastromal lenses are undergoing clinical trials for the treatment of presbyopia. The lenses are placed in the corneal pocket and create a multifocal effect. They can theoretically be adjusted or replaced. Patient acceptance is variable, and no peer-reviewed reports are available.

Scleral expansion

This newly described technique is based on the Schachar theory of accommodation, which remains unconfirmed. Expansion of the ciliary ring is postulated to increase zonular tension and is said to restore accommodation by an average of 3.25 D. Four scleral pockets are dissected 3.0–3.5 mm posterior to the limbus, and 2.0 mm by 4.0 mm segments are inserted. The serious complication of anterior segment ischemia has been reported. The device is undergoing a Phase I FDA clinical trial, and long-term peer-reviewed reports are not available.

Surgical Correction of Astigmatism

Transverse Keratotomy

The cylindrical component of the cornea's refracting power can be altered by many different surgical maneuvers, such as modification of previous incisions, resection of tissue with resuturing, application of heat or radiofrequency to produce stromal shrinkage, and use of the excimer laser with PRK or LASIK (see Figure 24-2).

Although a single radial incision will induce flattening in that meridian, overall flattening will also occur, resulting in a hyperopic shift. Arcuate or transverse incisions, on the other hand, produce concomitant steepening in the opposite meridian (coupling), thus inducing cylindrical change with less effect on the spherical equivalent of refraction. Cylindrical change can be increased by the following:

- Reducing the distance between the visual axis and a transverse keratotomy
- Increasing the length or depth of the incision
- Using multiple incisions
- Making radial cuts in the same meridian

Some authors argue that the *coupling ratio* (the ratio of desired flattening to induced steepening in the opposite meridian) can be modified by the type of incision (arcuate versus tangential) and the length and number of parallel incisions. Short, straight, or tangential incisions induce less steepening (higher ratio) in the opposite meridian than do arcuate or longer incisions. Modified Ruiz procedures (combination of nonintersecting radial and tangential incisions) produce the highest coupling ratios.

Paradoxically, higher coupling ratios have less effect on the opposite meridian but more effect on the spherical equivalent. A coupling ratio of 1:1 means no net effect on spherical equivalent. Procedures that result in a coupling ratio lower than 1:1 are inherently unstable (more effect in the nonoperated meridian, as with an arcuate cut greater than 100°) and should be avoided. Incisional surgeries can only reduce the power of the cornea and therefore correct plus cylinder. To date, there is no reliable nomogram to predict the coupling ratio and, consequently, the effect of astigmatic surgery on the spherical equivalent refraction of the eye.

PATIENT SELECTION The decision to correct astigmatism depends on patient needs and symptoms, the amount and axis of astigmatism, and anisometropia. Nomograms cover 1.00–6.00 D for congenital astigmatism. Predictability for an individual eye is not ideal with any current system.

SURGICAL TECHNIQUES Astigmatic keratotomy can be performed alone or in combination with RK or cataract surgery. As with RK, numerous tables and nomograms, as well as a variety of surgical equipment, are used for astigmatic keratotomy. AK can be performed in conjunction with other refractive surgery procedures, for example, after PRK or LASIK.

Arcuate keratotomy Limbal relaxing incisions (LRI) are a specific form of arcuate keratotomy that has become increasingly popular as a technique performed at the time of cataract or refractive surgery to reduce astigmatism (see BCSC Section 11, *Lens and Cataract*).

INSTRUMENTATION The instruments used are similar to RK with different diamond blade designs for specific nomograms. Thin trapezoid-shaped blades work better for tangential incisions. Front-cutting diamond blades allow better visibility of corneal marks. The Hanna arcuate trephine is specifically designed for making smooth curvilinear incisions of specified optical zone and arc length. With any system, accurate assessment of the both the visual axis, as in RK, and of the plus cylinder axis are essential. The axis should be identified preoperatively and verified intraoperatively.

VARIABLES AFFECTING OUTCOME As with RK, patient age and closeness to the visual axis increase the effect. Length, type (curvilinear versus straight), and number of incisions change the amount of flattening. Tangential incisions may be used in pairs along the steep meridian (maximum of two pairs, one on each side of the visual axis), no closer than the 4.0 mm optical zone and preferably farther away. Arcuate incisions are usually not placed inside the 5.0 mm optical zone, and conservative nomograms use a standard 7.0 mm optical zone to reduce glare and aberrations. Incisions to correct post-PK astigmatism may be placed in the graft, in the graft–host junction, or in the host, but this last provides minimal effect.

EFFICACY AND PREDICTABILITY Few large prospective trials exist. The ARC-T study (referenced below) showed reduction in astigmatism using a 7.0 mm optical zone and varying arc lengths of 1.6 D ±1.1 D from the preoperative mean of 2.8 D ±1.2 D. Other studies suggest final uncorrected visual acuity of 20/20 in 20%–33% and 20/40 in 65%–80% eyes with congenital astigmatism. Overcorrections occur in 4%–20% of patients.

POSTOPERATIVE REFRACTION, VISUAL ACUITY, AND CORNEAL TOPOGRAPHY Irregular astigmatism can occur or increase after AK.

STABILITY OF REFRACTION There are no reports longer than 6 months.

COMPLICATIONS Complications are similar to RK. Off-axis astigmatic keratotomy can lead to undercorrection or worsening of preexisting astigmatism. To avoid creating an isolated block or edge of cornea that swells and cannot be epithelialized, astigmatic incisions should not intersect other incisions (radial).

OCULAR SURGERY AFTER ASTIGMATIC KERATOTOMY AK can be combined with or done after cataract, RK, PRK, or LASIK surgery. PK can be done after extensive AK, but the wounds may have to be closed as in RK.

FUTURE DEVELOPMENTS Recently, full-arc depth-dependent AK has been described with placement of paired arcuate incisions 90° in length and with variable depth determined by nomogram. The technique may offer better corneal sphericity and less chance of corneal perforation than the current technique. Since its FDA approval, LASIK is the procedure of choice for correction of myopic astigmatism and hyperopic astigmatism.

Akura J, Matsuura K, Hatta S, et al. A new concept for the correction of astigmatism—full arc, depth dependent astigmatic keratotomy. *Ophthalmology*. 2000;107:95–104.

Faktorovich EG, Maloney RK, Price FW Jr. Effect of astigmatic keratotomy on spherical equivalent: results of the Astigmatism Reduction Clinical Trial. *Am J Ophthalmol*. 1999; 127:260–269.

Price FW, Grene RB, Marks RG, et al. ARC-T Study Group. Astigmatism reduction clinical trial: a multicenter prospective evaluation of the predictability of arcuate keratotomy. *Arch Ophthalmol*. 1995;113:277–282.

CHAPTER 26

Laser Procedures for Refractive Correction

The overwhelming advantage of photoablation is the submicron precision with which it removes tissue. This potential was first recognized in 1983 by Trokel and exploited in clinical trials in the United States beginning in 1988. The FDA granted approval for the use of photoablation in treatment of low myopia without significant astigmatism in 1995 and has since expanded its indications for use (Table 26-1).

> United States Food and Drug Administration—Center for Devices and Radiological Health Website. www.fda.gov/cdrh/LASIK/lasers.htm

Excimer Laser for Photorefractive Keratectomy (PRK)

The popularity of PRK has decreased with the increasingly widespread use of LASIK. Nevertheless, PRK has some advantages: because no flap is made, this procedure eliminates microkeratome-associated risks; it can also be used in thinner corneas because less corneal stroma is altered. In addition, PRK can be used for both refractive and therapeutic purposes in patients with map-dot-fingerprint dystrophy. Disadvantages of PRK compared to LASIK are longer initial visual recovery time and associated discomfort, greater difficulty of enhancement, and potential prolonged use of topical steroid medication.

PRK for Myopia

PATIENT SELECTION Despite the broader range of FDA approval, most surgeons confine use of PRK to mild and moderate myopia (less than 7 D). Patients should discontinue soft contact lenses for at least 1 week, and rigid gas-permeable contact lenses for at least 4 weeks, before refraction and topography are performed in order to achieve corneal stability. Patients should be counseled about realistic expectations: unrealistic patient expectations are an absolute contraindication to refractive surgery. Prepresbyopic and presbyopic patients should be informed about loss of near vision and offered the option of undercorrection for one eye (monovision).

Correction of tear deficiency should be carefully considered before PRK to reduce problems of haze and regression. Patients with significant connective tissue disease, active corneal disease, or corneal thinning disorders such as keratoconus or pellucid marginal degeneration should not have PRK. Although keloid formation has been thought to be

Table 26-1 FDA-Approved Lasers for Refractive Surgery (as of January 2004)

Company and Model	Approval Number and Date	Approved Indications (D = Diopters)
Lasers for LASIK		
Alcon: LADARVision	P970043/S10 10/18/02	Wavefront-guided LASIK: Myopia up to −7.0 D with or without astigmatism less than 0.5 D
Autonomous Technology: LADARVision	P970043/S5 5/9/00	Myopia less than −9.0 D with or without astigmatism from −0.5 to −3.0 D
Bausch & Lomb Surgical: Technolas 217a	P990027 2/23/00	Myopia from −1.0 to −7.0 D with or without astigmatism less than −3.0 D
Bausch & Lomb Surgical: Technolas 217a	P990027/S2 5/15/02	Myopia less than −11.0 D with or without astigmatism less than −3.0 D
Bausch & Lomb Surgical: Technolas 217a	P990027/S4 2/25/03	Hyperopia between 1.0 and 4.0 D with or without astigmatism up to 2.0 D
Bausch & Lomb Surgical: Technolas 217z	P990027/S6 5/15/02	Wavefront-guided LASIK: Myopia up to −7.0 D with or without astigmatism up to −3.0 D
LaserSight: LaserScan LSX	P980008/S5 9/28/01	Myopia from −0.5 to −6.0 D with or without astigmatism up to 4.5 D
Nidek: EC5000	P970053/S2 4/14/00	Myopia from −1.0 to −14.0 D with or without astigmatism less than 4.0 D
Summit Autonomous: LADARVision	P970043/S7 9/22/00	Hyperopia less than +6.0 D with or without astigmatism less than −6.0 D
VISX: Star S2 & S3	P930016/S12 4/27/01	Hyperopia between +0.5 and +5.0 D with or without astigmatism up to +3.0 D
VISX: Star S2 & S3	P930016/S14 11/16/01	Mixed astigmatism up to 6.0 D; cylinder is greater than sphere and of opposite sign
VISX: Star S3 (EyeTracker)	P990010/S1 4/20/00	Same as S2, except with eye tracker
VISX: Star S4 & WaveScan WaveFront System	P930016/S16 5/23/03	Wavefront-guided LASIK: Myopia up to −6.0 D with or without astigmatism up to −3.0 D
WaveLight: ALLEGRETTO WAVE	P020050 10/07/03	Myopia up to −12.0 D with or without astigmatism up to −6.0 D
WaveLight: ALLEGRETTO WAVE	P030008 10/10/03	Hyperopia up to +6.0 D with or without astigmatism
Lasers for PRK and other refractive surgeries		
Bausch & Lomb Surgical: KERACOR 116	P970056 9/28/99	PRK; Myopia from −1.5 to −7.0 D with or without astigmatism less than −4.5 D
LaserSight: LaserScan LSX	P980008 11/12/99	PRK; Myopia from −1.0 to −6.0 D with or without astigmatism less than 1.0 D

(Continued)

Table 26-1 FDA-Approved Lasers for Refractive Surgery (as of January 2004) (Continued)

Company and Model	Approval Number and Date	Approved Indications (D = Diopters)
Nidek: EC5000	P970053/S1 9/29/99	PRK; Myopia from −1.0 to −8.0 D with or without astigmatism from −0.5 to −4.0 D
Refractec: ViewPoint CK System	P010018 4/11/02	Conductive keratoplasty; Hyperopia from +0.75 to +3.25 D with or without astigmatism up to 0.75 D
Summit: Apex Plus	P930034/S9 3/11/98	PRK; Myopia from −1.0 to −6.0 D with or without astigmatism from −1.0 to −4.0 D
Summit: Apex Plus	P930034/S12 10/21/99	PRK; Hyperopia from +1.5 to +4.0 D with or without astigmatism less than −1.0 D
Summit Autonomous: LADARVision	P970043/S8 7/11/00	Name change only
Sunrise: Hyperion	P990078 6/30/00	Laser thermokeratoplasty (LTK); Hyperopia from +0.75 to +2.5 D with or without astigmatism less than 0.75 D
VISX: Model B & C (Star & Star S2)	P9300163/S3 4/24/97	PRK; Myopia from 0 to −6.0 D with or without astigmatism from −0.75 to −4.0 D
VISX: Model B & C (Star & Star S2)	P930016/S5 1/29/98	PRK; Myopia from 0 to −12.0 D with or without astigmatism from 0 to −4.0 D
VISX: Star S2	P930016/S7 11/2/98	PRK; Hyperopia from +1.0 to +6.0 D
VISX: Star S2 & S3	P930016/S10 10/18/00	PRK; Hyperopia from +0.5 to +5.0 D with or without astigmatism +0.5 to +4.0 D
VISX: Star S2 & S3	P9300116/S13 3/19/01	Add myopia blend zone; increase overall ablation zone from 6.5 to 8.0 mm

(Adapted from United States Food and Drug Administration website: www.fda.gov/cdrh/LASIK/lasers.htm. See website for updates.)

a contraindication to PRK, one recent study found that African Americans with history of keloid formation did well after PRK. Patients with epithelial basement membrane dystrophy (EBMD; eg, map-dot-fingerprint dystrophy) considering refractive surgery are good candidates for PRK rather than LASIK because PRK may be therapeutic. Female patients who are pregnant should wait 3–6 months after completing nursing before having PRK because of the possibility of regression from hormonal effects.

The surgeon should anticipate the patient's post-PRK keratometric readings and exclude anyone whose keratometric readings would be too flat or too steep after PRK. The post-PRK cornea should probably not be flatter than 35 D or steeper than 48–50 D because of potential adverse effects on visual quality and/or acuity. The cornea flattens approximately 0.8 D for every diopter of myopia treated.

SURGICAL TECHNIQUES Patients should be educated about the surgery, including the sights, sounds, and odors to be anticipated during the procedure. The laser is calibrated, then the patient is aligned under the instrument. The optical zone (typically 6.0–6.5 mm centered around the visual axis) may be marked depending on the mode of epithelial removal. Epithelium is carefully and completely removed in this zone by one of the following methods:

- Mechanically scraping with spatula or blade, with or without topical 20% ethyl alcohol
- Using an automated brush
- Using the laser to reduce the thickness and then scraping the residue
- Using the laser to completely remove epithelium to Bowman's layer

The optical zone does not need to be marked if laser ablation of the epithelium is being performed.

The optical zone must be free of epithelial cells, debris, and excess fluid before ablation. Ablation typically takes 20–60 seconds for broad-beam excimer lasers and two to three times longer for scanning and flying-spot lasers. The patient fixates with verbal encouragement from the surgeon, aided by tracking devices available on some lasers. Mechanical fixation is used in the presence of poor patient cooperation. Some lasers require an erodible masking material to improve the smoothness of the postoperative surface (see Figure 24-5). Immediately postoperatively, topical nonsteroidal agents and antibiotics are used to reduce pain and combat potential infection. Although limited use of topical anesthetic has been reported for postoperative analgesia, this technique is still not considered standard of care. Bandage contact lenses or patching may be used, and the patient is followed until the epithelium heals. Some surgeons use topical steroids for up to 3 months postoperatively.

INSTRUMENTATION Broad-beam and scanning lasers have been FDA approved for PRK.

VARIABLES AFFECTING OUTCOME Surgical variables include method of epithelial removal, type of laser, size of optical zone, and depth of ablation. Patient variables include wound-healing response, age, attempted correction, and pregnancy (effect could be decreased during pregnancy).

EFFICACY AND PREDICTABILITY Almost all patients show a reduction in myopia and an increase in uncorrected visual acuity (UCVA). Predictability varies by degree of myopia; greatest accuracy occurs with a target correction of less than 3.00 D. Overall, refractive outcome is within 0.50 D in approximately 50%–68% of patients and within 1.00 D in 77%–92% at 1 year. UCVA is 20/20 in approximately 50%–72%, and 20/40 in 85%–98%, of patients (with myopia up to 6.00 D). For patients with myopia greater than 6.00 D, 20%–60% are within 1.00 D of emmetropia. UCVA is 20/40 or better in 60%–90% of higher myopes. Choice of laser, size of optical zone, and use of multizone/multipass technique (see Figure 24-10) can affect these results.

CORNEAL TOPOGRAPHY AFTER PRK Topography has been used to estimate decentration of ablation and to study central islands. Decentration of 1.0 mm or more is associated with increased symptoms of ghosting, induced astigmatism, and monocular diplopia.

Central islands are defined as 1.00–3.00 D elevations of 1–3 mm diameter occurring at least 1 month postoperatively and associated with visual symptoms or refractive changes. Central islands occur in up to 17% of patients, depending on the diligence of interpretation of the computerized videokeratography and choice of laser (they are not reported with scanning lasers). No consensus exists on the cause of the islands, but they may be related to epithelial hyperplasia or incomplete ablation secondary to the collection of stromal fluid from acoustic shock wave or ablation plume. Nonhomogeneous laser beams may be a possible cause as well. Despite the introduction of central island pre-treatment programs for broad-beam lasers, central islands still occur. Symptomatic central islands that do not spontaneously resolve after 6 months can be treated with a transepithelial approach.

CHANGE IN BEST-CORRECTED VISUAL ACUITY Gain or loss of one line of best-corrected visual acuity is within normal variation of Snellen testing. Loss of two lines or more occurs in 2%–4% of patients at 1 year but declines to less than 1% at 2 years.

STABILITY OF REFRACTION In general, a 1-month low hyperopic response (planned over-correction) is followed by regression of 0.50–1.00 D toward myopia over 6–12 months and then no significant change for up to 6 years. Absolute values should be verified for each laser. No reports of long-term hyperopic drift, as seen in RK, have been recorded.

COMPLICATIONS Complications may be related to deviations from planned correction, postoperative medication, wound healing, or mechanical factors. *Undercorrection* occurs much more frequently at higher degrees of myopia: 65% of extreme myopes (greater than 10.00 D) will be undercorrected (more than -1.00 D myopic) at 1 year, in contrast to 10%–20% of myopes less then -6.00 D. Regression is associated with smaller optical zones and deeper ablations and is reduced by multizone treatment and zone sizes of 6.0 mm and larger. Undercorrection is associated with loss of uncorrected visual acuity and may respond temporarily to increased steroid use. It may require retreatment if symptomatic, as reported in 9%–15% of patients.

Overcorrection of more than $+1.00$ D at 1 year is much less frequent, occurring in less than 5% of all myopes. It may be related to age (>40 years). Overcorrection does not always respond to the withdrawal of steroids and may require hyperopic retreatment. Use of topical nonsteroidals or soft contact lenses may decrease small overcorrections.

More than 1.00 D of *induced astigmatism* occurs in 2%–5% of patients at 1 year. It can be treated with myopic or hyperopic astigmatic PRK or LASIK or with astigmatic keratotomy peripheral to the ablation zone.

Tear secretion test values have been noted to decrease after PRK or PARK and may be caused by the temporary decrease in corneal sensation that occurs after the procedure.

Steroid-induced glaucoma occurs in 1.5%–3.0% of patients using fluorometholone but in up to 25% using dexamethasone or stronger steroids. Because of changes in corneal curvature and/or corneal thickness, Goldmann tonometry readings after PRK are artificially reduced. Measurement of IOP from the temporal rather than central cornea may be more accurate, and Tonopen readings also are more reliable. *Steroid-induced herpes simplex virus keratitis* is a rare event that requires withdrawal of steroid and initiation of antiherpetic treatment (known ocular herpes is a relative contraindication to PRK). *Steroid-induced ptosis* usually resolves on discontinuation of the steroid. *Steroid-induced cataract* has been reported with steroids other than fluorometholone used 4 or more times per day for more than 3 months.

The use of therapeutic contact lenses to aid in epithelial healing is associated with *sterile infiltrates*, especially in patients using topical nonsteroidal anti-inflammatory drugs (NSAIDs) for longer than 24 hours without concomitant topical steroids. Incidence of infectious keratitis has been reported as 0.2% (6 of 3000 PRKs); all infiltrates must be suspected to be infectious and managed appropriately.

Complications related to wound healing include *regression, recurrent corneal erosion, haze formation,* and *late scarring.* Although PTK is shown to be an effective treatment for traumatic recurrent corneal erosions, a small number of patients have had onset of erosions following PRK without demonstrated underlying dystrophy or additional trauma. These patients respond to standard treatments for recurrent corneal erosions.

Wound-healing patterns after PRK can be separated into three groups:

- Normal healers, who have trace to 1+ haze and refraction of 0 to +1.00 D at 1 month
- Inadequate healers, with no haze and refraction >+1.00 D at 1 month
- Aggressive healers, with 1+ or greater haze that increases in months 2 and 3 as refraction becomes myopic (regresses)

In addition, a group of very late (after 12 months) scar formers has been described.

Normally, haze peaks between 6 and 12 weeks and declines thereafter. Haze formation may be delayed and is possibly associated with ultraviolet exposure. The exact etiology of the haze is unknown, but it appears to be associated with increased cellular reflectivity from wound-healing keratocytes. Grade 2 haze, a reticular pattern easily detected over the ablation zone that interferes with refraction, occurs in 0%–17% of patients in different series, with increased frequency in deeper ablations. Treatment with steroids or reablation shows variable effect, and haze is known to resolve spontaneously with normal wound remodeling. Reablation should therefore be delayed for at least 6 months. Topical mitomycin (0.02%) has been used to prevent recurrence of subepithelial fibrosis after debridement.

Mechanical complications include central islands (discussed earlier under "Corneal Topography After PRK"), haloes and glare, and decentration of ablation zone. Haloes are associated with pupils that dilate beyond the ablation zone. Incidence of nighttime glare and haloes decreased from 75%–80% in patients with a 4.0 mm optical zone to 5% with a 6.0 mm optical zone and 0.5% with a 7.0 mm optical zone. However, a decrease in night vision was reported by 32% of patients in a recent publication surveying satisfaction in 690 patients who had PRK. Patients whose scotopic pupil size is larger than the ablation size are at increased risk for night vision problems.

Decentration averages 0.3–0.6 mm as determined from computerized topography and is associated with decrease in low-contrast visual acuity. Small amounts of decentration are asymptomatic, requiring no treatment.

OCULAR SURGERY AFTER PRK Retreatment with PRK, LASIK, RK, and AK has been done successfully. Cataract surgery and PK have been performed without unusual responses. IOL power for cataract surgery is calculated similarly to RK. Retinal detachment surgery has been performed after PRK. PRK has been found to be an effective method to correct anisometropia resulting from prior retinal detachment surgery.

Photoastigmatic Refractive Keratectomy (PARK)

There are two methods of performing surface ablation with moving shutters to treat regular astigmatism (but not irregular astigmatism):

- *Sequentially:* cylinder is removed from the flat or minus axis using a slit shutter with a transition zone followed by the spherical ablation with the iris shutter (or vice versa)
- *Elliptically:* simultaneous movement of the iris and the slit shutters corrects cylinder and sphere

Theoretical limits based on Munnerlyn's formula (see Chapter 24), the width of the ablation zone, and residual corneal thickness dictate the amount of astigmatism that can be treated relative to the spherical equivalent (Fig 26-1).

Ablation can also be achieved by using opaque masks with scanning slits, erodible masks, or patterns of flying spots. Handheld erodible masks have been supplanted by "in the rail" masks for more accurate and stable placement (Fig 26-2). No randomized prospective trials have compared these different technologies, many of which are proprietary and will be limited to certain lasers. Techniques to treat irregular astigmatism are likewise evolving and include topographically linked laser ablation and wavefront-guided laser ablation.

PATIENT SELECTION Congenital astigmatism of 1.00–6.00 D and postoperative astigmatism (following PK and cataract surgery) of up to 10.00 D have been treated. If the spherical equivalent is greater than 0 D, then hyperopic astigmatism techniques are required to avoid overcorrection.

SURGICAL TECHNIQUES Astigmatic correction is incorporated into the PRK program by the manufacturer. Accurate preoperative refraction and careful alignment on axis are critical, since a 15° offset in the treating axis can decrease effective cylinder change by 50% and result in a significant refractive axis shift.

INSTRUMENTATION In order to confirm accurate alignment of the patient under the laser, some surgeons preoperatively mark the horizontal corneal axis at the slit lamp.

VARIABLES AFFECTING OUTCOME PARK is similar to PRK.

EFFICACY AND PREDICTABILITY PARK is similar to PRK. However, low degrees of astigmatism are corrected more efficiently than moderate and high amounts. In a multicenter clinical trial for myopia up to -6.00 with cylinder from -0.75 D to -4.00 D, 91% of patients achieved 20/40 UCVA, and 40% of patients achieved 20/20 UCVA, by their last postoperative visit. Uncorrected visual acuity tends to be lower than with spherical PRK.

POSTOPERATIVE REFRACTION, VISUAL ACUITY, AND CORNEAL TOPOGRAPHY PARK corrects from 43% to 79% of preoperative cylinder, depending on amount of astigmatism and the laser used.

STABILITY OF REFRACTION Stability has been reported to be achieved within the first month with various broad-beam excimer lasers.

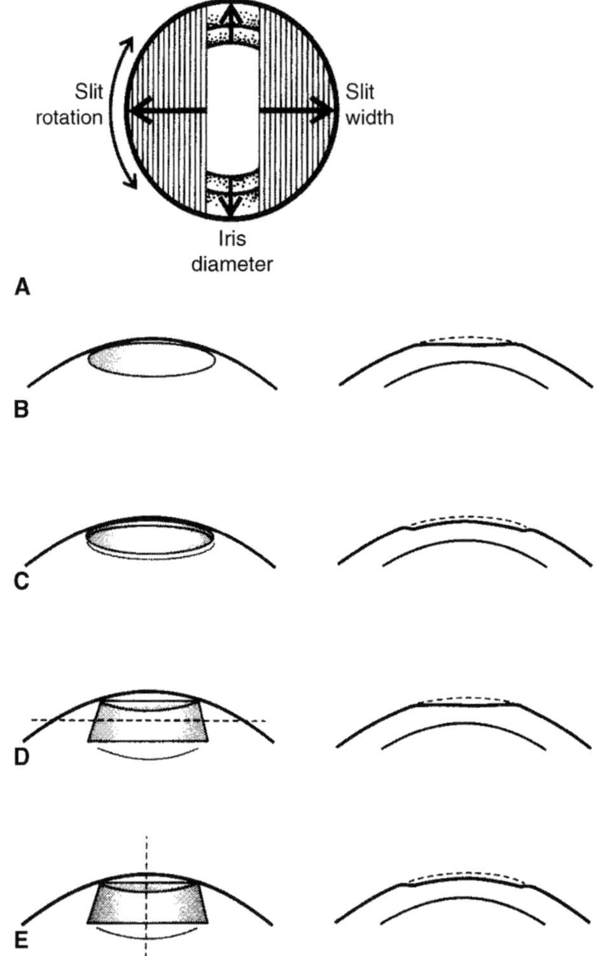

Figure 26-1 Photorefractive keratectomy for astigmatism (PARK). **A,** Schematic illustration of the method of creating cylindrical ablations by progressively widening the separation between parallel blades during the ablation. Variables that can be controlled include depth of ablation, width of ablation zone, and orientation of the slit. With blades oriented as shown, the cornea would be flattened in the horizontal meridian to correct an against-the-rule astigmatism. **B,** Comparison of myopic ablation in which the greatest amount of tissue is removed centrally and progressively less removed toward the periphery. **C,** PTK with small transition zone, in which a uniform amount of tissue is ablated without intended refractive change. **D, E,** cylindrical ablation for correction of against-the-rule astigmatism. Cross section through the originally steep meridian after ablation **(D)** is identical to myopic ablation **(B),** whereas a cross section through the originally flat meridian **(E),** in which no refractive change is intended, is identical to PTK **(C).** *(Reproduced with permission from Sietz B, McDonnell PJ. Astigmatism. In: Talamo JH, Krueger RR. The Excimer Manual: A Clinician's Guide to Excimer Laser Surgery. Boston; Little, Brown; 1997:94. Used by permission of Lippincott-Raven Publishers.)*

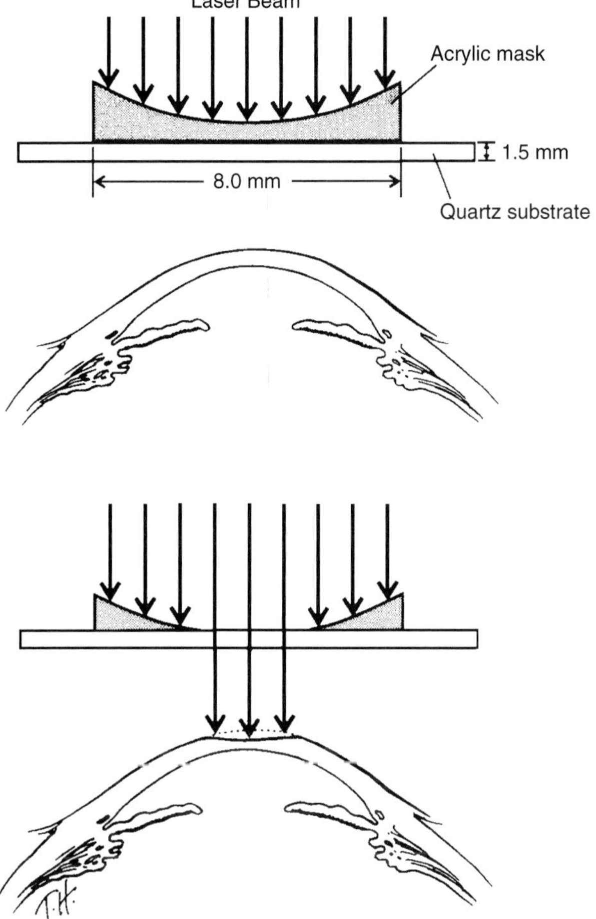

Figure 26-2 Erodible mask technique for PARK. The erodible plastic button adheres to a quartz substrate (transparent for 193 nm radiation). The shape of the mask is transferred by the wide-area laser beam inversely onto the cornea underneath the mask. When the mask is completely eroded, the greatest amount of tissue will have been ablated centrally, with progressively less tissue removed toward the periphery of the ablation zone, and more tissue ablated in the original steep meridian. *(Reproduced with permission from Sietz B, McDonnell PJ. Astigmatism. In: Talamo JH, Krueger RR. The Excimer Manual: A Clinician's Guide to Excimer Laser Surgery. Boston: Little, Brown; 1997:95. Used by permission of Lippincott-Raven Publishers.)*

COMPLICATIONS In addition to PRK complications, problems related to misalignment and the potential for inducing more irregular astigmatism must also be considered.

OCULAR SURGERY AFTER PARK Similar to myopic PRK.

Sietz B, McDonnell PJ. Astigmatism. In: Talamo JH, Krueger RR. *The Excimer Manual: A Clinician's Guide to Excimer Laser Surgery.* Boston: Little, Brown; 1997:92–102.

PRK for Hyperopia

PATIENT SELECTION PRK has been FDA approved for treatment of up to 6 D of hyperopia. Patients should be informed that hyperopic PRK is less predictable than myopic PRK and that the time to achieve stabilization is longer.

SURGICAL TECHNIQUES An area of epithelium slighter larger than 9 mm is removed prior to stromal ablation of a doughnut-shaped area with outside diameter of 9 mm and inside diameter of 5 mm.

INSTRUMENTATION Same as myopic PRK.

VARIABLES AFFECTING OUTCOME Same as myopic PRK.

EFFICACY AND PREDICTABILITY Stability is achieved between 3 and 6 months after surgery.

POSTOPERATIVE REFRACTION, VISUAL ACUITY, AND CORNEAL TOPOGRAPHY In a study of 124 patients with 1–6 D of hyperopia, UCVA was 20/40 in 91%, and 20/20 in 64%, of eyes at 1 year. Another study of 52 eyes demonstrated that by 6 months 95% achieved 20/40, and 67% were within ±0.5 D.

COMPLICATIONS Similar to myopic PRK. However, patients undergoing hyperopic PRK should be informed of a longer epithelial healing time because of the larger ablation zone as well as a temporary reduction in best-corrected visual acuity in the first week to month, which improves with time. Corneal epithelial iron ring has been reported after hyperopic PRK. Recently, 12 eyes of patients who underwent hyperopic PRK were reported to develop visually significant apical nodular scarring within 3 months of initial treatment that did not resolve spontaneously. Acute corneal necrosis after excimer laser keratectomy for hyperopia has been reported in one patient. After this patient underwent penetrating keratoplasty, light microscopy of the cornea revealed acute inflammation and keratocytes with apoptosis.

> Williams DK. One-year results of laser vision correction for low to moderate hyperopia. *Ophthalmology.* 2000;107:72–75.

PRK for Hyperopic Astigmatism

PATIENT SELECTION The FDA has approved hyperopic PRK for a spherical component from +0.5 to +5.0 with astigmatism of +0.5 to +4.0 D. Mean refractive spherical equivalent should be less than 6.0 D.

SURGICAL TECHNIQUES Similar to hyperopic PRK. The patient must be properly aligned under the laser to treat astigmatic axis accurately.

INSTRUMENTATION Same as myopic PRK.

VARIABLES AFFECTING OUTCOME Same as myopic PRK.

POSTOPERATIVE REFRACTION, VISION, AND CORNEAL TOPOGRAPHY At 12 months 61% of patients were ±0.50 D from emmetropia.

EFFICACY AND PREDICTABILITY In 276 eyes studied, 95% had UCVA ≥20/40 at 1 year; 49% were 20/20 at 6, 9, and 12 months. Stability was achieved in 97% of eyes by 12 months.

COMPLICATIONS Similar to myopic PRK. In addition, clinical trials revealed that a sub-population smaller than 5% of patients had unpredictable refractive results. These outliers occurred in all refractive categories and could not be identified preoperatively.

OCULAR SURGERY AFTER PRK Retreatment with PRK, LASIK, RK, and AK has been done successfully. Cataract surgery and PK have been performed without unusual responses. IOL power for cataract surgery is calculated similarly to RK. Retinal detachment surgery has been performed after PRK.

PRK for Mixed Astigmatism

No excimer lasers have been FDA approved to perform PRK for mixed astigmatism. The FDA has approved one laser for treatment of mixed astigmatism with LASIK (see Table 26-1).

Future Developments in PRK

The issue of whether live virus, particularly HIV, can withstand excimer laser ablation and remain infectious after aerosolization is still under investigation. Oral polio vaccine has been documented to survive excimer laser ablation.

New imaging techniques for studying the cornea in vivo will provide more information about the healing response to PRK. *Ocular coherence tomography* provides high-resolution cross-sectioning imaging of the cornea that may give more information about changes of thickness and curvature after PRK. *In vivo confocal microscopy* or *tandem scanning confocal microscopy* will also provide more information about healing in vivo. *Three-dimensional ultrasound* can determine whether steepening of the cornea was caused by epithelial hyperplasia or thickening of the stroma and, consequently, could guide the choice of retreatment regimens.

Wavefront technology can detect optical aberrations that distort a ray of light as it passes through the entire optical system. Custom laser ablation can then be performed with a small spot scanning laser equipped with a fast eye tracker and a device linking the wavefront analysis data with the laser ablation. For example, customized laser treatment, now in the early stages of development, offers the possibility of increasing the number of patients who see 20/20 or better after PRK.

Laser ablation introduces spherical aberration into the eye. Modifying the existing ablation algorithms to compensate for this induced aberration may improve postoperative visual performance. Wavefront lasers are being used for PRK to improve final visual acuity by treating aberrations; in addition, they have potential for treating irregular astigmatism.

See also "Future Developments in LASIK" later in this chapter.

L'Esperance FA Jr. Choosing the appropriate PRK patient. In: *Focal Points: Clinical Modules for Ophthalmologists.* San Francisco: American Academy of Ophthalmology; 1998: vol 16, no 9.

Sher NA. Postoperative management of the PRK patient. In: *Focal Points: Clinical Modules for Ophthalmologists.* San Francisco: American Academy of Ophthalmology; 1998: vol 16, no 10.

Laser In Situ Keratomileusis (LASIK)

LASIK (see Figure 24-7) was described by Pallikaris in 1990, with the first clinical results appearing in 1994. This procedure combines the accuracy of PRK with the healing advantages of ALK and the maintenance of an intact Bowman's layer–epithelial complex. However, LASIK adds the potential disadvantages of the complex automated keratectomy devices to the wound-healing complications of PRK. Recently, LASIK has become more popular than PRK because of high patient acceptance associated with low perioperative discomfort, rapid return of vision, and reduced need for long-term topical medications.

LASIK for Myopia

PATIENT SELECTION The maximum amount of myopia that can be treated depends on the surgeon, parameters of the chosen excimer laser, and corneal thickness. The upper limit of treatment is determined by the thickness of the remaining stromal bed after the flap thickness and ablation depth are subtracted. In addition, optical considerations must be taken into account: large optical zone ablation diameters remove more tissue than small optical zone ablation diameters. For most surgeons, the treatment limit is 15 D or less of myopia. LASIK should not be performed in patients with classic symptomatic epithelial basement membrane dystrophy (EBMD) because of the increased incidence of postoperative flap complications including flap epithelial ingrowth, flap keratolysis, and corneal scarring. In such patients, PRK can be used therapeutically for the EMBD as well as refractively to treat the myopia. Other contraindications are similar to those noted for PRK.

SURGICAL TECHNIQUES Similar to ALK, a single large-diameter (usually 8.5 mm or 9.5 mm) lamellar flap of 130–180 μm thickness is created in the standard manner. The diameter and thickness of the flap are determined by the surgeon based on such variables as the amount of refractive error to be treated (higher myopia will require a thinner flap to leave a large enough stromal bed behind), type of refractive error to be treated (hyperopic corrections require a larger flap), the corneal curvature and diameter (flatter corneas require a larger flap), and the surgeon's preference. Again as in ALK, careful attention to the maintenance, assembly, and operation of the manual or automated keratome is essential. The flap is hinged nasally or superiorly and folded back, and the stroma is ablated to the appropriate depth. The flap is repositioned after irrigation of the interface, allowed to dry, and verified to be adherent. The eye is shielded (not patched) and treated with antibiotics with or without nonsteroidal anti-inflammatory drops.

INSTRUMENTATION Microkeratomes can be automated or manual, have varying speeds of blade oscillation, use a nasal or superior flap hinge location, and have a blade angle of 25°–26°. Water jet and laser microkeratomes (Intralase femtosecond) have been introduced. Flap thickness can range from 80 μm to 220 μm (most commonly 130–180 μm). Flap diameter can range from 8 mm to 11 mm. Newer keratomes may decrease intraoperative flap complications.

VARIABLES AFFECTING OUTCOME The size of the optical zone and depth and profile of the laser ablation determine the theoretical correction. Some lasers overcorrect and some undercorrect using PRK nomograms. Treatment may have a greater effect on older patients, and this variable is included in many LASIK nomograms.

EFFICACY AND PREDICTABILITY As with PRK, accuracy depends on the initial amount of myopia. Data at 6 months suggest that 40%–60% of patients are within 0.50 D of emmetropia, and 70% are within 1.00 D. UCVA of 20/20 is obtained by 30%–40% of patients, and 20/40 by 80%–90%. Reoperation rate is 5%–10% for undercorrection, with overcorrections occurring less frequently.

POSTOPERATION REFRACTION, VISUAL ACUITY, AND CORNEAL TOPOGRAPHY Loss of two lines of best-corrected visual acuity is reported in up to 9% of patients at 6 months. Central islands are infrequent, but decentration does occur, with outcomes similar to PRK.

STABILITY OF REFRACTION Refraction shows myopic regression of magnitude similar to PRK up to 1 year.

COMPLICATIONS Complications after LASIK are related to the flap and/or laser treatment. *Microkeratome-related complications* include free flap, buttonhole of the flap, and incomplete flap. *Corneal perforation* caused by incorrect assembly of certain keratomes has been reported. Significant microkeratome complications causing abandonment of the planned LASIK procedure have been reported to occur in 0.6%–1.6% of cases; these complications are dependent on the experience of the surgeon and laser center because of the learning curve associated with microkeratome use. However, in such cases significant visual loss can be prevented if ablation is not performed at the time and the flap is allowed to heal down before another LASIK procedure is attempted months later. Some have advocated early PTK (within the first few weeks) for buttonholes.

Flap folds (Fig 26-3) are a major cause of decreased visual acuity after LASIK. Some 56% of flap folds occur on the first postoperative day, and 95% within 1 week. Although some superficial folds or microfolds are associated with flap–stromal bed mismatch in the correction of higher refractive errors, they are not visually significant and do not need to be treated. Visually significant stromal folds, microfolds, or macrofolds may result from misalignment of the corneal flap after flap replacement or movement of the corneal flap; such folds can cause hyperopic change in refraction, increased astigmatism, and/or irregular astigmatism. Lifting and refloating the flap will be more likely to eliminate the folds if they are identified and treated within 24 hours. Other techniques described to eliminate more fixed folds include removal of epithelium overlying folds prior to lifting

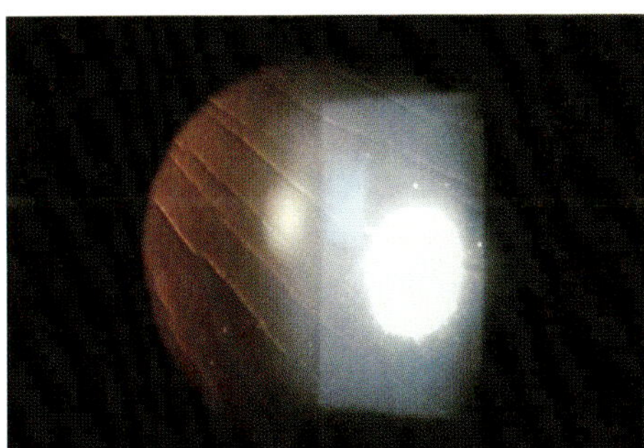

Figure 26-3 Microfolds in flap. *(Reproduced from External Disease and Cornea: A Multimedia Collection. San Francisco: American Academy of Ophthalmology; 2000.)*

the flap, hydration of the underside of the flap with deionized water or isotonic or hypotonic solution, or suturing the flap down after lifting.

Flap subluxation (Fig 26-4) has been reported to occur in up to 1.4% of eyes. If this problem is detected early, the flap should be immediately repositioned, which usually yields an excellent visual prognosis. Lost, miscut, or displaced flaps are reported to occur in 1%–3% of eyes. *Late flap dehiscence* from blunt trauma has been reported more than 1 year after LASIK.

Epithelial erosions during LASIK have been reported to occur in up to 10% of patients. Higher epithelial erosion rates may occur in older patients and patients with preexisting dry eyes or EBMD. This complication may be microkeratome, blade, or laser-center dependent. Techniques suggested to decrease the erosion rate include limitation of toxic topical medication, increase in corneal lubrication, meticulous microkeratome maintenance, and elimination of suction on the microkeratome reverse pass. Erosions may require temporary use of a bandage contact lens and can be associated with slower visual recovery or increased chance of epithelial ingrowth.

Epithelial ingrowth and implantation in the interface is reported to occur in less than 3% of eyes and is increased following enhancement procedures (Fig 26-5). Ingrowth may be related to type of keratome, angle of keratectomy blade, and surgeon experience. It can result in loosening of the flap, necrosis of the overlying flap, or significant opacity. Visually significant epithelium should be mechanically removed. Adjunctive measures have also been described, such as application of 20% alcohol to the stromal bed or underside of the flap to destroy remaining epithelial cells or suturing of the flap.

Because of changes in corneal contour and thickness, *Goldmann tonometry readings* may be inaccurately low after LASIK. Tonopen readings appear to be more accurate.

Corneal sensation is reduced in the area of ablation for at least 3 months and returns to normal in 6–12 months. This finding may be the cause of the temporary decrease in tear function that has been noted after LASIK.

An unusual syndrome, *diffuse lamellar keratitis* (DLK, sands of the Sahara, SOS) with diffuse interface haze, may occur at postoperative day 1–6 and cause decrease in vision (Fig 26-6, Table 26-2).

The condition appears to be a nonspecific inflammatory response to a variety of toxic insults. It has been reported in association with epithelial defects that occur during primary LASIK or enhancement or months after the LASIK procedure. Other reported

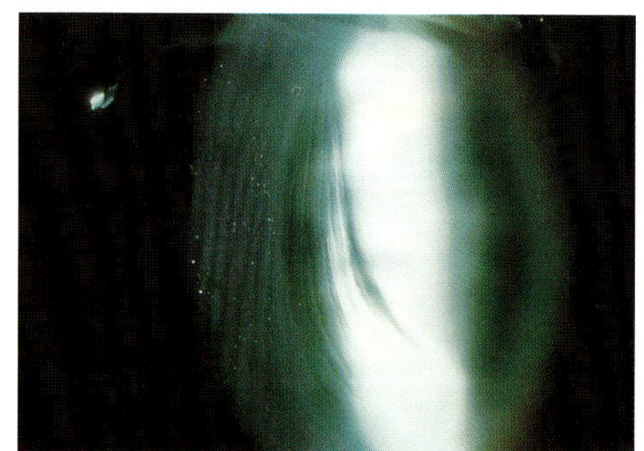

Figure 26-4 Flap subluxation. *(Reproduced from* External Disease and Cornea: A Multimedia Collection. *San Francisco: American Academy of Ophthalmology; 2000.)*

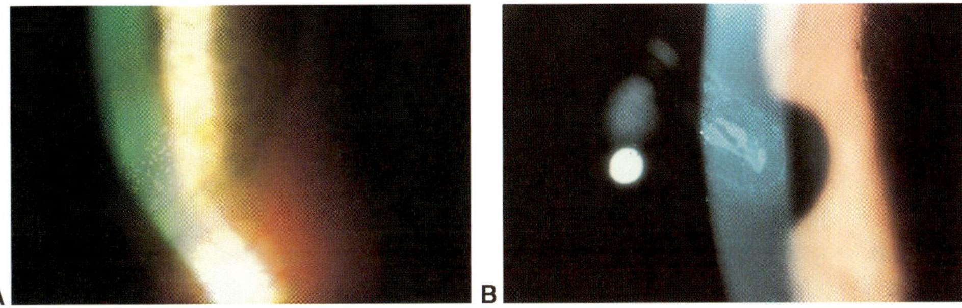

Figure 26-5 Epithelial ingrowth. **A,** Early; **B,** severe. *(Reproduced from External Disease and Cornea: A Multimedia Collection. San Francisco: American Academy of Ophthalmology; 2000.)*

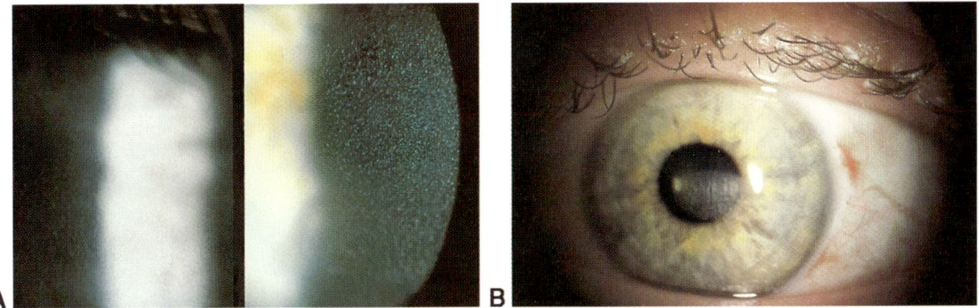

Figure 26-6 Diffuse lamellar keratitis. **A,** Stage 1 DLK. **B,** Stage 4 DLK with central scar and folds. *(Part A reproduced from External Disease and Cornea: A Multimedia Collection. San Francisco: American Academy of Ophthalmology; 2000. Part B courtesy of Jayne S. Weiss, MD.)*

Table 26-2 Staging of DLK

Stage	Findings
1	Peripheral WBCs, granular appearance
2	Central WBCs, granular appearance
3	Central dense clump of WBCs in visual axis
4	Permanent scarring or stromal melting

(WBCs = white blood cells)

inciting factors include foreign material on the surface of the microkeratome blade or motor, meibomian gland secretions, povidone-iodine solution, substances produced by laser ablation, contamination of the sterilizer with gram-negative endotoxin, and red blood cells in the interface. Although stages 1 and 2 usually respond to frequent topical steroids, stages 3 and 4 usually require lifting the flap and irrigating, followed by intensive topical steroid treatment. Systemic steroids may be used adjunctively in severe cases. Recovery of vision is usually excellent if the condition is managed early.

Infections have been reported with *Staphylococcus epidermidis, Pneumococcus, Streptococcus viridans, Mycobacterium chelonae, Nocardia asteroides, Aspergillus flavus, Scedos-*

porium apiospermum, and *Curvularia* (Fig 26-7). The infiltrates, which should be distinguished from DLK, can occur at the flap interface. A flap infection should be cultured and aggressively treated with topical antibiotics. Sterile peripheral keratitis has also been reported after LASIK.

Iatrogenic keratectasia can develop after LASIK if there is insufficient remaining stromal bed. Most surgeons leave 250–300 μm of cornea untouched by laser ablation or corneal flap dissection. In addition, corneal thinning disorders such as keratoconus, suspected keratoconus, or pellucid marginal degeneration are contraindications to LASIK. Although keratectasia is usually considered when LASIK is performed for higher myopic corrections, in thin corneas, or in patients who have had multiple laser ablations, the condition has also been reported to occur in eyes with less than 4 D of myopia. Gas-permeable contact lenses or penetrating keratoplasty may be required for treatment. Intracorneal ring segments (Intacs) are being investigated as a possible treatment.

Corneal perforation occurring during laser ablation has been reported from inaccurately calculating or assuming the stromal thickness.

Rare complications include optic nerve ischemia, premacular subhyaloid hemorrhage, and macular hemorrhage associated with preexisting lacquer cracks or choroidal neovascularization.

LASIK for Myopic Astigmatism

PATIENT SELECTION FDA-approved parameters depend on the particular laser, but up to approximately 14 D of myopia and 5 D of astigmatism can be treated.

SURGICAL TECHNIQUES Similar to LASIK for myopia except that the patient should be positioned meticulously to align the laser treatment accurately. The axis of astigmatism can be marked.

INSTRUMENTATION Similar to myopic LASIK.

VARIABLES AFFECTING OUTCOME Similar to myopic LASIK.

EFFICACY AND PREDICTABILITY In one study, at 6 months 52.8% of eyes had UCVA of 20/20 or better, and 93.6% of eyes had UCVA of 20/40 or better. Another study at 6 months showed 47.4% with UCVA of 20/20 or better, and 84.4% with UCVA of 20/40 or better.

POSTOPERATIVE REFRACTION, VISUAL ACUITY, AND CORNEAL TOPOGRAPHY At 6 months one study reported 73.2% of eyes within ±0.50 D of intended manifest refraction spherical equivalent (MRSE), and 96% of eyes within ±1.00 D of intended MRSE.

STABILITY OF REFRACTION Most of the stabilization occurs in the first month, with complete stabilization achieved between 3 and 6 months postoperatively.

COMPLICATIONS Similar to myopic LASIK, but at 6 months 15% of eyes that had LASIK for myopic astigmatism encountered difficulty with night driving, as compared to 6% of eyes that had LASIK for myopia alone.

LASIK for Hyperopia

PATIENT SELECTION LASIK has been FDA approved for correction of hyperopia up to 6 D.

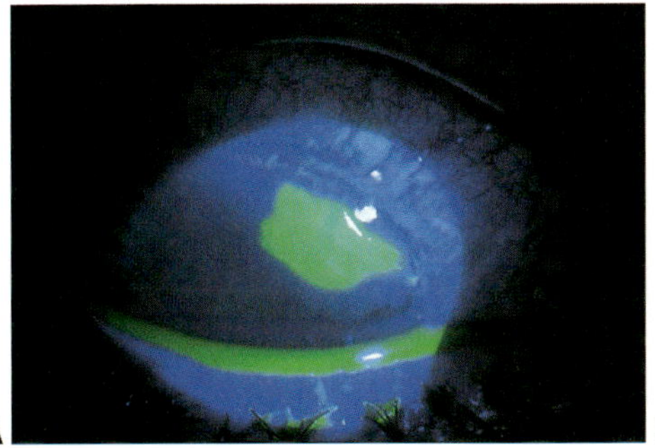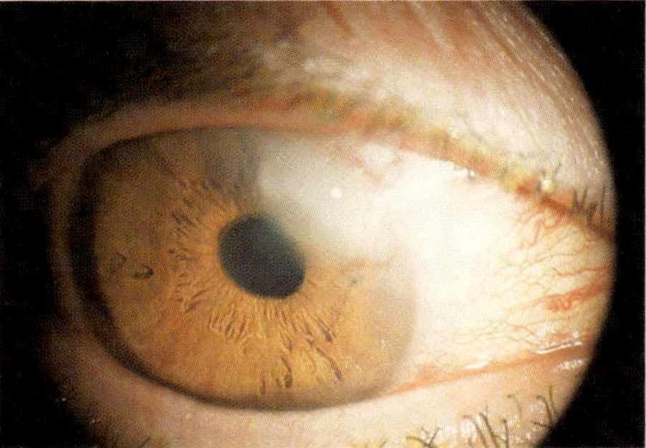

Figure 26-7 Corneal flap infection after LASIK. **A,** Fluorescein staining epithelial defect. **B,** Corneal flap infiltrate. *(Photographs courtesy of Jayne S. Weiss, MD.)*

SURGICAL TECHNIQUES A flap of at least 9.5 mm is made with the microkeratome in preparation for the laser treatment at 9.5 mm. Because of the larger laser treatment area compared to myopic LASIK, the flap hinge must often be protected during the ablation. Centration is critical during ablation.

INSTRUMENTATION Similar to LASIK for myopia.

VARIABLES AFFECTING OUTCOME Similar to LASIK for myopia.

EFFICACY AND PREDICTABILITY At 6 months, 20/40 UCVA was achieved by 95% of patients with hyperopia of less than 3.0 D, and by 78% with hyperopia of 3.0–5.0 D. Retreatment was performed in 20% of low hyperopes and 33.3% of moderate hyperopes.

POSTOPERATIVE REFRACTION, VISUAL ACUITY, AND CORNEAL TOPOGRAPHY At 6 months after hyperopic LASIK, UCVA of 20/20 was achieved by 64% of patients with 1.0–1.99 D of hyperopia, 48% of patients with 2.0–2.99 D of hyperopia, 33% of patients with 3.0–3.99 D of hyperopia, and 40% of patients with 4.0–4.99 D of hyperopia. Only 11.1% of patients with 5.0–6.0 D of hyperopia achieved 20/20, with 10% of patients in the highest hyperopia group losing 2 lines of best-corrected acuity. Hyperopic LASIK has been performed successfully for consecutive hyperopia after PRK, ALK, RK, and LASIK.

Higher amounts of hyperopic treatments result in a smaller central area of steepening and increased likelihood for loss of best-corrected visual acuity with small decentrations. Consequently, despite the larger range of FDA approval, some surgeons do not treat hyperopia greater than 3–4 D.

STABILITY OF REFRACTION Because of regression after hyperopic treatment, the patient should initially be overcorrected or myopic immediately after treatment to allow for full correction of hyperopia after stabilization.

COMPLICATIONS Loss of best-corrected visual acuity is not uncommon within the first month after treatment. At 1 month after hyperopic LASIK, only 72% of patients were corrected to 20/20 with their glasses, but this improved to 87% at 6 months.

Small treatment decentration can result in decentration of central steepening on topography and associated loss of visual acuity. Poor topographic results with poor visual acuity are more frequent at higher levels of hyperopic treatments.

LASIK for Hyperopic Astigmatism

PATIENT SELECTION Hyperopic astigmatic correction is FDA approved for hyperopia less than 6.0 D with astigmatism less than 6.0 D.

SURGICAL TECHNIQUES Similar to LASIK for hyperopia.

INSTRUMENTATION Similar to LASIK for myopia.

VARIABLES AFFECTING OUTCOME Similar to LASIK for myopia.

EFFICACY AND PREDICTABILITY Of the 66 eyes followed at 9 months, 95% had UCVA of 20/40 or better, and 57.6% had UCVA of 20/20 or better. Efficacy was decreased with higher refractive errors. For example, at 6 months 36.7% of eyes with 1.0–1.99 D spherical equivalent achieved 20/20, but only 17.6% of eyes with 4.0–4.99 D spherical equivalent achieved 20/20.

POSTOPERATIVE REFRACTION, VISUAL ACUITY, AND CORNEAL TOPOGRAPHY At 6 months, 50% of eyes were within ±0.50 D of intended MRSE, and 89% were within ±1.00 D of intended MRSE.

STABILITY OF REFRACTION Although most stabilization occurred in the first month, there was a small, continued regression up to 9 months.

COMPLICATIONS Similar to myopic LASIK. Although 12% of eyes lost two lines of best-corrected visual acuity at 1 month, only 4% of eyes showed this change at 9 months.

OCULAR SURGERY AFTER LASIK Elevation of the flap and retreatment with the excimer laser has been successfully done beyond 12 months. Cataract surgery, astigmatic keratotomy, PRK, PTK, ICR placement, and retinal detachment surgery have also been successfully performed after LASIK.

Future Developments in LASIK

Some subclinical changes have been noted after LASIK and PRK that could have future implications. Malondialdehyde (MDA) was increased in the rabbit lens after LASIK but not after PRK, so this finding is probably related to use of the microkeratome in LASIK. Higher MDA levels may suggest oxidative events that could be associated with subsequent cataractogenesis. Aqueous flare is increased after LASIK and PRK but not after intracorneal rings. Retinal nerve fiber layer thickness decreases after LASIK. However, there are no publications documenting the clinical relevance of these observations.

Continued improvements in microkeratomes should lead to better LASIK results by decreasing complications. The *femtosecond laser* can be used to create a corneal flap, but published results are not available.

Wavefront-guided laser ablation may improve visual results by inducing less higher-order aberration than conventional excimer laser. In one study, higher-order aberrations increased 20% after wavefront-guided LASIK compared to 77% after conventional LASIK; and 52.5% of wavefront-guided patients had uncorrected visual acuity equal to or better than the preoperative best-corrected visual acuity.

Recent published results on *topographically guided LASIK* to treat corneal irregularities demonstrated improved uncorrected vision and regularity in patients with severe corneal irregularities from decentered optical zone after LASIK or irregular astigmatism after keratoplasty or trauma. Poorer results were found in patients with small irregularities such as central islands. Topographically guided LASIK could be indicated in scarred or extremely irregular corneas with so much distortion that wavefront measurement would be too rough for custom corneal ablation.

The *Nd:YLF picosecond laser* has been used in clinical trials in nonsighted eyes to create an instrastromal lenticule that is removed by lifting an anterior flap in the cornea.

In *laser-assisted subepithelial keratomileusis (LASEK)*, laser ablation is performed under an epithelial flap. The epithelium is trephined and peeled back after focal placement of 20% ethanol onto the trephination site through a well. This procedure may offer both decreased risk because no stromal flap is created and increased comfort because the corneal epithelium is preserved.

Although LASIK has rapidly surpassed PRK in popularity for treatment of many refractive errors, visual results are actually very similar between the procedures. A study of patients treated for myopia of −1.00 D to −9.50 D showed equal refractive outcomes. Another study of treatment of myopia between −6.00 D and −15.00 D showed slightly less tendency for postoperative optical symptoms in LASIK eyes compared to PRK eyes. Potential complications of LASIK are more severe than with PRK, including the possibility of corneal perforation associated with certain microkeratomes and endophthalmitis. However, common problems related to PRK are reduced with LASIK (epithelial healing, topical steroids for months, haze formation), and reoperations may be easier for the patient.

See also "Future Developments in PRK" earlier in this chapter.

Dastgheib KA, Clinch TE, Manch EE, et al. Sloughing of corneal epithelium and wound healing complications associated with laser in situ keratomileusis in patients with epithelial basement membrane dystrophy. *Am J Ophthalmol.* 2000;130:297–303.

Linebarger EJ, Hardten DR, Lindstrom RL. Diffuse lamellar keratitis: diagnosis and management. *J Cataract Refract Surg.* 2000;26:1072–1077.

Pallikaris IG, Siganos DS. Excimer laser in situ keratomileusis and photorefractive keratectomy for correction of high myopia. *J Refract Corneal Surg.* 1994;10:498–510.

Pop M, Payette Y. Photorefractive keratectomy versus laser is situ keratomileusis: a control-matched study. *Ophthalmology.* 2000;107:251–257.

Price FW. LASIK. In: *Focal Points: Clinical Modules for Ophthalmologists.* San Francisco: American Academy of Ophthalmology; 2000: vol 18, no 3.

Zadok D, Tran DB, Twa M, et al. Pneumotonometry versus Goldmann tonometry after laser in situ keratomileusis for myopia. *J Cataract Refract Surg.* 1999;25:1344–1348.

Laser Treatment of Presbyopia

There are no FDA-approved excimer laser procedures for presbyopia treatment. Techniques are still in evolution, with few published results.

Both decentration of excimer laser myopic ablation and zonal excimer laser using a specially designed mask have been reported for treatment of presbyopia. One publication reported that inferior decentration of 1 mm caused steepening of the inferior cornea, resulting in good distance and near visual acuity with no loss of spectacle-corrected vision at 22 months. Long-term studies in a large cohort are not available.

Thermokeratoplasty

The noncontact holmium-YAG laser can heat and shrink corneal stroma *(laser thermokeratoplasty)*, thus producing corneal steepening and correction of hyperopia or hyperopic astigmatism. The contact holmium-YAG laser was withdrawn from the market because of regression and unpredictability of effect. Clinical investigations are continuing into the use of diathermy for correction of hyperopia.

PATIENT SELECTION Noncontact holmium-YAG laser has been FDA approved for correction of hyperopia of at least 0.75 D to 2.50 D in patients who are 40 years and older with 0.75 D or less of astigmatism.

SURGICAL TECHNIQUES The patient is given topical anesthetic and waits for a standardized period of drying. One set of 8 laser treatment spots is delivered to the cornea at a 6 mm optical zone, and an additional 8 spots are applied at a 7 mm optical zone (Fig 26-8).

INSTRUMENTATION The Sunrise Hyperion LTK is the only FDA-approved device currently available for thermokeratoplasty.

VARIABLES AFFECTING OUTCOME Patient variables include age and amount of hyperopia. Surgical variables include optical zone of spot placement, number of spots placed, and millijoule power applied by the laser for each spot. The treatment nomogram is based on the patient's age and hyperopia to program the millijoules of energy applied to each of the 16 laser spots.

EFFICACY AND PREDICTABILITY A total of 612 eyes were enrolled in the U.S. trials; 2-year followup was available for 72 patients. At 2 years, UCVA was 20/40 or better in 68%, 20/25 or better in 47%, and 20/20 or better in 20%.

STABILITY OF REFRACTION Overcorrection or myopia is expected over the first 6 months. Appropriate correction was achieved by 6–12 months. However, smaller amounts of regression still occurred over the 2 years of study. Little data is available on timing and efficacy of repeat treatments.

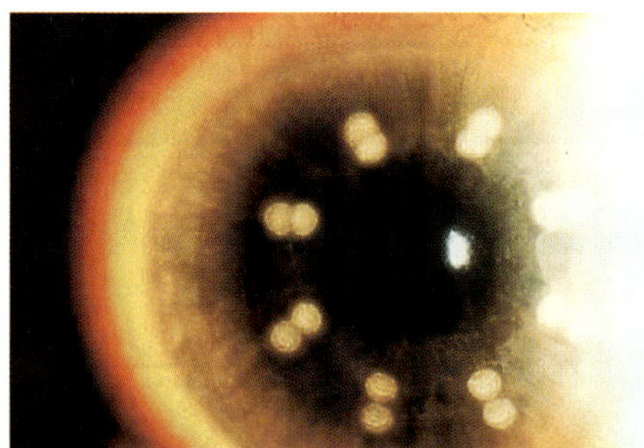

Figure 26-8 Peripheral white thermokeratoplasty spots. *(Reproduced from* External Disease and Cornea: A Multimedia Collection. *San Francisco: American Academy of Ophthalmology; 2000.)*

COMPLICATIONS The central visual axis is not treated by the laser, and the complication rate is low. Less than 1% of eyes in the clinical trials lost 2 or more lines of vision after 3 months. When vision loss did occur, it was associated with other conditions such as cataract formation. Although 3.5% of eyes had more than 2 D of induced cylinder at 1 month, this number had decreased to 0.2% at 12 months. However, 5% of patients still had 1 D of induced cylinder at 12 months. Patients should not have enhancement surgery until stability is achieved.

The advantages of laser thermokeratoplasty are the low complication rate, excellent safety, and ease of the procedure. The disadvantage is the variability of effect caused by regression. Holmium laser thermokeratoplasty has been reported to be useful for treatment of overcorrection after PRK despite a low predictability. There are no publications concerning the results of laser thermokeratoplasty after LASIK, although the effect has been noted to be enhanced after lamellar corneal cutting.

Ismail MM, Perez-Santonja JJ, Alio JL. Laser thermokeratoplasty after lamellar corneal cutting. *J Cataract Refract Surg.* 1999;25:212–215.

Conductive Keratoplasty

Conductive keratoplasty, which uses radiofrequency waves to cause corneal steepening, has been approved by the FDA for the correction of hyperopia of at least 0.75 D to 3.00 D with 0.75 D or less of astigmatism.

Basic Texts

Cornea and External Disease

Albert DM, Jakobiec FA, eds. *Principles and Practice of Ophthalmology.* 6 vols. 2nd ed. Philadelphia: Saunders; 2000.

Arffa RC, ed. *Grayson's Diseases of the Cornea.* 4th ed. St Louis: Mosby; 1997.

Brightbill FS. *Corneal Surgery: Theory, Technique, and Tissue.* 3rd ed. St Louis: Mosby; 1999.

Catania LJ. *Primary Care of the Anterior Segment.* 2nd ed. Norwalk, CT: Appleton & Lange; 1995.

Corbett M, Rosen ES, O'Brart DP. *Corneal Topography: Principles and Applications.* London: BMJ Books; 1999.

Coster DJ. *Cornea.* Fundamentals of Clinical Ophthalmology. London: BMJ Books; 2002.

Kaufman HE, Barron BA, McDonald M, eds. *The Cornea.* 2nd ed. Boston: Butterworth-Heinemann; 1998.

Krachmer JH, Mannis MJ, Holland EJ, eds. *Cornea.* 3 vols. St Louis: Mosby; 1997.

Krachmer JH, Palay DA. *Cornea Color Atlas.* St Louis: Mosby; 1999.

Leibowitz HM, Waring GO III, eds. *Corneal Disorders: Clinical Diagnosis and Management.* 2nd ed. Philadelphia: Saunders; 1998.

Murray PR. *Manual of Clinical Microbiology.* 7th ed. Washington, DC: ASM Press; 1999.

Ostler HB, Ostler MW. *Diseases of the External Eye and Adnexa: A Text and Atlas.* Baltimore: Williams and Wilkins; 1993.

Pepose JS, Holland GN, Wilhelmus KR, eds. *Ocular Infection and Immunity.* St Louis: Mosby; 1996.

Seal DV, Bron AJ, Hay J, eds. *Ocular Infection: Investigation and Treatment in Practice.* London: Martin Dunitz; 1998.

Smolin G, Thoft RA, eds. *The Cornea: Scientific Foundations and Clinical Practice.* 3rd ed. Boston: Little, Brown; 1994.

Related Academy Materials

Focal Points: Clinical Modules for Ophthalmologists

Dubord PJ. Scleritis and episcleritis (Module 9, 1995).

Dunn SP. Iris repair: putting the pieces back together (Module 11, 2002).

Gans LA. Surgical treatment of pterygium (Module 12, 1996).

Garcia-Ferrer FJ, Schwab IR. New laboratory diagnostic techniques for corneal and external disease (Module 9, 2002).

Heidemann DG. Atopic and vernal keratoconjunctivitis (Module 1, 2001).

Helm CJ. Melanoma and other pigmented lesions of the ocular surface (Module 11, 1996).

Hodge W, Hwang DJ. Antibiotic use in corneal and external disease (Module 10, 1997).

Koch DD. Cataract surgery after refractive surgery (Module 5, 2001).

L'Esperance FA. Choosing the appropriate PRK patient (Module 9, 1998).

Maguire LJ. Computerized corneal analysis (Module 5, 1996).

Margo CE. Nonpigmented lesions of the ocular surface (Module 9, 1996).

Mets MB, Noffke AS. Ocular infections of the external eye and cornea in children (Module 2, 2002).

Parrish CM. Herpes simplex virus eye disease (Module 2, 1997).

Raizman MB. Update on ocular allergy (Module 5, 1994).

Schultze RL, Singh GD. Neurotrophic keratitis (Module 2, 2003).

Sher NA. Postoperative management of the PRK patient (Module 10, 1998).

Stein RM, Stein HA. Corneal complications of contact lenses (Module 2, 1993).

Zloty P. Diagnosis and management of fungal keratitis (Module 6, 2002).

Publications

Lane SS, Skuta GL, eds. *ProVision: Preferred Responses in Ophthalmology,* Series 3 (Self-Assessment Program, 1999; reviewed for currency 2001).

Skuta GL, ed. *ProVision: Preferred Responses in Ophthalmology,* Series 2 (Self-Assessment Program, 1996; reviewed for currency 2001).

Wang MX. *Corneal Dystrophies and Degenerations: A Molecular Genetics Approach* (Ophthalmology Monograph 16, 2003).

Wilson FM II, ed. *Practical Ophthalmology: A Manual for Beginning Residents* (1996).

Slide-Scripts

Fong DS. *Eye Care for the Elderly* (Eye Care Skills for the Primary Care Physician Series, 1999).

Mead MD, Shingleton BJ. *Eye Trauma and Emergencies* (Eye Care Skills for the Primary Care Physician Series, 1996; reviewed for currency 1999).

Continuing Ophthalmic Video Education

Al-Torbak AA. *Capsulorrhexis in Mature Cataract;* Dewey SH, Werner L, Apple DJ, et al. *Cortical Removal by J-Cannula Irrigation to Reduce Posterior Capsule Opacification;* Assi AC, Lacey A, Aylward B. *Basic Properties of Intraocular Gases;* Busin M, Arffa RC. *Deep Suturing Techniques for Penetrating Keratoplasty;* Teichmann KD, Al-Rajhi AA. *Maximum Depth Lamellar Keratoplasty for Keratoconus With Anwar's Big Bubble* (2001).

Farrell TA, Alward WLM, Verdick RE. *Fundamentals of Slit-Lamp Biomicroscopy* (1993; reviewed for currency 2000).

Multimedia

Donnenfeld ED, Holland EJ, Pflugfelder SC, et al. *LEO Clinical Update Course on Cornea and External Disease* (CD-ROM, 2003).

Eye Care Skills on CD-ROM (all seven titles from the Eye Care Skills for the Primary Care Physician Series) (2001).

Lane SS, Hardten DR, Probst LE, et al. *LEO Clinical Update Course on Refractive Surgery* (CD-ROM, 2001).

Sher NA, ed. *External Disease and Cornea: A Multimedia Collection With Refractive Surgery Supplement* (1994, 2000).

Skuta GL, Fransen SR, eds. *ProVision Interactive: Clinical Case Studies on CD-ROM.* Volume 1, Cornea and Neuro-Ophthalmology (1996; reviewed for currency 2001).

Preferred Practice Patterns

Preferred Practice Patterns Committee, Cornea/External Disease Panel. *Bacterial Keratitis* (2000).

Preferred Practice Patterns Committee, Cornea/External Disease Panel. *Blepharitis* (2003).

Preferred Practice Patterns Committee, Cornea/External Disease Panel. *Conjunctivitis* (2003).

Preferred Practice Patterns Committee, Cornea/External Disease Panel. *Corneal Opacification and Ectasia* (2000).

Preferred Practice Patterns Committee, Cornea/External Disease Panel. *Dry Eye Syndrome* (2003).

Ophthalmic Technology Assessments

Ophthalmic Technology Assessment Committee. *Corneal Endothelial Photography* (1996).
Ophthalmic Technology Assessment Committee. *Corneal Topography* (1999).

Ophthalmic Technology Assessment Committee. *Epikeratoplasty* (1995).

Ophthalmic Technology Assessment Committee. *Excimer Laser Photorefractive Keratectomy (PRK) for Myopia and Astigmatism* (1999).

Ophthalmic Technology Assessment Committee. *Intrastromal Corneal Ring Segments for Low Myopia* (2001).

Ophthalmic Technology Assessment Committee. *Laser In Situ Keratomileusis for Hyperopia, Hyperopic Astigmatism, and Mixed Astigmatism: Safety and Efficacy* (2003).

Ophthalmic Technology Assessment Committee. *Laser In Situ Keratomileusis for Myopia and Astigmatism: Safety and Efficacy* (2002).

Ophthalmic Technology Assessment Committee. *Punctal Occlusion for the Dry Eye* (1996).

To order any of these materials, please call the Academy's Customer Service number at (415) 561-8540, or order online at www.aao.org.

Credit Reporting Form

Basic and Clinical Science Course, 2005–2006
Section 8

The American Academy of Ophthalmology is accredited by the Accreditation Council for Continuing Medical Education to provide continuing medical education for physicians.

The American Academy of Ophthalmology designates this educational activity for a maximum of 40 category 1 credits toward the AMA Physician's Recognition Award. Each physician should claim only those hours of credit that he/she actually spent in the activity.

The American Medical Association has determined that non-US licensed physicians who participate in this CME activity are eligible for AMA PRA category 1 credit.

If you wish to claim continuing medical education credit for your study of this section, you may claim your credit online or fill in the required forms and mail or fax them to the Academy.

To use the forms:

1. Complete the study questions and mark your answers on the Section Completion Form.
2. Complete the Section Evaluation.
3. Fill in and sign the statement below.
4. Return this page and the required forms by mail or fax to the CME Registrar (see below).

To claim credit online:

1. Log on to the Academy website (www.aao.org).
2. Go to Education Resource Center; click on CME Central.
3. Follow the instructions.

Important: These completed forms or the online claim must be received at the Academy within 3 years of purchase.

I hereby certify that I have spent _______ (up to 40) hours of study on the curriculum of this section and that I have completed the Study Questions.

Signature: ____

                                                                                    Date

Name: ____

Address: ____

City and State: ____ Zip: _____________

Telephone: (_________) _________________ Academy Member ID# _______________
              area code

Please return completed forms to: **Or you may fax them to:** 415-561-8575
American Academy of Ophthalmology
P.O. Box 7424
San Francisco, CA 94120-7424
Attn: CME Registrar, Customer Service

2005–2006
Section Completion Form

Basic and Clinical Science Course

Answer Sheet for Section 8

Question	Answer	Question	Answer	Question	Answer
1	a b c d	16	a b c d	31	a b c d
2	a b c d	17	a b c d	32	a b c d
3	a b c d	18	a b c d	33	a b c d
4	a b c d	19	a b c d	34	a b c d
5	a b c d	20	a b c d	35	a b c d
6	a b c d	21	a b c d	36	a b c d
7	a b c d	22	a b c d	37	a b c d
8	a b c d	23	a b c d	38	a b c d
9	a b c d	24	a b c d	39	a b c d
10	a b c d	25	a b c d	40	a b c d
11	a b c d	26	a b c d	41	a b c d
12	a b c d	27	a b c d	42	a b c d
13	a b c d	28	a b c d	43	a b c d
14	a b c d	29	a b c d		
15	a b c d	30	a b c d		

Section Evaluation

Please complete this CME questionnaire.

1. To what degree will you use knowledge from BCSC Section 8 in your practice?

   ☐ Regularly

   ☐ Sometimes

   ☐ Rarely

2. Please review the stated objectives for this BCSC Section 8. How effective was the material at meeting those objectives?

   ☐ All objectives were met.

   ☐ Most objectives were met.

   ☐ Some objectives were met.

   ☐ Few or no objectives were met.

3. To what degree is this BCSC Section 8 likely to have a positive impact on health outcomes of your patients?

   ☐ Extremely likely

   ☐ Highly likely

   ☐ Somewhat likely

   ☐ Not at all likely

4. After you review the stated objectives for BCSC Section 8, please let us know of any additional knowledge, skills, or information useful to your practice that were acquired but were not included in the objectives. [Optional]

5. Was BCSC Section 8 free of commercial bias?

   ☐ Yes

   ☐ No

6. If you selected "No" in the previous question, please comment. [Optional]

7. Please tell us what might improve the applicability of BCSC to your practice. [Optional]

Study Questions

Although a concerted effort has been made to avoid ambiguity and redundancy in these questions, the authors recognize that differences of opinion may occur regarding the "best" answer. The discussions are provided to demonstrate the rationale used to derive the answer. They may also be helpful in confirming that your approach to the problem was correct or, if necessary, in fixing the principle in your memory. Where relevant, additional references are given. The following study questions and discussions were submitted by Deepinder Dhaliwal, MD, on behalf of the Self-Assessment Committee.

1. Which of the following associations is incorrect?

   a. Mesectoderm—corneal endothelium

   b. Mesectoderm—corneal stroma

   c. Type IV collagen—Bowman's layer

   d. Type IV collagen—Descemet's membrane

2. The patient with which of the following diagnoses would likely have the best visual acuity?

   a. Primary familial amyloidosis

   b. Reis-Bücklers dystrophy

   c. Lattice dystrophy, type I

   d. Central cloudy dystrophy of François

3. A 55-year-old patient presents in your office with complaints of decreased vision. On examination, you detect severe anterior basement membrane dystrophy and a cataract. Which one of the following tests would be *most* helpful to you to determine whether the main cause of decreased vision is the corneal pathology or the cataract?

   a. Potential acuity meter

   b. Corneal topography

   c. Contact lens overrefraction

   d. Glare testing

4. Follicular conjunctivitis is associated with all of the following conditions except:

   a. Herpes simplex virus conjunctivitis

   b. Adult inclusion conjunctivitis

   c. Drug-induced conjunctivitis

   d. Allergic conjunctivitis

5. Which of the following statements regarding topical fluorescein is false?

   a. It is a nontoxic, water-soluble dye.

   b. It is used to detect disruption of intercellular junctions.

   c. It can be used to detect subtle epithelial irregularity even without an epithelial defect.

   d. It has antiviral properties.

6. Which of the following statements regarding the cornea is true?

   a. The cornea is a spherical surface with an average central refractive power of 43 D.

   b. The refractive index of the corneal stroma is 1.336.

   c. The tear–cornea interface is responsible for most of the eye's refractive power.

   d. A keratoscopic image of high with-the-rule astigmatism would appear as an ellipse with the long axis oriented horizontally.

7. Which of the following statements regarding the ocular surface is false?

   a. The mucin layer is the innermost layer of the tear film, is hydrophobic, and is produced by conjunctival goblet cells.

   b. Ocular rosacea results in a decreased tear breakup time.

   c. Blinking is important in the release of meibomian gland lipid.

   d. The tear film provides the cornea with essential nutrients and oxygen, and leukocytes gain access to the cornea through the tear film.

8. All of the following suggest aqueous tear deficiency except:

   a. Decreased tear lysozyme levels

   b. Decreased lactoferrin levels

   c. Decreased tear film osmolarity

   d. Tear meniscus between the globe and the lower eyelid of 0.3 mm

9. Which of the following is the *most* common corneal finding of sarcoidosis?

   a. Calcific band keratopathy

   b. Nummular keratitis

   c. Thickening of Descemet's membrane

   d. Deep stromal vascularization

10. Patients who complain of increased symptoms first thing in the morning could have any of the following conditions except:

    a. Anterior basement membrane dystrophy

    b. Fuchs endothelial dystrophy

    c. Floppy lid syndrome

    d. Keratoconjunctivitis sicca

11. In the U.S., all of the following conditions could cause xerophthalmia except:

    a. Chronic alcoholism

    b. Cystic fibrosis

    c. Bowel resection

    d. Glomerulonephritis

12. All of the following organisms can invade an intact corneal epithelium except:

    a. *Neisseria meningitidis*

    b. *Corynebacterium diphtheriae*

    c. *Shigella*

    d. *Pseudomonas aeruginosa*

13. Which of the following viruses is transmissible even after medical instrumentation is cleaned with alcohol?

    a. Herpes simplex virus

    b. Adenovirus

    c. Human immunodeficiency virus

    d. Epstein-Barr virus

14. Which of the following statements regarding *Acanthamoeba* is false?

    a. Two potentially infectious forms of *Acanthamoeba* exist: the motile trophozoite and the dormant cyst.

    b. *Acanthamoeba* can be grown on blood agar.

    c. *Acanthamoeba* can be visualized with calcofluor white, acridine orange, or the Giemsa stain.

    d. *Acanthamoeba* keratitis can appear as a pseudodendrite early in its course.

15. All of the following can be seen with ocular adenoviral infection except:

    a. Preauricular lymphadenopathy

    b. Large central geographic corneal erosions

    c. Multifocal subepithelial infiltrates

    d. Enlarged corneal nerves

16. Which of the following statements regarding the Herpetic Eye Disease Study (HEDS) is false?

    a. It demonstrated that topical corticosteroids given together with a prophylactic antiviral reduce persistence or progression of stromal inflammation and shorten the duration of herpes simplex stromal keratitis.

    b. It showed that long-term suppressive oral acyclovir therapy reduces the rate of recurrent HSV keratitis and helps to preserve vision.

    c. It showed some additional benefit of oral acyclovir in treating active HSV stromal keratitis in those patients also receiving concomitant topical corticosteroids and trifluridine.

    d. It demonstrated that oral acyclovir did not appear to prevent subsequent HSV stromal keratitis or iritis when it was given briefly along with trifluridine during an episode of epithelial keratitis.

17. A healthy 60-year-old man presents with a 2-day history of a painful rash on the right side of his forehead extending down to the eyelids. A vesicular skin lesion is also seen near the tip of his nose. Which of the following therapies would be most appropriate?

    a. Topical trifluridine 1% drops 8 times per day for 14 days

    b. Oral famciclovir 500 mg two times per day for 10 days

    c. Oral valacyclovir 1000 mg three times per day for 10 days

    d. Oral acyclovir 800 mg three times per day for 10 days

18. A 9-year-old boy with a history of atopy presents with a seasonally recurrent bilateral conjunctivitis and complains of blurred vision for 1 week. Giant papillae are seen upon lid eversion. All of the following could also be seen on the slit-lamp exam except:

    a. Vascular pannus and punctate epithelial erosions involving the superior cornea

    b. An oval epithelial ulceration with underlying stromal opacification in the central cornea

    c. Limbal follicles

    d. Conjunctival symblephara

19. Which of the following statements regarding graft-versus-host disease (GVHD) is false?

    a. It is a relatively common complication of allogeneic bone marrow transplantation in which the grafted cells can attack the patient's tissues.

    b. Conjunctival inflammation and severe sicca are the main features.

    c. Cicatricial lagophthalmos can occur.

    d. Aggressive lubrication is adequate even in severe cases of GVHD.

20. Which of the following infectious agents can be linked to interstitial keratitis?

    a. Herpes simplex virus

    b. Herpes zoster virus

    c. *Chlamydia trachomatis*

    d. All of the above

21. Which of the following associations regarding location of stem cells is incorrect?

    a. Cornea—limbus

    b. Conjunctiva—basal conjunctival epithelium most concentrated in the bulbar conjunctiva

    c. Epidermis—rete ridges

    d. All are correct

22. Which of the following conditions has been associated with limbal stem-cell dysfunction?

    a. Aniridia

    b. Contact lens wear

    c. Atopic keratoconjunctivitis

    d. All are correct

23. Surgical treatment of squamous cell carcinoma should include all of the following except:

    a. Excision of conjunctiva 1 mm beyond the clinically apparent margins of the tumor

    b. Resection of a thin lamellar scleral flap beneath the tumor

    c. Treatment of the remaining sclera with absolute alcohol

    d. Cryotherapy applied to the conjunctival margins

24. A 25-year-old Japanese woman presents with slate gray pigmentation of the episclera of the right eye with associated pigmentation of the periocular skin. Which of the following statements applies to her?

    a. Malignant melanoma can develop in the skin, uvea, or orbit, but not in the conjunctiva.

    b. Her lifetime risk of uveal melanoma is about 1 in 400, significantly greater than the risk of the general population.

    c. The risk of malignant transformation is the same in all patients regardless of their complexion.

    d. This condition is always unilateral.

25. Which of the following would signal possible malignant transformation of primary acquired melanosis?

    a. Nodularity

    b. Enlargement

    c. Increased vascularity

    d. All of the above

26. Confirmed ocular teratogens with effects on the anterior segment other than cataract include all of the following except:

    a. Maternal diabetes

    b. Radiation

    c. Maternal ingestion of antiseizure medications and retinoic acid

    d. Maternal use of topical Viroptic in the first trimester

27. Which of the following statements regarding nanophthalmos is false?

    a. Patients have a crowded anterior segment, which can lead to angle-closure glaucoma.

    b. Peripheral choroidal effusions can occur spontaneously.

    c. Large choroidal effusions occur during anterior segment surgery, possibly secondary to impaired venous outflow through the vortex veins as a result of scleral inelasticity.

    d. An extremely low power intraocular lens is required in these patients to achieve emmetropia.

28. All of the following conditions result in corneal clouding at birth except:

    a. Congenital glaucoma

    b. Congenital hereditary endothelial dystrophy with autosomal recessive inheritance (CHED2)

    c. Congenital hereditary endothelial dystrophy with autosomal dominant inheritance (CHED1)

    d. Birth trauma

29. Which of the following corneal dystrophies recurs most frequently in a corneal graft?

    a. Granular

    b. Macular

    c. Lattice

    d. Fuchs

30. Which of the following statements regarding Schnyder crystalline corneal dystrophy is false?

    a. It is a rare, slowly progressive, autosomal dominant stromal dystrophy.

    b. Central subepithelial crystals are seen in nearly 100% of patients later in life.

    c. Decreased corneal sensation also occurs.

    d. Dense corneal arcus lipoides is characteristic.

31. Which of the following is not a cause of calcific band keratopathy?

    a. Hereditary transmission

    b. Juvenile rheumatoid arthritis

    c. Hypercalcemia caused by sarcoidosis

    d. Decreased serum phosphorus with normal serum calcium

32. All of the following medications or diseases can be associated with cornea verticillata except:

    a. Chlorpromazine

    b. Chloroquine

    c. Gaucher disease

    d. Fabry disease

33. What is the best treatment course for a patient on amiodarone with cornea verticillata?

    a. Immediate cessation of the drug

    b. Concomitant administration of a steroid drop to decrease corneal pathology

    c. Placement of punctal plugs

    d. Observation

34. Which of the following can be related to spontaneous hyphema?

    a. Herpetic disease

    b. Retinoblastoma

    c. Juvenile xanthogranuloma

    d. All of the above

35. A 33-year-old man was involved in a motor vehicle accident that resulted in a broken windshield. Slit-lamp examination reveals multiple glass foreign bodies embedded at various levels of the stroma. All wounds were Seidel negative. Which of the following is the most appropriate treatment strategy?

    a. The patient should be taken to the operating room and all superficial and deep fragments should be removed immediately.

    b. All exposed glass fragments should be removed and deeper fragments left in place.

    c. Ointment should be placed in the eyes since superficial and deep fragments will eventually be extruded with time.

    d. Eyes should be patched, with follow-up the next day.

36. The principal indications for a conjunctival flap include all of the following except:

    a. Neurotrophic keratopathy

    b. Stromal herpes simplex viral keratitis

    c. Painful bullous keratopathy in a patient who is not a good candidate for penetrating keratoplasty

    d. Small corneal perforation

37. All of the following are contraindications for use of donor cornea tissue except:

    a. Posterior choroidal melanoma

    b. Leukemia

    c. Previous PRK for correction of 2 D of myopia

    d. Active septicemia

38. All of the following are appropriate therapeutic approaches to deal with a small wound leak (with no anterior chamber shallowing) seen on the first postoperative visit after penetrating keratoplasty except:

    a. Patching

    b. Resuturing of wound

    c. Use of aqueous inhibitor

    d. Placement of therapeutic contact lens

39. All of the following may be signs of corneal graft rejection except:

    a. Radial perineuritis

    b. Subepithelial infiltrates

    c. Linear keratic precipitates

    d. Elevated linear epithelial ridge

40. Currently, the most prevalent refractive surgery is:

    a. Myopic LASIK

    b. Hyperopic LASIK

    c. LASEK

    d. Cataract removal with intraocular lens implantation

41. Which of the following statements regarding incisional refractive surgery is true?

    a. Radial incisions lead to flattening in both the meridian of the incision and 90° away.

    b. Tangential incisions lead to steepening in the meridian of the incision and flattening in the meridian 90° away (known as coupling).

    c. The larger the optical zone, the greater the effect.

    d. For optimum effect, the incision should be at 50% depth.

42. What is the approximate amount of corneal tissue that would be ablated in a 3 D myope having PRK using a 6 mm optical zone and a broad-beam laser?

    a. 9 μm

    b. 18 μm

    c. 36 μm

    d. 48 μm

43. In a post-LASIK patient with diffuse lamellar keratitis, which of the following signs would prompt immediate flap lift with irrigation as opposed to medical management?

    a. Peripheral white blood cells (WBCs)

    b. Central and peripheral WBCs

    c. Only central WBCs with associated cell clumping in visual axis

    d. All of the above

Answers

1. Answer—c. During development of the anterior segment, the surface ectoderm forms the lens placode and gives rise to the corneal and conjunctival epithelium. Both the corneal endothelium and stroma are formed by two separate waves of mesectoderm. Bowman's layer is not a true basement membrane and is not made up of type IV collagen. Instead, Bowman's layer consists of compact stromal fibers containing collagen types I, V, and VI.

2. Answer—d. In general, visual acuity is reduced earlier when there is corneal surface irregularity as opposed to diffuse clouding with a smooth epithelial surface. Therefore, dystrophies such as primary familial amyloidosis, where amyloid occurs as subepithelial deposits; Reis-Bücklers dystrophy, which affects Bowman's layer; and lattice dystrophy, where amyloid is deposited most heavily in the anterior stroma and subepithelial area, would all cause some vision difficulty by the second decade of life. Central cloudy dystrophy of François, on the other hand, appears as deep, polygonal, gray areas with an unaffected anterior stroma and smooth epithelium. Vision is typically not reduced by this condition.

3. Answer—c. If corneal surface irregularity from severe anterior basement membrane dystrophy is the main cause of decreased visual acuity, overrefraction with a rigid gas-permeable contact lens will mask the surface irregularity and improve visual acuity. Potential acuity meter testing does not isolate the area of pathology. Corneal topography will demonstrate irregular astigmatism if the corneal pathology was visually significant; however, the visual acuity does not always correlate to the degree of irregularity. Glare testing is of no benefit since both corneal pathology and cataract can manifest decreased vision with glare testing.

4. Answer—d. Common causes of follicular conjunctivitis include herpes simplex virus conjunctivitis, adult inclusion (chlamydial) conjunctivitis, drug-induced or toxic conjunctivitis, molluscum contagiosum blepharoconjunctivitis, and adenoviral conjunctivitis. Allergic conjunctivitis is papillary rather than follicular.

5. Answer—d. Although fluorescein has no antiviral properties, rose bengal, a halide derivative of fluorescein, has antiviral and other toxic effects.

6. Answer—d. The cornea is an aspheric surface with the central cornea typically about 3 D steeper than the periphery. The refractive index of air is 1.000, aqueous and tears is 1.336, and the corneal stroma is 1.376. The air–tear interface of the cornea is responsible for most of the eye's refractive power.

7. Answer—a. Although the mucin layer is the innermost of the three layers and is secreted by conjunctival goblet cells, it is a *hydrophilic* layer that overlies the hydrophobic ocular surface.

8. Answer—c. In lacrimal gland dysfunction states, the normal production of proteins by the lacrimal gland is diminished. A decreased tear lysozyme or lactoferrin level is highly suggestive of dry eye. Tear film osmolarity has been shown to be increased in patients with aqueous tear deficiency as well as those with meibomian gland dysfunction. The tear meniscus is normally 1.0 mm in height and convex. A tear meniscus 0.3 mm or less is considered abnormal.

9. Answer—a. Sarcoidosis is a multisystem disorder of uncertain etiology. After pulmonary involvement, ocular involvement is the most common manifestation, seen in up to 50% of affected patients. Although all of the findings listed in the question can occur in sarcoidosis, the most common corneal manifestation is calcific band keratopathy, often associated with chronic uveitis or elevated serum calcium levels.

10. Answer—d. Patients with anterior basement membrane dystrophy could have symptoms such as tearing, photophobia, and foreign body sensation related to recurrent erosion upon awakening. Patients with Fuchs dystrophy often experience blurred vision first thing in the morning due to increased corneal edema secondary to eyelid closure. Patients with floppy eyelid syndrome complain of increased foreign body sensation upon awakening because of eversion of the lax upper lid during sleep. In contrast, patients suffering from keratoconjunctivitis sicca notice that their symptoms get worse as the day progresses, with prolonged use of the eyes, or with exposure to environmental extremes.

11. Answer—d. Vitamin A deficiency leads to xerophthalmia. Worldwide, xerophthalmia usually represents a dietary deficiency caused by low intake of this fat-soluble vitamin. In the U.S., however, it is more likely to occur from decreased absorption of vitamin A, sometimes associated with chronic alcoholism or with diseases that cause lipid malabsorption (particularly cystic fibrosis, biliary cirrhosis, and bowel resection). Glomerulonephritis does not affect lipid absorption.

12. Answer—d. Most bacteria must rely on a break in epithelial barrier function to invade the cornea. Organisms that can overcome an intact corneal epithelium include *Neisseria gonorrhoeae*, *Neisseria meningitidis*, *Corynebacterium diphtheriae*, and *Shigella* species.

13. Answer—b. The viral envelope lipid bilayer is vulnerable to damage by ultraviolet light, detergents, alcohols, and general-use antiseptics. Thus, enveloped viruses such as herpes simplex virus, Epstein-Barr virus, and human immunodeficiency virus are intrinsically susceptible to the external environment, and their infectivity is short-lived outside the host. Alcohol treatment of medical instrumentation is generally sufficient to prevent iatrogenic infection. In contrast, nonenveloped viruses such as adenoviruses are relatively resistant to environmental insult and, in some cases, can persist for weeks outside the human host. The application of dilute (1%) bleach to tonometer tips for at least 10 minutes is recommended to prevent transmission of adenoviruses.

14. Answer—a. The *Acanthamoeba* life cycle includes the motile trophozoite and the dormant cyst forms. Free-living amoebae are found in both forms, but only the trophozoite is infectious. Both forms are found in infected human tissues.

15. Answer—d. EKC is the only adenoviral syndrome with significant corneal involvement. The infection is bilateral in a majority of patients and may be preceded by an upper respiratory infection. Photophobia and reduced vision from adenoviral subepithelial infiltrates may persist for months to years. It is not associated with enlarged corneal nerves, which are seen in such conditions as MEN syndrome and leprosy.

16. Answer—c. HEDS showed no additional benefit of oral acyclovir in treating active HSV stromal keratitis in patients also receiving concomitant topical corticosteroids and trifluridine. When given briefly along with trifluridine during an episode of epithelial keratitis, acyclovir also did not appear to prevent subsequent HSV stromal keratitis or iritis.

17. Answer—c. These symptoms are pathognomonic of herpes zoster ophthalmicus (HZO). The current recommendation for HZO is oral famciclovir 500 mg three times per day, valacyclovir 1000 mg three times per day, or acyclovir 800 mg five times per day for 7–10 days, best if started within 72 hours of the onset of skin lesions. Topical antiviral medications are not effective. Intravenous acyclovir therapy is indicated in patients at risk for disseminated zoster due to immunosuppression.

18. Answer—d. This boy's signs and symptoms indicate vernal keratoconjunctivitis. Depending on the severity of the condition, all of the signs listed in answers a, b, and c may occur. However, conjunctival symblephara do not form in vernal keratoconjunctivitis.

19. Answer—d. Graft-versus-host disease is a relatively common complication of allogenic bone marrow transplantation performed most commonly for hematopoietic malignancies. Conjunctival inflammation in GVHD can be severe and even associated with limbal stem-cell deficiency and secondary corneal scarring, but the latter is a rare complication. Typical presentations include conjunctival and corneal epithelial erosions, aqueous tear deficiency, and cicatricial lagophthalmos. Aggressive lubrication and punctal occlusion are the mainstays of local therapy. Severe filamentary keratopathy can be additionally treated with mucolytic agents (10% acetylcysteine) as needed. Severe ocular surface disease in GVHD may be associated with active nonocular (often skin) GVHD and may require increased systemic immunosuppression by cyclosporine or tacrolimus (FK506).

20. Answer—d. Although congenital syphilis was the first infection to be linked with interstitial keratitis, many other agents can also cause IK.

21. Answer—b. Stem cells for skin and mucous membranes reside in basal epithelial layers, in locations relatively sheltered from environmental insults. Conjunctival epithelial stem cells reside in the basal conjunctival epithelium with concentrations in the fornix and just posterior to the lid margin.

22. Answer—d. Several disorders can be associated with limbal stem-cell dysfunction, including aniridia, contact lens–induced keratopathy, atopic keratoconjunctivitis, ocular cicatricial pemphigoid, Stevens-Johnson syndrome, chemical injuries, and keratitis associated with multiple endocrine neoplasia (MEN IIb or III).

23. Answer—a. The conjunctiva should be excised 4 mm beyond the clinically apparent margins of the tumor.

24. Answer—b. The combined ocular and cutaneous pigmentations seen in this patient are referred to as *oculodermal melanocytosis.* Approximately 5% of cases are bilateral. Malignant transformation is possible but rare and seems to occur only in patients with a fair complexion. Malignant melanoma can develop in the skin, conjunctiva, uvea, or orbit. The lifetime risk of uveal melanoma in a patient with ocular melanocytosis is about 1 in 400, significantly greater than the risk of 1 in 13,000 of the general population.

25. Answer—d. Malignant transformation should be suspected when a lesion shows nodularity, enlargement, or increased vascularity. Small typical areas of primary acquired melanosis can be observed and biopsy delayed until progression is observed.

26. Answer—d. No topically administered ophthalmic medication is suspected or confirmed to produce a teratogenic effect.

27. Answer—d. Nanophthalmos is characterized by a small, functional eye with relatively normal internal organization and proportions. Patients have a high degree of hyperopia (7–15 D) due to a short axial length (15–20 mm). Extremely high intraocular lens powers are required to achieve emmetropia.

28. Answer—c. Corneal clouding at birth has many different etiologies, including congenital glaucoma, birth trauma, sclerocornea, Peters anomaly, or CHED2. Two forms of CHED are recognized. The more common autosomal recessive type (CHED2) presents at birth, remains stationary, and is accompanied by nystagmus. The bluish white cornea may be two to three times normal thickness and have a ground-glass appearance, but this finding is not associated with tearing or photophobia. The dominant form (CHED1) presents in the first or second year of life, although expressivity is variable. It is slowly progressive and accompanied by pain, photophobia, and tearing, but nystagmus is not present. The cornea exhibits a diffuse blue-gray ground-glass appearance.

29. Answer—c. The frequency of regraft is highest in lattice dystrophy, followed by granular dystrophy and then macular dystrophy. Fuchs dystrophy does not typically recur in the graft.

30. Answer—b. Features of this rare, slowly progressive autosomal dystrophy include central subepithelial crystals (seen only in 50% of patients), central corneal opacification, dense corneal arcus lipoides, midperipheral corneal opacification, and decreased corneal sensation.

31. Answer—d. This calcific degeneration of the superficial cornea involves mainly Bowman's layer. There are six main causes: chronic ocular disease; hypercalcemia caused by hyperparathyroidism, vitamin D toxicity, milk-alkali syndrome, sarcoidosis, and other systemic disorders; hereditary transmission; elevated serum phosphorus with normal serum calcium; chronic exposure to mercurial vapors or to mercurial preservatives in ophthalmic medications; and silicone oil instillation in an aphakic eye.

32. Answer—c.

33. Answer—d. The development of deposits with amiodarone therapy is not an indication to stop this medication, since it is unusual for these deposits to result in reduction of acuity or ocular symptoms.

34. Answer—d. Spontaneous hyphema should alert the examiner to the possibility of clotting abnormalities, herpetic disease, intraocular lens problems, or rubeosis iridis in adults. Juvenile xanthogranuloma, retinoblastoma, and leukemia are associated with spontaneous hyphema in children.

35. Answer—b. If several glass foreign bodies are present, all of the exposed fragments should be removed. Fragments that are deeply embedded in the cornea are often inert and can be left in place. Careful gonioscopic evaluation of the anterior chamber is essential to ensure that the iris and the angle are free of any retained glass particles.

36. Answer—d. Conjunctival flap surgery is performed less frequently now than in the past because of more effective medical and surgical treatment modalities. However, this procedure remains an effective method for managing inflammatory and structural corneal disorders when restoration of vision is not an immediate concern. It should not be used for active microbial keratitis or corneal perforation since residual infectious organisms may proliferate under a flap if an ulcer is not sterilized first. A corneal perforation must first be sealed, because otherwise it would continue to leak under the flap.

37. Answer—a. Eyes with posterior choroidal melanoma may be considered acceptable; however, most medical eye bank directors decline their usage. All other conditions exclude the donor cornea.

38. Answer—b. The wound is always checked carefully for leakage on postoperative visits. Small wound leaks that do not cause anterior chamber shallowing frequently close spontaneously. Patching, therapeutic contact lenses, and use of inhibitors of aqueous production may hasten wound closure. Resuturing is advised for leaks lasting longer than 3 days.

39. Answer—a. Corneal transplant rejection takes three clinical forms—epithelial, subepithelial, and stromal—which may occur either singly or in combination. In epithelial rejection, lymphocytes cause an elevated, linear epithelial ridge that advances centripetally. In subepithelial rejection, subepithelial infiltrates are seen, sometimes accompanied by a cellular anterior chamber reaction. Isolated stromal rejection is not common but can be seen as stromal infiltrates and neovascularization. In very aggressive severe or prolonged bouts of graft rejection, the stroma can become necrotic. Endothelial rejection is the most common and serious form of corneal transplant rejection. Inflammatory precipitates are seen on the endothelial surface

in fine precipitates, in random clumps, or in linear form (Khodadoust line). Inflammatory cells are usually seen in the anterior chamber as well.

40. Answer—d. Refractive surgery encompasses a broad range of procedures to change the refraction of the eye. Such procedures can involve the cornea or the lens. Currently, the most prevalent refractive surgery is cataract removal with intraocular lens implantation.

41. Answer—a. Tangential incisions (arcuate or linear) lead to flattening in the meridian of the incision and steepening in the meridian 90° away. The closer radial incisions approach the visual axis (ie, the smaller the optical zone), the greater their effect. For optimum effect, the incision should be 85%–90% deep to allow an intact posterior lamellae and maximum anterior bowing of the other lamellae.

42. Answer—c. For low amounts of correction (<7 diopters), the amount of tissue to remove centrally is estimated by Munnerlyn's formula: Ablation depth in micrometers equals diopters (D) of myopia divided by 3 times the square of the optical zone (mm). In this case,

$$3 \text{ D} / 3 \text{ multiplied by (6 mm squared)} = 1 \times 36 = 36 \text{ μm}$$

43. Answer—c. An unusual syndrome, diffuse lamellar keratitis (DLK, sands of the Sahara, SOS) with diffuse interface haze, may appear on postoperative day 1–3 with possible decrease in vision. The condition appears to be a nonspecific inflammatory reaction in response to a variety of toxic insults. Central or peripheral WBCs with granular appearance usually respond to frequent topical steroids; however, when dense clumps appear in the visual axis, lifting the flap and irrigating, followed by intensive topical steroid treatment is usually required. For severe cases, systemic steroids may be used adjunctively.

Index

(*i* = image; *t* = table)

Ablepharon, 271
Abnormal polarity, definition/implication of, 234*t*
Abrasions, corneal, 381–382
Absidia, ocular infection caused by, 121
ACAID. *See* Anterior chamber–associated immune
 deviation
Acanthamoeba, 121–122, 122*i,* 176
 cytologic identification of, 61*i*
 keratitis/ocular infection caused by, 121–122, 122*i,*
 176–178, 176*i*
 herpes simplex keratitis differentiated from, 177
 isolation techniques for diagnosis of, 127
 treatment of, 177–178
 stains and culture media for identification of, 127*t,*
 177
Acanthosis, definition/implication of, 234*t*
Accommodation, Schachar theory of, scleral expansion
 for presbyopia correction and, 474
Acetylcysteine, for filamentary keratopathy, 80
Acid, ocular injuries caused by, 367
Acid-fast staining, 57*t*
ACL syndrome, congenital corneal keloids in, 284
Acne rosacea, 65–67, 66*i,* 67*i*
Acquired immunodeficiency syndrome. *See* HIV
 infection/AIDS
Acridine orange staining, 57*t*
Acrocephalopolysyndactyly, 333*t*
Actinic (Labrador) keratopathy (spheroidal
 degeneration), 345–346
Actinomyces, 118
Acute hemorrhagic conjunctivitis, 134
Acyclovir
 for herpes simplex virus infections, 137*t,* 139,
 142–144
 for herpes zoster infections, 149
ADCC. *See* Antibody-dependent cell cytotoxicity
Adenoviruses
 epidemic keratoconjunctivitis /ocular infection
 caused by, 110, 130–134, 132*i,* 133*i*
 pharyngoconjunctival fever caused by, 131
Adherence, as microbial virulence factor, 106
Adhesins, 106
Adnexa. *See* Ocular adnexa
Adrenochrome deposition, corneal pigmentation
 caused by, 354, 354*t,* 355*i*
Advancement flaps, 413
Aggrecan, 12
Aging
 of conjunctiva, 341
 of cornea, 341–342
 of sclera, 342
 stromal corneal degenerations and, 346–348
AHC. *See* Acute hemorrhagic conjunctivitis
AIDS. *See* HIV infection/AIDS
AK. *See* Arcuate keratotomy
AKC. *See* Atopic keratoconjunctivitis
ALK. *See* Automated lamellar keratoplasty

Alkalis (alkaline solutions), ocular injuries caused by,
 365, 366*i*
Alkaptonuria, 328
 corneal pigmentation and, 354*t*
 gene linkage of, 293*t,* 328
Alleles, 291
Allergic conjunctivitis, 195–196
Allergic reactions. *See also specific type and*
 Hypersensitivity reactions
 anaphylaxis as, 186–188, 187*i,* 187*t*
 conjunctivitis, 195–196
 contact lens wear and, 97–99, 98*i,* 201–204, 203*i*
 in eyelid
 contact dermatitis, 194*i,* 195
 contact dermatoblepharitis, 193–195, 194*i*
 vernal keratoconjunctivitis, 197–199, 198*i,* 199*i*
Allografts
 corneal, 425. *See also* Keratoplasty, penetrating
 rejection of, 437–440, 438*i,* 439*i,* 444. *See also*
 Rejection (graft)
 limbal, 408–409, 410–411*i*
 for chemical burns, 368
 indications for, 400*t*
Alloplastic intracorneal implants, 456, 457*i,* 470–472,
 471*i,* 472*t*
Amebic keratitis. *See Acanthamoeba,* keratitis caused by
Amicar. *See* Aminocaproic acid
Amikacin, for bacterial keratitis, 171*t*
Amino acids, corneal changes in disorders of, 325–328
Aminocaproic acid/ε-aminocaproic acid, for hyphema,
 377
Amiodarone, cornea verticillata caused by, 353
Amniotic membrane transplantation, 401
 for chemical burns, 368
 indications for, 400*t*
Amorphous corneal dystrophy, posterior, 281–282
Amphotericin B, for fungal keratitis, 175
Amyloid AA, 330, 331
Amyloid AL, 330
Amyloid degeneration, 349–350. *See also* Amyloidosis/
 amyloid deposits
Amyloidosis/amyloid deposits, 328–331, 329*t*
 conjunctival, 329*t,* 330–331, 330*i*
 corneal, 328–331, 329*t*
 in gelatinous droplike dystrophy, 304, 304*i,* 329*t,*
 330
 in lattice dystrophy, 299*t,* 301–302, 302*i,* 329*t,* 330
 primary familial (gelatinous droplike dystrophy),
 304, 304*i,* 329*t,* 330
 primary localized, 329*t,* 330–331, 330*i*
 primary systemic, 329*t,* 331
 secondary localized, 329*t,* 331, 349–350
 secondary systemic, 329*t,* 331
ANA. *See* Antinuclear (antineutrophil) antibodies
Anaerobes, as normal ocular flora, 105*t*
Anaphylactic hypersensitivity reaction, 186–188, 187*i,*
 187*t*
 ocular, 193–195, 194*i*

Biomicroscopy
slit-lamp, 14–18
clinical use of, 17–18
illumination system of
direct illumination methods and, 14–16, 15*i*,
16*i*
indirect illumination methods and, 16–17
recurrent corneal erosions seen with, 91
ultrasound, 34
Bipedicle (bucket handle) flap, 412–413
Birth trauma, corneal edema caused by, 285, 286*i*
Bitoric ablation, 457, 458*i*
Bitôt spot, 83–84, 84*i*
BKS technique. *See* Barraquer-Krumeich-Swinger
technique
Blepharitis
infectious, 109*t*, 152–157, 153*t*, 153*i*
in meibomian gland dysfunction, 64, 152, 153*t*
seborrheic, 67–68, 152, 153*t*
staphylococcal, 152–157, 153*t*, 153*i*
marginal infiltrates in, 154, 155*i*, 217
types of, 153*t*
Blepharoconjunctivitis
contact, 193–195
herpes simplex virus causing, 135–136, 135*i*, 136*i*,
137
marginal corneal infiltrates associated with, 154,
155*i*, 216–217
staphylococcal, 152–154, 155–156
keratitis and, 154–156
Blepharoptosis. *See* Ptosis
Blindness
congenital anomalies causing, 269
river (onchocerciasis), 44*t*, 123
Blinking (blink reflex), 47
in external eye defense, 103
in meibomian gland lipid release, 49, 50
Blood, cornea stained by, 375*i*, 376, 376*i*
Blue nevus, 249–250
Blue sclera, 273–274
in Ehlers-Danlos syndrome, 274
in keratoglobus, 316
in Marfan syndrome, 335
in osteogenesis imperfecta, 274
Bony orbit. *See* Orbit
Borrelia burgdorferi, 119
Bowman's layer/membrane, 9*i*, 10
bp. *See* Base pair
Bradykinin, as inflammatory mediator, 186*t*
Bridge flap, 412
Broad-beam lasers, for photoablation, 461
Brush marks, in meibomian gland dysfunction, 63
Bucket handle (bipedicle) flap, 412–413
Bucrylate. *See* Cyanoacrylate adhesives
Bulbar conjunctiva, 8. *See also* Conjunctiva
Bulla
of cornea, 22*t*
of eyelid, 21*t*
Burns
chemical. *See* Chemical injury
thermal, 363–364
Butylcyanoacrylate tissue adhesive, 416

C-reactive protein, in immune-mediated disease, 191*t*
C5a peptidase, in ocular infections, 114
Calcific band keratopathy (calcium hydroxyapatite
deposition), 350–352, 351*i*
in sarcoidosis, 69–70
Calcofluor white staining, 57*t*
CALT. *See* Conjunctiva-associated lymphoid tissue
Canaliculitis, 109*t*
Cancer, corneal nerve enlargement and, 338, 338*t*
Candida (candidiasis)
albicans, 120*i*
keratitis/ocular infection caused by, 119–121, 120*i*,
175
as normal ocular flora, 105, 105*t*
Candidate gene screening, 292
Canthoplasty, for persistent epithelial defects, 94
Capsid (viral), 108
Carbohydrates, disorders of metabolism of, corneal
changes in, 318–320, 319*t*
Carbon, corneal deposits caused by, 354*t*
Carcinoma, definition of, 233
Carcinoma in situ, of conjunctiva, 242, 243*i*
Carotid artery, eyelids supplied by, 7
Carpenter syndrome, 333*t*
Caruncle, 8
Cat-scratch disease, 166
Cataract, steroid-induced, after photorefractive
keratectomy, 481
Cataract surgery
corneal endothelial changes caused by, 395
in nanophthalmos, 273
after radial keratotomy, 368
Catarrhal (marginal corneal) infiltrates,
blepharoconjunctivitis and, 154, 155*i*, 216–217
Cationic protein, as inflammatory mediator, 188*t*
Cats, *Bartonella henselae* transmitted by, 117
Cautery, thermal
for punctal occlusion, 81, 82*i*
in cicatricial pemphigoid, 210–211
for superior limbic keratoconjunctivitis, 90
Cavernous sinus, eyelids drained by, 7
Cefazolin, for bacterial keratitis, 171*t*
Cefotaxime, for gonococcal conjunctivitis, in neonates,
162
Ceftazidime, for bacterial keratitis, 171*t*
Ceftriaxone
for bacterial keratitis, 171*t*
for gonococcal conjunctivitis, 160
in neonates, 162
Cell-adhesion molecules, as inflammatory mediators,
186*t*
Cell death, programmed (PCD/apoptosis), 233*t*
Cell-mediated immunity. *See* Cellular immunity
Cell turnover, 232
Cellular atypia, definition/implication of, 234*t*
Cellular immunity (cell-mediated immunity), 187*i*,
188*t*, 189
Cellulitis, preseptal, *Haemophilus* causing, 117
Centering procedures, for keratorefractive surgery, 463
radial keratotomy outcome affected by, 466
Central cloudy dystrophy of François, 306–307, 307*i*
gene linkage of, 294*t*

Henderson-Patterson bodies, 111
HEP. *See* Hepatoerythropoietic porphyria
Heparan sulfate
  in microbial adherence, 106
  in mucopolysaccharidoses, 318
Heparin, as inflammatory mediator, 188*t*
Hepatoerythropoietic porphyria (HEP), 336
Hepatolenticular degeneration (Wilson disease),
  336–337, 337*i*
Herbert's pits, 163, 164*i*
Hereditary hemorrhagic telangiectasia (Osler-Weber-
  Rendu disease), 72
Hereditary sensory neuropathy, neurotrophic
  keratopathy and, 85–86
Herpes simplex virus, 134–145
  blepharoconjunctivitis caused by, 135–136, 135*i*,
    136*i*, 137
  iridocyclitis caused by, 144
  keratitis caused by, 44*t*, 137–144
    Acanthamoeba keratitis differentiated from, 177
    epithelial, 137–140, 138*i*, 140*i*
    interstitial, 141, 141*i*
    neurotrophic keratopathy/ulcers and, 85, 86*i*, 145
    steroid-induced, after photorefractive keratectomy,
      481
    stromal, 141–144, 141*i*, 143*i*, 144*i*
  ocular infection/inflammation caused by, 44*t*,
    134–145
    complications of, 144–145
    pathogenesis of, 134–137
    after photorefractive keratectomy, 481
    primary, 135–136, 135*i*, 136*i*
    recurrent, 136–144
    treatment of, 136, 137*t*, 139–140, 142–144
    varicella-zoster virus infection differentiated from,
      146, 146*t*
  type 1, 134
  type 2, 134
Herpes zoster, 145–149
  ophthalmic manifestations in, 85, 147–148, 147*i*,
    149*i*
Herpes zoster ophthalmicus, 147–149, 147*i*, 149*i*
  neurotrophic keratopathy in, 85
Herpesviruses, 110. *See also specific type*
Herpetic Eye Disease Study, 142–144
Heterogeneity, genetic, 291
Heterozygote/heterozygous alleles, 291
Hexagonal cells, specular photomicroscopy in
  evaluation of percentage of, 33
Hexagonal keratotomy, 473
Hib. *See Haemophilus, influenzae,* type b
Highly active antiretroviral therapy (HAART), 112
Histamine, as inflammatory mediator, 186*t*, 188*t*
Histiocytes, cytologic identification of, 59
Histiocytoma, fibrous (fibroxanthoma), 256
Histocompatibility antigens. *See* Human leukocyte
  (HLA) antigens
Histocryl. *See* Cyanoacrylate adhesives
History, family, pedigree analysis and, 292
HIV (human immunodeficiency virus), 112. *See also*
  HIV infection/AIDS
  testing for antibody to, 112
  viability of after excimer laser ablation, 487

HIV infection/AIDS, 112
  corneal microsporidiosis in, 178
  diagnosis of, 112
  Kaposi sarcoma in, 112, 256–257, 257*i*
  molluscum contagiosum in, 129
  ocular infection/manifestations and, 112
HLA antigens. *See* Human leukocyte (HLA) antigens
Holmium-YAG laser, for thermokeratoplasty, 496
Homogentisic acid, corneal lesions of in alkaptonuria,
  328
Homologous antigens, 421
Homoplastic keratomileusis, 469
Homozygote/homozygous alleles, 291
Hordeolum, 156–157
  external (stye), 156
  internal, 156–157
Horner-Trantas dots, 197
Host defenses, in ocular infection, 107–108
HPV. *See* Human papillomaviruses
HSV. *See* Herpes simplex virus
Hudson-Stähli line, 354*t*, 355
Human Genome Project, 290
Human herpes virus 8, Kaposi sarcoma caused by, 130,
  256
Human immunodeficiency virus (HIV), 112. *See also*
  HIV infection/AIDS
  testing for antibody to, 112
Human leukocyte (HLA) antigens, 421
Human papillomaviruses, ocular infection caused by,
  111, 129–130, 240
Human transforming growth factor β–induced gene
  mutation
  in granular dystrophy, 300
  in lattice dystrophy, 301
  in Reis-Bücklers dystrophy, 298
Hunter syndrome, 318, 319*t*
Hurler syndrome, 318, 319*t*
  congenital/infantile corneal opacities in, 283
Hurler-Scheie syndrome, 318
Hurricane (vortex) keratopathy, 370
Hyaluronic acid, for dry eye, 80
Hyaluronidase, in ocular infections, 114
Hybridization, 292
Hydrogen peroxide, as inflammatory mediator, 186*t*
Hydrops, in keratoconus, 312
  management of, 314
Hydroxyapatite deposition (calcific band keratopathy),
  350–352, 351*i*
  in sarcoidosis, 69–70
Hypercalcemia, corneal changes in, 338. *See also* Band
  keratopathy
Hyperemia, conjunctival, 21*t*
  causes of, 71
Hyperkeratosis, definition/implication of, 234*t*
Hyperlipidemia, in Schnyder crystalline dystrophy, 305
Hyperlipoproteinemias, 320–321, 321*t*
  in Schnyder crystalline dystrophy, 305, 321
Hyperopia
  cornea plana and, 276
  microcornea and, 274
  nanophthalmos and, 273
  surgical correction of, 472–474
    automated lamellar keratoplasty for, 455, 455*i*, 473

surgical correction of, 474
Preseptal cellulitis, *Haemophilus* causing, 117
Preservatives, in ocular medications
    allergic reactions to, 98, 98*i*, 203, 370–371
    demulcents, 78–80
    persistent corneal defects caused by (toxic ulcerative
        keratopathy), 86, 93–94
    toxic keratoconjunctivitis caused by, 97, 370–371
Pressure patching, for corneal abrasion, 382
Primary acquired melanosis, 251–252, 252*i*, 252*t*
Primary endothelial failure, after penetrating
    keratoplasty, 432, 433*i*
Prions, 124
PRK. *See* Photorefractive keratectomy
PRNG. *See* Penicillin-resistant *N gonorrhoeae*
Proband, 292
Programmed cell death (PCD/apoptosis), 233*t*
Prokaryotic cells, 112–113. *See also* Bacteria
Propamidine, for *Acanthamoeba* keratitis, 177–178
Propionibacterium acnes
    as normal ocular flora, 105, 105*t*
    ocular infection caused by, 116, 116*i*
Prostaglandins, as inflammatory mediators, 188*t*
Proteases
    corneal, as inflammatory mediators, 186*t*
    microbial, in ocular infections, 106–107
Protein AF, 330
Protein AP, 330
Proteinaceous (spheroidal) degeneration, 345–346
Proteins, disorders of metabolism of, corneal changes
    in, 328–331, 329*t*
Proteoglycans
    corneal, 10
    scleral, 12
Proteus, keratitis caused by, 117
Protozoa, ocular infection/inflammation caused by,
    121–123, 122*i*
Proximal illumination, for slit-lamp biomicroscopy, 16
Pseudocryptophthalmos, 271, 272
Pseudoepitheliomatous hyperplasia, 242
Pseudoguttatae, inflammatory, 26
Pseudo–Hurler polydystrophy, 324
Pseudomembrane, conjunctival, 21*t*, 22*t*
Pseudomonas
    aeruginosa, 116, 117*i*
    ocular infection/inflammation caused by, 116
        keratitis, 168, 169*i*
Pseudopemphigoid, 207, 371
Psychotropic drugs, tear production affected by, 76*t*
Pterygium, 344, 344*t*
    conjunctival transplantation for, 406*i*, 407–408
    excision of, 344, 405, 406*i*
        bacterial scleritis after, 179, 180*i*
    gene linkage of, 293*t*
PTK. *See* Phototherapeutic keratectomy
Ptosis (blepharoptosis)
    mechanical, 20
    steroid-induced, after photorefractive keratectomy,
        481
Public health ophthalmology, 44, 44*t*
PUK. *See* Peripheral keratitis, ulcerative
Punctal occlusion
    for cicatricial pemphigoid, 210–211

for dry eye, 80–81, 81*i*, 82*i*
Punctate epithelial defects/erosions
    conjunctival, 21*t*
    corneal, 21–22*t*, 27*i*, 30*t*
Punctate epithelial keratitis, 21*t*, 27–28*i*, 30*t*
    superficial Thygeson, 212–213, 212*i*
Punctate epithelial keratopathy, 25, 27–28*i*
    exposure causing, 87
    microsporidial, 167
    staphylococcal blepharoconjunctivitis and, 154, 155*i*
Punctate staining patterns (fluorescein), 18, 19*i*
Purine bases, 289
Purines, disorders of metabolism of, hyperuricemia
    caused by, 335–336
Pustule, of eyelid, 21*t*
Pyogenic granuloma, 255–256, 256*i*
Pyrimidine bases, 289

Rabies virus, ocular infection caused by, 151
Racquet (single pedicle) flaps, 413
Radial incisions, for keratorefractive surgery, corneal
    biomechanics affected by, 454–455
Radial keratotomy (RK), 451*t*, 465–469, 465*i*
    complications of, 467–468
    corneal topography and
        postoperative, 41, 42*i*, 466–467
        preoperative, 41, 42*i*
    efficacy and predictability of, 466
    iron lines associated with, 355
    ocular surgery after, 468–469
    preoperative evaluation for, 465
    refraction after, 466–467
        stability of, 467
    surgical techniques for, 466
    variables affecting outcome of, 466
    visual acuity after, 466–467
Radial perineuritis, *Acanthamoeba* keratitis and, 176
Radiation, anterior segment injury caused by, 364
Radius of curvature, 8–9
    instantaneous (tangential power), 38, 38*i*
    keratometry in measurement of, 36–37
RANTES, as inflammatory mediator, 186*t*
Rapid plasma reagin (RPR) test, 118–119
RB. *See* Reticulate body
Reactive arthritis (Reiter syndrome), 215–216
Reactive hyperplasia. *See* Lymphoid hyperplasia
Rebleeding, after traumatic hyphema, 375–376, 375*i*,
    376*i*
Recessive inheritance (recessive gene/trait), 291
Recipient eye, preparation of for penetrating
    keratoplasty, 427–428
Recurrent corneal erosion, 90–93, 93*i*
Red blood cells, cytologic identification of, 59
Reflex tear arc, 49
Refraction
    clinical, 13
    after intracorneal lens/ring placement, 471
        stability of, 472
    after laser in situ keratomileusis (LASIK)
        hyperopia correction and, 493
        hyperopic astigmatism correction and, 494
        myopia correction and, 489
        myopic astigmatism correction and, 492